Textbook
of
Orthopedics

1

2

3

4

Textbook
of
Orthopedics

Dr. Rajesh Malhotra MS

Additional Professor,
Deptt. of Orthopedics, AIIMS, New Delhi

Dr. Surya Bhan MS, FRCS (Ed)

Professor & Head,
Deptt. of Orthopedics, AIIMS, New Delhi

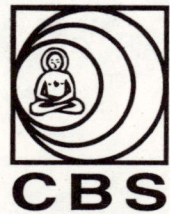

CBS

CBS PUBLISHERS & DISTRIBUTORS
NEW DELHI • BANGALORE

TEXTBOOK OF ORTHOPEDICS

ISBN: 81-239-1153-X

First Edition 2004

Published by:
Satish K. Jain for CBS Publishers & Distributors
4596/1A, 11, Darya Ganj, New Delhi-110 002 (India)
E-mail : cbspubs@del3.vsnl.net.in
Website : http://www.cbspd.com

Branch Office:
Seema House, 2975, 17th Cross, K.R. Road,
Bansankari 2nd Stage, Bangalore - 560070
Fax : 080-6771680, E-mail : cbsbng@vsnl.net

Publishing Director : Vinod K. Jain

Laser typesetting by:
NS Computers, New Delhi

Printed at:
Meenakshi Art Printers,

Preface

Myriads of textbooks are available on the orthopaedic medicine yet the authors have constantly felt an urge to create a work, which outline the principles of orthopaedics and is able to answer the questions, which arise in the minds of undergraduates and postgraduates. The book is directed at the advanced student or clinician who wishes to gain a deeper understanding of the diagnoses and management of orthopaedic conditions. The book presents clinical information necessary to make an accurate diagnosis, integrate basic science principles with clinical management, and clearly illustrate treatment protocols and guidelines with plenty of algorithms and clinical pathways. Each chapter opens with a brief description of relevant anatomy, history, examination and special clinical tests as relevant to the system and the special investigations. This makes up the basis for a scientific approach to assessment and the treatment of orthopaedic conditions. The emphasis in this book has been on providing a better understanding of the subject with abundance of figures, illustrations and clinical pictures and the work carries within it the vast clinical experience garnered by the authors during their long careers. It is an attempt by us to contribute to the education of the present generation of physician and we hope that you will enjoy going through this book.

Rajesh Malhotra
Surya Bhan

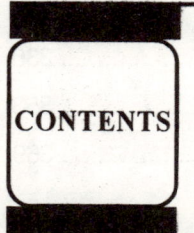

Contents

Section I
General Orthopedics

Section II
Regional Orthopedics

Section III
Trauma

General Characteristics

Miscellaneous

SECTION I
General Orthopedics

Bone : Normal Structure and Development

- Components
- Zones
- Structure
- Cells
- Matrix
  Collagen
  Proteoglycans
  Matrix proteins (non collagenous)
- Mineralization Front
- Tissues Surrounding Bone
- Bone Circulation
- Bone Development
  Endochondral
  Intramembranous
- Bone Remodelling
- Markers of Bone Turnover

Components

Bone is made of two main components: the cortical bone and cancellous bone. Each bone has a limiting surface shell known as the cortex. Cortical bone forms 80% of the skeleton. Cortex encloses plates and rods of bone tissue called cancellous or trabecular bone. Long bones have thick cortical bone in the middle to resist bending forces. Cancellous bone is designed to resist compressive forces and is present in vertebral bodies and in expanded ends of long bones. According to the Wolff's law, "Architecture of the bone reflects its functions" (Fig. 1.1). It means, cancellous and cortical bones modify their structure in response to the type of loading. Bone formation occurs on the compressive side and resorption occurs on the tensile side.

Zones

The bones are often divided morphologically into the following three zones (Fig. 1.2).

1. **Epiphysis** or bone end is the region above the growth plate in children and above the epiphyseal scar in adults. It is covered by articular (hyaline) cartilage and forms the joint surfaces.

2. **Metaphysis** is the region below the growth plate. It is the area of growth and most active remodelling area of bone during growing years.

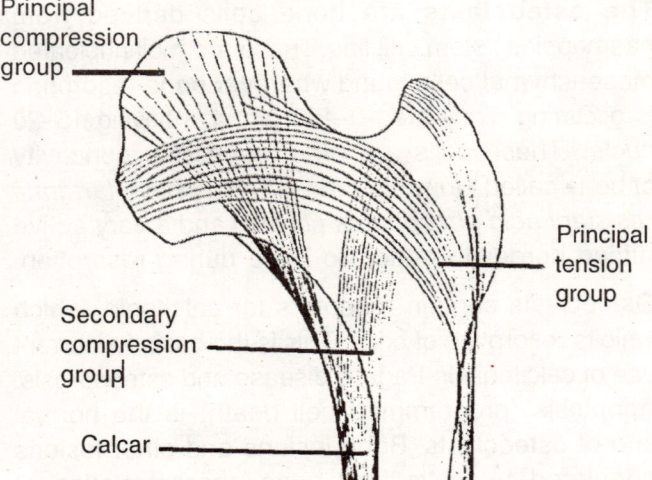

Principal compression group

Principal tension group

Secondary compression group

Calcar

Fig. 1.1. Wolff's law: demonstrated in neck of femur (compressive trabeculae near the calcar are much more prominent)

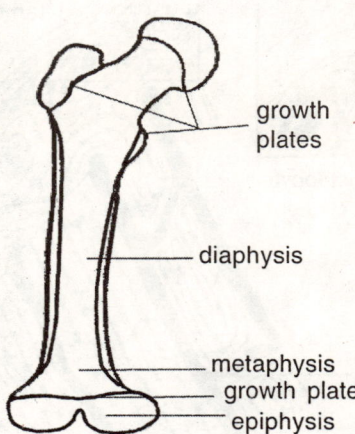

growth plates

diaphysis

metaphysis
growth plate
epiphysis

Fig. 1.2. Morphologic classification of a long bone (e.g. femur)

It is composed predominantly of cancellous bone.

3. **Diaphysis** is the region between the metaphyseal ends of a long bone.

Many diseases have predilection for one or another of these zones.

Structure

Bone consists of mesenchymal cells and an extracellular matrix, which undergoes mineralization. The basic structural unit of organized bone is the Haversian system or an osteon (Fig. 1.3). Osteon consists of a series of concentric lamellae 4–12 μm thick surrounding a central canal approximately 20 μm in diameter. Between these lamellae there are more irregularly arranged layers of bone called the interstitial lamellae. Within the interstitial lamellae, there are small oval cavities or lacunae joined by fine branching canaliculi. Each lacuna contains an osteocyte with its fine protoplasmic processes extending in the canaliculi to form a true cellular syncytium. The central canal is about 3–9 mm in length and contains interlacing reticular tissue, osteoblasts in various stages of activity and a neurovascular bundle. The Haversian systems follow longitudinal axis of the bone and branch and interconnect to each other to varying degrees. Haversian systems also connect to horizontal Volkmann's canals, which pass through the endosteal surfaces.

At the periphery of each osteon is a cement line, a narrow area containing ground substance primarily composed of glycosaminoglycans. Neither canaliculi nor collagen fibers cross the cement line. Biomechanically cement line is the weakest link in microstructure and microfractures often start and propagate along cement lines.

Cells in bone

The osteoblasts are bone cells of mesenchymal origin, which are found at sites of ossification. These are cuboidal cells, 20–30 μm in size with fine cytoplasmic processes between them. An osteoblast has a large and vesicular eccentric nucleus and marked presence of rough endoplasmic reticulum.

Osteoblasts synthesize both type I collagen (the extracellular bone matrix) and non-collagenous proteins. They contain receptors for parathormone; thus, they indirectly regulate osteoblastic bone resorption.

Reduced osteoblastic activity is seen in osteoporosis. Intrinsic inability of osteoblasts to produce normal bone is seen in *hypophosphataemic vitamin D resistant rickets*. Osteogenesis imperfecta results from genetic defect in production of pro-alpha collagen chains by osteoblasts.

The osteocytes are cells lying within a lacuna and surrounded by calcified bone matrix. Osteocytes have processes (5–7 nm in diameter) that extend through apertures of the lacunae into canaliculi in bone. These processes allow osteocyte to maintain the open pathways in bone and participate in transfer of ions and nutrients between blood and bone. Osteocytes express *CD44,* a transmembrane glycoprotein, which may act as a marker for osteocyte.

The osteoclasts are bone cells derived from haemopoietic stem cell line. These are multinucleated mesenchymal cells found wherever bone resorption is occurring. They are 10–100 μm size having 15–20 nuclei. These cells are often seen in a concavity of bone called *Howship's lacuna.* They have *tartarate resistant acid phosphates (TRAP)* and a very active ruffled border to attach to bone during resorption.

Osteoclasts contain receptors for calcitonin, which inhibits resorption of bone. This is the basis for current use of calcitonin in Paget's disease and osteoporosis. Apoptosis (programmed cell death) is the normal fate of osteoclasts. Bone lesions and other lesions populated by cells that have characteristics of osteoclasts include giant cell tumour, giant cell variants, and epithelial tumours including breast, lung, liver and thyroid.

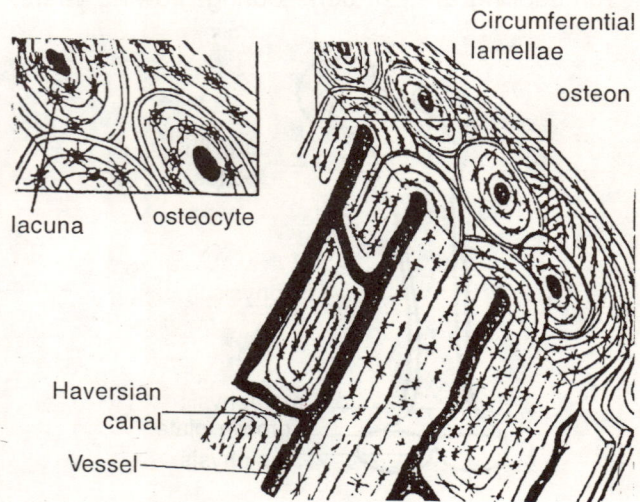

Fig. 1.3. Microstructure of bone: Osteon (Inset)

Structural Composition of Matrix

Bone matrix is a composite consisting of two types of material:

(i) Organic extracellular matrix containing collagen (30–35% of dry weight). This provides flexibility and resilience to bone.

(ii) Mineral, consisting of calcium and phosphorus salts especially hydroxyapatite [$Ca_{10}(PO_4)_6(OH)_2$] (65–70% of dry weight). This provides brittleness and hardness to bone. The ratio of calcium to phosphorus in bone is 2:1.

Collagen is the principal extracellular component of connective tissue. It provides a scaffold on which mineral is deposited. It is made up of bundles of fibrils about 280 nm long (Fig. 1.4). Each collagen molecule is a triple helix made of polypeptide chains. The three procollagen chains are stabilized by disulfide bridges. Fourteen types of collagen molecules are known. Type I is the most common type and is found in skin, fascia, tendon and bone. Type II collagen is unique to hyaline cartilage in articulations and is a marker of differentiated chondrocytes. Collagen mutations associated with clinical syndromes include:

(i) Osteogenesis imperfecta (type I collagen defect).

(ii) Ehlers-Danlos syndrome (type VII).

Lysine-derived cross-links connect and stabilize strands of collagen. Cross-linking of collagen is critical for the physical and structural stability of extracellular matrix. Abnormalities of cross-linking are associated with:

(i) Lathyrism

(ii) Osteogenesis imperfecta

The cross-links pyridinoline and deoxypyridinoline, which are formed during collagen synthesis, are secreted in urine and form the basis of urinary analysis of bone turnover.

Proteoglycans

Proteoglycans are composed of glycosaminoglycans (GAG) protein complexes. They contribute to compressive strength of bone.

Matrix proteins (non-collagenous proteins) promote mineralization. Examples are osteocalcin, osteonectin and osteopontin.

Osteocalcin attracts osteoclasts and regulates bone density. Osteocalcin levels in serum and urine are raised in Paget's disease, renal osteodystrophy and hyperparathyroidism.

Mineralization front (calcification front)

The collagenized protein produced by osteoblasts is called osteoid which normally undergoes minerali-

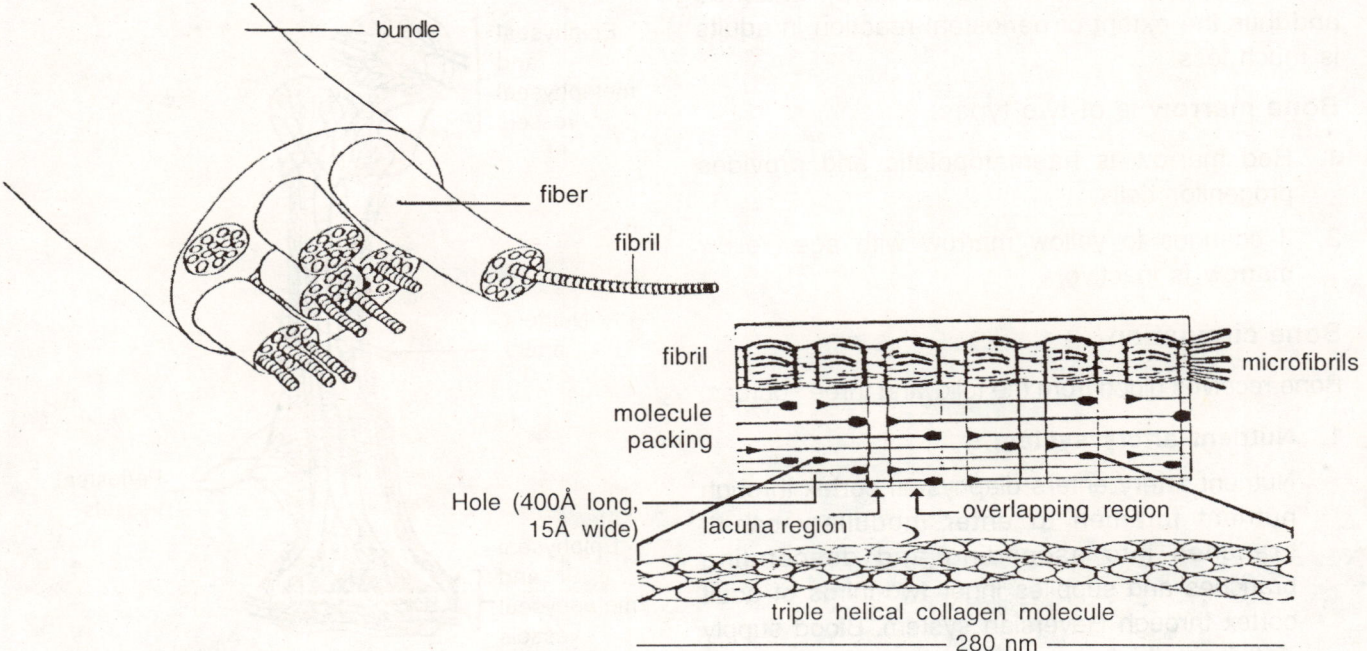

Fig. 1.4. Structure of Collagen (showing hole regions 400Å long in which mineral crystals are deposited in bone)

zation to become bone. Normally 20% of bone surfaces are covered by osteoid, which is 10 μm thick and constitutes 2% of structural bone. Osteoid begins to get calcified 10 days after deposition, i.e. mineralisation takes place at the rate of 1 μm/day. This is known as *mineralization lag time.*

Clinical Significance

Mineralization front is the site for deposition of:

1. Bone scanning agents, such as technetium methyl diphosphonate. Thus a bone scan is hot because mineralization is taking place.

2. Bone labeling agents such as tetracycline; hence, tetracycline labeling is used in investigating metabolic bone disease.

3. Mineralization inhibitors such as aluminium; aluminium-induced osteomalacia is seen in renal disease related bone disease where phosphate-binding aluminium gels are used.

Tissues Surrounding Bone

Periosteum is connective tissue membrane, which covers bone. It consists of outer fibrous layer and inner cambium layer which is loose, vascular and osteogenic. Periosteum is attached to surface of bone by Sharpey's fibers. In children, periosteum is loosely attached to bone, and is functionally more active and increases diameter of bone with growth. In adults periosteum is firmly attached and thus the extent of periosteal reaction in adults is much less.

Bone marrow is of two types:

1. Red marrow is haematopoietic and provides progenitor cells.

2. It changes to yellow marrow with age. Yellow marrow is inactive.

Bone circulation

Bone receives blood from the following three sources.

1. **Nutrient artery system**

   Nutrient artery enters diaphyseal cortex through nutrient foramen to enter medullary canal, branches into ascending and descending branches and supplies inner two-thirds of adult cortex through Haversian system. Blood supply is through high-pressure *centrifugal* (inside to outside) blood flow.

2. **Metaphyseal-epiphyseal system** is formed by genicular arteries forming periarticular vascular plexus around joints.

3. **Periosteal system** is a low-pressure system comprised of capillaries supplying the outer one-third of the mature cortex. Bones with tenuous blood supply include scaphoid, talus, femoral head and odontoid. This renders them more susceptible to non-union and avascular necrosis of part or whole of the bone.

Venous system

Venous flow is *centripetal* (outside to inside) in adult bone where the cortical capillaries drain to venous sinusoids and hence to emissary veins.

Centripetal arterial flow is seen in children who have rich periosteal vascularity and in adults following fracture when nutrient system is disrupted.

The blood supply of a long bone is given in Fig. 1.5.

Bone Development

Bone is created by two mechanisms: first, by formation of bone in the cartilage (endochondral ossification) and second, by direct transformation of fibrous tissue into bone (intramembranous ossification).

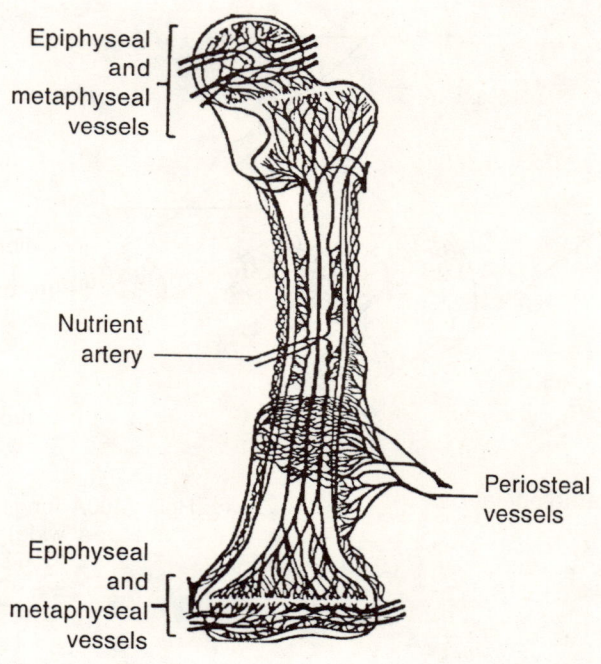

Fig. 1.5. Blood supply of a long bone

Endochondral ossification consists of mineralisation of preformed cartilage model. Examples are long bones of skeleton except clavicle. Hyaline cartilage matrix consists mainly of proteoglycan and type II collagen. A calcified collar developing at middiaphysis is the primary centre of ossification. Secondary centre of ossification forms at the epiphyseal ends. Growth plates are these cartilaginous epiphyseal plates which contribute to length of bone from infancy until maturity. There are 5 zones or phases of epiphyseal plate with characteristic appearance of cartilage cells namely, phase of resting cells, phase of proliferation, phase of maturation, phase of hypertrophy and the phase of provisional calcification.

Clinical Significance

Matrix is being removed rapidly in hypertrophic cell zone to prepare for further calcification, therefore it is the weakest zone and can fracture easily. Disturbance of cell multiplication and differentiation of cartilage occurs in Achondroplasia. Disturbance in mineralization of matrix occurs in rickets and osteomalacia. Though endochondral ossification at growth plate ceases at skeletal maturity, it is still seen in reparative response to fracture repair in callus, growth of loose bodies in joint, in cartilage cap of osteochondroma and in synovial chondromatosis (Table 1.1).

Intra membranous ossification

Bone is formed by transformation of fibrous tissue into bone. There is no "*Intervening cartilaginous step*". Examples are skull, ilium, and clavicle. Diaphysis of developing bones increase in width by membranous ossification occurring in periosteum. The osteoid consists mainly of type I collagen. These bones grow only by apposition of new bone on surface.

Blastema bone is membranous bone formation in young children with amputations or resections.

Bone remodelling occurs throughout life. Bone remodels in response to change in mechanical function or stress according to *Wolff's law*. The compression side forms bone while bone resorption occurs on the tensile side. Changes in piezoelectric charge affect bone formation, e.g. electronegativity forms bone. Cortical bone remodels by osteoclastic tunneling, laying of cement line, layering of osteoblasts and deposition of lamellae until tunnel size has narrowed to diameter of central canal of osteon. Cancellous bone remodels by osteoclastic resorption, followed by osteoblasts, which lay down new bone.

Markers of Bone Turnover

Serum Markers

Biochemical markers of bone formation are:

    Bone alkaline phosphatase

    Osteocalcin (*GLA protein*)

    Collagen related products

Procollagen I extension peptides [amino terminal (N), carboxy terminal (C)]

Biochemical markers of bone resorption are:

    Bone tartarate resistant acid phosphatase (TRAP)

    Free gamma carboxyglutamic acid

    Collagen related products

        Hydroxyproline,

        Pyridinoline cross-links (pyd),

        Deoxypyridinoline cross-links (dpd),

        Hydroxylysine glycosides, N-telopeptides

Urinary Markers for Bone Turnover

    Urinary calcium in fasting state

    Urinary hydroxyproline

    Urinary cross-links (pyd and dpd)

Table 1.1. Sites of Endochondral Ossification

Endochondral Ossification

    Physiological
- Bone Development

    Repair Response
- Fracture Callus
- Osteophyte Formation in Osteoarthritis

    Pathological
- Cartilage Cap of Osteochondroma
- Synovial Chondromatosis
- Growth of Osteocartilaginous Loose Bodies in Joints
- Osteopetrosis

CHAPTER 2

Abnormalities of Growth

Embryology

The primitive streak appears 12 days after conception. Mesenchyme develops from mesoderm and gives rise to connective tissues, muscles, vessels, blood cells and genitourinary system. Overall 42–44 pairs of somites develop from mesoderm and line both sides of notochord. Each somite develops into a lateral dermatome (forms skin), a medial myotome (forms muscle) and a ventral sclerotome (forms bones). The limb buds appear between 4 and 6 weeks. Upper limbs form quickly and rotate externally. Lower limbs develop after a few days and eventually rotate internally.

Bones (except skull, scapula, ilium and part of clavicle) form through mesenchymal aggregation into a cartilage model that is replaced systematically by bone (endochondral ossification) (Fig. 2.1).

Clavicle is the first bone to ossify during intrauter-ine life. It is the only long bone which ossifies by intramembranous ossification.

Primary centres of ossification appear in the diaphysis of bones between 7 and 12 weeks.

Distal femur is the only secondary ossification centre present at the time of birth.

Genetic disorders

Genetic disorders can be due to chromosomal disorders (e.g. Down's syndrome), single gene disorders or polygenic or multi-factorial disorders (such as, congenital hip dislocation, clubfoot and scoliosis).

Chromosomes have been mapped and location of defective genes that cause orthopaedic disorders have been identified e.g. Gaucher's syndrome is associated with disorder of chromosome 1, Mucopoly-saccharidoses syndrome VI and Cri du chat with chromosome 5, MPS VII, Ehler-Danlos VII, and

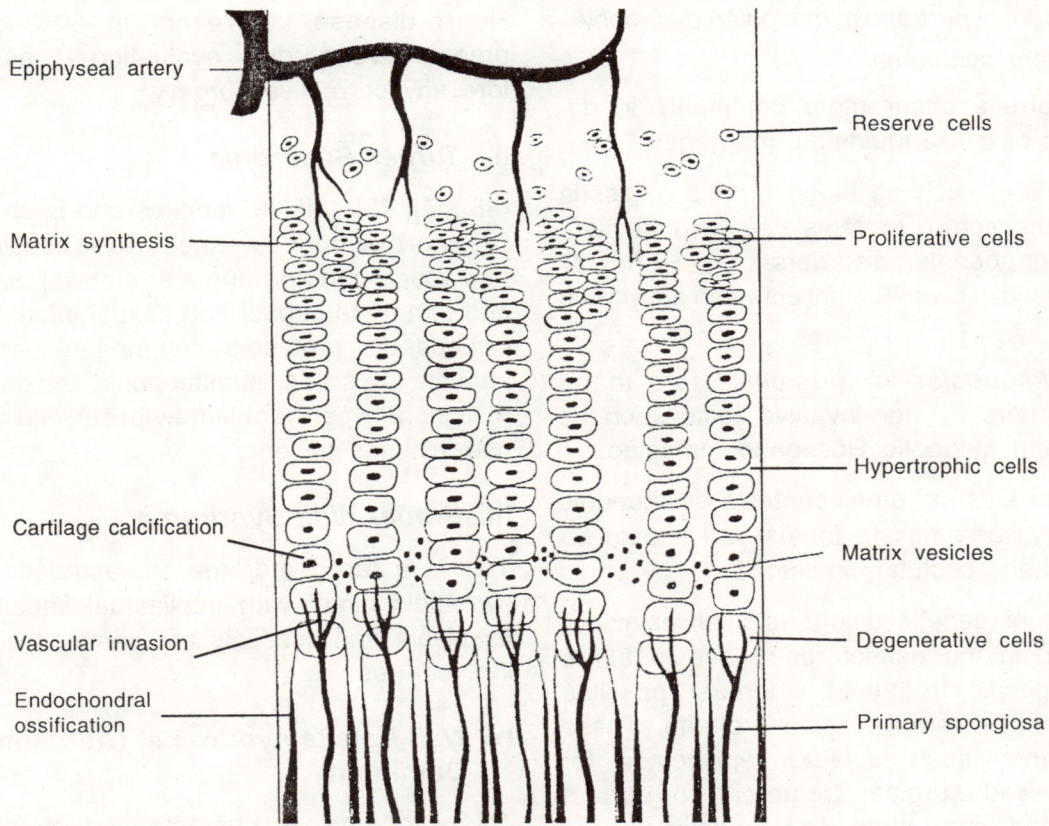

Fig. 2.1.   Endochondral ossification in a growth plate

some Marfan's are associated with disorders of chromosome 7, Nail Patella syndrome is associated with disorder of chromosome 9, and Prader Willi syndrome with chromosome 15 abnormality.

Chromosomal abnormalities are transmitted by several mechanisms:

Autosomal Dominant   Single abnormal gene causes the disorder. These are usually structural defects such as:

> Achondroplasia
> Cleidocranial dysostosis
> Hereditary multiple exostosis
> Marfan's syndrome
> Neurofibromatosis
> Osteogenesis imperfecta (type I and IV)
> Polydactyly

Variable expressivity and incomplete penetration can suppress expression of dominant inheritance of genetic disorders.

Autosomal Recessive Inheritance These disorders are expressed only if both genes of the genetic pair are affected. These are usually biochemical or enzymatic defects such as:

> Gaucher's Disease
> Hurler's Syndrome
> Homocystinuria
> Morquio's syndrome
> Osteogenesis imperfecta (Type II and III)
> Ochronosis
> Sanfilippo syndrome
> Schie's syndrome
> Hypophosphatasia

X-linked Inheritance

This involves only X-chromosomes; so in males even recessive abnormal genes are expressed due to genetic inactivity of Y-chromosomes. In females, presence of one abnormal gene causes a carrier state while rare occurrence of both genes of genetic pair being abnormal causes the disease.

Examples are

X-linked dominant

> *Vitamin D Refractory Rickets*

X-linked recessive

> *Haemophilia*

Pseudo hypertrophic muscular dystrophy
Hunters syndrome

Genetic disorders occur more commonly in off-springs born of consanguineous marriages.

Genetic markers such as blood groups or tissue types or some serum proteins can help in diagnosing certain genetic disorders, e.g. HLA B27 positivity is found in over 90% patients with ankylosing spondylitis.

Prenatal diagnosis is possible for many genetic disorders by non-invasive tests such as ultrasound and Magnetic Resonance Imaging.

Invasive tests such as amniocentesis or chorionic villous biopsy carry risk to foetus and should be used only when absolutely indicated.

Management of genetic disorders involves counselling including the risk of recurrence in future offspring. Specific treatment wherever possible can be given to improve quality of life. These include treatment such as factor replacement for haemophilia and surgical treatment to correct deformities and limb length discrepancies.

Common Genetic Disorders

I. *Down Syndrome* (Trisomy 21)

This is the commonest chromosomal abnormality. The incidence increases with maternal age. Orthopaedic problems include atlantoaxial instability, scoliosis, spondylolisthesis, hip instability, slipped capital femoral epiphysis, patellar dislocation and planovalgus feet.

Heart disease is present in 50% cases and preoperative cardiac evaluation is essential before any corrective surgery.

II. *Turner Syndrome*

(45 XO): This affects females and is characterised by short stature, webbed neck, cubitus valgus (increased carrying angle at elbows), short fourth and fifth metacarpals and sexual infantilism. Other orthopaedic problems commonly seen in these patients are scoliosis, osteopenia and genu valgum. Malignant hyperthermia may occur with anaesthetic use in these patients.

III. *Prader Willi Syndrome*

This is a rare syndrome characterised by floppy, hypotonic infant with intellectual impairment. Hip dysplasia and scoliosis are common accompanying features.

IV. *Nail Patella syndrome* (Autosomal Dominant)

This syndrome is characterised by absence or hypoplasia of the nails and patellae (Fig. 2.2a-d),

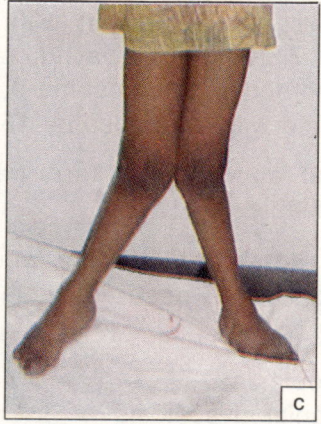
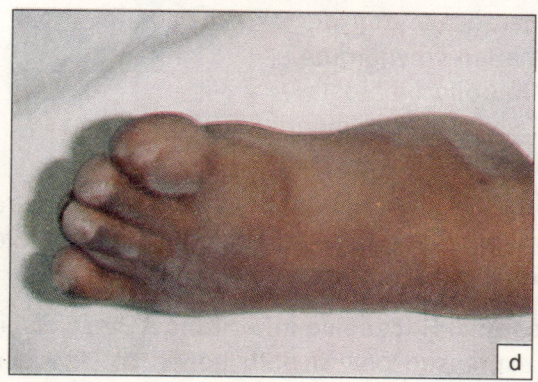

Fig. 2.2c,d. Clinical photographs showing genu valgum and absent nail in the big toe.

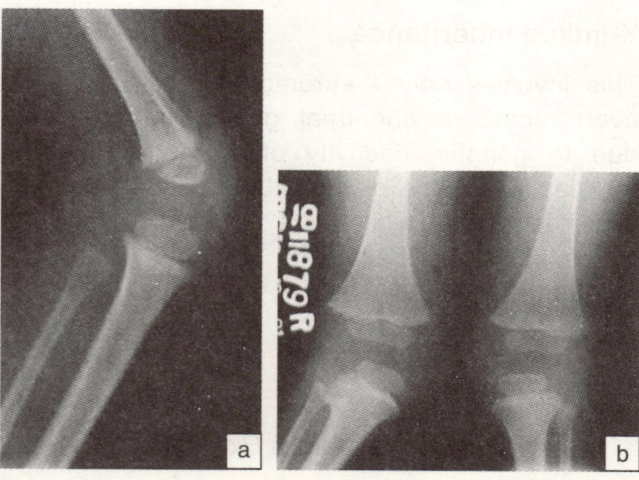

Fig. 2.2a,b. X-rays of patient with nail-patella syndrome showing absent patella with genu valgum.

bilateral iliac horns, dislocation of radial heads and small scapulae. Renal dysfunction occurs commonly in middle age in these patients.

Bone Dysplasias

Dysplasia refers to deformities caused by intrinsic bone disturbances.

Classification There are many ways to classify dysplasias:

- According to presence or absence of dwarfism (Fig. 2.3)
- According to zone of bone where growth is affected (Fig. 2.4)
- According to presence of sclerosis

1. *According to presence or absence of dwarfism*

A. **Without dwarfism**

B. **With dwarfism**

Dysplasias with dwarfism can be further sub-divided into two types:

(a) Proportionate dwarfism - displays symmetrical decrease in both truncal and limb length e.g.

Mucopolysaccharidoses

Metaphyseal chondrodysplasia

Multiple epiphyseal dysplasia

Pyknodysostosis

(b) Disproportionate dwarfism

  i) **Short limbed** dwarfism

   1. Achondroplasia
   2. Chondroectodermal dysplasia (Ellis-Van - Crevald syndrome)
   3. Diastrophic dysplasia
   4. Diastrophic dwarfism

  ii) **Short trunk** dwarfism

   1. Kniest syndrome
   2. Spondyloepiphyseal dysplasia

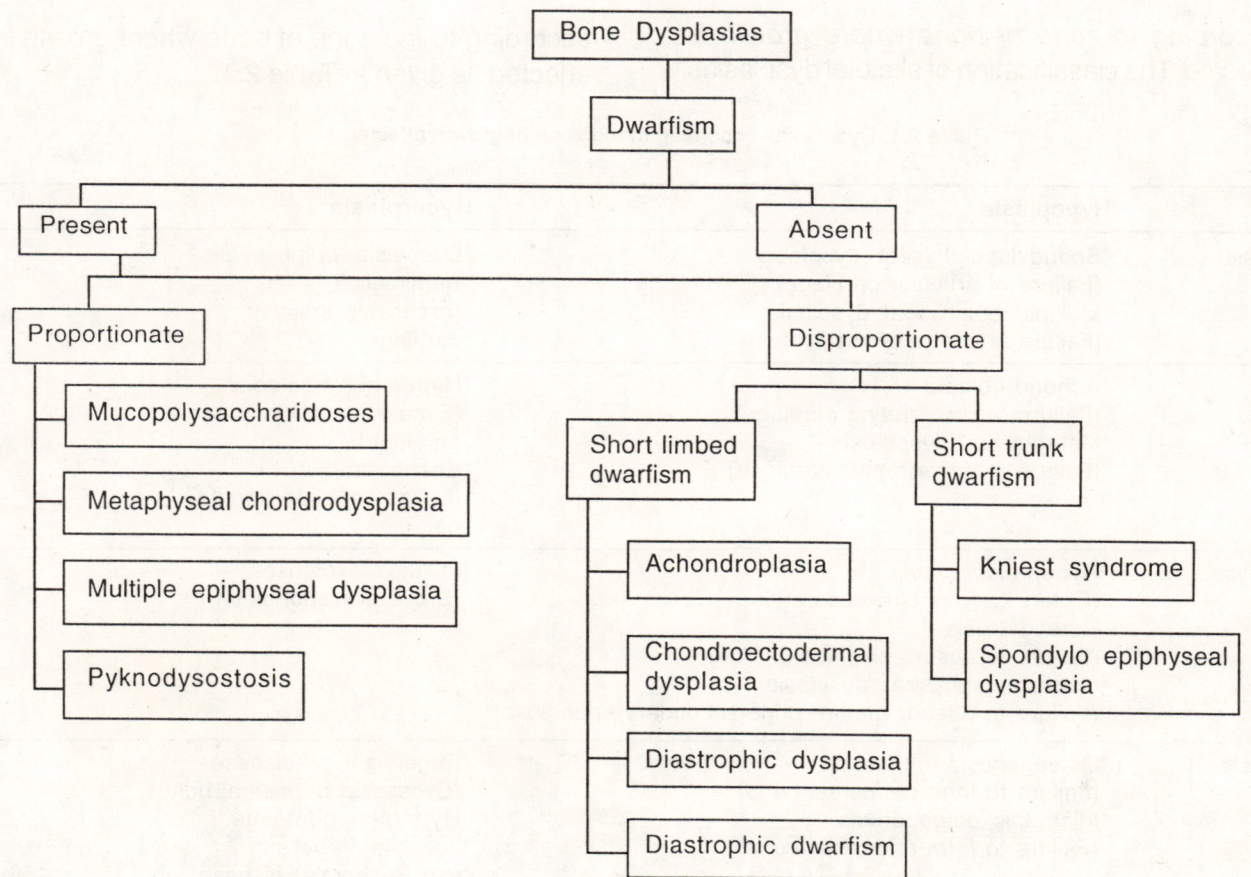

Fig. 2.3. Classification of Bone dysplasias with dwarfism

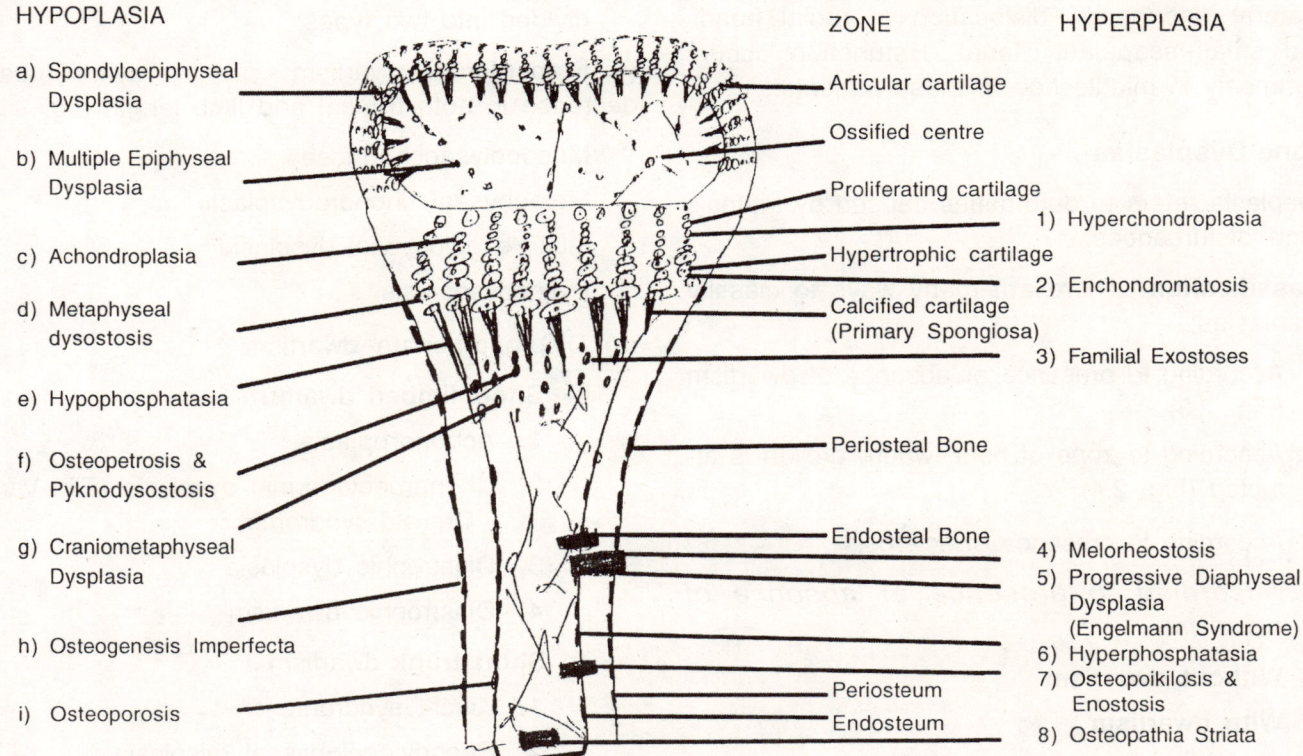

HYPOPLASIA

a) Spondyloepiphyseal Dysplasia

b) Multiple Epiphyseal Dysplasia

c) Achondroplasia

d) Metaphyseal dysostosis

e) Hypophosphatasia

f) Osteopetrosis & Pyknodysostosis

g) Craniometaphyseal Dysplasia

h) Osteogenesis Imperfecta

i) Osteoporosis

ZONE

Articular cartilage

Ossified centre

Proliferating cartilage

Hypertrophic cartilage

Calcified cartilage (Primary Spongiosa)

Periosteal Bone

Endosteal Bone

Periosteum

Endosteum

HYPERPLASIA

1) Hyperchondroplasia

2) Enchondromatosis

3) Familial Exostoses

4) Melorheostosis
5) Progressive Diaphyseal Dysplasia (Engelmann Syndrome)
6) Hyperphosphatasia
7) Osteopoikilosis & Enostosis
8) Osteopathia Striata

Fig. 2.4. Dysplasias of Bone according to zone of growth affected

2. *According to zone of bone where growth is affected:* The classification of skeletal dysplasias according to the zone of bone where growth is affected is given in Table 2.1.

Table 2.1. Dysplasias according to the zone of growth affected

Zone	Hypoplasia	Hyperplasia
Epiphysis	*Spondyloepiphyseal dysplasia (Failure of articular cartilage) *Multiple epiphyseal dysplasia (Failure of centre of ossification)	*Dysplasia epiphysealis hemimelica (excessive articular cartilage)
Physis	*Achondroplasia (Failure of proliferating cartilage) *Metaphyseal dysostosis (Failure of hypertrophic cartilage)	*Hyperchondroplasia (Excess of proliferating cartilage) *Enchondromatosis (Excess of hypertrophic cartilage)
Metaphysis	*Hypophosphatasia (Failure to form calcified cartilage) *Osteopetrosis (Failure to absorb calcified cartilage) *Craniometaphyseal dysplasia (Failure to absorb mature bone-secondary spongiosa)	*Multiple exostoses (Excessive spongiosa)
Diaphysis	*Osteogenesis imperfecta (Failure to form periosteal bone) *Idiopathic osteoporosis (Failure to form endosteal bone)	*Engelmann's disease (Excessive periosteal bone) *Hyperphosphatemia *Juvenile Paget's *van Buchem's disease (excessive endosteal bone)

3. *According to presence of sclerosis*

   a) Non sclerosing

   b) Sclerosing

   > Osteopetrosis
   >
   > Pyknodysostosis
   >
   > Enostosis (bone island)
   >
   > Osteopoikilosis
   >
   > Osteopathia striata
   >
   > Camurati Engelmann Disease
   >
   > Melorheostosis

Some Important bone dysplasias

Achondroplasia: This is the commonest form of disproportionate dwarfism. This is an autosomal dominant condition characterised by defective endochondral ossification. The defect is in the proliferative zone of the physis. It is caused by a mutation of FGFR-3 (Fibroblast Growth Factor Receptor-3) gene on human chromosome 4.The skull is abnormal; the transverse diameter of foramen magnum is markedly reduced (base of skull forms by endochondral ossification). The patient has a normal trunk, short limbs, prominent forehead, button noses, small nasal bridge and trident hand (extended middle and ring fingers cannot be approximated). The spinal abnormalities include thoracolumbar kyphosis (commonest deformity), lumbar canal stenosis (short pedicles with reduced interpedicular distance) and excessive lordosis. Other common features include radial head subluxation, broad and short iliac wings (*Champagne glass pelvic outlet*), metaphyseal flaring with inverted V shaped distal femoral physis, coxa valga, genu varum, and radial or tibial bowing. The patients have normal intelligence and sexual function. They commonly work as circus dwarfs. Patients may need surgery for spinal cord decompression, correction of spinal deformities, correction of genu varum or limb lengthening.

Spondyloepiphyseal Dysplasia (SED)

This condition leads to short trunk dwarfism. Involvement of vertebrae (beaking) and epiphyseal centres is commonly seen. The congenital variety has autosomal dominant inheritance. Tarda variety has variable inheritance.

The large joints like hip and shoulder are commonly involved resulting in premature osteoarthritis of these joints. Scoliosis is a common feature of this condition (Fig. 2.5a-c).

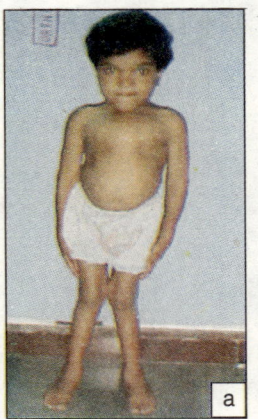

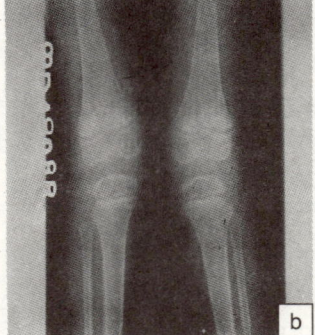
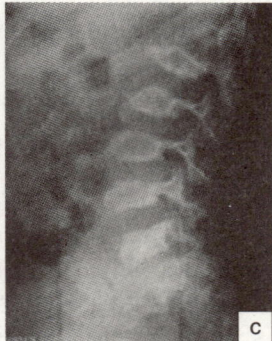

Fig. 2.5.   (a) Spondyloepiphyseal Dysplasia-Clinical photograph, (b, c) Radiographs showing bilateral genu valgum and beaking of vertebrae.

Other manifestations include delayed appearance of epiphysis, flattened facies, platyspondyly, odontoid hypoplasia, coxa vara, and genu valgum.

Associated retinal detachment and myopia may be seen. Patients usually have a normal life span.

Multiple Epiphyseal Dysplasia

This is an Autosomal Dominant disorder characterised by stunted growth in children, joint pains and progressive deformity. It is usually confined to lower limbs principally affecting the hips. The face, skull and spine are normal (cf. SED).

Early osteoarthritis commonly of the hip joints may be seen. Radiologically, irregular epiphyseal ossification is seen. The radiologic appearance may mimic Perthes' disease (Fig. 2.6).

Treatment consists of corrective osteotomy or joint replacement when indicated.

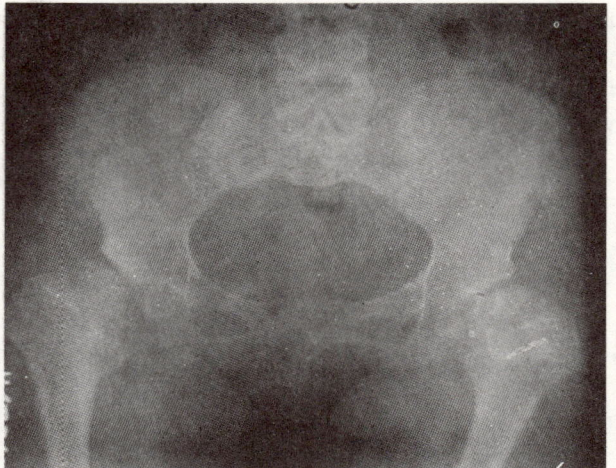

Fig. 2.6.   Pelvis x-ray in a patient with multiple epiphyseal dysplasia showing involvement of both hips

Osteogenesis Imperfecta (Brittle Bone Disease)

This is one of the commonest heritable bone disorders (1: 20,000 births) characterised by fragility of bones but with wide variation in severity.

The disease is caused by abnormal collagen synthesis (failure of cross-linking) due to mutation in genes that produce type I collagen. Osteogenesis imperfecta is classified into four types:

Type I	Mild
Type II	Moderately severe
Type III	Progressive deforming
Type IV	Severe (often stillbirths)

Type I and II are autosomal dominant while Type III & IV are autosomal recessive. Salient features are due to involvement of bones, teeth, ligaments or sclerae.

The condition is characterised by excessive fragility of bones, blue sclerae, osteoporosis, excessive joint laxity, bowing of bones and crumbling teeth or *dentinogenesis imperfecta* (Fig. 2.7). Other features are herniae, deafness (both conductive and sensorineural), and undue ease of bruising with poor scar formation. Deformities, especially scoliosis, chest deformities, trefoil pelvis, biconcave vertebrae and basilar invagination may be seen. X-rays show wormian bones in suture lines, beaded ribs, osteoporosis, thinned cortices and deformities due to malunited fractures. Metaphyses appear expanded. Occasionally a cystic or *popcorn*

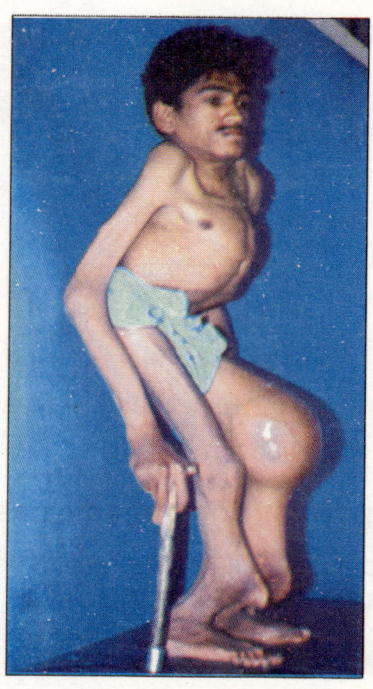

Fig. 2.7.   Clinical picture of Osteogenesis Imperfecta. Note the bowing of bones

appearance is seen due to irregular (curliform) ossification adjacent to the epiphyseal metaphyseal region. *Hyperplastic callus* is seen sometimes after fractures. Fractures unite readily and nonunion is not a problem. The tendency to fractures reduces with age. The life expectancy can be normal in mild variety whereas severely affected subjects die before reaching adulthood.

Osteogenesis imperfecta (OI) should be differentiated from child abuse (battered baby syndrome). Children with OI have wormian bones, generalised osteoporosis, expansion of metaphysis and metaphyseal fractures (cf. diaphyseal fractures in child abuse. The multiple fractures in battered baby syndrome show different stages of healing). Histologically, there is increased diameter of haversian canals and osteocytic lacunae, increased number of cells and replicated cement lines.

Management comprises of prevention of fractures and correction of deformity whenever indicated. Soffield osteotomies (sheekh kabab bone with intramedullary fixation) are sometimes required for progressive bowing of long bones.

Diaphyseal Aclasis (Hereditary Multiple Exostosis)

This is the commonest skeletal dysplasia and shows autosomal dominant inheritance. It is characterised by a defect of remodelling with disturbance in the rate of endochondral ossification. This leads to shortening, uneven length of limbs and deformities at forearm, knee and ankle (Fig. 2.8a-c).

Multiple osteochondromas (bony excrescence covered with cartilaginous caps in metaphyseal region of one bone or at multiple sites in multiple bones) are seen.

The involvement can sometimes be bilaterally symmetrical. Bony lumps in early childhood are the commonest presentation. Nerve compression (e.g. of lateral popliteal nerve) or fracture of osteochondroma are occasional presenting features. Bursitis over the prominent osteochondroma may occur (Fig. 2.8d,e).

Osteochondromas grow only with growth of child and stop growing at skeletal maturity. Any increase in size after maturity may suggest malig-

nant change to chondrosarcoma. Malignant transformation is reported in approximately 10% cases (range 5–28%){cf. 1% in solitary osteochondroma}. Chondrosarcoma is the most common malignancy. Malignant change is more likely in exostoses of flat bones than in those affecting long bones.

Dwarfism or shortening is the most difficult aspect of the syndrome to manage.

Treatment involves removal of only the particular osteochondroma, which becomes painful, causes deformity of limb or subluxation of neighbouring joint (Fig. 2.8f,g) or the one, which has undergone malignant transformation.

Dyschondroplasia (Ollier's disease, enchondromatosis)

This is a non-hereditary developmental disorder where unossified cartilage remains in the metaphysis and diaphysis, often forming large tumor masses.

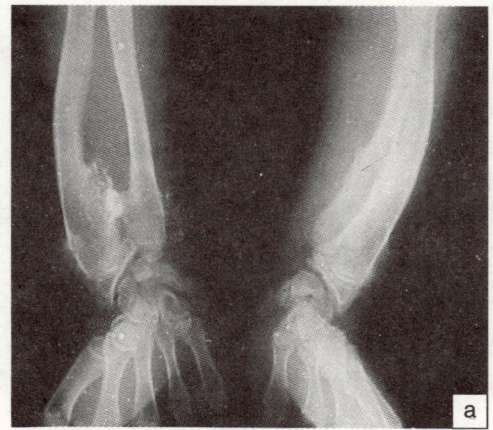 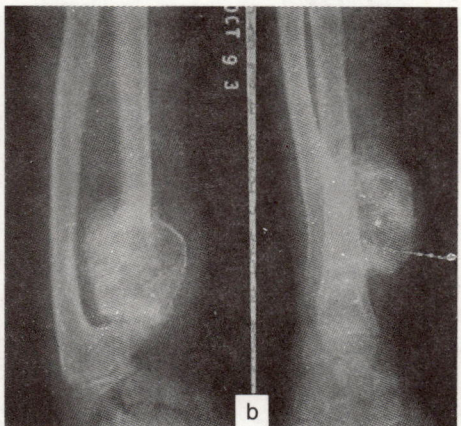 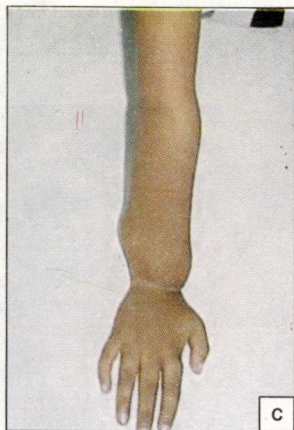

Fig. 2.8a-c. Diaphyseal aclasis involving lower end of forearm bones causing deformities

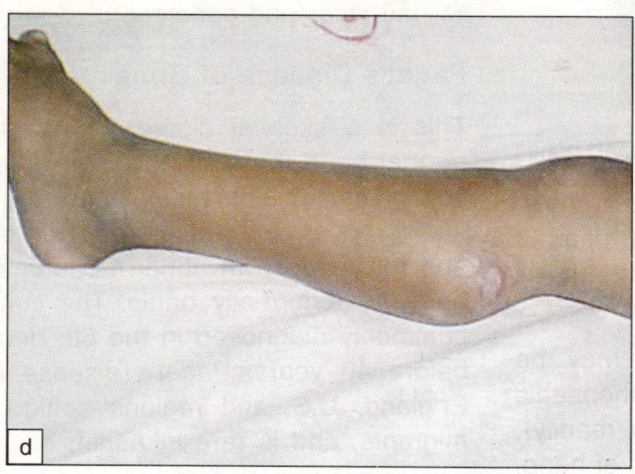 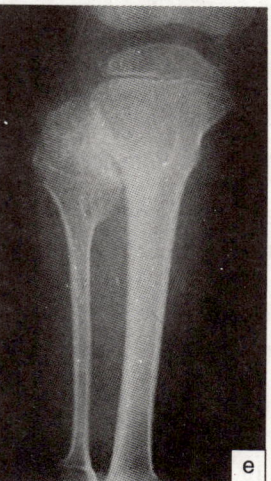

Fig. 2.8d,e. Bursitis arising from proximal fibular exostosis

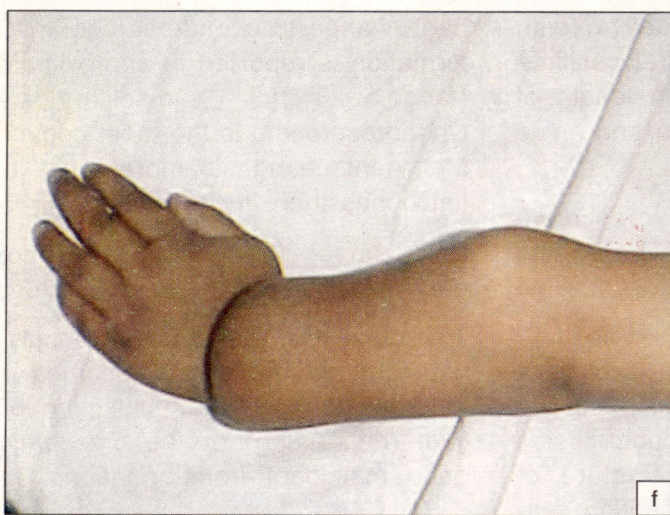
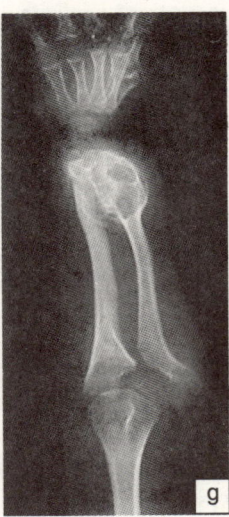

Fig. 2.8f,g.   Dislocation of radial head due to distal radial exostosis

This condition is often asymmetric with unilateral involvement of one extremity. It presents usually with bony lumps in childhood. The femur and tibia are the most commonly affected bones. Ilium and bones of hands (Fig. 2.9) and feet are also commonly involved.

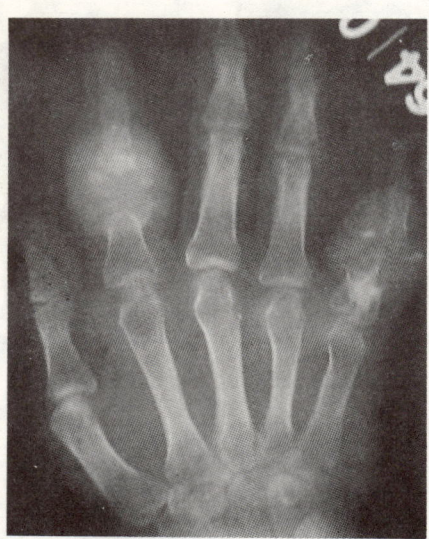

Fig. 2.9.   Multiple enchondromatosis involving hand bones

On x-rays, affected bones show irregular translucent areas in metaphysis, with streaks of areas of calcification. Density of bone between streaks is increased.

The affected bones are short. There may be asymmetrical limb shortening. Other orthopaedic complications include fractures (which heal readily), angular deformity and marked deformities of hand. The most serious complication is transformation into malignant tumors. Chondrosarcoma may occur in nearly 30% patients.

Maffucci's Syndrome

This is a congenital, non-hereditary syndrome, which is characterised by enchondromas along with haemangiomas of the soft tissues and viscera. The condition is usually diagnosed at about 5 years of age and is generally unilateral. The risk of tumor development is 100%. The malignancies in Maffucci's syndrome are:

1. Chondrosarcoma may arise in underlying enchondromas.

2. Malignant vascular tumors such as angiosarcoma and lymphangiosarcoma

3. Epithelial and mesenchymal tumors such as thyroid, pituitary, central nervous system (astrocytomas), ovary, breast and gastrointestinal (liver and pancreas).

Paget's Disease of Bone

This is a skeletal disorder characterised by abnormal bone remodelling. There is intense activation of osteoblasts and osteoclasts with high tissue turnover in the skeleton. Bones are enlarged and thickened with abnormal internal architecture and are abnormally brittle. The condition is most commonly diagnosed in the 5th decade. It is rare before 40 years. Paget's disease is common in England, U.S. and regions settled by European migrants, and is rare in Asians.

It may be monostotic or polyostotic. The polyostotic

form frequently shows involvement of the vertebrae. The condition is often asymptomatic. Although pain is the most common presentation, other features are frequent fractures, deafness, platybasia and basilar invagination, degenerative joints, calcific periarthritis, uremia, hypercalcaemia, nephrolithiasis and high output cardiac failure. Patients with skull involvement feel increased hat size.

X-rays show deformity, thickening of cortical bone (lytic lesion in early stages and in skull) and coarsening of bone trabeculae (Fig. 2.10a,b). "*Osteitis circumscripta*" refers to osteolytic skull / calvarium involvement (Fig. 2.10c).

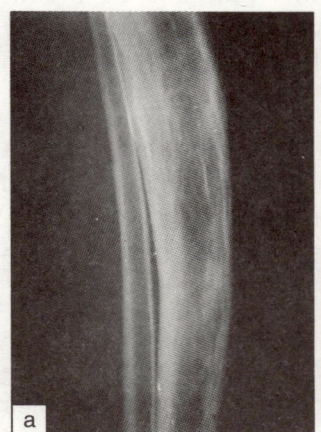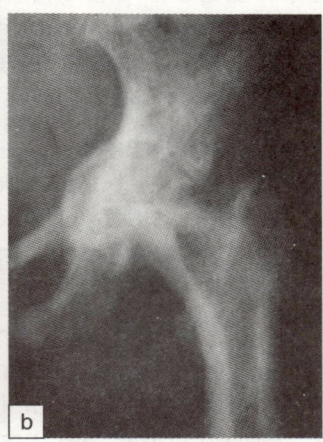

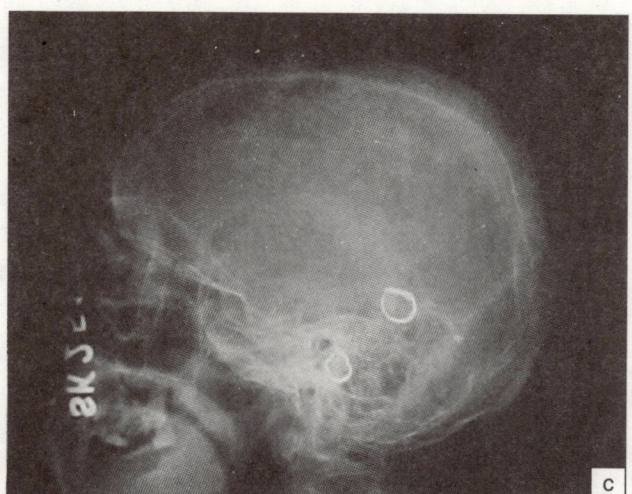

Fig. 2.10a-c. Pagetic involvement of tibia, hip joint and skull

When sclerotic areas are present in skull, they are often poorly outlined and likened to "*Cotton Balls*". Osteolytic lesions are also common in vertebrae. There may be increased density in the periphery of the vertebral body with accentuation in the central portion of the body ("*Picture Frame Vertebrae*" / "*Window Frame*").

Renal angioid streaks and blindness may occur.

Thickening of vertebrae can cause spinal stenosis and neural encroachment.

Fractures in Paget's heal in irregular fashion *(Osteitis Deformans)*

Differential Diagnosis

Hyperphosphatasia is a genetic disorder, which is rare and has microscopic similarities with Paget's disease. Hyperphosphatasia occurs in younger patients, is generalised and symmetric and causes severe disfigurement.

Laboratory Tests

Laboratory tests in Paget's disease show high tissue turnover. There is raised alkaline phosphatase (indicating increased osteoblastic activity) and increased excretion of collagen in urine (urinary hydroxyproline or pyridoline cross-links) indicating high rate of breakdown of bone.

Histologically, active Paget's disease is characterised by osteoclast remodelling (normally less than 20% of bone surface), fibrosis and abnormally wavy, irregular and *curliform cement lines.*

In inactive stages, presence of curliform cement lines may be the only hallmark.

Treatment

Treatment for Paget's disease is based on ability of drugs to slow down bone remodelling activity. Calcitonin is widely used. Bisphosphonates (such as alendronate and etidronate) bind to bone mineral, thereby inhibiting both the formation of and dissolution of calcium phosphate crystals. Pamidronate, available only for intravenous use, does not inhibit bone formation and is extremely useful.

Treatment may be required for persistent bone pains, fractures, neurological complications and high output cardiac failure.

Orthopaedic surgery in Paget's disease may be complicated by excessive haemorrhage due to increased vascularity.

Paget's Sarcoma

About 3% of osteosarcomas reportedly arise in

Pagetic bone. It is the most common cause of secondary osteosarcoma in elderly. The most frequent location is humerus, followed by pelvis and femur. The patients present with new acute pain in an area of recent lytic destruction in a patient with longstanding disease (15–25 years).

Metastases are very frequent-often at initial presentation. It has extremely poor prognosis. Treatment includes ablative surgery, chemotherapy and radiotherapy.

Benign Tumors in Paget's: Benign tumors may occur in Paget's disease. The examples are

i)   Giant cell tumors (*Avellino Tumor*)

ii) Desmoplastic fibroma

Fibrous Dysplasia

Fibrous dysplasia is a developmental disorder characterised by replacement of normal bone and marrow by tissue composed of fibrous tissue and minute spicules of woven bone.

It has several clinical pathologic variants. The monostotic variety involves one bone and is more common in females. The most common sites are mandible, rib and femur. In the polyostotic form many bones are involved, often in one limb or one half of body. The involvement is throughout the skeleton including hands and feet.

Albright or McCune Albright Syndrome

It is a genetic non-heritable disorder and is seen nearly exclusively in females. It is characterised by a triad of localised hyperpigmentation of the skin (*cafe au lait*), *polyostotic fibrous dysplasia* and hyperfunctional endocrinopathies such a *precocious puberty.* Other endocrine abnormalities may occur such as hyperthyroidism, hypercortisolism, increased growth hormone and hypophosphatasia. Diabetes Mellitus or Gigantism may result from these endocrine dysfunctions. Vaginal bleeding may occur in early childhood.

Variant with skull and facial bone involvement

This is called "*Cherubism*" or "*leontiasis - osseum*". Skull (especially base) and mandible are often involved in this condition. There is marked facial asymmetry resulting from unilateral involvement.

Obliteration of air sinuses and cranial nerve foramina may occur. Proptosis and paralysis of II, VII and VIII nerves may occur.

Myxomas of soft tissues (especially intramuscular myxomas) may be seen in association with fibrous dysplasia (*Mazabraud's syndrome*).

Clinically, fibrous dysplasia presents with skeletal deformities, fractures or pain and pigmented areas on skin, often on one half of body, commonly on trunk and thigh and mucous membrane in mouth. The margins of skin lesions are smooth and known as *coastline of Maine* (cf. Neurofibromatosis: irregular margins-*coastline of California*) There may be coxa vara or diminished neck shaft angle in proximal femur (*'Shepherd's Crook"* deformity). Unilateral involvement of limb may result in enlargement of limb and limb length discrepancy.

Radiologically, x-rays in fibrous dysplasia have a fine, granular, homogenous appearance (*Ground Glass Appearance*). Other areas may have densities or lucencies in the marrow of the bone (Fig. 2.11a,b).

Histologically, the lesion is characterised by fibrous tissue replacement of bone, sparse cellularity along with an admixture of irregular spicules of woven trabecular bone. Bony spicules are of

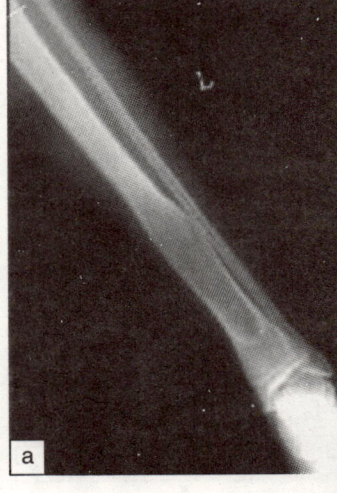
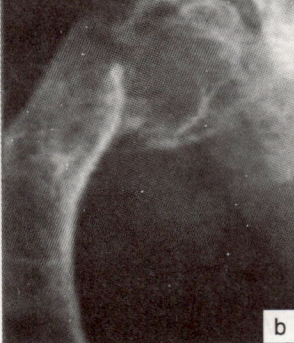

Fig. 2.11. (a) Fibrous Dysplasia of the tibia showing ground glass appearance (b) Pathological fracture due to fibrous dysplasia

uneven size and shape and mimic alphabet soup ("*Chinese Alphabet*"). Occasionally "calcified spherules", 0.1 to 0.2 mm diameter (round or oval structures), exhibiting concentric lamellations may appear instead of woven bone.

Clinical course usually progresses till epiphyseal closure. The localised forms progress slowly and have a favourable outcome. Extensive involvement early in life is deforming and commonly causes fractures. Late reactivation of monostotic lesion may occur in later life or pregnancy.

Laboratory Investigations are normal except raised serum alkaline phosphatase in one-third cases.

Differential Diagnosis

Fibrous dysplasia should be differentiated from hyperparathyroidism (latter diagnosis favoured by hypercalcaemia and absence of skin pigmentation).

Treatment

The treatment aims at prevention and treatment of fractures and deformities. Curettage and bone grafting can be undertaken for small lesions. Resection of bone (e.g. of rib) may have to be undertaken sometimes. Lesions in upper extremity can often be treated satisfactorily by conservative means.

Complications

The commonly encountered complications include fracture, deformity especially coxa vara (*shepherd crook*), endocrine problems (McCune - Albright) and sarcomas. Sarcomas are seen in 0.5% cases, more commonly in polyostotic than monostotic

forms. The common sites are skull, facial bones and femur. Osteosarcoma is the commonest malignancy although fibrosarcoma, chondrosarcoma, and malignant fibrous histiocytoma may also occur. Malignant change is suggested by pain, swelling and definite radiological changes, and carries a poor prognosis.

Cleido-Cranial Dysplasia (Cleido-Cranio Dysostosis) is an autosomal dominant disorder affecting the membrane bones, principally the clavicles, skull, scapulae, pelvis and terminal phalanges. It is the only dysplasia in which growth of membrane bones alone is affected. It has been mapped to chromosome 6p21 in mice.

The head shape is a characteristic feature. Patients have a large head with prominent frontal and parietal bones. Delayed fusion of cranial sutures and fontanelles with multiple wormian bones is commonly seen. Partial or complete aplasia of clavicles is seen (Fig. 2.12a,b).

Shoulder joints can be approximated anteriorly. Other features are drooping shoulders with small scapulae, short terminal phalanges with hypoplastic nails and teeth abnormalities (disordered eruption; deciduous teeth persist long; supernumerary teeth). Intelligence and life expectancy are normal.

The condition should be differentiated from Pyknodysostosis, which may have short, or absent clavicles, wormian bones and dysplastic terminal phalanges but bones are dense and abnormally fragile.

Note Wormian bones are sutural bones seen in

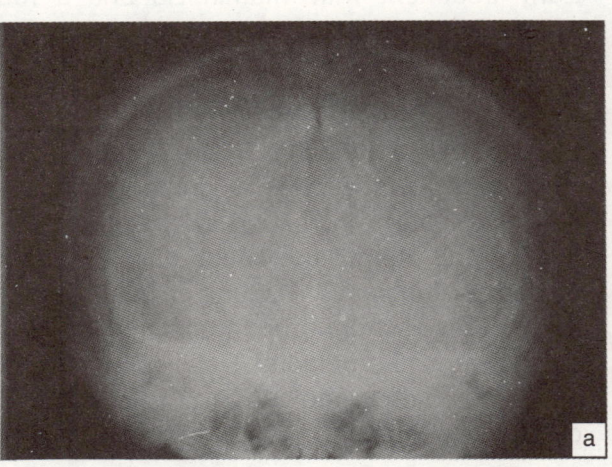 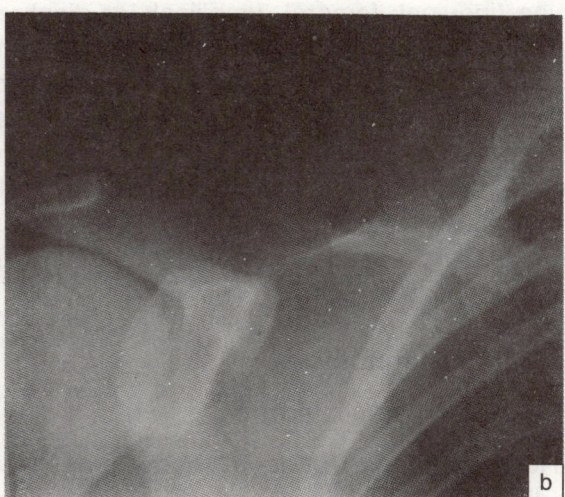

Fig. 2.12a,b. Cleidocranial Dysostosis. Note the wormian bone in skull (a) and absence of clavicle (b)

irregular sinewy sutures of skull bones seen classically in osteogenesis imperfecta but are also are present in cleido-cranial dysostosis and pyknodysostosis.

Connective Tissue Syndromes

Marfan's Syndrome is an autosomal dominant disorder of collagen synthesis (possibly alpha one sub unit). Incidence is 1 in 1.5 million. The syndrome is characterised by:

i)   Excessive height with unequal body proportions The lower segment (Pubis to heel) is more than upper segment (head to pubis). The normal ratio is 1:1. The arm span (distance between fingertips with arms horizontal) is more than height (normally 1:1).

ii) Arachnodactyly: Long slender metacarpals and phalanges (*"sedia"* fingers) is a distinguishing feature.

iii) Ocular abnormalities include dislocated lens (usually in superior direction), detached retina, cataract and myopia.

iv) The cardiac abnormalities seen are aortic dilatation and aneurysm, pulmonary dilatation, cardiac arrhythmias and valvular abnormalities.

Other features are high arched palate, excessive joint laxity and rarely contractures in hand joints. Skeletal deformities include recurrent dislocation of patella, dislocation of hip, radial head and clavicle. Genu recurvatum, severe genu varum, severe scoliosis (in 50% cases) refractory to bracing, chest deformities and narrow shoulder girdle are the other skeletal deformities seen. Herniae (inguinal, femoral, umbilical or diaphragmatic), dural ectasia, meningocele and spontaneous pneumothorax may occur. The radiological findings are not striking. Overgrowth of long bones, especially distal segments, scoliosis on lateral radiographs, sometimes abnormally tall vertebrae, pelvis with wide cavity and vertical ilia and coxa valga (increased neck shaft angle) are the features commonly seen.

Differential Diagnosis

It should be differentiated from

(a) Homocystinuria (unequal body proportions with dislocated lens), which is an autosomal recessive condition presenting with mental retardation and osteoporosis. The lens usually dislocates inferiorly. Homocystine can be found in urine of these patients.

(b) Congenital contractural arachnodactyly presents with congenital symmetrical contractures. There is no generalised laxity, dislocation of lens or heart disease.

Ehlers–Danlos Syndrome is an autosomal dominant disorder of connective tissue affecting skin, ligaments and blood vessel walls. The condition is characterised by hyperextensible *"cigarette paper"* skin. Skin splits easily and leaves pigmented tissue paper scars. Joint hypermobility and dislocation, soft tissue/ bone fragility and soft tissue calcification is also seen. Increased vascular fragility (tendency to bruising, aneurysm formation and spontaneous vessel rupture) and increased incidence of visceral tears are seen. Treatment consists of physical therapy, orthotics andarthrodesis.

Homocystinuria is an autosomal recessive inborn error of methionine metabolism due to reduced enzyme cystathionine b synthetase. Patients show Marfanoid habitus and high arched palate but joint laxity is uncommon. Over half the patients are mentally retarded. The lens dislocation is usually inferior (cf. Marfans). Osteoporosis is common and may lead to flat or biconcave vertebrae appreciated on lateral x-ray of spine. *Spontaneous thrombotic episodes* may be precipitated by anaesthesia or minor surgery in these patients.

This condition is differentiated from Marfans by autosomal recessive inheritance, mental retardation, osteoporosis and inferior dislocation of lens.

Early treatment with vitamin B6 and a reduced methionine diet may help.

Sclerosing Bone Dysplasias

Osteopetrosis (*Marble Bone Disease / Albers Schönberg Disease*) is a group of bone disorders that lead to increased sclerosis and obliteration of the medullary canal due to decreased osteoclast function (a failure of bone resorption). It may result from abnormality of the immune system (thymic defect). Deficiency of carbonic anhydrase isoenzyme 2 (CA-2) is associated with clinical appearance of osteopetrosis.

Two main types of osteopetrosis are defined clinically:

Severe congenital/infantile form is autosomal recessive and often, termed 'malignant variant'. It is apparent at birth or early infancy (may be stillborn in severely affected cases). The bone is fragile and pathological fractures are common (Fig. 2.13a,b). Fractures heal normally but at times lead to deformity such as coxa vara. Failure to remodel skeleton into cortical and medullary bone does not allow appropriate degree of haemopoiesis. This leads to anaemia, leucopenia and thrombocytopenia. Extramedullary haemopoiesis leading to hepatosplenomegaly ensues. Bleeding tendencies, infections and failure to thrive are seen.

Skull shows thickened vault and base with absence of air cells and sinuses. Cranial nerves compression (II, VII, VIII) leading to deafness and blindness is also seen. Sometimes hydrocephalus may be present due to reduced size of foramen magnum. Dentition is delayed and teeth are small.

These patients often die in infancy due to complications.

Milder Tarda form/Adult type is autosomal dominant. This disease form may be asymptomatic or may present with bone pains and increased fractures. It is compatible with normal life span.

Histology

Osteoclasts in osteopetrosis lack the normal ruffled border. Marrow spaces are filled with necrotic calcified cartilage that has not remodelled into mature lamellar bone.

Radiology

Marble bones (obliteration of distinction between cortex and medulla) and *bone within bone* (when remodelling is abnormal intermittently and leads to a defined radiographic anatomical outline of skeleton within another bone) especially in metacarpals and phalanges are seen. (Fig. 2.13c)

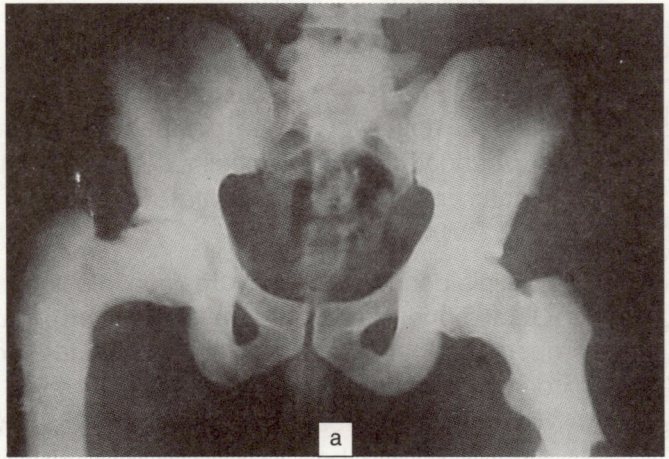 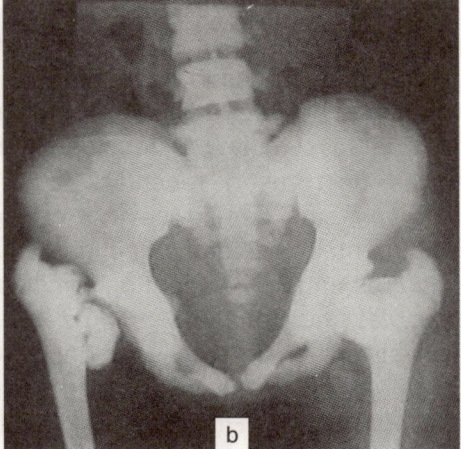

Fig. 2.13a,b.   X-Rays of patients with osteopetrosis. Note the pathologic fractures

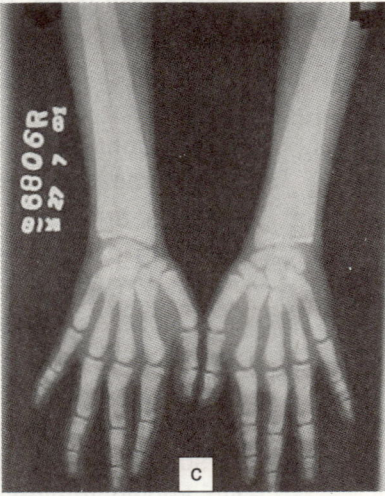

Fig. 2.13c.   Osteopetrosis involving forearm and hand

Metaphysis of long bones are expanded and club shaped. This may lead to "*Erlenmeyer flask*" deformity at proximal humerus/distal femur metaphysis. Skull is thick and sclerotic with absent air cells and sinuses. Vertebral bodies are uniformly dense or have a sandwich appearance or a classical "*Rugger Jersey*" spine where segments of increased density above and below are separated by a band of more translucent bone. Transverse or longitudinal striations may be seen in less severe cases with fluctuating activity of the disease. Ilium may have arcuate bands occasionally. Involvement of mandible is rare but when present, leads to *osteomyelitis of mandible* following dental work. Osteomyelitis of maxilla may also occur rarely.

Laboratory investigations reveal no consistent abnormality except anemia, thrombocytopenia and leukopenia.

Treatment

Medical therapy has included prednisone to improve hematologic function but it slows growth. Other agents used are high dose calcitriol and parathormone to stimulate osteoclasts. Interferon gamma has been used recently. *Bone Marrow Transplantation* can be life saving during childhood. Treatment of skeletal affections is prevention of fractures and consequent deformities. Whenever possible, the fractures should be treated conservatively. When internal fixation is required, plating for fracture should be preferred to intramedullary nailing. However, risk of infection after surgery in these cases is high.

Pyknodysostosis is an autosomal recessive disorder which is characterised by short limb dwarfism, persistent open fontanelles with wormian bones, osteosclerosis with increased bone fragility, hypoplastic acromial ends of clavicle and short digits with hypoplastic terminal phalanges. (Classical appearance of skull, clavicle and hands). Dysplastic facial bones and mandible, large calvarium, frontal bulging and small face are seen. Maxillae are small and angle of mandible is more obtuse than normal. Face is small and jaw recedes. The other features are:

- Dental abnormalities (premature or delayed eruption).
- Osteosclerotic or undermodelled ribs.

- Clavicles may sometimes be absent.
- Kyphosis, scoliosis, increased density of vertebrae
- Genu valgum.

X-rays show increased sclerosis with incomplete remodelling of tubular bones and multiple fractures.

Differential Diagnosis

1. Osteopetrosis (Pyknodysostosis is an autosomal recessive condition with typical appearance of skull, clavicle and hands, delayed fontanelle closure, without striped osteosclerosis and haemopoietic complications).

2. Cleido-Cranial dysostosis has no increased bone density or fragility and is autosomal dominant.

Prognosis is good with normal life expectancy in this disorder.

Enostosis (Bone Island)

Bone Island is a well-circumscribed round or oval sclerotic focus of dense compact haversian bone surrounded by host cancellous bone. It is typically small and is an incidental finding on X-rays (Fig. 2.14a,b).

Multiple bone islands may be seen in osteopoikilosis. Giant bone islands (more than 2 cm) may show increased uptake on bone scan and should be distinguished from osteosarcoma. A benign looking lesion that increases more than 25% within 6 months should be biopsied to rule out low-grade osteosarcoma. An enostosis itself needs no treatment.

Osteopoikilosis (Spotted Bone Disease) is an autosomal dominant, rare, clinically benign, symptomless condition in which bones show multiple, discrete or clustered foci of uniform radiodensity giving bone a spotted appearance. The disorder is symmetrical, epiphyseal and metaphyseal in location and involves *small bones of hands and feet* and articular ends of long bones commonly. About 10% patients have skin papules (cutaneous skin nodules, usually fibrous tissue pathologically such as fibromatosis, scleroderma like lesions, keloids) called as "*Dermatofibrosis lenticularis disseminata*". Histologically, the lesion is identical to solitary bone island. It follows a benign course. No known malignant degeneration is reported.

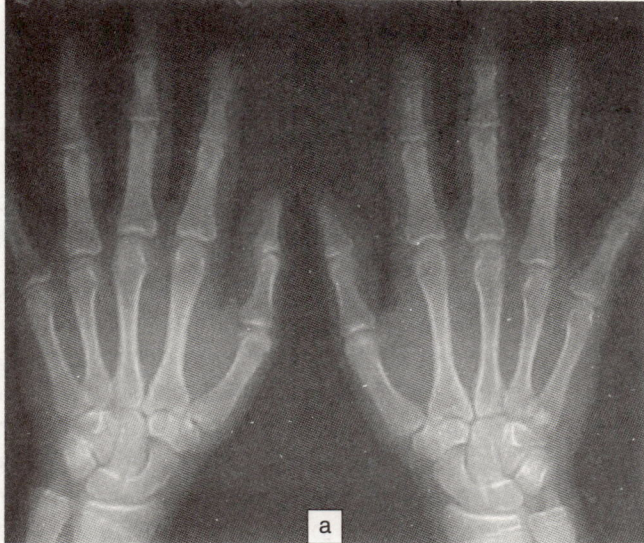
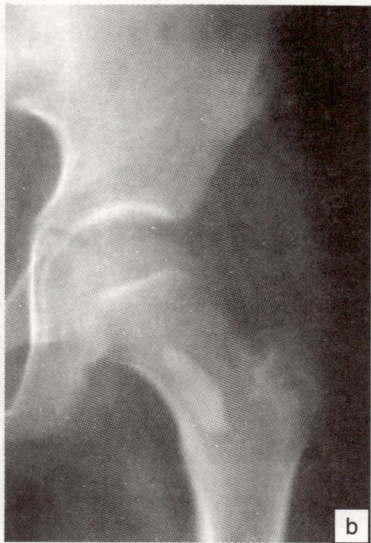

Fig. 2.14a,b. Bone island incidentally discovered in (a) base of fifth metacarpal, and (b) proximal femur

Osteopathia Striata is an autosomal dominant, benign, asymptomatic dysplasia characterised by symmetrical metaphyseal radiodense striations. The striations are oriented parallel to the long axis of bone and are thick near the epiphysis and tapering into the diaphysis. A characteristic fan like pattern is seen in the pelvis. It may be associated with sclerosis of skull and dermal hypoplasia. The condition may occur along with osteopoikilosis or melorheostosis.

Melorheostosis is rare, non-familial, asymmetric, usually unilateral bony disorder. The affected bones display peculiar linear streaks of hyperostosis along the main axes of long bones likened to melting wax dripping down the sides of a candle (Fig. 2.15a,b).

There may be associated pain, soft tissue contractures (palmar and plantar fascia contractures), fibrosis and skin abnormalities. The affected limb is short; there are often deformities and limitation of joint motion. Ectopic bone or soft tissue melorheostosis may be present in para-articular locations. Soft tissue tumors such as lipomas and fibrous lesions have been reported in association with melorheostosis. In children attempts at surgical management of contractures are unrewarding. Pain usually subsides over years. Radiologic progression is not usually observed in adults. Malignant change has not been reported in this condition.

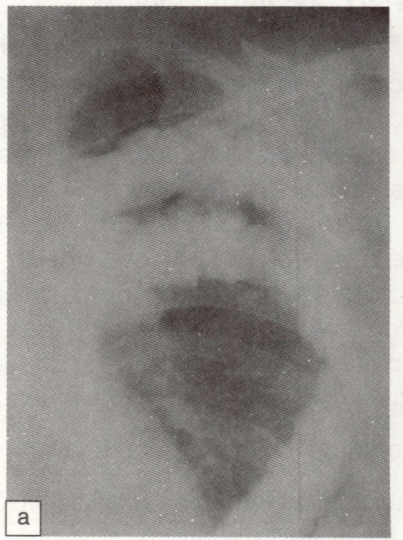
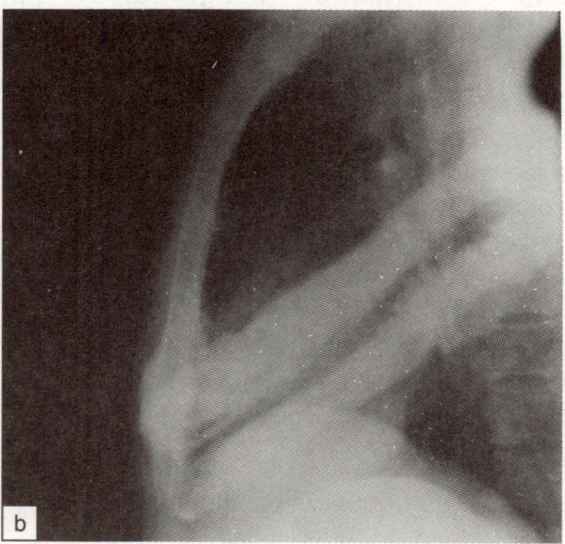

Fig. 2.15a,b. Radiographic appearance of Melorheostosis

Progressive Diaphyseal Dysplasia (Camurati-Engelmann Disease) is an autosomal dominant disorder characterised by progressive symmetrical hyperostosis of diaphyseal part of long bones and occasionally skull. Clinically, leg pain, waddling gait, wasting of muscle, hypotonia and easy fatigability are common features. The condition presents in infancy and the affected children are "late walkers". Lower limbs involvement is commonly seen including tibia and femur (followed by humerus). Bones formed by membranous ossification (periosteum and endosteum) are affected more than the bones developed essentially through endochondral ossification (epiphysis and metaphysis). The skull shows thickened vault and base with narrowed foramina. There may be pressure on optic and auditory nerves. The serum alkaline phosphatase may be raised. X-rays show fusiform thickening of diaphyseal cortices. Contours of bone are smooth (unlike melorheostosis). Differential diagnosis includes:

1. Paget's disease (asymmetrical involvement; end of bone is always involved).

2. Melorheostosis (hot candle wax dripping appearance of bone).

3. Infantile cortical hyperostosis (occurs at younger age and regresses).

This is a self-limiting condition, which regresses with age. Corticosteroids have been used to stimulate osteoclasts, reduce bone deposition and relieve pain.

Fibrodysplasia Ossificans Progressiva (Myositis Ossificans Progressiva) is a rare disorder, which is autosomal dominant but most cases arise by spontaneous mutation. There is progressive heterotopic ossification of tendons, ligaments, fasciae and skeletal muscle associated with over expression of *bone morphogenetic protein 4*. Characteristically, a short hallux (more rarely thumb) is present at birth. Other stigmata at birth may be microdactyly (esp. hypoplasia of terminal phalanx), synostosis of phalanges of first digit or hallux valgus. Rarely first metacarpal and metatarsal are also short. The onset is usually before the age of 4 years.

The disorder begins as rubbery, painful, tender, often erythematous deep nodules initially in head, shoulder, back and posterior neck and later in limbs. These lesions subside after a few weeks and after 3 months turn into hard non-tender nodules. Some swellings are cystlike and on occasion break down and discharge. Some lesions regress while many undergo endochondral ossification (Fibrous tissue-cartilage-calcified cartilage-woven bone-lamellar bone) to form mature bone.

There is progressive immobility and extra-articular ankylosis. Early symptoms may only be of some discomfort with restriction of movements. Torticollis may be the presenting sign due to neck tissue involvement. Scoliosis may also occur. Masseter is involved early. Tongue, facial muscles other than masseter, diaphragm, levator ani, sphincters, muscles of larynx and eye and heart muscle are spared. Deafness has also been reported. Shoulder and chest are the most commonly involved sites (Fig. 2.16a,b). Other sites in decreasing order of occurrence are hip, elbow, abdomen, knee, jaw, neck and ankle (involvement is rare distal to elbow and knee).

The most common cause of death is pneumonia due to involvement of the thoracic cage. Any trauma, infection or surgery may lead to the formation of heterotopic bone. The disease is progressive if onset is early and death occurs before 20 years of age. Milder cases may have exacerbation or remissions over a longer period. Diphosphonate sodium etidronate has been used with limited success in this disease.

Inborn Errors of Metabolism

Mucopolysaccharidoses

These are lysosomal storage disorders due to genetic deficiencies of enzymes (such as lysosomal acid hydrolases) that breakdown glycosaminoglycans (mucopolysaccharides) resulting in their intralysosomal accumulation. The disease affects zones of maturation and degeneration in the physis. The effect on skeletal growth and development is marked leading to proportionate dwarfism. Radiological signs are common in all groups and differ only in severity and age of onset and are collectively called "*dysostosis multiplex*".

The common salient features are:

1. Radiological features : Skull is thick ; sella turcica is enlarged (J shaped)

2. Broad clavicles: especially medially

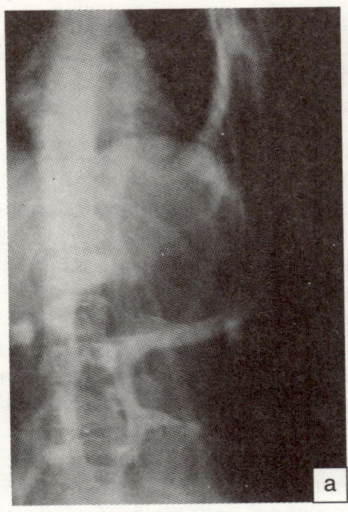
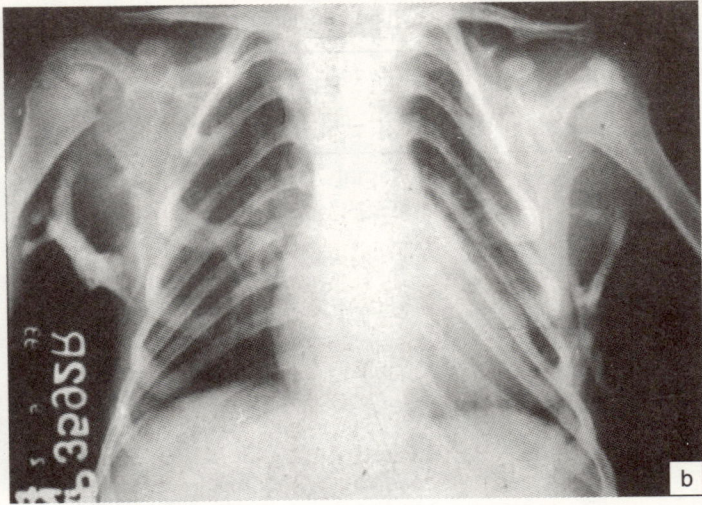

Fig. 2.16a,b. X-rays of patient with Fibrodysplasia Ossificans Progressiva

3. Ribs are narrow posteriorly and broad anteriorly (paddle shaped)

4. Scoliosis is common.

5. Anterosuperior part of the vertebral body is deficient giving rise to 'hook' vertebrae. (Fig: 2.17)

6. Wide flat pelvis and acetabular roof obliquity; coxa valga is commonly seen.

7. Second to fifth metacarpals are pointed proximally.

8. Bullet shaped phalanges (short and stubby).

9. Sloping lower ends of radius and ulna giving rise to inverted V shaped deformity.

The distinctive radiological features of Morquio's disease (Type IV) are:

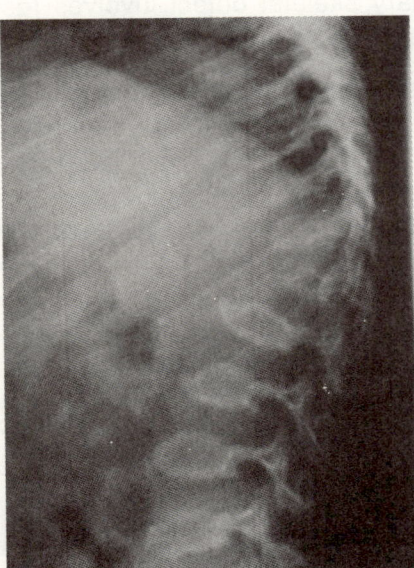

Fig. 2.17. X-ray showing beaking of vertebrae in Mucopolysaccharidoses

- Vertebral bodies have anterior beak and platyspondyly

- Capital femoral epiphysis becomes irregular and disappears.

- Coxa vara is common

- Odontoid hypoplasia with C_1–C_2 instability.

- Metacarpals and phalanges have central constriction

Characteristic features of common types are seen in Table 2.2.

Mucolipidoses are a group of storage diseases with some skeletal findings similar to Mucopolysaccharidoses but without excessive mucopolysaccharides in urine.

GM1 Gangliosidosis Type I

This is an autosomal recessive, severe disorder similar to Hurler's syndrome, which presents at birth (unlike Hurler's). It results from the deficiency of enzyme β–galactosidase. It is characterised by coarse facies, mental retardation, hepatosplenomegaly, stiff joints and failure to thrive. There is a cherry red spot in macula in about half the patients. X-ray changes are similar to Hurler's except excessive periosteal bone formation around shafts of long bones (*Cloaking*).

The disease has a poor prognosis and patients die within 2 years.

Mucolipidosis II

This is an autosomal recessive disorder similar to gangliosidosis type I (I-cell disease) and Hurler's syndrome clinically and radiologically but the disease

Table 2.2. Characteristic features of common Mucopolysaccharidoses

MPS Type	Syndrome	Enzymatic Defect	Inheritance	Age At Onset	Acid MPS in Urine	Salient Clinical Features
IH	HURLER	α- L Iduronidase	Autosomal Recessive	First few months (<2 years)	Dermatan sulfate and Heparan sulfate	Coarse Facies (Gorgoylism), early corneal clouding. Severe skeletal changes: kyphoscoliosis, short mandible with missing condyles. Hepato-splenomegaly, mental retardation, death before 10-15 years due to cardio-respiratory complications.
IS	SCHEIE	α- L Iduronidase	Autosomal Recessive	Later childhood	Dermatan sulfate and heparan sulfate	Late corneal clouding, joint contractures, may be normal radiologically, normal intelligence, normal life expectancy.
II	HUNTER	Iduronate 2-Sulfatase	X-Linked recessive	6–12 months (<4 years)	Dermatan sulfate and heparan sulfate	No corneal clouding, no kyphoscoliosis, skeletal changes mild, progressive deafness, mental retardation, only males are affected. Live upto second or third decade. Die due to cardiorespiratory complications.
III	SAN FILIPPO	N-heparan sulfatase or α-N acetyl glucosamini-dase	Autosomal Recessive	Early childhood (after 2 years)	Heparan sulfate	Minimal physical abnormalities; may be normal radiologically, Progressive dementia
IV	MORQUIO SYNDROME	Galactose 6-sulfatase	Autosomal Recessive	2–4 years	Keratan sulfate	Corneal clouding, severe skeletal changes; dwarfing with platyspondyly, Genu valgum, progressive spinal cord damage, myelopathy, atlantoaxial instability due to odontoid hypoplasia; thin tooth enamel, Joint laxity, protruding sternum (manubrio-sternal angle 90°). Premature osteoarthritis; normal intelligence: survive into adulthood.
VI	MAROTE AUX LAMY	N-acetyl gelactosa-mine 4 – sulfatase	Autosomal Recessive	Early - late childhood	Dermatan sulfate	Corneal clouding, severe skeletal changes; cardiopulmonary failure. Normal intelligence, variable survival

Note: *Hurler's syndrome has most prominent coarse facies (GORGOYLISM)

presents earlier in life. A number of lysosomal enzymes are deficient. Cultured cells show dense inclusion granules (hence the name I-cell disease). The prognosis is poor and most children die within first year of life.

Sphingolipidoses

Sphingolipidoses arise due to deposition of sphingolipids. These disorders generally have less effect on skeleton. Only Gaucher's disease has significant skeletal involvement.

Gaucher's Disease

This is an autosomal recessive storage disease caused due to reduced enzyme glucocerebrosidase. Accumulation of glucocerebrosides occurs in large reticulo-endothelial cells (*Gaucher cells*) in spleen, skeleton and liver.

The primary skeletal defect involves resting layer of the cartilage.

Weakness, anaemia and hepatosplenomegaly are common. The skeletal manifestations are osteoporosis, osteolysis by Gaucher cells and bone infarction. Avascular necrosis of femoral head and humeral head may be seen. Pathological fractures may occur and take long time to heal. The bones show expanded "flask-shaped" metaphyseal regions with periosteal new bone formation.

The diagnosis is made by finding Gaucher cells (large, multinucleated cells with wrinkled cytoplasm, pale staining with strong acid phosphatase reaction).

Currently no specific treatment is available. Splenectomy may be indicated for hypersplenism. Treatment and prevention of fractures is important.

CHAPTER 3

Bone and Joint Infections

Introduction

Bone and joint infections are serious clinical problems. One quarter of the patients with bone and joint infections used to die in pre-antibiotic era. Mortality has come down in the present day (due to antibiotics) but morbidity remains high. The presentation of infections in bone can be protean. A careful correlation of clinical, radiologic, and histological findings is must for proper diagnosis and treatment.

Difference between bone and soft tissue infections

Bone has unique architecture and compartmentalised hypervascular milieu, which provides ideal nidus for growth of organisms and chronic infection.

The pathological reaction to infection in bone is considerably modified by loss of blood supply. The *endosteal* blood supply is compromised due to infection, thrombosis of vessels and pressure necrosis and the *periosteal* due to stripping of periosteum by abscess. Formation of sequestra due to devitalization of bone by infection defies attempts to obtain adequate concentration of antibiotics at the site of infection. Even after the focus of infection has been sterilised by antibiotics the mineralised structure of bone creates special problems of healing.

Osteomyelitis in the presence of implants is associated with development of a biofilm that coats the bacteria and protects them from macrophages and antibiotics.

Osteomyelitis often occurs in growing children and especially in lower limbs. Therefore disabling sequelae such as partial or complete epiphyseal growth arrest with resultant deformities and limb length inequalities are common.

Osteomyelitis

Acute Hematogenous Osteomyelitis is bone and bone marrow infection caused by blood borne organisms. It commonly affects children. Boys are affected more often than girls. **Staphylococcus aureus (coagulase positive) is the commonest pathogen** causing acute osteomyelitis. E. coli and Group B streptococci cause osteomyelitis in neonates. However, anaerobic infections may also be seen (Peptococcus magnus, bacteroides). Hemophilus influenzae commonly causes osteomyelitis in children three months to four years old.

Metaphysis is the initial site of infection because it presents an extremely vascular area. Branches of nutrient artery provide network of vessels for zones of endochondral ossification in this area. Most vessels do not anastomose and terminate in venous sinusoids i.e. they are end-arteries. They have hairpin bends, which leads to vascular congestion. Venous sinusoids are ideal bed for bacterial seeding (Fig. 3.1). Large calibre of metaphyseal veins in children leads to marked slowing of blood flow and thus predisposes them to post-traumatic thromboses and colonisation by blood borne bacteria. Also, trauma often localises to metaphysis and bacteraemia may infect resultant haematoma. Metastatic infection may occur in spine following genitourinary infections by gram negative rods gaining access to spine via venous plexuses (Batson's plexuses) which lack valves and anastomose freely with segmental systemic veins and portal system (Fig. 3.2).

Sources of infection in a long bone
(Fig. 3.3)

Factors predisposing to osteomyelitis have been listed in Table 3.1.

Pathogenesis

Once infection occurs it spreads to adjacent cancellous bone and through cortex, via haversian canals, to the periosteum. Periosteum reacts by forming new bone (involucrum) occa-

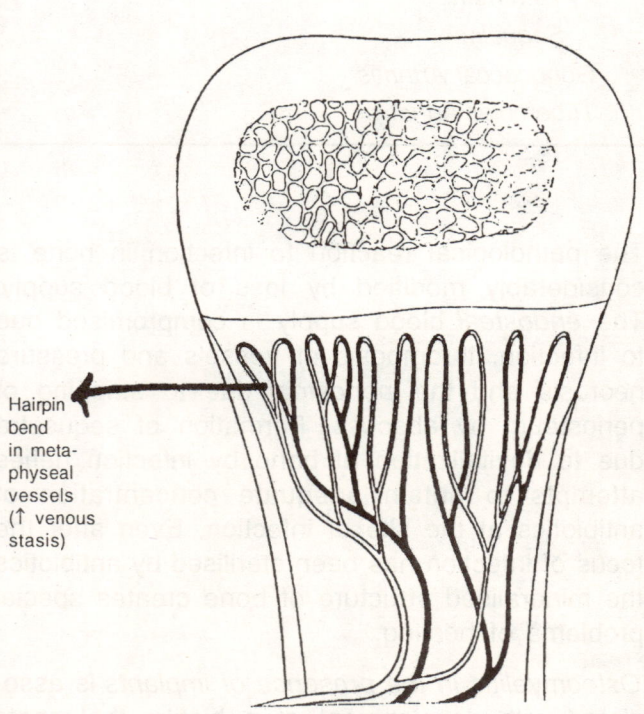

Fig. 3.1. Vascular supply of metaphysis

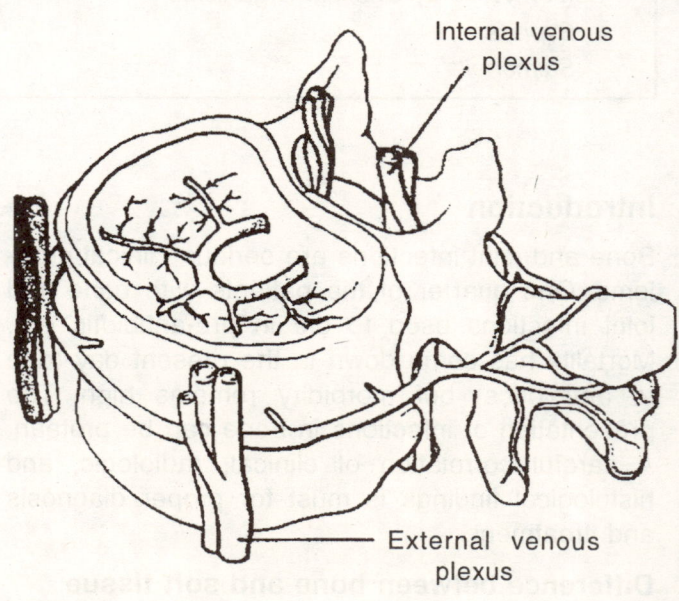

Fig. 3.2. Batson's Venous Plexus

Table 3.1. Factors predisposing to osteomyelitis

1. Host susceptibility due to :
   ☆ Predisposing trauma, surgery
   ☆ Loss of natural barriers (decubitus ulcers, dental procedures)
   ☆ Underlying receptive pathophysiology
      • Post splenectomy
      • Sickle cell disease
   ☆ Deficient host defence (neutrophil depletion/dysfunction)
   ☆ Overwhelming of host defences, antibiotic resistance and chronic disease
   ☆ IV drug users
2. Virulence of infecting organism or its by-product (e.g. endotoxin)
3. Combination of these (as in diabetes)

sionally and may rupture. Infection leads to vascular compromise and leads to bone necrosis (sequestrum formation). Epiphyseal growth plate offers a barrier to spread of infection to the joint. However, intraarticular location of metaphysis may lead to spread of infection to joint. Some examples are given in Table 3.2.

Table 3.2. Examples of joints with intraarticular metaphysis

Joint	Intra-articular metaphysis
Hip	(upper femoral)
Shoulder	(upper humeral)
Elbow	(radial neck)
Ankle	(lower fibular)

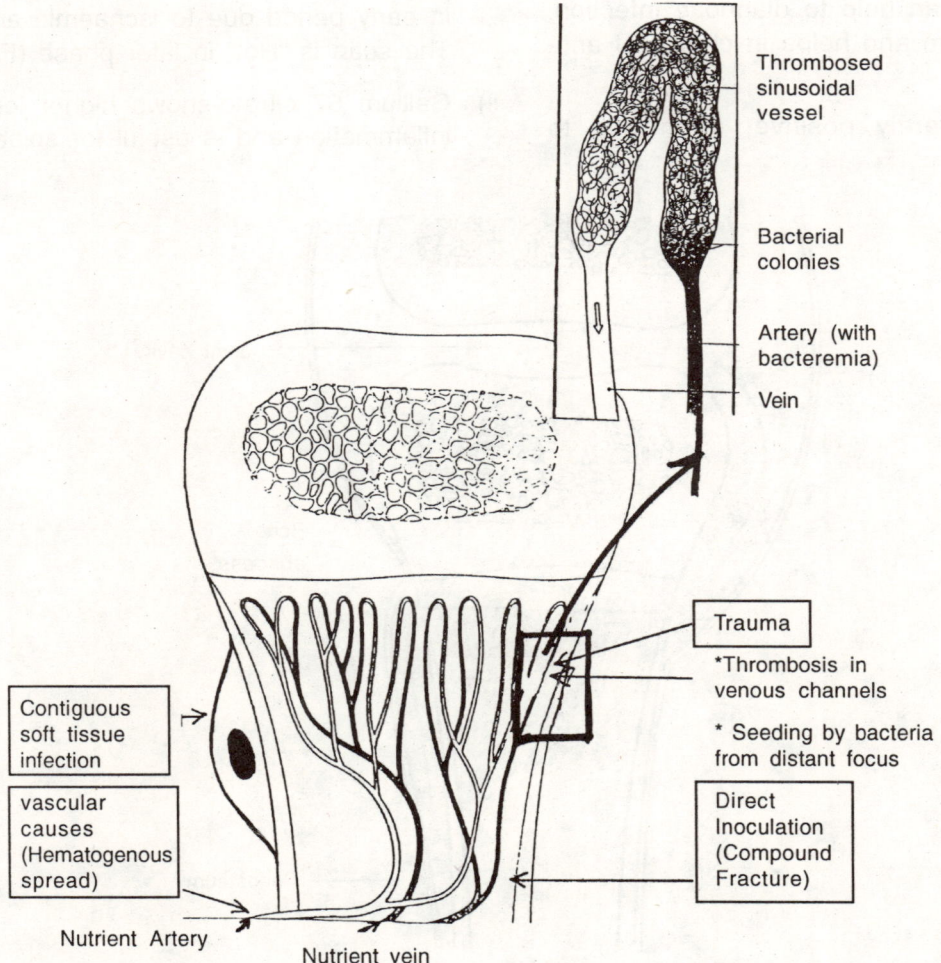

Fig. 3.3.   Sources of infection in a long bone. *Inset* Stasis in metaphyseal vessel with bacterial colonisation

Rarely, joint may be involved by pus tracking under the periosteum (outside the bone) and entering the joint (Fig. 3.4).

Clinically, acute osteomyelitis is characterised by chills, fever, pain, erythema, swelling and tenderness. Pain is often the only symptom in adult osteomyelitis.

Empirical antibiotic treatment may mask the symptoms and delay diagnosis. The infection is most common in metaphysis of long bones (lower limbs more commonly than upper limbs). An effusion may be seen in an adjacent joint (*sympathetic effusion*). It is a sterile response and clinically the movements at joint are not restricted.

Investigations

The leukocyte count may be raised with a shift to the left. Erythrocyte sedimentation rate (ESR) and levels of C-reactive protein (CRP) are usually raised. Aspiration can help to diagnose infection, identify the organism and helps in choice of antibiotics.

Blood culture is rarely positive, often due to empirical antibiotic therapy initiated by primary physician.

Imaging

X-ray changes appear late and are non-specific. First 7–10 days may show muscular oedema and *obliteration of soft tissue (fat) planes. Periosteal reaction (elevation) is the earliest bone change* and is seen at around 10 days (Fig. 3.5a). Demineralisation of bone is seen at 10–14 days. Skeletal changes such as periostitis, sequestrum formation and involucrum formation take 3–6 weeks to appear.

Radionucleide scans

Bone scans are sensitive and positive early, after 24–48 hours. Commonly used scans are:

i) Tc 99^m diphosphonate scan-localises vascularity and new bone formation. It may be negative in early period due to ischaemia and necrosis. The scan is "Hot" in later phase (Fig. 3.5b,c).

ii) Gallium 67 citrate-shows higher localisation in inflammation and is useful for spine infections.

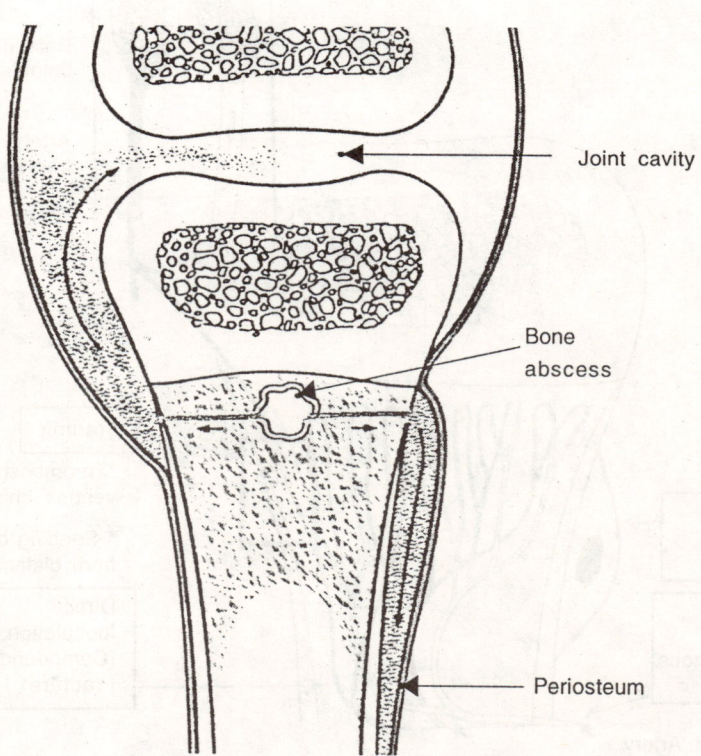

Fig. 3.4.   Joint involvement by acute osteomyelitis

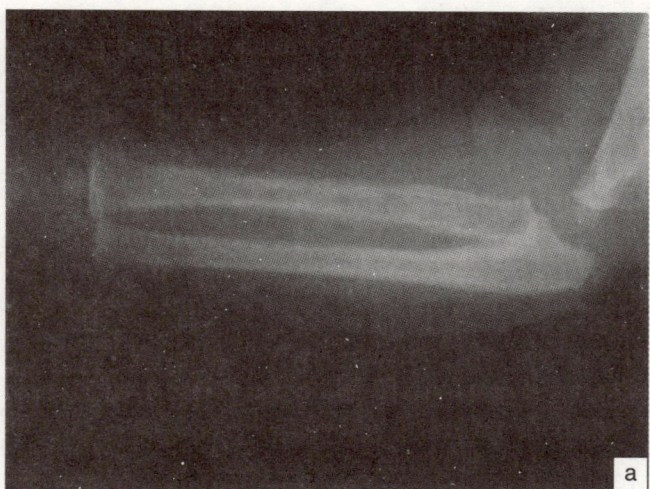

Fig. 3.5a. X-Ray showing periosteal reaction in the radius following acute osteomyelitis

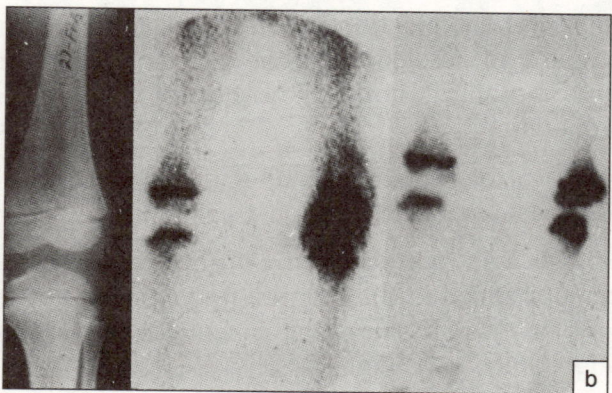

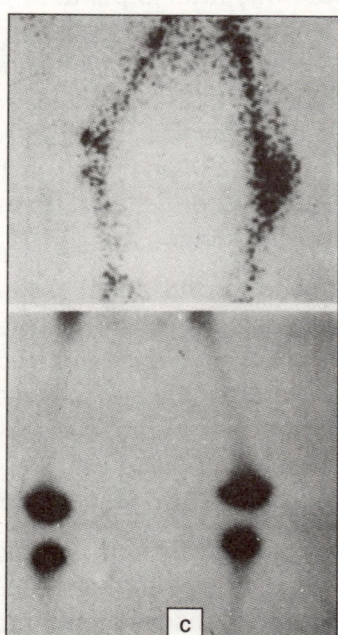

Fig. 3.5b,c. Bone scan showing increased uptake around left knee

iii) Indium 111-labelled leukocyte scan-localises neutrophils and is useful for extremities.

Ultrasound may localise deep-seated soft tissue swellings. Magnetic Resonance Imaging (MRI) helps in diagnosis and defining the extent of the involvement.

Differential diagnosis

Osteomyelitis should be considered in differential diagnosis of all orthopaedic afflictions with ambiguous clinical and radiographic findings. The parents often give the history of trauma but it should not allow the orthopaedist to miss the septic process. It is extremely important especially in paediatric patients to rule out neoplastic lesions especially Ewing's sarcoma. The differential diagnosis of osteomyelitis is shown in Table 3.3.

Treatment

Acute hematogenous osteomyelitis can be treated successfully with rest (splintage) and antibiotics if started early. Parenteral third generation cepha-

Table 3.3. Differential diagnosis of osteomyelitis

---

1. Tumours
    a) Benign lesions
        Osteoid osteoma
        Osteoblastoma
        Eosinophilic granuloma
    b) Malignant lesions
        Round cell tumours (especially Ewing's sarcoma)
        Lymphoma
2. Inflammatory conditions
    a) Septic arthritis
        Swelling and tenderness at the joint
        Any attempted movement at the joint is painful
        Aspiration of joint reveals pus
    b) Rheumatic fever
        Insidious onset
        Less intense symptoms
        Differentiated from the osteomyelitis by fleeting arthritis
3. Scurvy
4. Congenital Syphilis (with syphilitic osteitis and periostitis)
5. Trauma with fracture

---

losporin or penicillinase resistant synthetic penicillin is drug of choice. Choice of intravenous antibiotics should be decided by expected sensitivity of most likely pathogen, which may be modified if necessary, once culture report is available. The patient is monitored closely, clinically and with total and differential leukocyte counts. Intravenous antibiotics are continued till patient is afebrile. This is followed by oral antibiotics for a total of 6 weeks.

Surgical Treatment

Conservative treatment should be abandoned and patient operated when:

- the response to antibiotic is not rapid, which is evident by continuing fever, leucocytosis and severe pain;

- patient presents late (for drainage of pus and debridement of infected tissues).

Surgery consists of drainage of abscess. If no pus is found after incising the periosteum, holes should be drilled in the cortex to localise the site of infection. A window of cortex is removed from the metaphyseal region to allow free drainage. Extensive curettage of medullary cavity should **not** be done routinely. Wound is closed over a drain, which is removed within few days to avoid secondary bacterial contamination.

Course

Complete resolution of acute hematogenous osteomyelitis is possible with early, effective, intravenous antibiotic therapy. Long-term morbidity occurs in almost one-fourth patients where the disease leads to chronic osteomyelitis. Chronic osteomyelitis and recurrences are more common in patients who are diagnosed late.

Neonatal Osteomyelitis is caused by hematogenous infection. The common organisms are Group-B streptococcus (commonest), Staphylococcus aureus and Escherichia coli. Group-B streptococcus is commonly found in vagina and infection occurs during delivery and commonly involves one bone. Staph. aureus and E. coli can cause polyostotic involvement in the newborns. Immunological incompetence of the newborn may delay clinical diagnosis in some patients due to absence of systemic symptoms. Combination of penicillinase

resistant synthetic penicillin and third generation cephalosporin is the primary antibiotic regimen.

Post traumatic osteomyelitis

Post traumatic osteomyelitis occurs following compound fractures, surgery and puncture wounds. Direct inoculation of bacteria occurs through the wounds. Polymicrobial infections are common in road traffic accident cases. Gram negative organisms (including pseudomonas) are often present in addition to staphylococcus and streptococcus. *Pseudomonas is the most common organism in infections of heel/calcaneus following puncture wounds* (*Thorn in tennis sneakers*). The site of involvement in post traumatic osteomyelitis is at the site of inoculation and the diaphyseal involvement is most common (cf. metaphyseal involvement in haematogenous osteomyelitis). Significant amount of foreign material including cloth, dirt and metallic debris may be found in these wounds.

Removal of all foreign matter and dead tissue is the most important step in treatment.

When associated with fracture, complete immobilisation of the fracture fragments is mandatory for reestablishment of vascular supply to deal adequately with infection.

Subacute Osteomyelitis is primarily a radiological diagnosis. The condition most often involves femur and tibia. The patient may have pain without systemic/local signs or symptoms. It occurs following partially treated acute osteomyelitis. Total leukocyte count and blood cultures are often normal in this condition. ESR, radiographs and cultures from bone may help in making the diagnosis.

Brodie's abscess (Bone abscess) is a localised form of subacute osteomyelitis. The onset is insidious and systemic manifestations are mild or absent. Radiographic features consist of localised radiolucency usually seen in the metaphysis of long bones. It is typically elongated with well-demarcated margin and surrounded by reactive sclerosis.

Sequestra are always absent. A radiolucent tract may be seen extending from the lesion into the growth plate. (Bone abscess may cross the epiphyseal plate and extend into epiphysis unlike acute osteomyelitis). Epiphyseal osteomyelitis is caused exclusively by Staphylococcus aureus.

Differential Diagnosis

Brodie's abscess may mimic an osteoid osteoma radiologically and clinically. Presence of radiolucent tract from the lesion into the growth plate favours infection. When present in epiphysis, it should be differentiated from chondroblastoma.

Treatment

Treatment of Brodie's abscess in metaphysis includes surgical curettage. Epiphyseal osteomyelitis is treated with antibiotics. Drainage is indicated if pus is present.

Chronic osteomyelitis may arise following inappropriately treated acute hematogenous osteomyelitis or inadequate surgical debridement of necrotic bone in exogenous osteomyelitis following trauma or surgery. The necrotic bone is walled off by periosteal new bone (involucrum) and fibrous tissue. Each cavity thus formed contains a piece of dead bone surrounded by granulation tissue (sequestrum) and harbours bacteria. Skin and soft tissues are often involved and get scarred, oedematous and poorly vascularised. Fistulous tracts form. Sequestrum/sequestra may be extruded through the sinus tract. Cavities containing sequestra may remain quiescent for variable intervals. Periods of quiescence are often followed by acute exacerbations. If drainage persists over many years, epidermoid carcinoma may develop in 1% patients (may occur 30–40 years after original infection). A *Marjolin's ulcer* is ulceration developing in epidermoid carcinoma of sinus tract. Complications of chronic osteomyelitis are enumerated in Table 3.4.

Table 3.4. Sequelae and complications of chronic osteomyelitis

→ Acute exacerbation
→ Pathological fracture (Fig. 3.6a)
→ Limb length discrepancy
 • Shortening of bone (epiphyseal damage) (Fig. 3.6b)
 • Lengthening of bone (epiphyseal hyperaemia) (Fig. 3.6c)
→ Angular deformities (Partial closure of epiphysis). (Fig. 3.6d)
→ Metastatic abscesses
→ Contractures and joint stiffness
→ Scarring of the skin
→ Epidermoid (squamous cell) carcinoma of sinus tract
→ Amyloidosis.

Chronic osteomyelitis is rare in healthy adults. It is seen in immunosuppressed hosts, in the presence of major nutritional or systemic disorder, diabetics, and in patients with peripheral vascular disease and IV drug abusers.

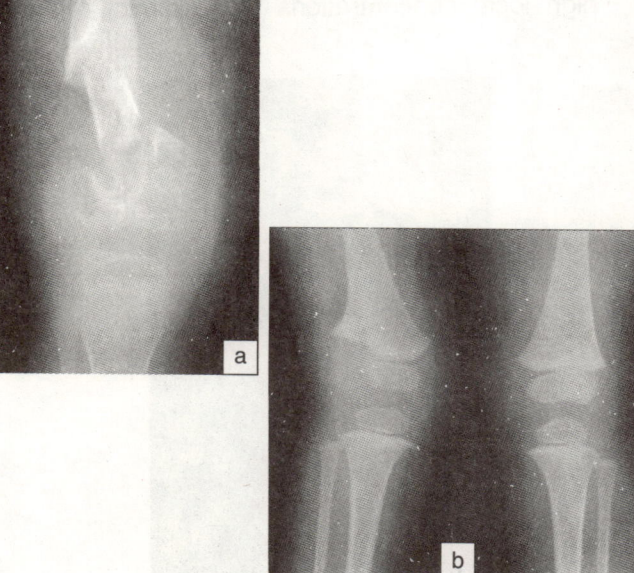
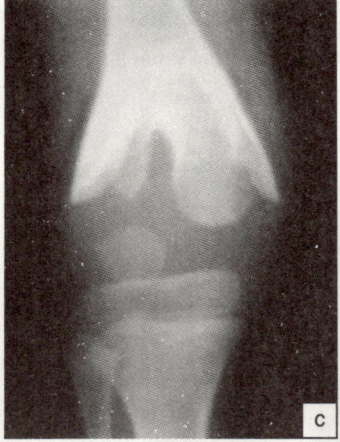
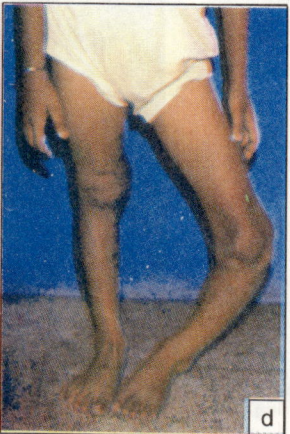

Fig. 3.6a. Pathologic fracture
Fig. 3.6b. Epiphyseal damage
Fig. 3.6c. Epiphyseal damage with growth arrest
Fig. 3.6d. Genu varum as a complication of asymmetric growth arrest left knee

Diagnosis

Diagnosis is readily made with presence of drainage and x-ray changes which include thickening and irregularity of bone, dense sequestrae surrounded by zone of lucency, cavities and radiolucent tracts in the bone, and presence of involucrum (reactive periosteal new bone) (Figs. 3.7a-c). Radionucleide studies may help in subtle cases without drainage. Attempt to isolate the offending organism should be made by taking *cultures from deeper areas or cavity during surgery* as drainage fluid has abundant contaminants. Bone scan (in the presence of implants) and Magnetic Resonance Imaging (MRI) (when implants are absent) are extremely valuable in establishing vascularity of segments of diaphysis with doubtful vascularity.

Treatment

Treatment consists of a wide range of procedures ranging from drainage of abscess and sequestrectomy to extensive debridement. The basic principles of surgical treatment of chronic osteomyelitis are:

i) **Sequestrectomy and Saucerization** Debridement with excision of dead, necrotic, infected tissues and sequestrae (sequestrectomy) till bleeding surfaces of bone and removal of the sinus tracts is done. Dense reactive bone, though not necrotic, is removed, as it is often poorly vascularised. Deroofing of the osteomyelitis cavity (saucerization) is done to facilitate drainage.

ii) **Obliteration of the dead space** (with an attempt to increase vascularity and promote healing) by :

–**Cancellous bone grafts**/vascularised bone grafts.

–**Antibiotic impregnated bone cement** Polymethylmethacrylate (PMMA or bone cement) beads impregnated with antibiotics (Fig. 3.8) are used to obliterate dead space and provide high local concentrations of antibiotics without

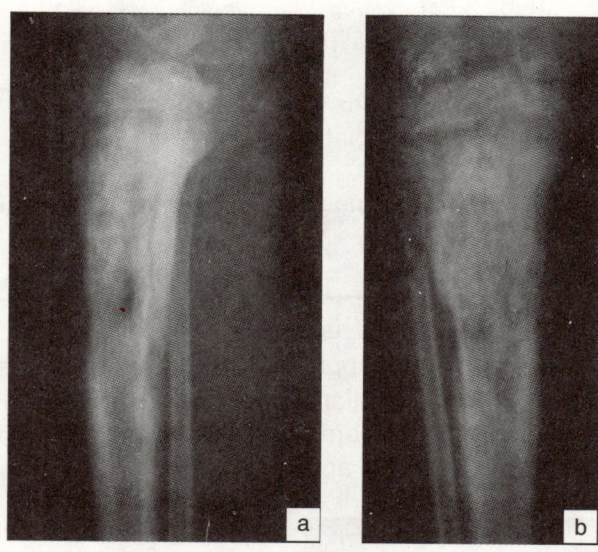

Fig. 3.7a,b.   AP and lateral x-rays of the proximal tibia showing chronic osteomyelitis

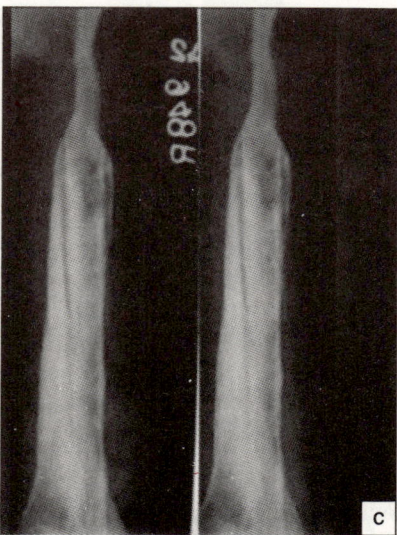

Fig. 3.7c.   X-rays showing tubular sequestrum

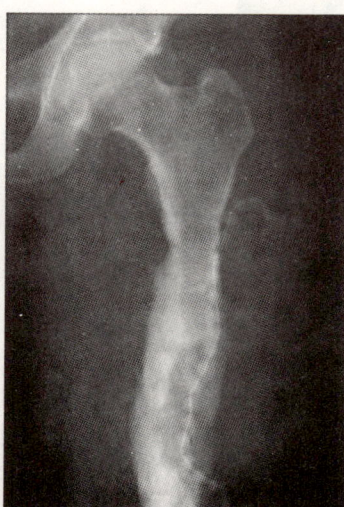

Fig. 3.8.   Chronic osteomyelitis of femur treated by sequestrectomy, saucerization and gentamycin beads

systemic ill effects. Antibiotics elute from beads within 2 weeks and their local antibiotic levels are insignificant by 6–8 weeks and the beads should then be removed.

–**Surrounding muscle**: When antibiotic laden PMMA beads are not available local muscle flaps can be used to obliterate dead space.

iii) **Soft tissue coverage**: is often required. The various methods include:

- **Skin grafting**
- **Local Myocutaneous flaps**
- **Fasciocutaneous flaps**
- **Distant free flaps**

The treatment of infected nonunions is very difficult. Extensive debridement with concomitant antibiotic therapy is the most often performed operation. All necrotic bone with surrounding granulation tissue is removed. External fixation is the most useful method for skeletal stabilisation in the presence of infection. Hyperbaric oxygen has been used as adjuvant treatment in gas gangrene and chronic osteomyelitis.

Amputation may be required following multiple unsuccessful surgical procedures in patients with severe soft tissue scarring, joint contractures and infected nonunions or in those with malignancy of sinus tract.

Garre's Chronic Sclerosing Osteomyelitis is an unusual form of osteomyelitis affecting diaphysis of long bones in adolescents. Anaerobes have been implicated as causative organisms. The disease is probably caused by organisms of low virulence and/or occurs in hosts with good resistance/immune response. The onset is insidious with localised pain and tenderness. Intense proliferation of periosteum occurs causing bony deposition, which is seen as dense progressive sclerosis on x-rays. Malignancy must be ruled out. Biopsy must be performed in cases where the diagnosis is doubtful. Surgery and antibiotics are ineffective in providing cure.

Chronic Recurrent Multifocal Osteomyelitis (CRMO) is a variant of osteomyelitis seen in children and young adults. The etiology of this condition is unknown. The onset is insidious with low-grade fever, swelling and pain in the affected bones. Systemic symptoms may be absent. Occasionally, concomitant pustulosis palmoplantaris, or acne may be present.

Diagnosis

The laboratory values are normal except raised ESR. Multiple metaphyseal lytic lesions are seen in metaphysis of tubular bones (especially distal tibia and distal femur) and medial side of clavicle (Fig. 3.9). The involvement of bones is sometimes symmetrical. Periosteal new bone in the region of clavicle may raise the suspicion of round-cell malignancy. Bone scan may reveal multiple asymptomatic sites of involvement. Cultures for bacterial, fungal and viral organisms are negative. The histopathological findings suggest subacute or chronic osteomyelitis. The clinical

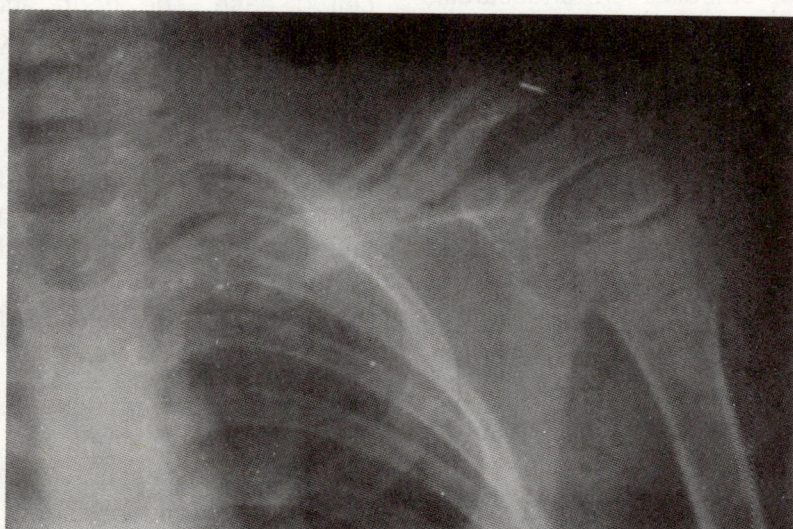

Fig. 3.9.   Chronic Recurrent Multifocal Osteomyelitis involving the clavicle

course is characterised by remissions and exacerbation over a period of several years and eventual resolution – so only symptomatic treatment is recommended.

Osteomyelitis in Special Situations

Diabetic Foot

Unsuspected underlying osteomyelitis is present in majority of diabetic foot ulcers. Chronic infections are common. The aetiology is polymicrobial and may be due to anaerobic organisms. Peripheral neuropathy and vascular insufficiency contribute to osteomyelitis. Decreased sensation predisposes to repeated trauma and vascular insufficiency (due to microangiopathy) predisposes to delayed healing and infection. Extensive debridement or amputation is often required. The antibiotic regimen includes ciprofloxacin and clindamycin.

Intravenous Drug Abusers

Pseudomonas aeruginosa is the organism responsible in most cases (alone or in combination with other organisms). The axial skeleton is predominantly involved. Spine, especially lumbar spine (> 50% cases), or pelvis followed by sternal sites (such as manubriosternal or sternoclavicular joints or even sternum) are the commonly involved areas. Occasionally shoulder, knee, hip and tibia may be involved by osteomyelitis/arthritis. Fever and chills are conspicuously absent and local pain is often the only clinical finding. The other associated morbid conditions are thrombophlebitis, septic embolization, endocarditis and hepatitis. ESR is often raised. Radiographs are often normal but technetium bone scan is almost always positive. Antibiotics are the mainstay of treatment and surgical debridement is usually not required.

Sickle Cell Disease

Recurrent attacks of bone infection are common in sickle cell disease. Vascular insufficiency and bone infarcts are the underlying causes. **Staphylococcus aureus is the most common causative agent,** though salmonella may also be isolated. Patients with sickle cell anemia are ten times more susceptible to salmonella osteomyelitis as compared with normal population. Other diseases leading to ischaemia and infection are Gaucher's disease (after biopsy) and osteopetrosis (Jaw osteomyelitis via tooth infection).

Post Splenectomy

Patients are prone to streptococcal infections due to the presence of poor host response especially to capsulated organisms.

Osteomyelitis by Unusual Organisms

Syphilitic osteomyelitis

Syphilis is a chronic systemic infection caused by Treponema palladium

A. **Congenital syphilis** is transmitted from mother to infant. Osteochondritis, periostitis and osteitis are the typical features. Destruction at the medial aspect of the metaphysis of a long bone (*Wimberger sign*) is characteristic. It is most classically seen in tibia. In the late stages, involvement of tibia results in characteristic anterior bowing deformity known as "*Saber-Shin*" deformity.

B. **Acquired syphilis** may present as chronic osteitis with extensive sclerosis of medullary canal or syphilitic abscesses (*Gumma*). Sequestrae are **never** seen.

Salmonella Osteomyelitis is mostly caused by serotypes other than S. typhi. It is common in sickle cell disease (but it is **not** the commonest organism causing osteomyelitis in sickle cell disease). It may occur in subjects without sickle cell disease. The bone affection occurs during convalescence 4 to 6 weeks after enteric fever. Diaphyseal involvement is common especially in femur. Vertebrae and ribs are also involved. Infection of tibia, fibula, humerus and clavicle has also been reported. Multiple sites of infection are commonly seen. After one to two weeks radiographs show multiple punched out destructive lesions throughout the metaphysis and diaphysis with extensive subperiosteal bone formation and irregular sclerosis.

Treatment The treatment includes antibiotics (e.g. chloramphenicol, ampicillin or ciprofloxacin) for six weeks. Abscesses should be drained. Recurrences are commonly seen.

• **Pseudomonas** (more commonly) and **Serratia**

marcescens infections occur in IV drug abusers and involve axial skeleton.

- **Brucella osteomyelitis** occurs in meat handlers and involves spine (commonest site) and flat bones.

Anaerobic Osteomyelitis Bacteroides and anaerobic streptococci are the most common pathogens causing anaerobic osteomyelitis. Others include actinomyces infections, which are seen typically in the vicinity of jaw (mandible more than maxilla); Propionibacterium acnes seen in prosthetic joint infections and clostridia seen in lower limb compound fractures. Vascular disease, peripheral neuropathy, diabetes, human bites, trauma and presence of prosthetic joints are predisposing factors for anaerobic osteomyelitis.

Fungal osteomyelitis is also seen in immunocompromised patients. Actinomycosis is the commonest fungal infection. It usually involves soft tissues of head and neck. The mandible is involved in head and neck infection, vertebrae and ribs are involved in lung infection while spread to pelvic bones occurs from colon and appendix. Multiple abscesses and sinuses are commonly found. Yellow sulfur granule like fungal colonies are typically discharged from the sinuses. X-rays show much more soft tissue involvement than bony involvement. Irregular, patchy destruction and sclerosis of bones is a prominent feature. Treatment is by high dose antibiotics/antifungals administered for prolonged periods up to several months. In localised infections, surgical excision of expendable bone can be done.

Predisposing conditions for other fungal infections are given in Table 3.5.

Parasitic osteomyelitis

Echinococcus osteomyelitis

Skeletal involvement is rare in hydatid cyst disease (0.5–4% cases). Spine is involved most commonly (50% cases) followed by pelvis and femur.

Radical excision wherever possible is the treatment of choice.

Viral osteomyelitis (Varicella osteomyelitis) was usually caused by small pox virus. Infections are extinct now, though, sequelae of previous infections are seen sometimes. The infection usually involves children and adolescents. Elbow, tibia and fibula are commonest sites and feet may sometimes be involved. Infections are often bilateral. Disease manifests as periarticular swelling and painful restriction of joint movements. Deformity, ankylosis of joint, epiphyseal separation and growth disturbance of affected bones may result. Antibiotics and surgical treatment do not help and are not indicated.

Tubercular Osteomyelitis Commonest involvement by tubercular osteomyelitis is in vertebral bodies. Metacarpals and phalanges (Tubercular dactylitis) are sometimes involved. Multiple bones may be involved and the affected bones become swollen and fusiform. The appearance is called *'spina ventosa'*. X-ray shows expansion of bone, rarefaction leading to cystic appearance and periosteal reaction. Tubercular dactylitis should be differentiated from enchondroma, rheumatoid arthritis and syphilitic dactylitis. In long bones, tubercular osteomyelitis involves metaphyseal

Table 3.5. Predisposing factors for fungal infections

Pathogenic organism	Predisposing factors	Salient features
Candida infection	Immunocompromised hosts	Common sites: Spine, femur, sternum
Aspergillosis	Corticosteroid use, Alcohol abuse, Cirrhosis	Lung involvement by aspergilloma common
Coccidiomycosis	Pulmonary exposure	Spine commonly involved
Mucormycosis	Diabetes	Rhino cerebral involvement
Cryptococcosis	Immunocompromised patients: Lymphoma, AIDS	Pneumonia common in AIDS patients

regions. (Fig. 3.10a,b) New bone formation does not occur except in vertebrae and in small bones of hands and feet. Juxta articular metaphyseal lesions may discharge into the adjacent joint and lead to tubercular arthritis. Treatment consists of antitubercular chemotherapy. Surgery (curettage of lesion) is indicated for juxta articular lesion to prevent arthritis of adjacent joint.

Infectious Arthritis

Relevant Anatomy

Orthopaedic surgery is concerned mainly with

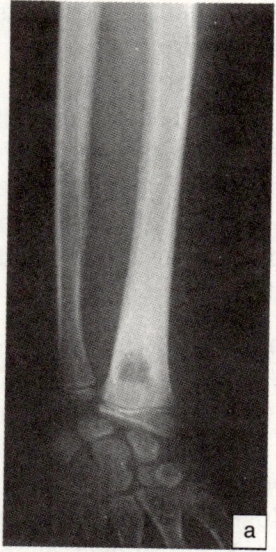

Fig. 3.10a. Tubercular involvement of lower end of Radius

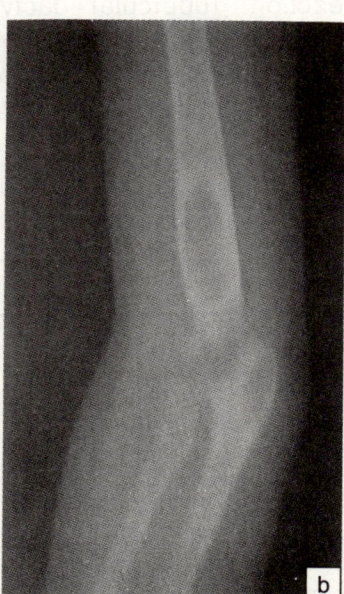

Fig. 3.10b. Tuberculosis involving the Elbow joint.

synovial joints. Other types of joints are synostosis (bony), syndesmosis (fibrous) or synchondrosis/ symphysis (cartilage). The ends of bones in synovial joint are covered with hyaline cartilage. Hyaline cartilage consists of chondrocytes embedded in matrix of collagen fibres and proteoglycans. Articular cartilage has zones like physis and a mineralization / calcification front at the junction between calcified cartilage and normal articular cartilage called *Tidemark*. Articular cartilage gets its nutrition by diffusion of metabolites from synovial fluid, as the cartilage has no neurovascular supply. The cartilage in adult cannot grow or repair itself. Defects resulting from injury are repaired by fibrocartilage or fibrous tissue.

Synovial membrane is a smooth, glistening membrane, which surrounds the joint cavity and produces synovial fluid. It has rich vascularity and cells specialised in phagocytosis and hyaluronic acid production. Synovial fluid is a dialysate of plasma with the addition of hyaluronic acid produced by synovial membrane. External to synovium, thick fibrous capsule surrounds the joint. Capsule has special thickenings to form ligaments of the joint. Nerve endings in the capsule transmit proprioception, pain and pressure sensation.

Pyogenic Arthritis

Source of Infection

Infection of the joint is most commonly caused by Staphylococcus aureus.

The bacteria can gain entrance in to the joint by following routes:

i) Hematogenous spread usually occurs from a distant focus of infection. It occurs most commonly in patients with underlying illness and immune deficiency. Chronic illnesses such as rheumatoid arthritis, intravenous drug abuse and local joint trauma may predispose adults to hematogenous infection.

ii) Direct extension from adjacent focus of infection

 a) Infection in newborn and infants can extend from metaphysis to the joint by transphyseal vessels (which get obliterated after infancy).

 Infection cannot cross the physis so septic arthritis is less common in children.

b) Extension of metaphyseal osteomyelitis can occur where metaphysis is intra-articular, most commonly at hip. Other joints include shoulder (upper humeral epiphysis), ankle (distal fibular epiphysis) and elbow (radial neck).

c) Contiguous soft tissue infection can extend and cause septic arthritis.

d) Umbilical vein sepsis in newborn can lead to pyogenic arthritis.

iii) Direct inoculation is seen following penetrating/ open joint injuries and following diagnostic or therapeutic procedures (e.g. aspiration of joint fluid, intra-articular injections, arthroscopy). Femoral venipuncture may also lead to septic arthritis of hip in infants.

Prosthetic joint surgery is another source of direct inoculation.

Pathogenesis

The presence of bacteria in the joint incites an intense local reaction. The synovial membrane becomes hyperaemic, oedematous and prolifer- ates. It produces purulent fluid containing mark- edly increased leukocytes. Articular cartilage gets destroyed by:

a) Proteolytic enzymes released by bacteria and disintegrating inflammatory cells

b) Pressure necrosis by raised intra-articular pres- sure

c) Interference with chondrocyte nutrition and

d) Invasion of matrix and enzymatic degradation by proliferating synovium.

The various sources of infection to a joint include hematogenous spread, from contiguous soft tis- sue infection, spread from focus of ostesmyelitis in adjacent bone and direct inoculation through a penetrating wound (Fig. 3.11).

Infection spreads to underlying bone and can destroy the growth plate resulting in limb length discrepancies and / or angular deformities in growing children. Infected synovial membrane eventually is replaced by granulation tissue. Marked distension of joint, destruction of carti- lage, capsule and ligaments and spasm of the neighbouring muscles may culminate in patho- logical dislocation of the joint (most commonly hip). In neglected cases, multiple discharging sinuses may form. The eventual outcome of the joint depends on the virulence of the organism, age of the patient and the state at which thera- peutic intervention is done.

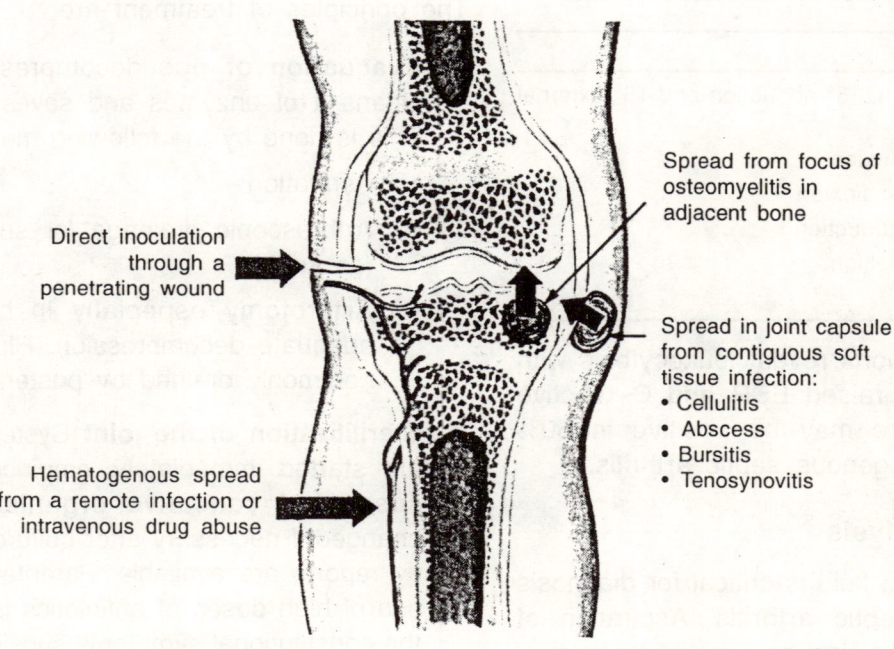

Direct inoculation through a penetrating wound

Hematogenous spread from a remote infection or intravenous drug abuse

Spread from focus of osteomyelitis in adjacent bone

Spread in joint capsule from contiguous soft tissue infection:
• Cellulitis
• Abscess
• Bursitis
• Tenosynovitis

Fig. 3.11. Sources of infection to a joint

In newborns and infants the femoral head is mainly cartilaginous and is rapidly destroyed by the infection. Marked destruction gives rise to a *hypermobile* joint *(Tom-Smith's Arthritis)* with exaggerated movements and marked shortening. In young children the infection results in bony ankylosis. In adolescents and adults, the joint destruction by septic process may be followed by fibrous ankylosis.

Clinical Features

Pyogenic arthritis is usually monoarticular infection and most commonly involves hip in infants and young children and knee in older children and adults. The onset is acute with constitutional symptoms and high fever. Fever may sometimes be absent in infants. The child is apprehensive, anxious and anorexic. The chief complaint is swelling, pain and limitation of motion of involved joints. Affected joint is warm, erythematous, tender, distended and has reduced range of motion with pain on attempted movements. Spasm of surrounding muscles is often quite obvious. Patient holds the joint in the position of maximum capacity to reduce intra-articular pressure and thus minimise pain.

The position of maximum intra-articular volume of various joints is given in Table 3.6.

Table 3.6. Position of maximum intra-articular volume

Joint	Position
Hip	60° Flexion, 15° abduction and 15° external rotation
Knee	30°–60° flexion
Ankle	15° plantar flexion
Shoulder	30°–60° abduction
Elbow	30°–60° flexion
Wrist	Neutral

Laboratory investigations reveal leukocytosis with shift to the left and raised ESR and C–reactive protein. Blood culture may be positive in 50% patients with hematogenous septic arthritis.

Synovial Fluid Analysis

Evaluation of synovial fluid is critical for diagnosis and treatment of septic arthritis. Aspiration of joint fluid is done following an aseptic technique. Wide bore needle is used for aspiration and as much fluid as possible is removed from the joint (to decompress the joint). Aerobic and anaerobic cultures should be taken. Tubes containing heparin or EDTA should be used for collecting fluid for cell examination. In septic arthritis, the synovial fluid shows the following abnormalities (Table 3.7). These along with positive culture clinch the diagnosis.

Imaging Studies

Early X-ray changes may be subtle and comparison with opposite (normal) joint helps to distinguish subtle changes. An effusion with distension of capsule may appear as soft tissue swelling. The earliest bony change is rarefaction of bone. This is followed by erosion of juxta–articular bone. In later stages, joint space is diminished due to destruction of articular cartilage. Bone scan, CT scan and MRI can help in early diagnosis in cases with ambiguous clinical signs.

Differential Diagnosis

Septic arthritis should be differentiated from acute osteomyelitis, haemophilia, gouty arthritis and tuberculosis.

Treatment

Septic arthritis should be treated as an emergency

The principles of treatment are:

1. **Evacuation of pus** decompresses the joint, cleans it of enzymes and saves the cartilage. This is done by the following methods:

   - Aspiration

   - Arthroscopic drainage for superficial joints (as knee)

   - Arthrotomy especially in hip to ensure adequate decompression. Hip joint is most commonly drained by posterior approach.

2. **Sterililization of the joint** Systemic antibiotics are started immediately, empirically based on suspected causative organism. They are changed if necessary after culture and sensitivity reports are available. Parenteral administration of high doses of antibiotics is continued till the constitutional symptoms subside. Once ESR comes down / fever settles, switch to oral therapy for 4–6 weeks.

Table 3.7. Synovial fluid analysis in septic arthritis

Analysis	Normal	Septic arthritis
Gross appearance		
Colour	Straw or clear yellow	Serosanguinous or purulent (Yellow-white, grey)
Volume	1–4 ml	Increased
Clarity	Clear	Turbid
Viscosity and mucin		
Clot Viscosity	High (1" long string between thumb and forefinger)	Very Low
Mucin clot	Good	Poor
Microscopic Examination		
Leukocytes (cells/ml)	<300	>50,000
Neutrophils	<25%	>80%
Bacteria	Negative	Positive
Biochemistry		
Serum/synovial fluid glucose ratio	0.8–1.0 (20 mg/100 ml less than serum)	< 0.5 (50–100 mg/100 ml less than serum)
Protein (g/dl)	2	≤ 8
Culture	Negative	Positive

3. **Splinting the joint** Splinting provides rest for expeditious recovery and prevents occurrence of deformity.

4. **Restoration of function** The joint is mobilised to regain movement. Correction of residual deformities helps in restoring function.

Sequelae of Septic Arthritis

1. Ankylosis of joint: fibrous or bony

2. Instability of joint/pathological dislocation: Hypermobile joint (Tom Smith arthritis) (Fig. 3.12).

3. Degenerative arthritis (secondary)

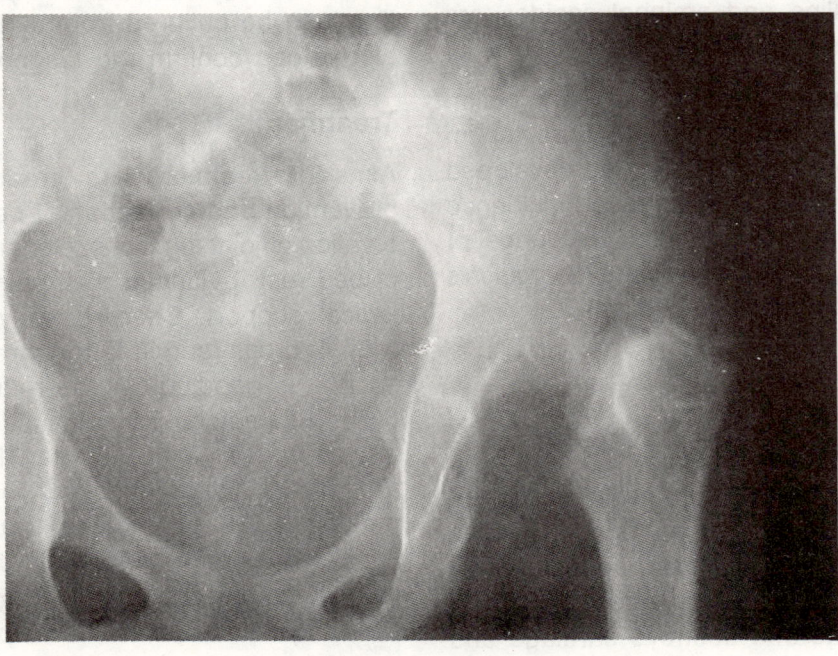

Fig. 3.12. Tom Smith arthritis with pathological dislocation

4. Sepsis
   - Septicaemia
   - Metastatic abscesses
   - Osteomyelitis
5. Soft tissue contractures
6. Epiphyseal damage
   - limb length discrepancies
   - Angular deformities
7. Death

Gonococcal Arthritis

Neisseria gonorrhoea is a common cause of bacterial arthritis, which affects young, healthy adults. It is usually monoarticular and the knee is involved most commonly. Polyarthritis is much more common than in other infections. Wrists, interphalangeal joints of hands and feet may be involved. Polyarthralgias, tenosynovitis and dermatitis are seen in majority of patients. Gonococcal arthritis may be migratory and disseminated (classical triad-tenosynovitis, polyarthralgia, purpuric skin lesions).

Diagnosis Gonococcus is a fastidious organism and difficult to isolate. Blood cultures are positive only in 10% (cf. 50% in non-gonococcal arthritis) and positive joint fluid culture in 25% (cf. 85–95% in non-gonococcal arthritis).

Treatment: Penicillins and aminoglycosides are the antibiotics of choice.

Tubercular Arthritis is a granulomatous infection caused by human or bovine strain of Mycobacterium tuberculosis. It is very common in underdeveloped and developing countries. The increased incidence of HIV has given rise to increased incidence of tuberculous infection, multidrug resistant tuberculosis and tuberculosis by atypical organisms.

Pathology

The infection reaches the joint either by hematogenous route or rarely by spread from adjacent bone. Disease is usually synovial initially. Synovium proliferates and hypertrophies and gets studded with tubercles. Joint effusion occurs. Tubercular granulation tissue covers articular cartilage as a pannus and destroys cartilage and subchondral bone. If untreated, necrotic material and synovial exudates perforate the capsule and form a cold abscess. Secondary pyogenic infection through the sinus tracts may further destroy the joint.

Clinical features

Clinically, tuberculosis presents as monoarticular arthritis in children and young adults. Superficial joints such as knee readily divulge effusion and synovial thickening. Marked muscular atrophy is seen around the joint and joint is held in position of deformity due to effusion and muscle spasm. Night cries and night sweats may be present. Fixed joint deformities develop in later stages due to destruction of cartilage and subchondral bone. Cold abscess and sinuses may be present in late stages.

Diagnosis

X-rays show increased joint space followed by rarefaction of bone as the earliest feature. Joint space narrowing occurs subsequently with destruction of cartilage. Reactive new bone is absent. Sequestrae are rare.

Blood examination shows anaemia and elevated erythrocyte sedimentation rate. Synovial fluid is straw coloured and has raised leukocyte count, low sugar content and forms poor mucin clot. Tubercular bacilli are rarely seen. Sometimes they can be cultured from synovial fluid. Synovial biopsy can confirm the diagnosis.

Treatment

Aims of treatment are eradication of disease, prevention and correction of deformities and preservation of joint functions. General measures consist of bed rest, balanced diet, pain relief and psychological support. Chemotherapy is usually started with 4 drugs and if after three months, the response is good, it can be reduced to two. HRZE (INH, Rifampicin, Pyrazinamide and Ethambutol) regime is used initially while HR can be continued after initial period is over. The total duration of therapy is 12–18 months. Traction in these patients, either domiciliary or in the hospital relieves pain, counters spasm and prevents and corrects deformity at the joint. It also provides rest to the joint. Deformities may sometimes have to be assessed under anaesthesia to evaluate contribution by muscle spasm. A deformity, which corrects under anaesthesia, may be kept splinted in plaster or PVC splints. Gentle active and passive exercises for mobilisation of the joint should be started as soon as the disease activity has reduced and pain has abated. Surgical treatment may be required to confirm diagnosis, reduce disease load, improve vascularity (and hence penetration of chemo-therapeutic agents), and correct deformities. Synovectomy and joint debridement are indicated when joint space is not compromised and useful range of motion is expected.

In markedly damaged and disorganised joints, arthrodesis in the functional position may be undertaken to eliminate pain, correct deformity and provide stable, functional joint.

Non-Infectious Disorders of the Joints

- Relevant Anatomy
- Arthrocentesis and Synovial Fluid Analysis
- Lubrication in Normal Synovial Joint
- Non Inflammatory Arthritides
  Degenerative Joint Disease
    Osteoarthritis
    Neuropathic Arthropathy
  Acute Rheumatic Fever
  Alkaptonuria
- Inflammatory Arthritides
  Rheumatoid Arthritis
  Systemic Lupus Erythematosus (SLE)
  Spondyloarthropathies / Enthesopathies / Seronegative Arthritides

  Ankylosing Spondylitis
  Psoriatic Arthropathy
  Reiter's Syndrome ("Reactive" arthritis)
- Crystal-Induced Arthritis
  Gout
  Chondrocalcinosis
  Hydroxyapatite Crystal Deposition Disease
- Hemorrhagic Arthropathy
  Hemophilic Arthropathy
- Synovial Disorders
  Pigmented Villonodular Synovitis (PVNS).
  Synovial Chondromatosis
  Synovial Sarcoma

A normal joint has three functions namely stability, motion and load distribution. The geometry of opposed articulating surfaces, mechanical properties of the cartilage and other connective tissues and integrity of the soft tissue structures (ligaments, muscles and tendons) are the features which determine the function of the joint. A joint dysfunction is evident clinically by instability, loss of motion and uneven distribution of load leading to pain.

Relevant Anatomy

Synovial joints are characterised by articulation between the bone ends covered by articular cartilage. Joint capsule made of fibrous connective tissue envelops the joint while the inside of the joint is lined by the synovial membrane. The synovium consists of a thin intimal layer (1 to 2 cell deep) of synovial cells (or synoviocytes) overlying a richly fibrovascular subintimal layer. Two types of cells are found in synovium, the type A (demonstrating macrophage function) and type B (fibroblast like cells). Type A cells are mainly phagocytic while type B cells secrete the hyaluronate-protein of the synovial fluid. Synovial cells have gaps between

them because of the lack of basal lamina and this ultrastructural feature allows interchange between synovial fluid and blood.

Synovial fluid is a dialysate of plasma containing small amounts of hyaluronic acid. Latter accounts for the high viscosity of the synovial fluid. In addition, synovial fluid contains cells, mostly mononuclear phagocytes and neutrophils. Synovial fluid has fewer proteins than plasma while the glucose, lactic acid and uric acid content of the synovial fluid is same as plasma.

Synovial fluid provides nutrition to the articular cartilage and also provides lubrication between the articulation.

In a normal joint the volume of synovial fluid is very small (0.2 ml for the knee).

Arthrocentesis and synovial fluid analysis

Arthrocentesis is the procedure where synovial fluid is tapped under aseptic conditions (to minimise the risk of infection). Synovial fluid analysis is very useful in diagnosing crystal induced synovitis,

(Gout, Calcium Pyrophosphate Crystal Deposition disease or hydroxyapatite crystal deposition), hemorrhagic synovitis (trauma, pigmented villonodular synovitis) or infection in the joint. Findings of synovial fluid analysis in various afflictions of the joint are shown in Table 4.1.

Lubrication in Normal Synovial Joint

The coefficient of friction for the normal adult human hip is 0.003–0.01. The various factors which reduce the coefficient of friction in the joint include elastic deformation of articular cartilage, synovial fluid, fluid film formation and oozing of fluid from the cartilage. The various mechanisms of lubrication in human synovial joints are:

(1) *Boundary lubrication*

In this mechanism, chemical adsorption of a layer of lubricant molecules occurs on the articulating surfaces. These lubricant molecules slide over each other during motion and protect the articulating surfaces. This mechanism is effective in low load situations. Since this layer of molecules is quite thin and the surface is largely nondeformable, the surfaces are not always entirely separated. Therefore, boundary lubrication is often called "thin film" or imperfect lubrication. Typical coefficients of friction in this mechanism are 0.01 to 0.10.

(2) *Fluid film lubrication*

In these types of lubrication, a much thicker film of lubricant (in contrast to the molecular size of the lubricant in boundary lubrication) causes a relatively large separation of the two bearing surfaces. Pressure in this fluid film supports the load on the bearing.

a) *Hydrostatic lubrication* : In this type of lubrication the pressure in the fluid film is generated by extrinsic pressure application.

b) *Hydrodynamic lubrication* : In this type of lubrication, the pressure in the fluid film between the bearing surfaces is generated by tangential movement of the bearing surfaces with respect to each other.

Coefficients of friction for modern hydrodynamic systems are from 0.002 to 0.01.

c) *Elastohydrodynamic lubrication*

This is the most prevalent mechanism during the dynamic joint function. The lubrication here is provided by the deformation of the articular surfaces as well as thin film of joint lubricant separating the bearing surfaces. The deformation of the bearing surfaces alter the contact area, fluid film geometry, restrict fluid escape

Table 4.1. Synovial fluid analysis in various arthritides

Condition	Colour	Mucin Clot	Fibrin Clot	Viscosity	WBC per mm³	Glucose	Protein	Others
Normal	Clear	Firm	None	High	200 (<25% neutrophils)	50-100 mg/dl	2g/dl	
Non inflammatory	Yellow	firm	Small	High	Low: 200-2000 (<25% neutrophils)	Low: <10mg/ 100ml	Low: <3 g/dl	Cartilage debris(+)
Chronic inflammatory/ crystal induced	Yellow or white	Friable	Large	Low	2000-75000 (>50% neutrophils)	>25mg/ 100 ml	Elevated: >3g/dl	Synovial fluid complement (C_2 and C_4) low, Rheumatoid Factor can be detected in RA. Crystals can be identified under polarised light in crystal induced effusion.
Septic	Yellow green	Friable	Large	Very Low	>100,000 (>75% neutrophils)	Low: 1–5 mg/dl	Elevated: >3g/dl	Culture & Gram's stain (+), Increased synovial lactate
Hemorrhagic	Reddish brown	–	–	Low	2000 – 10,000 >25% neutrophils	50–100 mg/dl	Elevated >3g/dl	–

and are associated with large increases in load carrying capacity of the joint.

d) *Squeeze film lubrication*

This type of lubrication is useful when high loads are applied for short duration. In this mechanism the bearing surfaces move perpendicularly towards each other. Pressure is generated in the fluid film to squeezes the fluid (lubricant) out from the gap between the two surfaces and this pressure keeps the bearing surfaces apart. If load is applied for long period, the bearing surfaces will eventually come in contact. Therefore, this mechanism is not sufficient for prolonged loading.

(3) "Mixed" mode of lubrication This mechanism results from combination of boundary lubricated solid contacts and pressure in the fluid film.

(4) Lubrication resulting from movement of fluid into or out of the bearing surfaces.

a) *Boosted lubrication or* fluid entrapment occurs when synovial fluid is trapped between the regions of bearing surfaces, which are in contact. The fluid flows out of the synovial fluid into the pores in the surrounding cartilage. Resulting increased concentration of hyaluronic acid and increased viscosity of the trapped synovial fluid boost the lubrication in these cases.

b) *Weeping lubrication* In this mechanism, the fluid flows out of loaded cartilage into the synovial fluid in the area of contact. This fluid provides a hydrostatic pressure to keep the bearing surfaces apart. This mechanism works best under high loads.

Non Inflammatory Arthritides

1. Degenerative Joint Disease

a) Osteoarthritis

Osteoarthritis is the commonest form of arthritis. Osteoarthritis is a non-inflammatory, functional disorder of joints characterised by loss of articular cartilage and formation of osteophytes. The aetiology is unknown in most cases. The disease is often categorised into primary and secondary forms. Primary osteoarthritis occurs in older age groups and develops insidiously without any known cause. Secondary osteoarthritis can occur at a younger age group and may arise secondary to

trauma, avascular necrosis, congenital disorders (hip dysplasia), inflammatory diseases, infectious diseases, metabolic diseases (gout, ochronosis) or haemorrhagic disorders (e.g. hemophilia) [Table 4.2].

Pathologic Features

Earlier stages of osteoarthritis are characterised by focal swelling and softening of the cartilage matrix. Hypercellularity of chondrocytes is seen. Tidemark is thin and wavy in early disease. The water content of the osteoarthritic cartilage is increased (as compared to reduction of water content in cartilage seen with ageing). The proteoglycan synthesis is increased with increased chondroitin sulfate to keratin sulfate ratio. Decreased synthesis of proteoglycans occurs in late stages with reduced proteoglycan-hyaluronic acid aggregates. Disruption of collagen (by the action of collagenase) is seen. Metalloproteinases (collagenase, gelatinase, stromelysin and cathepsins B and D) are found in high concentrations in the osteoarthritic cartilage.

In the late stages, chondrocyte cloning (more than one chondrocyte per lacuna), reduplication and breakdown of shiny tidemark, fissuring, destruction of cartilage and eburnation of subchondral bone occur. Grossly, in the earliest

Table 4.2. Conditions leading to secondary osteoarthritis

Conditions	Examples
Congenital	Hip dysplasia, congenital dislocation or subluxation of hip.
Developmental	Epiphyseal dysplasia (Spondyloepiphyseal, Multiple Epiphyseal) Perthes' Disease, Slipped capital femoral epiphysis.
Traumatic	Intra-articular fractures, Traumatic dislocations
Inflammatory	Non infectious inflammatory arthritides
Metabolic	Gout, Pseudogout (CPPD deposition disease), Ochronosis
Vascular	Avascular necrosis Caisson's Disease Steroid therapy Sickle cell disease Alcoholism Trauma, etc.
Radiation damage Paget's disease	

stages, the cartilage loses its shining smooth, bluish white appearance and becomes pale, soft and lustreless. Compressibility of the matrix is lost and minute fractures of the matrix occur with fibrillation and fissuring. Further deterioration leads to formation of clefts. Osteophyte formation occurs in an attempt to repair the articular cartilage and to broaden the weight-bearing surface. Osteophyte formation starts with the formation of granulation tissue at the site where capsule attaches to peripheral articular cartilage. Granulation tissue matures to fibrocartilage and then undergoes endochondral ossification to become bony and breakdown of osteochondral junction occurs next. Complete disintegration of the cartilage with subchondral microfractures lead to eburnation of the subchondral bone. Minute fractures of subchondral trabeculae with necrosis and resorption lead to the formation of subchondral cysts, which contain gelatinous material.

Synovial membrane proliferation and hypertrophy occurs. Capsule becomes thick and fibrosed due to extensive fibrous tissue proliferation.

Clinical Features

Clinically osteoarthritis has four recognised patterns of the disease. The first three of these are non-inflammatory in their clinical presentation.

1. **Disease limited to a single large (weight, bearing) joint** usually hip or knee, sometimes bilateral.

2. **Generalised process** involving distal inter-phalangeal (DIP) (Fig. 4.1a,b) and proximal interphalangeal (PIP) joints of the hand, first carpometacarpal (CMC) joint, knees, hips and metatarsophalangeal joints.

3. **Charcot's joints** seen in association with neurological deficit. There is a rapidly destructive osteoarthritis with marked instability and formation of multiple loose bodies. The joints are usually painless.

4. **Erosive osteoarthritis** usually affects the DIP or PIP joints but occasionally may involve large joints. Rapid destruction of the joint is seen and radiologically the disease resembles an inflammatory arthritis.

Knee is the most common joint affected in osteoarthritis. Patients with osteoarthritis are usually elderly, often obese, who experience an insidious onset of pain and stiffness.

Initially pain occurs following activity but later in the course of disease, rest pain (or "night pain" ostensibly due to the intra osseous hypertension) appears.

Stiffness ("gelling") occurs after a period of rest or immobilisation. Loss of movements occurs as the disease progresses. Deformities develop due to cartilage and bone destruction and contracture of the soft tissues. Mechanical symptoms such as locking or instability are common in knee joint due to loose bodies, degeneration of the meniscus or incompetence of anterior cruciate ligament (ACL). Baker's cyst in the popliteal fossa is a common presenting feature in osteoarthritis of

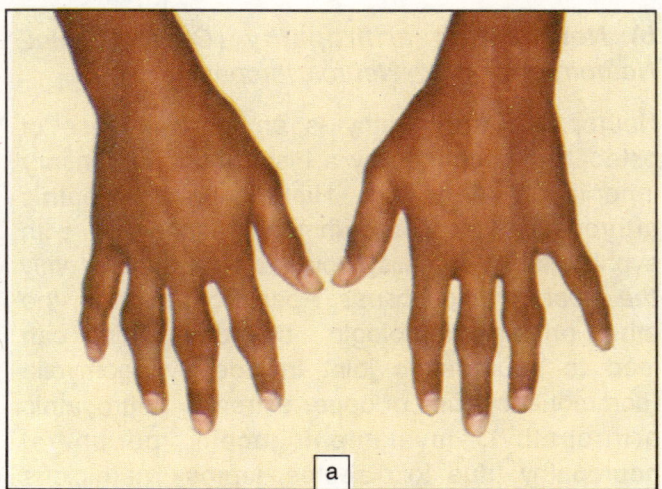

Fig. 4.1a.   OA with PIP involvement

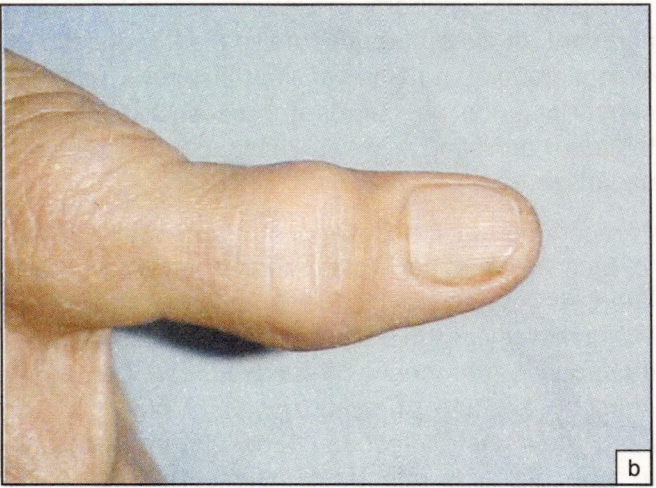

Fig. 4.1b.   OA involving DIP joints – Heberden's node

the knee. Heberden's nodes and Bouchard's nodes are seen in the hands.

On examination, the joint has "bony" swelling (usually synovial proliferation is not a prominent feature). Tenderness may be elicited at the site of joint line, capsular attachments, over the osteophytes or over the hamstring tendons. Palpable and audible crepitations are a common finding.

Decreased range of joint movement and fixed deformities are notable features.

Radiological Features

The most characteristic feature on x-rays is the loss of the joint space. Subchondral sclerosis (increased density of subchondral bone on both sides of the joint), bony osteophytes around the periphery of the joint and subchondral cysts may be seen. Loose bodies are seen in the joint at times. Bony erosions, subluxation and deformity are evident in advanced disease.

Laboratory Findings

No specific diagnostic tests for osteoarthritis are available at present. Laboratory parameters including blood tests, urinalysis or synovial fluid analysis (vide supra) are normal and serve to rule out the infectious or inflammatory disorders as the cause of symptoms.

Treatment

Aim of treatment in osteoarthritis is to relieve pain, improve function and prevent deformity. Another aim still in experimental stages is to modify the disease by discovering drugs to inhibit metalloproteinases such as modified tetracyclines, colchicine etc. General measures useful for management of osteoarthritis are patient education, weight reduction, lifestyle modification, use of supports (such as cane) or braces and physiotherapy consisting of heat, massage and regular exercises.

Paracetamol, in the dosage of 1 gm orally three to four times a day (maximum 4 gms/day) has been recommended by the American College of Rheumatology as the drug of choice for osteoarthritis. Inadequate therapeutic responses can be managed by addition of small doses of NSAIDs (to keep their gastrointestinal, renal, haematological and hepatic side effects to minimum).

Availability of selective cyclooxygenase II inhibitors (Valdecoxib, Rofecoxib, Celecoxib) has reduced the incidence of adverse effects associated with NSAIDs use. Opiates have also been used to relieve pain.

Glucosamine and Chondroitin Sulfate have been used as dietary supplements and are believed to increase the glycosaminoglycans synthesis in the articular cartilage. Glucosamine is also believed to be an antioxidant. Almost two thirds of the patients taking these supplements experience some amelioration of symptoms.

Intra articular Hyaluronic Acid has been approved by FDA as an instrument and not a drug. It is indicated when other conservative measures have failed and the patient has painful synovial effusion. Intra articular administration of five injections (one week between consecutive injections) provides relief to 60–65% patients. The relief, however, is not durable and symptoms recur after a period of a few months.

Surgical Treatment

The surgical treatment is indicated to relieve pain (most common indication), improve function and correct deformity when the conservative treatment has failed. A plethora of surgical options is available for the treatment of osteoarthritis ranging from arthroscopic removal of loose bodies and/ or debridement of joint to total joint replacement arthroplasties.

The indications, contra indications and technique of these procedures are described in the subsequent chapters pertaining to the specific joints.

b) *Neuropathic arthropathy* (*Charcot Joint, Neurotrophic joint, Neuroarthropathic joint*)

Neuropathic arthropathy is an extreme case of osteoarthritis caused by a disturbance in sensory innervation of a joint. Historically neuropathic arthropathy is most commonly associated with syphilis (tabes dorsalis) though *diabetes is currently the most common cause*. Apart from syphilis, the other primary neurologic disorders which can lead to neuropathic joint include syringomyelia (commonest cause of upper extremity neuropathic arthropathy), myelomeningocele, peripheral neuropathy (due to diabetes, leprosy, pernicious anaemia, peroneal muscular atrophy) or peripheral nerve injuries, congenital insensitivity to pain etc.

Clinically, patients are usually elderly, often diabetic, who present with swollen, painless and unstable joints. The joints may be warm and erythematous. Effusion may be bloody.

Diabetics often present with neuropathic joint following trauma or surgery. Characteristic changes in the neuropathic joint are marked destructive changes on both sides of the joint. This is evident in x-ray as bony sclerosis, cyst formation, debris, osteophyte formation and multiple bony pieces in the soft tissues. Heterotopic ossification commonly occurs. Joint appears distended with fluid and is often disorganised (subluxated/dislocated). There may be rapid disintegration of joint with absence of segments of bone (Fig. 4.2a-c).

Histology shows large amounts of cartilage and bone detritus with synovial hyperplasia and a variable degree of inflammation associated with giant cells.

Treatment of Charcot's joint aims to prevent further damage to the joint by limitation of activity and appropriate bracing. Arthrocentesis can be attempted in an attempt to reduce effusion with consequent distension and disorganisation of the joint. The procedure should be followed by pressure bandage application.

Charcot's joint is usually a contraindication to joint replacement or use of metallic implants due to very high incidence of failure and infection. Arthrodesis can be attempted in suitable cases but is thwarted by the twin risks of infection and difficulty in achieving fusion in these cases.

2. Acute Rheumatic Fever

Acute Rheumatic Fever is a disease which follows Group-A – β hemolytic streptococcus infection. Arthritis is one of the major criteria (Jone's criteria) for diagnosis while arthralgia is a minor criteria.

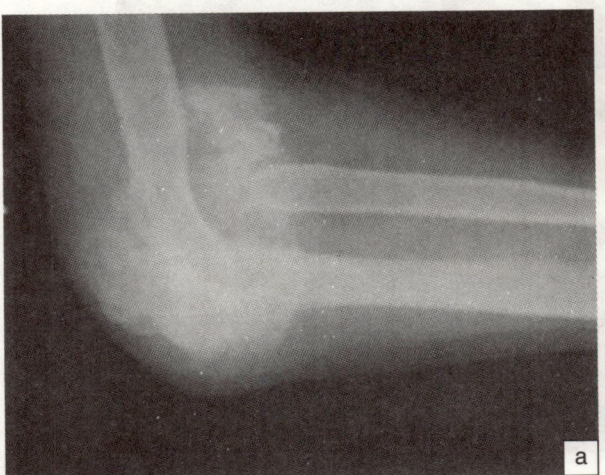
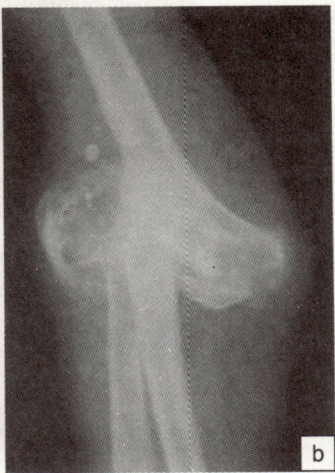

Fig. 4.2a,b. Charcot's joint elbow

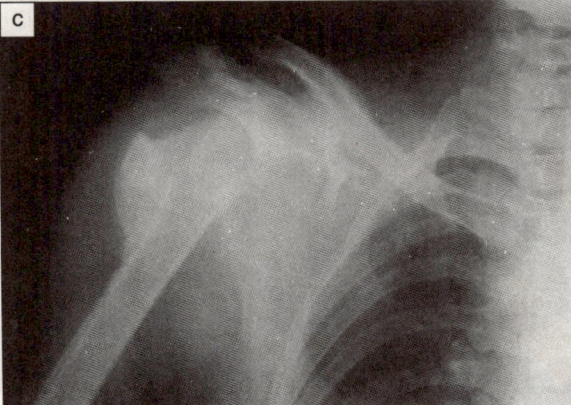

Fig. 4.2c. Charcot's joint shoulder

Patients are usually children who may have had recurrent sore throats and present with acute onset of tender, erythematous and painful effusion of the joint. The arthritis is migratory ("Fleeting"). It involves multiple large (knee, ankle) joints but at one time only one joint is affected. Subsidence of arthritis in the affected joint is followed by involvement of another joint.

Acute rheumatic arthritis should be differentiated from acute septic arthritis or acute osteomyelitis. Compared to pyogenic infections, the rheumatic fever has more insidious onset and produces less intense local and constitutional symptoms. History of migratory arthritis or the presence of systemic manifestations of rheumatic fever (carditis, erythema marginatum, subcutaneous nodules or chorea) clinches the diagnosis.

Laboratory Investigations

Throat swab may grow streptococci. Erythrocyte sedimentation rate is raised. PR interval is increased on ECG. Antistreptolysin "O" titres are raised (>1:160 dilution) in almost 80% of the patients.

Treatment of Rheumatic fever is best done by the paediatricians. Salicylates and penicillins remain the mainstay of treatment.

3. **Alkaptonuria** (*Ochronosis*) Ochronosis is an autosomal recessive inborn error of metabolism. The disease results from the defect of homogentisic acid oxidase enzyme system leading to deposition of excess homogentisic acid in the joints.

The disease is characterised clinically by degenerative arthritis, urine, which turns black on exposure or alkalinization and black pigmentation of tissues (especially fibro-cartilage) (Fig. 4.3a-c). Patients usually present in the fourth decade and disease usually progresses. Disease leads to arthropathy, genitourinary

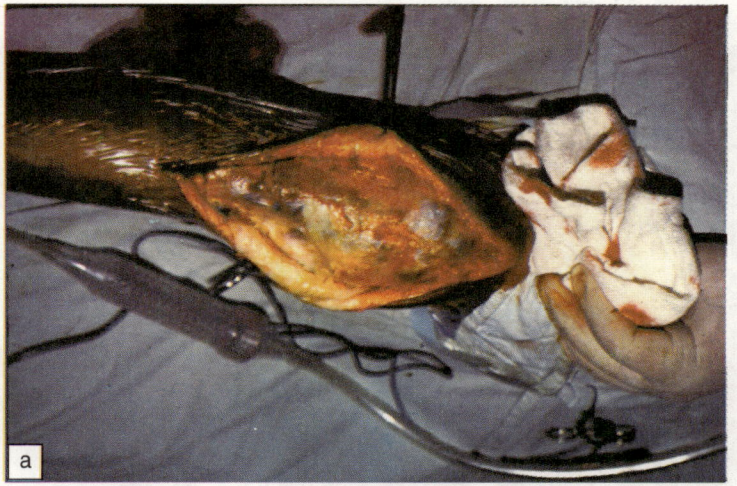

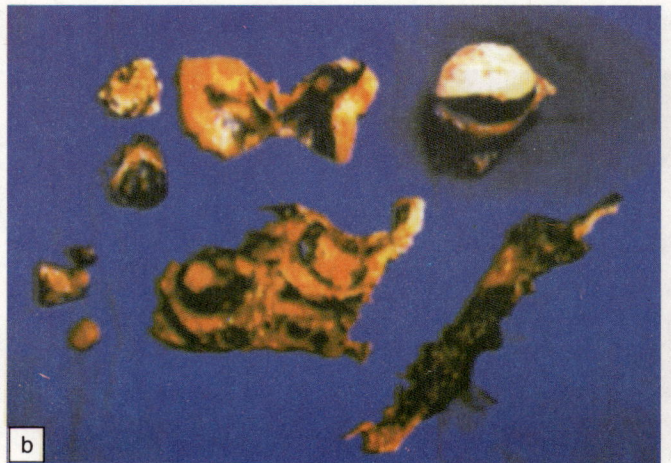
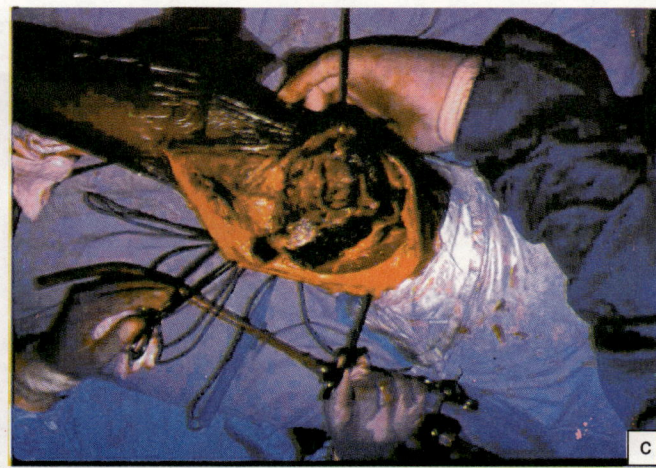

Fig. 4.3a-c. Intraoperative pictures of a patient with alkaptonuria. Note the black staining of the tissues

obstruction (by ochronotic calculi), ocular ochronosis, cutaneous ochronosis and cardiac involvement (due to deposition of homogentisic acid polymers in endocardium or heart valves). Pigment deposition leads to black discoloration of sclerae, ears, nose, cheeks and cartilage. Large peripheral joints (knees, shoulders, and hips) are most commonly affected by arthropathy. Radiological changes seen in large diarthrodial joint are indistinguishable from osteoarthritis with subchondral bone sclerosis and osteophyte formation (Fig. 4.3d). Ochronotic spondylitis leads to progressive degenerative changes in spine including vertebral osteophyte formation, diminished disc space and *calcification of intervertebral discs.*

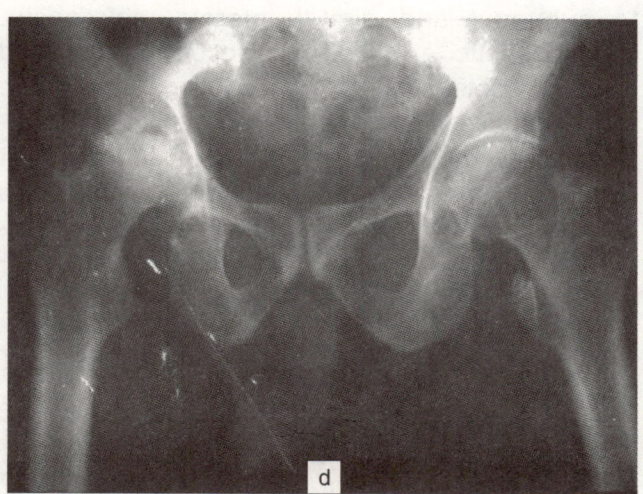

Fig. 4.3d. Alkaptonuria with right hip involvement

There is no treatment for alkaptonuria. Degenerated joints can be replaced by total joint arthroplasty when indicated and feasible.

Inflammatory Arthritides

Inflammatory arthritides are characterised by marked erosive destruction on both sides of the joint and marked morning stiffness.

1. Rheumatoid Arthritis

Rheumatoid arthritis (RA) is a chronic systemic inflammatory disorder of unknown aetiology that frequently involves the synovial lining of the peripheral joints. RA is the commonest form of inflammatory arthritis. Incidence has been reported to be 0.3 to 1.5% (with most reports agreeing to average 1% in the population). The disease occurs in all age groups but the incidence rises with advancing age, with a peak between the fourth and the sixth decades. Females are affected more commonly than males (M:F ratio = 9:1). Aetiology of RA is unknown. The disease probably arises in response to a pathogenic agent in a genetically predisposed host. The genetic predisposition is suggested by the fact the 70-80% of the affected individuals test positive for HLA DW4 and/or DR4. Also, there is an 8-fold risk of RA developing in an identical twin if the other sibling develops the disease. The risk is only 3-fold in dizygotic twins.

Possible pathogenic factors include infectious agents such as Mycoplasma, bacteria (Mycobacteria, enteric bacteria, bacterial cell wall), or viral (Epstein Barr Virus, Parvovirus BI9, Retrovirus) infections. Other triggering factors include endogenous antigens in the form of immunoglobulins (Rheumatoid factor), heat shock proteins, and cartilage antigens (Type II collagen, gp39, cartilage link protein, proteoglycans).

Destruction of the joint in RA is mediated by various factors such as cellular elements (mainly mononuclear cells), cytokines (especially interleukin 1, tumor necrosis factor alpha), immune complexes, enzymes (proteases), oxygen radicals and nitric oxide.

Pathologic Features Early rheumatoid arthritis is characterised by a local inflammatory response with accumulation of mononuclear cells. Chronic inflammation of the synovium is accompanied by hypertrophy and hyperplasia of the synovial lining cells. Papillary pattern forms on the surface of the synovium. The synovial membrane, normally 1 to 2 cell layers deep, may become 20 cell layers deep. Hypertrophied and inflamed synovium (pannus) extends over the articular surface and destroys the underlying cartilage leading to ankylosis of the joint. The pannus also invades and destroys the joint capsule and other inflamed periarticular supportive tissues. This process can lead to marked instability of the joint.

Clinical features

The onset of RA may by insidious over weeks or months (in 55–65% cases), intermediate (15–20%) or acute over days (in 8–15% cases). Affected patients complain of malaise, pain and stiffness of the joints and sometimes low-grade fever. The affected joints are warm, tender, erythematous, swollen, stiff and are painful to move. There is severe morning stiffness, lasting at least 45 minutes and gets relieved with movements and joint use. The most commonly involved joints are small joints of hands and feet (Fig. 4.4a). Other joints frequently involved are wrists, elbows, knees and ankles. Generally the disease is polyarticular, bilateral and symmetrical. Periarticular muscles undergo atrophy. Deformities develop quickly (especially in hands, feet and knees) unless efforts are made to prevent them.

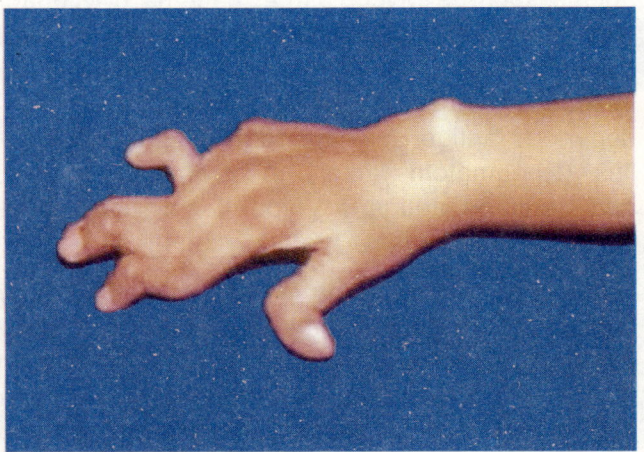

Fig. 4.4a. Rheumatoid involvement of the hand

Subcutaneous nodules develop in 25-30% patients of RA and are found on extensor aspect of the elbow (over proximal ulna) (Fig. 4.4b), occiput, over tendo Achilles and over sacrum. Nodes

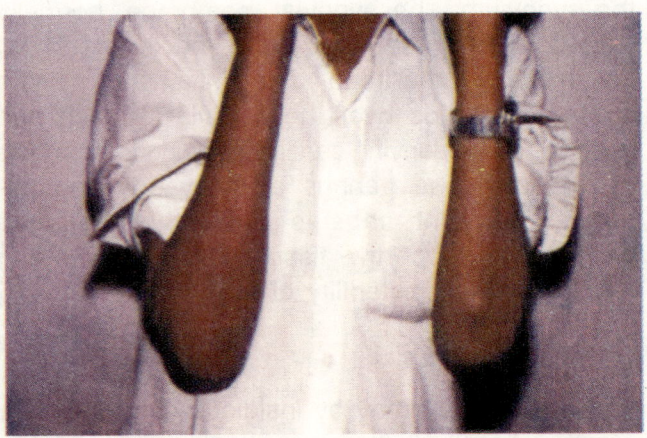

Fig. 4.4b. Rheumatoid nodule. Note the typical location on the extensor aspect of the forearm (left in this case)

in subcutaneous tissues may get sloughed and infected. Nodules are associated with positive serum rheumatoid factor and methotrexate therapy and may occur in viscera (e.g. lung, liver).

Tenosynovitis of tendons, triggering and rupture of tendons may occur. Entrapment of peripheral nerves (e.g. posterior interosseous nerve, ulnar nerve – both at elbow following synovitis) may occur.

Bursitis is common and student's elbow (olecranon bursitis) is the commonest bursal affliction.

Baker's cyst may form and may sometimes rupture early in the course of disease and may be confused with deep vein thrombosis ("pseudo-thrombophlebitis" syndrome). Vasculitis leading to subungul and digital infarcts may occur. "Pseudoseptic arthritis" may occur in RA and must be distinguished from septic arthritis. The former is a self-limiting condition wherein cultures of synovial fluid are negative and the joint becomes normal in 12–48 hours. No antibiotics are required. Raynaud's phenomenon may occur. Extraarticular manifestations of RA are enumerated in Table 4.3.

Table 4.3. Extraarticular manifestations of Rheumatoid Arthritis

Organ	Manifestation
Lungs	Effusion, nodules, interstitial disease, Bronchiolitis obliterans obstructive pneumonia (BOOP).
Eyes	Keratoconjuctivitis sicca, episcleritis, nodular episcleritis, scleritis, nodular scleritis, scleromalacia perforans
Nervous system	Peripheral nerves and cervical spine involvement (especially atlantoaxial instability).
Skin	Livido reticularis, purpura, skin infarcts, ulceration
Heart	Peri-, myo-, endo-carditis; coronary vasculitis

Various syndromes associated with RA are shown in Table 4.4.

Laboratory Investigations

A high titre (>1:160) of Rheumatoid Factor (most commonly IgM antibodies against autologous IgG) is present in almost 70% patients of RA. However serum Rheumatoid Factor may be elevated

Table 4.4. Syndromes associated with RA

Felty's Syndrome	Still's disease (acute onset juvenile RA), leucopenia and splenomegaly
Kaplan Syndrome	RA with pneumoconiosis
Sjogren's syndrome	Keratoconjunctivitis sicca complex (decreased salivary and lacrimal gland secretions and lymphoid proliferation)
Pseudothrombophlebitis syndrome	Ruptured Baker's cyst.
Brown Syndrome	Paralysis of upward and inward gaze due to involvement of superior oblique muscle.

in many rheumatic diseases (RA, SLE, Sjogren's etc), chronic bacterial infections (syphilis, tuberculosis, leprosy etc), viral diseases (Rubella, CMV, EBV, HIV etc), parasitic diseases, chronic inflammatory diseases (liver disease, sarcoidosis, pulmonary interstitial disease etc) and mixed cryoglobulinemias.

Slight leucocytosis with normal differential count is seen. Slight anaemia is seen in 30% patients. Serum complement level is normal or raised. Serum $\alpha 2$ and $\alpha 1$ globulins are raised.

Radiologic Features

Early radiologic changes include swelling of small peripheral joints, juxta articular osteoporosis and marginal bony erosions. These changes are followed by uniformly diminished joint space followed by destruction of the joint (Fig. 4.4c,d). There is no evidence of reparative activity and osteophytes and new bone formation are not seen. Advanced disease is seen on x-rays as bone resorption, deformity, fragmentation and disorganisation of the joint.

Treatment of RA is essentially multidisciplinary. Physician, orthopaedist, rehabilitation experts, physiotherapist, occupational therapist, psychologist and social worker have to work together to treat the patient. Involvement and support of the family is essential to achieve the goals of treatment.

Aims of the treatment are control of synovitis and pain, preservation of function and prevention of deformities. Drug therapy for RA is usually started with NSAIDs and subsequently disease modifying anti rheumatoid drugs (DMARD-including antimalarials, methotrexate, sulphasalazine, gold and d-penicillamine) are initiated if required. Immunosuppressive drugs (cyclophosphamide, azathioprine) are used if the patients do not respond to DMARDs. Steroids are used in patients with severe debilitating disease, patients with ocular involvement, patients with severe constitutional symptoms and in patients who do not respond to other drugs. Intra-articular steroids can alleviate acute inflammation in accessible large joints such as hip, knee or shoulder. Orthopaedic treatment of affected joints involves

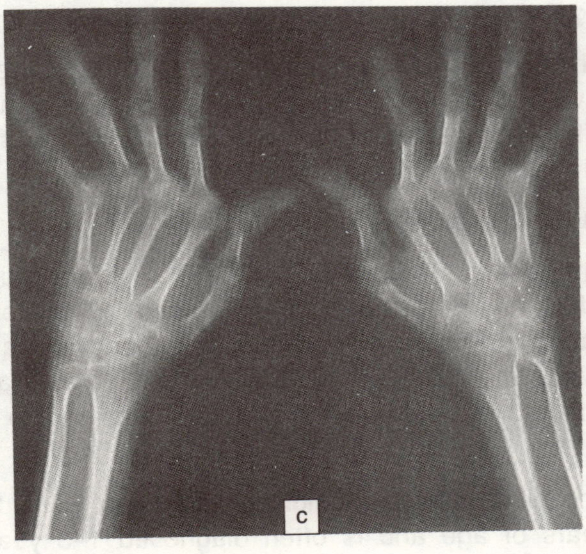

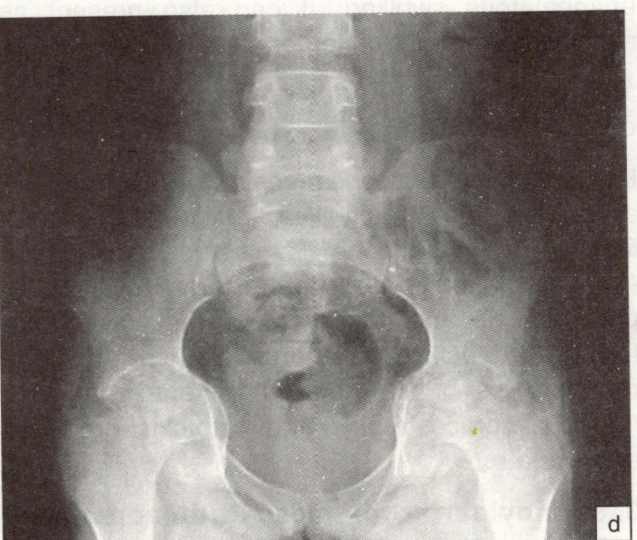

Fig. 4.4c. Anteroposterior radiograph of rheumatoid hand. Note the carpal coalition, ulnar drift at MCP and juxta articular osteoporosis

Fig. 4.4d. Bilateral hip joint involvement in Rheumatoid arthritis

splintage or traction to prevent/correct the deformity, physiotherapy including heat therapy and active and passive exercise and wedging casts to correct milder flexion deformities. Surgery should be undertaken only after cervical spine involvement and atlanto-axial instability has been ruled out preoperatively to prevent catastrophic complications. Surgery includes synovectomy (for failed conservative treatment in a large joint with preserved joint space when other joints are not involved), soft tissue procedures to correct deformities, corrective osteotomies, total joint replacement and sometimes, arthrodesis.

2. Systemic Lupus Erythematosus (SLE)

SLE is a chronic systemic inflammatory disease of unknown aetiology (possibly autoimmune) which usually affects women (Male: Female ratio 1:9) in the 2nd to 4th decades. Familial incidence of SLE is known (5% incidence among relatives of patients) and HLA DR2 and HLA DR3 predispose to the disease.

Clinically the disease is characterised by fever, skin lesions (butterfly malar rash, discoid rash) alopecia, mucosal lesions including non verrucous endocarditis, polyarthritis, synovitis, myositis, nephritis, carditis and pancytopenia. Renal involvement is the most common cause of death. Arthritis in SLE is the commonest feature and involves PIP, MCP and knee joints commonly. Joint involvement presents with tender and erythematous swelling. It can also present as avascular necrosis of femoral head (Fig. 4.4e,f).

The arthritis in SLE is non erosive and does not cause deformities.

Laboratory investigations reveal positive antinuclear antibodies (ANA), anti-DNA antibodies, antibodies to nuclear antigens, low serum complement (esp. C_2), lupus erythematosus (LE) cells, pancytopenia and raised ESR. Rheumatoid factor may be positive in serum. Treatment of SLE is on the lines of RA and drug therapy includes NSAIDs, corticosteroids and cytotoxic drugs as appropriate.

3. Spondyloarthropathies / Enthesopathies / Seronegative arthritides

Spondyloarthropathies are a clinically diverse group of conditions characterised by a negative

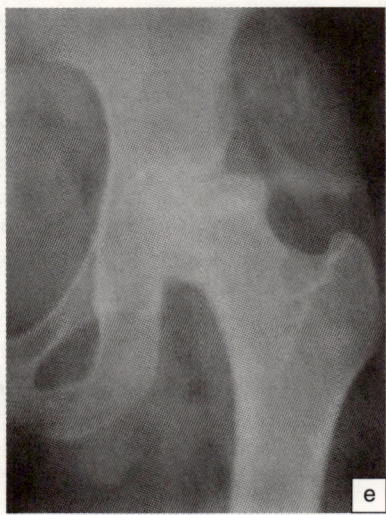

Fig. 4.4e. Avascular necrosis of left femoral head in a patient with SLE. Patient also received steroids

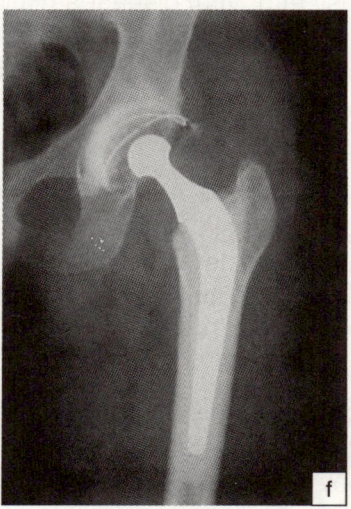

Fig. 4.4f. Same patient after total hip replacement

Rheumatoid factor, inflammatory polyarthritis typically involving sacroiliac joints, positive HLA B-27 and often, enthesopathy (bone formation at the site of insertion of ligaments into bone).

a) *Ankylosing Spondylitis*

Ankylosing Spondylitis (AS) is a seronegative inflammatory arthritis characterised by bilateral sacroiliitis often with associated spondylitis and uveitis in HLA B-27 positive patients. Males are affected more frequently (Male: Female ratio is 9:1).

The disease starts insidiously between 15 to 25 years of age and is often diagnosed 1–3 years after the onset. Low back pain with morning stiffness is the commonest presentation. Chest expansion is restricted due to involvement of the rib cage. Inflammatory arthritis of the peripheral joints occurs in 15-25% patients. Enthesopathy is seen as plantar fascitis, costochondritis and Achilles tendinitis. Temporo-mandibular joint involvement may lead to restriction of mouth opening. Spinal involvement starts at the thoracolumbar spine and eventually involves the whole spine (Fig. 4.5a,b). Patients often develop severe kyphotic deformity of the spine. Cervical spine involvement may (Fig. 4.5c) lead to chin on chest deformity of the spine. Hips are involved in about 50% cases of AS (Fig. 4.5d) and the involvement is bilateral in half the cases. Stiff spine along with fixed deformed hips makes the ambulation impossible. Extraskeletal involvement may occur in the form of dilatation of aorta, anterior uveitis and restrictive lung disease. Incidence of tuberculosis is higher in these patients due to restricted chest expansion.

Earliest involvement is seen in the bilateral sacroiliac joints (especially in the **inferior** part of the iliac side of the joints). Erosion, reactive bone formation and bony ankylosis of the sacroiliac joints is seen.

Spondylitis starts at the thoracolumbar junction where syndesmophytes first make their appearance. Squaring of the vertebrae and bamboo spine appearance is seen.

Pseudarthrosis (*"Anderson lesion", "Romanus lesion"*) of the spine is a complication of AS wherein fracture of the spine occurs (most commonly

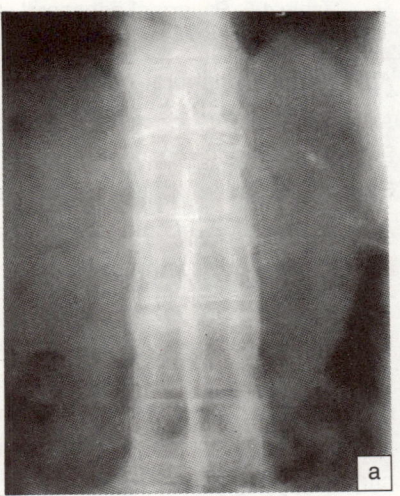
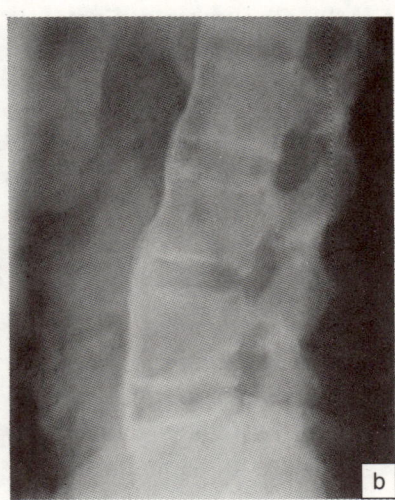

Fig. 4.5a,b. Bamboo Spine seen in Ankylosing Spondylitis

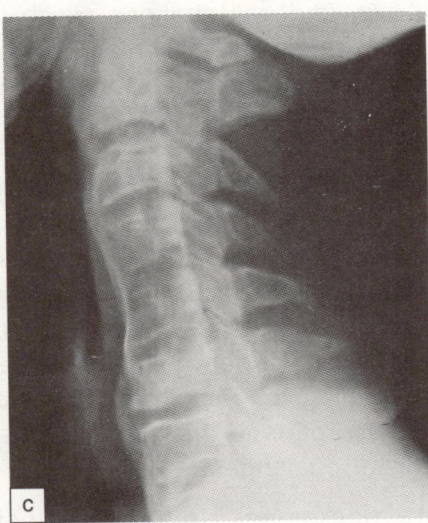
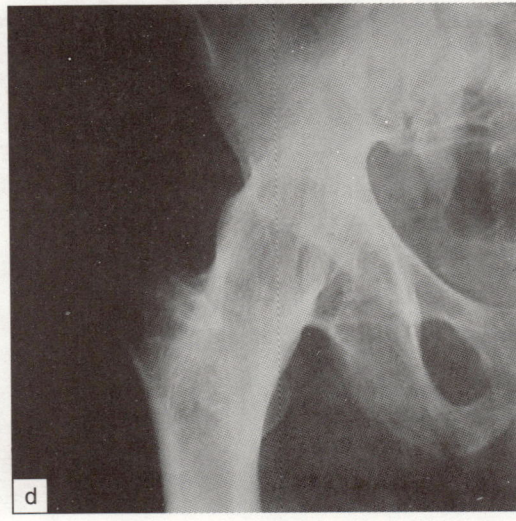

Fig. 4.5c. X-rays showing cervical spine involvement in Ankylosing Spondylitis. Note the fusion of spine

Fig. 4.5d. Bony ankylosis of hip in Ankylosing Spondylitis

through the discs and neural arches) due to stress and motion concentration, most commonly at the dorsolumbar junction. Pseudarthrosis is seen on the lateral radiographs as lucent area extending from anterior to posterior with significant adjacent sclerosis. Flexion and extension radiographs often demonstrate the spinal instability.

Atlanto-axial instability can sometimes occur in patients with AS.

Enthesopathy is evident by whiskering at the site of important ligament/tendinous insertions such as ischial tuberosity, ischial spine, calcaneus (Fig. 4.5e) etc. Ankylosis of hips and peripheral joints may be seen.

Laboratory Investigations HLA B27 is positive in >95% patients (though only 2% of patients with HLA B-27 get AS). Rheumatoid Factor is negative. ESR is raised.

Treatment of AS consists of NSAIDs and physiotherapy, especially breathing exercises, range of motion exercises, isometric exercises of the muscles and postural exercises. Hydrotherapy and/or swimming are especially useful.

Maintenance of proper posture (lie prone, use hard bed, don't use pillow) is extremely important to prevent ankylosis of spine in deformed position. Surgical treatment consists of total hip replacement when ambulation is difficult due to the involvement of hips and spine. Spinal surgery

may be indicated for correction of severe flexion deformity by spinal osteotomy (only after ensuring that hips are not affected or if affected, after hips are corrected) or stabilisation of spine with instrumentation in cases with pseudarthrosis or atlanto-axial instability.

b) *Psoriatic Arthropathy*

Psoriatic arthropathy is a seronegative inflammatory arthritis seen in 5–10% patients with psoriasis. Men and women are equally affected. It is primarily peripheral arthritis (DIP joints of fingers are commonly affected) though 20% patients may have spinal or sacroiliac involvement.

Five clinical types of Psoriatic arthropathy may occur (Table 4.5).

Table 4.5. Pattern of peripheral arthritis in psoriasis

Asymmetric peripheral polyarthritis (esp. DIP joints)
Arthritis Mutilans (destructive, deforming arthritis of fingers and toes)
Symmetrical polyarthritis (resembles RA but RF is absent)
Asymmetric oligoarticular (commonest)
Psoriatic spondyloarthritis (spine involvement)

Clinical course of psoriatic arthropathy is variable but distal joints (finger and toe joints) are most commonly involved. Asymmetric oligoarthritis leading to "*sausage*" digits is the commonest clinical type of arthritis. Back pain, stiffness and pain in other joints may occur.

Classical skin and nail changes clinch the diagnosis though rarely arthritis may appear before the obvious development of psoriasis in skin.

Radiologic features

Psoriatic arthropathy is characterised by severe erosive changes and destruction on both sides of the joint. Bone formation may coexist with erosive changes. Juxta articular osteoporosis is absent and DIP joints are involved (cf. Rheumatoid Arthritis). The phalangeal joints may be grossly destroyed leading to "*Pencil in cup*" deformity of DIP joint. Resorption of the terminal tufts may be seen in distal phalanges.

Bilateral sacroiliac joint ankylosis and syndesmophytes formation in the spine may be seen as in Ankylosing Spondylitis but unlike AS,

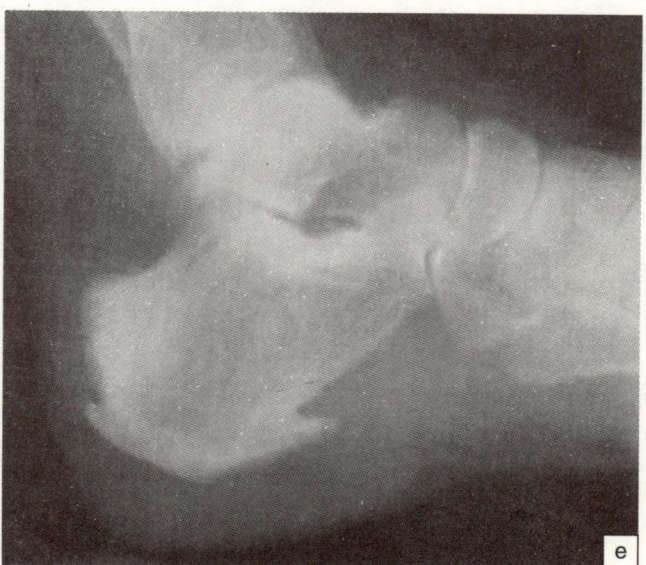

Fig. 4.5e. Enthesopathy in a patient with Ankylosing Spondylitis

these changes are often asymmetric in psoriatic arthropathy.

Laboratory Findings

HLA B-27 is positive in half the patients. ESR is raised.

Treatment consists of NSAIDs and physiotherapy. Disease modifying drugs (gold, antimalarials), steroids and immuno suppressive agents are often used as in the treatment of Rheumatoid Arthritis.

c) Reiter's Syndrome ("Reactive" arthritis)

Reiter's syndrome is characterised by the classical triad of urethritis, conjunctivitis and arthritis occurring in young males between 20 to 40 years of age.

The disease is often initiated following a gastrointestinal or genitourinary infection. History of sexual contact is often present. Chlamydia and salmonella have been implicated as the causative organisms.

Clinically, disease begins with urethritis, which is followed by conjunctivitis and arthritis. Skin lesions include circinate balanitis, keratoderma blenorrhagica and oral ulcers.

Arthritis is usually asymmetric, oligoarticular involvement of weight bearing joints which has an acute onset. Knees are most commonly affected followed by ankles and foot joints. Periosteal involvement, fascitis, enthesopathy or even ankylosis of joints may occur. Sacroiliac joint involvement (unilateral) may occur in almost half the patients with chronic disease.

Radiologic Features

X-rays show calcification of ligamentous insertions, periostitis in heel (calcaneum) and toes, erosion of metatarsal heads and even ankylosis of joints. Unilateral sacroilitis may be seen.

Laboratory Investigations

HLA B-27 is positive in almost 80% cases. Sterile pyuria may be seen. ESR is raised. Anaemia, leucocytosis and thrombocytosis may occur.

Treatment Reiter's syndrome is a self limiting disease and usually recovers in 6 weeks to 6 months. However, almost 50% cases recur. Physiotherapy and NSAIDs are the mainstay of treatment.

Crystal-Induced Arthritis

Crystal deposition disorders can present with rheumatologic or orthopaedic complications. Sodium urate (leading to gout) and calcium pyrophosphate (pseudogout) are two such particularly synoviotrophic crystals. Other crystals, which can be found in synovial fluid in association with arthritis, are hydroxyapatite crystals.

1. Gout

Gout is a painful clinical syndrome associated with the precipitation of monosodium urate crystals in the joints leading to synovitis and juxta articular destruction of the bone.

Gout is a disorder of nucleic acid metabolism and is caused by overproduction (lymphoproliferative or myeloproliferative disorders, hemoglobinopathies, enzyme defect e.g. X-linked disorder of high activity of enzyme PRPP synthetase - phosphoribosil pyrophosphate synthetase or excessive purine intake) or under-secretion (drugs, renal disease, lactic aciduria, ketoacidosis or idiopathic) of the uric acid. There may be a genetic predisposition to gout. Primary gout has a familial incidence in 6–18% cases. Diseases associated with gout include diabetes, hypertension, hyperparathyroidism, and hypothyroidism. Gout is also associated with surgeries, especially repetitive surgeries.

Clinically, the disease commonly affects males (90% cases) in the 5th decade of life. There is sudden onset of painful arthritis with red discoloration of the overlying skin. The first metatarsophalanageal joint is most commonly affected (Fig. 4.6a) followed by ankle, knee, wrist, finger joints and elbow. Fever and leucocytosis may occur. An acute attack may last from a few hours to several weeks. Recurrent chronic disease is characterised by crystal deposits as tophi (over olecranon, tendo achilles, helix of ears, eyelid), joint deformity and renal stones.

Bursitis, most commonly olecranon bursitis, often occurs in gout.

Radiologic Features

Soft tissue swelling and periarticular erosions with sclerotic overhanging margins are charac-

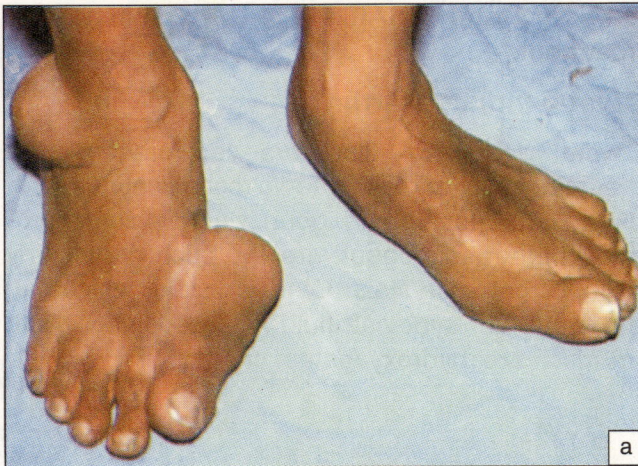

Fig. 4.6a. Gouty tophi of the foot

teristic (Fig. 4.6b,c). Calcified tophi may be seen on X-rays. Chronic gouty arthiritis is seen as narrowing of joint space, bone loss and deformity at the joint.

Laboratory Findings

Demonstration of monosodium urate crystals intracellularly (in WBCs) and extracellularly in the synovium is diagnostic. These crystal are thin, needle shaped and have a characteristic negative birefringence on polarised light microscopy (yellow coloured when oriented parallel to red filter and blue when perpendicular). Synovial fluid analysis also shows leucocytosis (10,000-25,000 WBC/cubic mm). Synovium shows a char-

acteristic granulomatous inflammatory response. Hyperuricemia (serum uric acid levels more than 7 mg/dl) is usually seen but is not essentially diagnostic (clinical gout may occur with normal serum uric acid levels while hyperuricemia may be present without clinical gout).

Treat ment

Indomethacin is used for initial treatment of acute gouty arthritis. Intravenous colchicine can be used in patients who cannot tolerate indomethacin.

Chronic gout is treated by drugs, which inhibit uric acid production such as allopurinol, which is xanthine oxidase inhibitor or uricosuric drugs which increase the renal excretion of uric acid such as probenecid.

Prophylaxis after recurrent attacks includes reduction of purine intake (reduced intake of meat and alcohol) and use of drugs such as colchicine, probenecid or allopurinol.

Surgery to excise painful tophi is sometimes indicated.

2. Chondrocalcinosis

Chondrocalcinosis is a condition where calcification of fibrocartilage and articular hyaline cartilage occurs. The causative conditions include calcium pyrophosphate dihydrate crystal deposition, ochronosis, hyper-parathyroidism, hypothyroidism, hemosiderosis and hemochromatosis.

Pseudogout or calcium pyrophosphate dihydrate

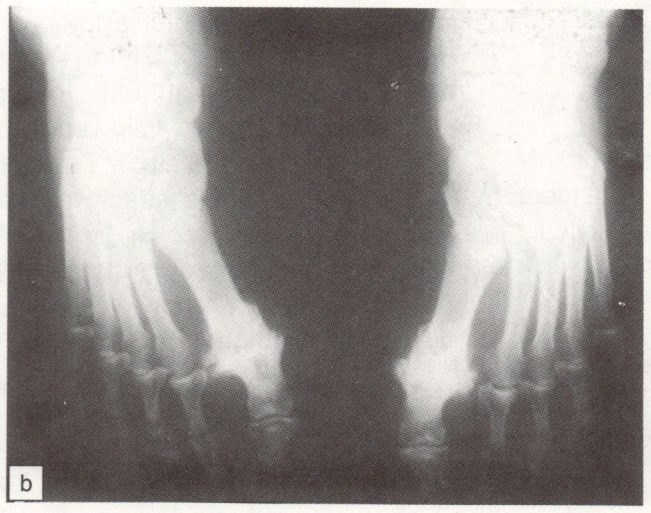
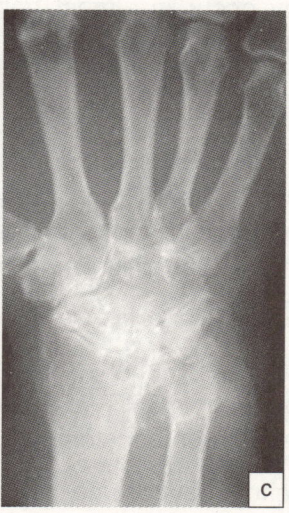

Fig 4.6b,c. Radiographic picture of gout
(b) Involvement of 1st MTP joint both sides; (c) Wrist involvement in gout

(CPPD) crystal deposition is seen in older people. Associated conditions include trauma, osteoarthritis, hyper-parathyroidism, hemochromatosis, neuropathic arthropathy and metabolic diseases such as hypomagnesemia and hypophosphatasia. Hereditary forms with autosomal dominant inheritance are reported. CPPD crystals are deposited in fibrocartilage, articular cartilage, synovium, tendons and ligaments. The crystals are phagocytosed by leucocytes and inflammation occurs. Characteristic sites of CPPD crystal deposition are knee, symphysis pubis, wrist, hip joint and the intervertebral disc.

Disease presents as acute arthritis or as chronic degenerative arthritis. Acute arthritis is often monoarticular (most commonly knee). Inflammatory synovitis and effusion is seen. The condition can sometimes be mistaken as septic arthritis.

Radiologic Features Calcification of menisci (diffuse) and hyaline cartilage (fine linear calcification) is seen on the x-rays. Bursae, ligaments and tendons may show calcifications. Calcification of symphysis pubis, triangular fibrocartilage and acetabular labrum may be seen.

Laboratory Investigations

Demonstration of short, blunt, rhomboid - shaped crystals in the neutrophils present in the synovial fluid is diagnostic. These crystals are weakly positively birefringent in polar light and appear yellow when perpendicular and blue when parallel to the red filter. Synovial fluid also shows leucocytosis in the range of 3000–5000 WBC/ cu mm. ESR is raised.

Treatment of the CPPD deposition disease is mainly with NSAIDs. Indomethacin is commonly used.

3. Hydroxyapatite Crystal Deposition Disease

Hydroxyapatite crystal deposition disease may present as primary crystal induced arthropathy or secondary to trauma or degenerative joint disease. Hydroxyapatite crystals are deposited in the soft tissues of joint space, rotator cuff tendons or bursa (leading to bursitis). Shoulder, knee and spine are most commonly involved. Rotator cuff tear arthropathy along with calcium hydroxyapatite crystal deposition is called "*Milwaukee shoulder*".

Spine calcification occurs in the form of calcification of intervertebral discs and paravertebral ligaments. Trochanteric bursitis may occur.

Hyroxyapatite crystals are non-birefringent and cause less inflammation than monosodium urate crystals and more inflammation than CPPD crystals.

Patients present with destructive arthropathy most commonly of the knee and shoulder. The disease occurs in later adult years with equal sex distribution.

Radiologically the disease appears as radiodense calcification in a local tumor mass like fashion or as subtle deposits in periarticular soft tissues.

Treatment of the hydroxyapatite crystal deposit disease is conservative with NSAIDs and physiotherapy. Large tumor mass like deposits may sometimes be treated with needling/aspiration or excision to relieve symptoms.

Hemorrhagic Arthropathy

Hemorrhagic arthropathy can be caused by a variety of conditions including trauma, hemophilia, synovial hemangioma, anticoagulant therapy, synovial tumors, idiopathic hemochromatosis, sickle cell disease or even pigmented villonodular synovitis.

Hemorrhage into the joint can damage the joint by macrophage activation with ensuing inflammation leading to destructive changes in the joint. Hemoglobin from the disintegrated red blood cells is broken down into hemosiderin, which is phagocytosed by macrophages or histiocytes. Intracellular hemosiderin leads to release of leucocyte and synovial derived chondrolytic enzymes. Also, the bleeding itself may directly lead to synovial proliferation and release of destructive enzymes (such as proteases).

Synovial fluid in hemorrhagic arthritis is characterised by reddish brown colour with reduced viscosity, moderate elevation of WBC (with more than 25% neutrophils), normal glucose and raised proteins. Excessive RBC's may be present in the cases with recent episode of hemorrhage.

Excessive hemosiderin deposit in the joint gives rise to brownish colour in these cases. Yellow colour may be seen in synovium due to the presence of abundant foamy (lipid laden) histiocytes.

Hemophilic Arthropathy

Hemophilia A is the commonest hereditary (sex linked recessive) coagulation disorder affecting 20 per 100,000 live male births and is caused by deficiency or malfunction of coagulation factor VIII. Hemophilia B (Christmas disease) is caused by lack of factor IX. Hemophilia C is a mild variety of disease caused by the deficiency of factor XI. It has autosomal dominant inheritance.

Normally very low serum levels of factor VIII are sufficient for adequate coagulation. Reduction of more than 75% in the serum levels (i.e. serum levels <25% of normal) leads to perceptible clinical illness. The disease is graded according to the severity of factor VIII deficiency into mild (serum factor VIII levels 5-25% of normal; moderate 1-5% and severe < 1%). Bleeding can be intraarticular, intrabursal or into the soft tissues. Repeated intra-articular bleeding leads to proliferative synovitis and extensive hemosiderin deposition.

Clinically, the disease presents with recurrent episodes of bleeding, especially in the joints. The disease usually presents in early childhood with discomfort, limitation of joint movement initially followed by pain and swelling. Contractures and deformities eventually occur. Knee is the most common joint involved (Fig. 4.7a) followed by elbow, ankle, shoulder and hip. The affected joint being swollen, warm and painful to move is often confused with septic arthritis and joint aspiration is needed to rule out infection. Bleeding into the

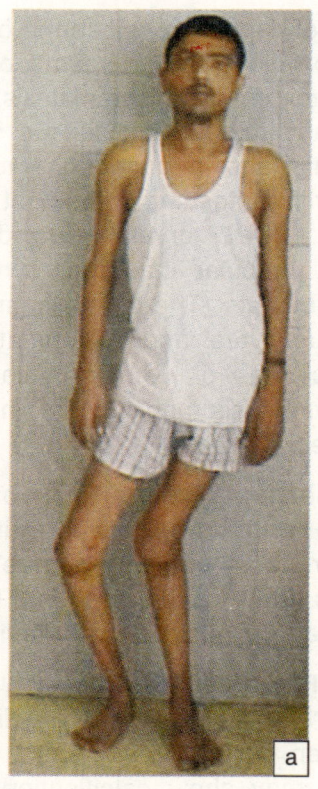

Fig. 4.7a. Knee joint involvement in hemophilic arthritis. Note the "wind swept" deformity (Genu varum right and Genu valgum left)

soft tissues can lead to neural deficit, the most classical example being femoral nerve palsy occurring due to hemorrhage in the iliacus muscle.

"Pseudotumors" are painless masses consisting of partially clotted blood surrounded by thick fibrous membrane resulting from juxta periosteal bleeding which mimic tumors clinically and radiologically (Fig. 4.7b,c). They occur in 1-2% cases of hemophilia. They are commonly seen in lower

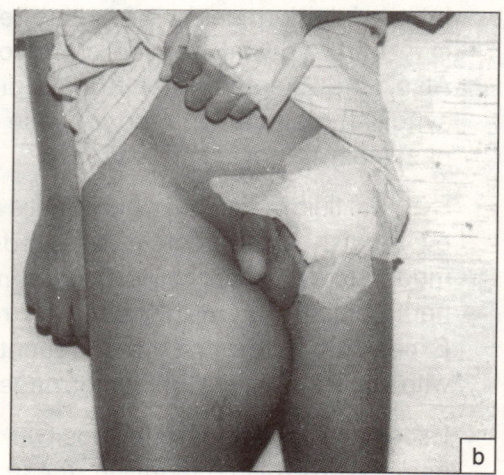

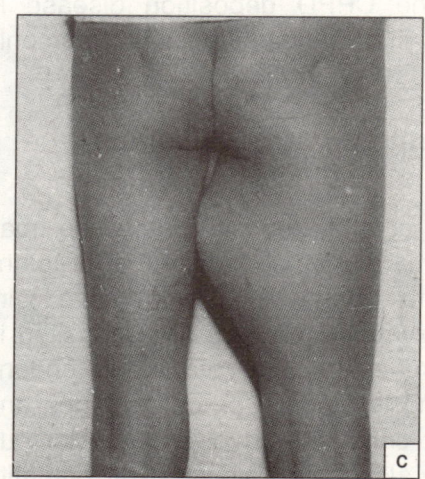

Fig. 4.7b,c. Clinical picture of pseudotumor of medial aspect of right thigh

limbs and pelvis. Pseudotumors can damage bone and muscles, can lead to infection or cause neuropathies.

Radiologic features

Early stages show soft tissue swelling. This is followed by osteoporosis. Further damage to the joint is seen as bony changes (squaring of patella, widened intercondylar notch of femur and enlarged femoral condyles in the knee, formation of subchondral cysts), joint space narrowing and loss of articular cartilage. Osteophyte formation is seen.

Pseudotumors are seen as cystic, expansile, lucent, soft tissue swellings eroding the cortex (Fig. 4.7d). MRI is classical with low signal on T_1 weighted images and high signal on T_2 weighted images.

Ultrasonography is useful to diagnose the intramuscular bleeds.

Laboratory investigations

Partial Thromboplastin Time (PTT) is elevated in hemophilia. Specified factor assays should be done to determine severity of the disease. Assays for factor VIII inhibitors (antibodies) should be done, as their presence is a contraindication to any surgical intervention.

Blood for HIV should be tested in hemophiliacs

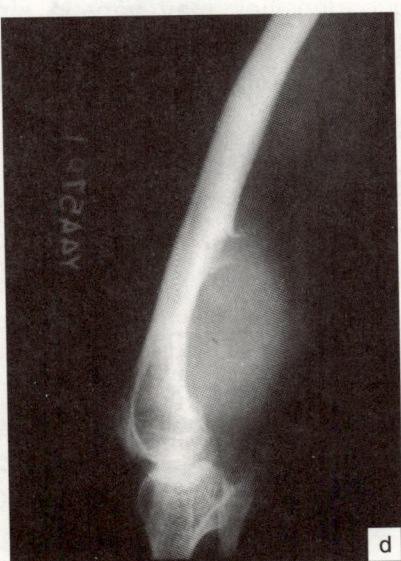

Fig. 4.7d. Radiographic picture of hemophilic pseudotumor with involvement of distal femur

as transfusion related AIDS is a well recognised complication of hemophilia (in up to 90% patients).

Treatment

Prophylaxis for hemophilia is extremely important and consists of avoidance of contact sports, physiotherapy and prophylactic administration of factor VIII whenever affordable.

Acute hemarthrosis is treated by splintage, compressive bandage, analgesics and replacement of factor VIII to bring the serum levels to 30-50 % of normal. Aspiration of the joint to relieve pain and swelling is useful within the first 24 hours when the antibodies to factor VIII are absent in the serum.

Fractures are usually managed conservatively in hemophilia with splintage/immobilisation. Factor replacement is done for the first 48-72 hours.

Hemorrhage in the muscles is managed by immobilisation, compression and factor VIII replacement. Synoviorthesis i.e. injection of a radioactive agent in the joint to destroy the synovium with radioactive phosphorus (^{32}P) is useful for chronic hemophilic synovitis.

Surgical management of chronic hemophiliac arthropathy includes synovectomy, correction of soft tissue contractures, arthrodesis and total joint replacement. Pseudotumors need excision but can be treated with radiotherapy and/or factor replacement sometimes.

Principles of surgery in hemophilia

1. HIV and inhibitors to factor VIII (antibodies) must be assayed in serum preoperatively.

2. Factors VIII replacement must start 45 minutes to 1 hour before surgery and continue till suture removal (or longer if indicated).

3. Factor VIII levels in the serum must be maintained at 100% (to normal levels) for the first week following surgery and at 50-75% during the second week.

4. Tourniquet should be used wherever possible.

5. Sharp dissection is preferred; blunt dissection should be avoided.

6. Meticulous hemostasis should be achieved.

Ligatures should be preferred and cautery should be used sparingly.

7. Wound should be closed with hemostatic continuous dexon sutures.

8. Drains should not be used.

9. Bulky compression dressing should be applied after surgery. Postoperative immobilisation in a splint is desirable.

10. Physiotherapy in the postoperative period should be performed under the cover of factor VIII replacement.

Synovial Disorders

1. Pigmented Villonodular Synovitis (PVNS)

PVNS is usually a localised, non neoplastic, monoarticular, fibrous-histocytic proliferation found in the synovial joints and tendon sheaths. Knee is the commonest joint affected while tendon sheaths of the digits of hand are the most commonly affected tendon sheaths (the so called "giant cell tumor of tendon sheath"). Lesion can also involve the hip joint, foot, wrist or shoulder.

The lesion can occur as an isolated discrete lesion of the tendon sheath, as localised nodular synovitis or as diffuse synovial disease with exuberant proliferation of villi and nodules (PVNS). The synovium in this condition is frequently brown due to deposition of hemosiderin.

Clinically the disease occurs in young adults and more commonly affects males. Painless insidious swelling without trauma and out of proportion to the degree of discomfort is typical.

Radiographs show joint swelling. Erosions, usually well defined, located on bare areas of bone and sometimes, even in subchondral areas are seen. Joint space is usually preserved, as the articular cartilage is not eroded. Hip joint is an exception where joint space narrowing may be the initial presentation.

Investigations

Synovial fluid may appear reddish brown in colour. Synovial biopsy shows reddish-brown, thickened nodular appearance. Villous proliferation of synovium is present with capillaries, multinucleated giant cells, foam cells (lipid laden histiocytes) and hemosiderin. Treatment of PVNS is surgical excision of the affected synovium or the tendon sheath (giant cell) tumor. Local recurrence is common.

2. Synovial Chondromatosis

Synovial chondromatosis is a condition resulting from synovial metaplasia to cartilage. This cartilage may undergo endochondral ossification.

The condition can arise de novo (primary synovial chondromatosis) or may occur in a broad range of disease such as degenerative joint disease, charcot's joints, osteochondritis dissecans, meniscal tears or following other injuries (osteochondral fractures, dislocations etc.). These cartilaginous or osteocartilaginous fragments often dislodge and become loose bodies causing mechanical symptoms. Interestingly these loose bodies continue to grow in size while lying free in synovial fluid.

Synovial osteochondromatosis, occurring de novo, is usually monoarticular affliction more common in males between the third to fifth decades. Knee is the most common joint involved (in two third cases) followed by elbow, ankle, hip and shoulder. Wrist and hand joint may be rarely involved.

Disease usually presents with swelling and mechanical derangement (clicking, locking or limitation of movements). Pain is often present.

Radiologic features include fine stippled calcification within the lobulated masses in the joint. Radiopaque densities may vary in size from a few millimetres to centimetres (Fig. 4.8a). Arthrography and MRI are invaluable in diagnosing noncalcified bodies.

The disease should be differentiated from tumoral calcinosis associated with scleroderma, dermatomyositis etc., chondrosarcoma and heterotopic ossification.

Laboratory investigations

Biopsy shows flake-like bodies in the synovium or irregular nodular contour of the synovium. The nodules are whitish or bluish-grey, are composed of hyaline cartilage and may be attached or floating in the synovial fluid.

Treatment is synovectomy and removal of loose bodies. Complications of synovial chondromatosis

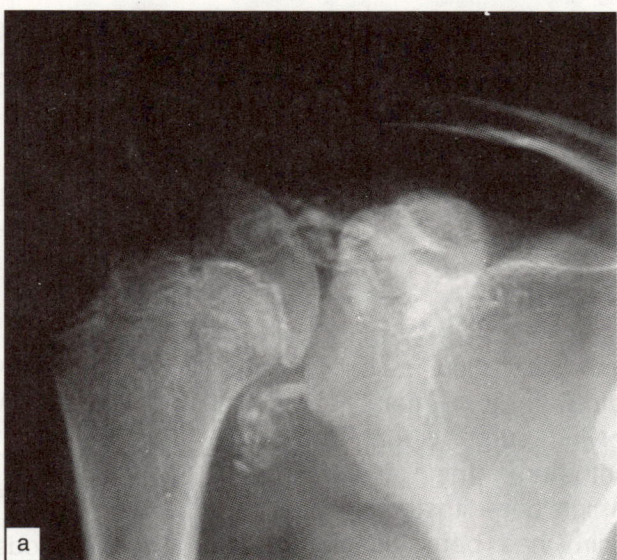

Fig. 4.8a.   X-ray showing synovial chondromatosis of the right shoulder

include recurrence after excision and malignant degeneration (to chondrosarcoma).

Synovial chondromatosis like changes may also involve bursae or tendon sheaths.

3. Synovial Sarcoma

Synovial sarcoma is a highly malignant mesenchymal tumor, which usually arises in close proximity of joints, most often in tenosynovial lining (tendon sheath, bursal sacs, fascial planes and joint capsule) but rarely arises from an intraarticular location (10%). It derives its name from microscopic appearance, which mimics the histologic appearance of the embryonic synovium. Synovial sarcoma is the fourth commonest soft tissue sarcoma, accounting for 10% of all malignant mesenchymal tumors.

Approximately 70% of synovial sarcomas occur in the lower extremity. Most frequently these tumors arise around the knee. These tumors also occur around shoulder, arm, elbow and wrist. Synovial sarcoma is the commonest soft tissue tumor in the foot.

Clinically, the tumor is most prevalent between 15 and 35 years of age. The most common presentation is of a painful, palpable soft tissue mass in the vicinity of a major joint. The tumor grows slowly initially but sometimes presents as a rapidly enlarging mass.

Radiologic appearance of the tumor is most often that of a soft tissue mass which shows dystrophic calcification or heterotopic ossification in about 50% cases. The calcifications can be dense, faint or punctuate. The soft tissue mass is juxta articular but usually outside the joint.

With growth the tumor eventually extends into the adjacent joint and invades and destroys the adjacent bones.

CT and MRI are useful diagnostic modalities for demonstrating soft tissue mass and its relationship with adjacent neurovascular structures, which are usually displaced but sometimes invaded by the tumor. CT images demonstrate the intralesional calcifications quite well. MRI is useful for demonstrating the dimensions of the tumor and areas of necrosis within the tumor.

Histologically, the tumor typically shows biphasic (fibroblastic and epithelial cells) cell population composed of epithelium like cells surrounded by malignant fibroblastic spindle cells. Epithelial cells form nests or glands, clefts, tubular structures and produce a mucinous material. Regional lymph nodes may be involved.

A monophasic form of synovial sarcoma has been described and consists of a dominant fibroblastic or epithelial cell pattern.

Course

Synovial sarcomas are high-grade lesions. They recur locally and spread by regional lymph nodes (involved in 20% cases) and through lung. Lung metastases are present in 75% patients while bone metastases occur in 10% cases. Synovial sarcoma is the commonest soft tissue sarcoma to metastasise to lymph nodes.

Prognostic factors for synovial sarcoma are shown in Table 4.6. Five years survivals may be as low as 25%.

Treatment

Traditionally these tumors are treated by radical surgery with adjuvant radiotherapy. Recently, multimodality approach involving surgery, radiotherapy and intensive chemotherapy (high dose cisplatin and doxorubicin or high dose ifosfamide and cisplatin with doxorubicin) has been used with encouraging results.

Table 4.6. Factors associated with poor prognosis of synovioma

- Size > 5 cm
- Monophasic variants
- Older Patients
- Epithelial gland cellularity > 50%
- Mitotic activity <15 mitoses per 10 high power fields (HPF)
- Mast Cells <20/HPF
- Tumor necrosis
- Presence of rhomboid cells
- High proliferating cell nuclear antigen (PCNA) score.

High dose ifosfamide chemotherapy has a role in the metastatic disease.

Regional lymph node involvement is treated by surgical excision followed by local radiation.

CHAPTER 5

Metabolic Bone Diseases

- *Calcium and Phosphorus Homeostasis and Remodeling*
- *The Calcitropic Hormones*
  Parathyroid Hormone (PTH)
  Vitamin D (Cholecalciferol)
  Calcitonin
- *Rickets*
- *Osteomalacia*

- *Primary Hyperparathyroidism*
- *Hypocalcemia*
- *Primary Hypoparathyroidism*
- *Pseudohypoparathyroidism (PHP)*
- *Pseudopseudohypoparathyroidism*
- *Osteoporosis*
- *Scurvy*

Metabolic bone diseases include a group of unrelated diseases affecting collagen or mineral deposition and hence adversely affecting bone.

It is important to understand the physiology of calcium and phosphorus homeostasis and action of calcitropic hormones in order to know how different pathological processes affect remodelling of bones.

Calcium and Phosphorus homeostasis and Remodelling

Adult human being has 1000 grams of calcium of which 99% is in the bone. Calcium in serum exists in three forms, namely protein (albumin) bound (40%), complexed (10%) and ionised (50%). Bone (endoskeleton) composed of hydroxyapatite $[Ca_{10}(PO_4)_6(OH)_2]$ serves as reservoir for the central pool of calcium. This central pool of calcium has large fluxes across three epithelia, namely, bone, intestine and kidney which are regulated by calcitropic hormones (mainly parathormone and 1,25 dihydroxy vitamin D). Average dietary intake of calcium is 500–1000mg daily of which 15–70% may be absorbed from the intestines. Absorptive efficiency may be increased by vitamin D, bile salts, acidic digestate and low calcium states whereas it is reduced by excessive phosphates or carbonates, fatty acids, alkaline medium, old age and oestrogen deficiency state at menopause.

Between 5 to 7 grams of calcium are filtered daily by kidneys and all except 250 mg (150–300 mg) is reabsorbed. In addition to excretion by kidneys, calcium is excreted by colon (500-mg daily approximately) and a small obligatory amount is lost from the skin in sweat (50–150 mg daily).

Only 1 gm of body calcium is present in the plasma and extracellular fluid. The normal serum calcium level is 8.8–10.8 mg/dl. The daily bone/plasma exchange is approximately 500 mg (Fig. 5.1). Adults with zero net calcium balance do not have net daily flux between central calcium pool and bone. Hence, urinary (plus sweat) calcium equals daily net calcium absorption from intestine. Major deviations from zero calcium balance occur during skeletal growth, bone senescence, lactation and during disease.

Almost 90% of total body phosphorus is found in the skeleton. In blood, the phosphorus is present in ionised as well as organic forms. The normal serum levels of phosphates are 3–4 mg/dl. The serum levels of phosphate are less tightly regulated than calcium. Changes in serum levels of phosphates are mainly due to changes in dietary intake.

Phosphorus homeostasis is mainly through control of its renal conservation, which is regulated by parathormone.

The Calcitropic Hormones
Parathyroid Hormone (PTH)

Parathyroid Hormone (PTH) is the major hormone

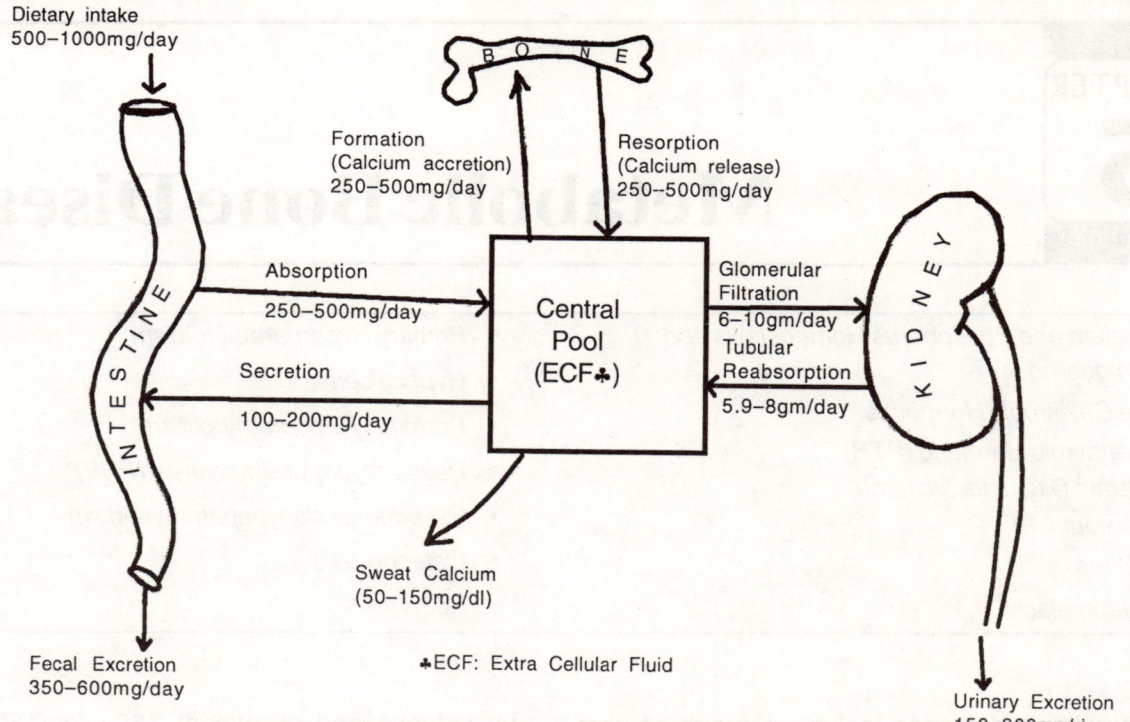

Fig. 5.1. Calcium homeostasis in the human body.

controlling calcium homeostasis. PTH is an 84 amino acid polypeptide hormone secreted by parathyroid gland, though, for full biological activity only 34 amino terminal acids are needed. Circulating parathyroid hormone is heterogeneous and consists mainly of inactive C-terminal fragments. PTH secretion is modulated mainly by plasma calcium with hypocalcaemia stimulating its secretion and hypercalcaemia suppressing it. Parathyroid hormone performs its function of maintaining calcium and phosphorus homeostasis by its action on the bone, renal tubule and renal 1–alpha hydroxylase system.

PTH increases plasma Ca^{2+} concentration in three ways : (Fig. 5.2)

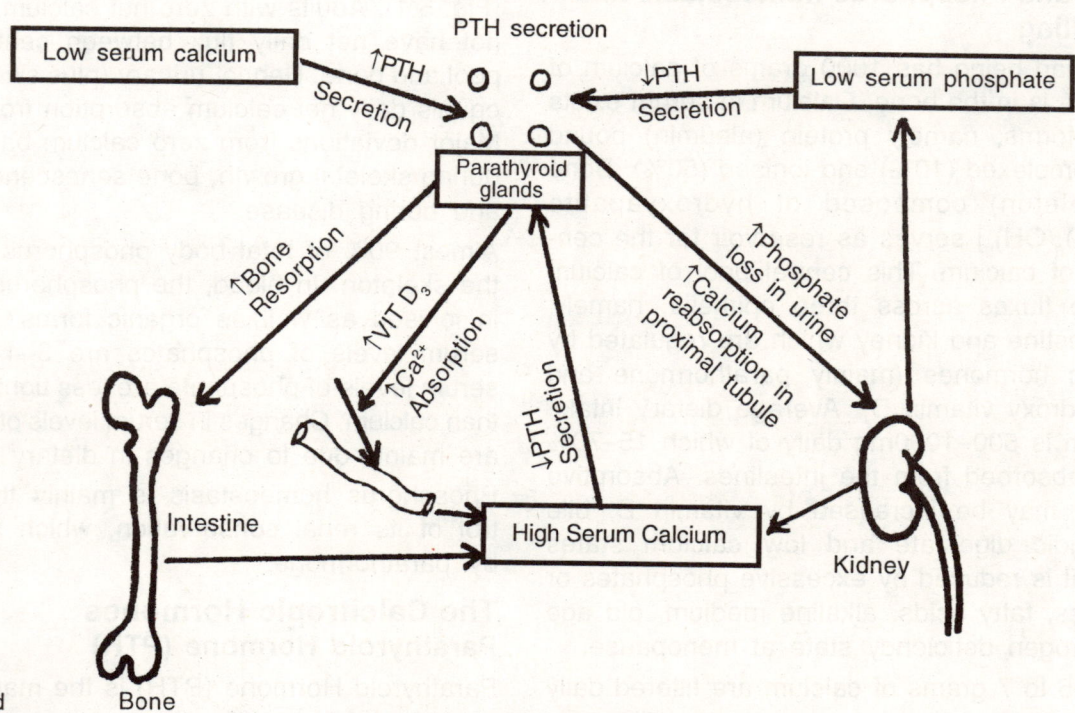

↑ : Increased
↓ : Decreased

Fig. 5.2. Secretion and actions of Parathyroid Hormone

- In presence of active vitamin D, it stimulates bone resorption resulting in release of calcium and phosphate.

- It enhances intestinal Ca^{2+} and phosphate absorption indirectly by promoting the production of calcitriol in the kidney.

- It augments active renal Ca^{2+} reabsorption in distal tubule.

PTH decreases plasma phosphate levels by reducing proximal tubular reabsorption of phosphate.

Vitamin D (Cholecalciferol)

Cholecalciferol (Vitamin D3) is a steroid hormone synthesised in skin from photochemical conversion of 7-dehydrocholesterol present in the skin from exposure to solar ultraviolet irradiation (wave band 280-305µ).

Ergo calciferol (vitamin D2) produced by ultraviolet irradiation of fungal steroid ergosterol is the dietary source and becomes important only when exposure of the skin to ultraviolet irradiation is absent.

Vitamin D3 is transported on a binding globulin to the liver where it undergoes 25 hydroxylation to form major circulating form and storage form in the body (25 hydroxy–D3). 25 hydroxy-D3 does not have biological activity at normal circulating levels in plasma but provides a reasonable measure of vitamin D status.

The major active metabolite 1,25 dihydroxy vitamin D (calcitriol) is formed by 1 alpha hydroxylation of 25 hydroxy vitamin D in the kidney.

The main regulators of calcitriol [1,25(OH)$_2$D3] synthesis are the serum concentrations of calcitriol itself, serum calcium levels, serum phosphate levels and serum PTH levels. PTH is the major inducer of the renal 25(OH) D3-1 alpha hydroxylase. Calcium regulates this enzyme directly as well as through regulation of PTH.

The principle effects of 1,25(OH)$_2$D3 are:

- Intestinal absorption of calcium and phosphate

- Renal tubular reabsorption of calcium

- Vitamin D is needed for bone mineralization but whether this effect is due to increased serum calcium and phosphate level or through stimulation of osteoblasts is not known.

Vitamin D3 also acts on other target organs such as.

- Parathyroids to suppress formation of PTH.

- Kidneys to down-regulate its own synthesis by suppression of 1 alpha hydroxylase as well as induction of 24 hydroxylase activity (to form inactive metabolite, 24, 25(OH)$_2$D3) which is the first step in the vitamin D catabolic pathway.

Calcitonin

Calcitonin is a 32 amino acid peptide secreted by parafollicular cells (C-Cells) of thyroid gland. Calcitonin is mainly an inhibitor of osteoclastic bone resorption. The major stimulus for calcitonin is calcium. Hypercalcaemia stimulates calcitonin production; the latter, in turn, directly inhibits calcium and phosphate resorption by the osteoclasts and reduces renal tubular reabsorption of calcium, thus bringing down serum calcium levels.

Osteoclastic inhibitory property of calcitonin is utilised in the treatment of Paget's disease, osteoporosis and hypercalcaemia of malignancy. Calcitonin also has profound analgesic effects in fractures and bone pains due to osteoporosis and widespread metastatic disease.

The key steps in the complex calcium homeostasis along with the role of key players is depicted in Fig. 5.3.

I) Levels of serum calcium regulate activity of parathyroids.

II) PTH regulates conversion of 25(OH) D3 to 1,25(OH)$_2$D3 in kidney

    * 1 hydroxylase activity is stimulated by increased PTH, decreased 1,25(OH)$_2$D3 and decreased serum phosphate.

    * 24-hydroxylase activity is stimulated by decreased PTH, decreased 1,25(OH)$_2$D3 and increased serum phosphate leading to formation of relatively inactive metabolite 24-25 (OH)$_2$ D3.

III) Calcium fluxes across distal kidney, bone and gut are regulated by concerted actions of PTH and vitamin D3.

IV) Negative feedback on 1,25(OH)$_2$D3 and PTH synthesis by increased serum 1,25(OH)$_2$D3 and calcium.

V) Calcitonin release in response to increased

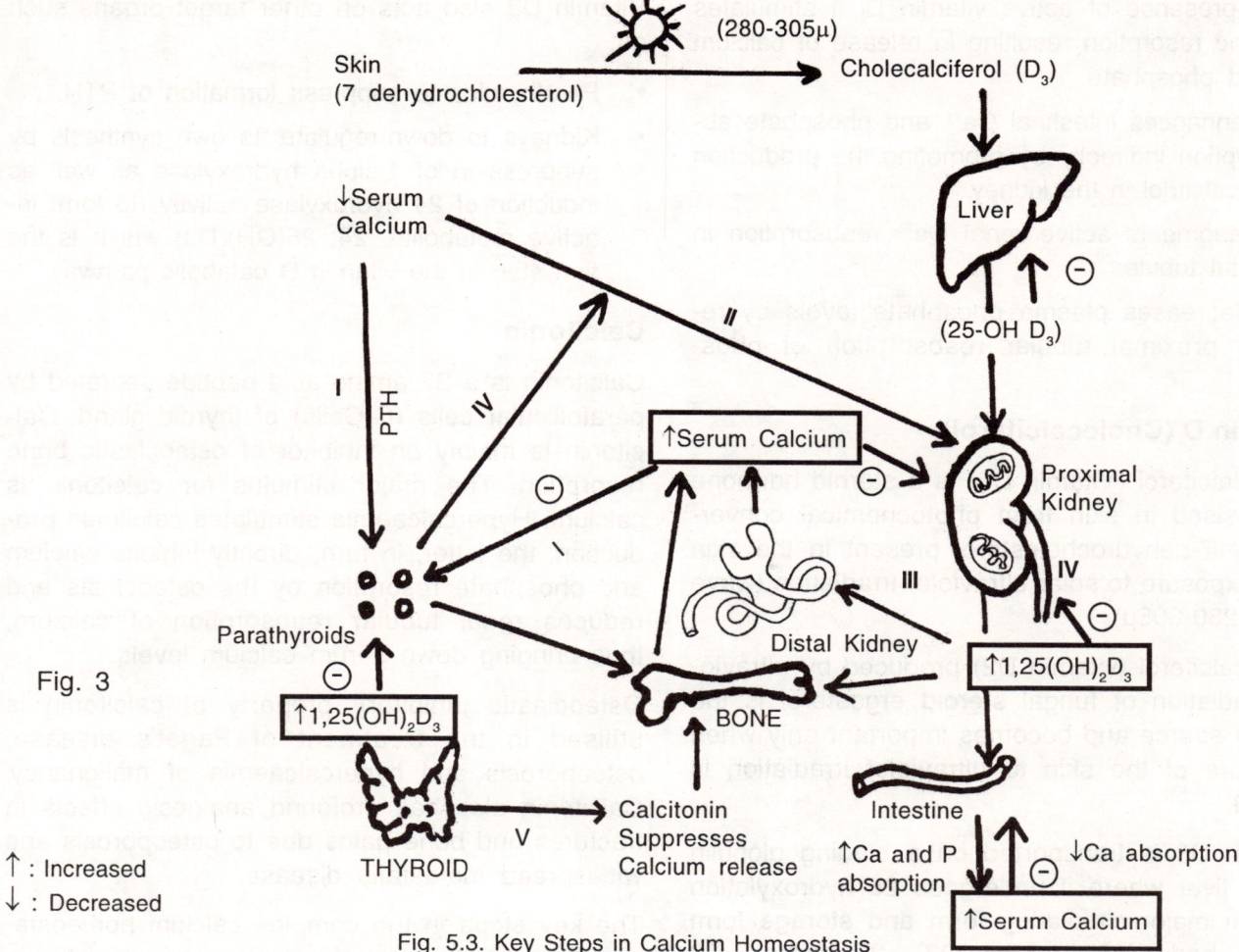

Fig. 5.3. Key Steps in Calcium Homeostasis

serum calcium levels leads to decreased calcium release by suppression of osteoclasts.

Rickets

Rickets is a disease of growing skeleton characterised by failure of mineralization leading to changes in the physis (increased width and disorientation) and bone (cortical thinning, bowing). Rickets is often divided into two types (viz. type I and II). In type I, there is primarily an abnormality or deficiency of calcium and/or vitamin D. The type II is caused by metabolic defects leading to deficiency of phosphates in the extracellular fluids, primarily due to excessive renal excretion resulting in the deficient mineralization of osteoid.

The causes of rickets are summarised in Table 5.1.

Vitamin D Deficiency Rickets (Nutritional Rickets)

Nutritional rickets occurs due to deficiency states,

in patients with dietary peculiarities, inadequate exposure to sunlight, premature infants, those with malabsorption or chronic parenteral nutrition. Decreased absorption of calcium and phosphates leads to secondary hyperparathyroidism (in response to hypocalcaemic state).

Vitamin D deficiency rickets usually manifest in the latter half of the first year or in the second year. Rickets is unusual below the age of 3 months.

In the normal bone, cartilage cells proliferate in parallel columns, hypertrophy and then degenerate. Mineralization occurs in the zone of degenerating cartilage. However, in the face of deficiency of calcium and phosphate which are necessary for mineralization of osteoid, the cartilage cells continue to proliferate with little or no mineralization. Poor mineralization leads to softening of bone. The epiphyseal plate appears widened and irregular on x-rays and the shafts of bone are easily deformed or fractured.

Table 5.1. Cause of Rickets

---

1. **Nutritional deficiency**
   - Vitamin D deficiency
   - Calcium deficiency–Phytate or oxalate chelation of dietary calcium
   - Phosphate deficiency–Antacid abuse

2. **Gastrointestinal absorption defects**
   - Absorption defects
   - Coeliac disease
   - Inflammatory bowel disease
   - Post gastrectomy

3. **Renal defects**
   - Renal Tubular defects (Renal Phosphate leak)
   - X linked Dominant Hypophosphatemic vitamin D Resistant Rickets (VDRR)
   - Fanconi's syndrome
   - FHVDRR with amino aciduria and glycosuria
   - Late onset Vitamin D resistant rickets
   - Vitamin D Dependent Rickets
     Type I–Renal tubular 1–alpha hydroxylase deficiency
     Type II–end organ resistance to 1,25 $(OH)_2D_3$
   - Renal Tubular Acidosis
     Proximal RTA
     Distal
     Combined RTA
   - Renal glomerular defects (Renal Osteodystrophy)

4. **Hepatic Factors**
   - Liver damage–absent 25 hydroxylation of D3
   - Hepatic microsomal enzymes stimulation following prolonged anticonvulsant therapy.

5. **Miscellaneous causes**
   - Oncogenous (Fibrous dysplasia, neuro-fibromatosis etc.)
   - Heavy metal intoxication
   - Hypophosphatasia
   - Drugs-fluorides

Clinical manifestations of rickets are protean. Hypotonia, generalized muscular weakness, lethargy and irritability are early symptoms. Craniotabes is seen over occipital or parietal bones in the newborn where compression and release of the soft membranous bones gives the feeling of ping pong ball. Bossing of frontal and parietal bones and delayed closure of anterior fontanelle are other findings in skull. There is widening at the wrists, knees and ankles due to enlarged epiphyses. Chest shows multiple deformities namely, "pigeon breast" due to sternum projecting forwards, prominence of costochondral junctions ("rachitic

rosary"), a horizontal depression along the lower border of chest corresponding to insertion of diaphragm ("Harrison's sulcus") and thoracic spine deformities such as kyphosis and scoliosis.

Dental disease is commonly seen in the form of delayed eruption of primary teeth and eruption of dysplastic teeth. Angular deformities of long bones occur after one year of age when the child starts weight bearing. Anterior bowing of legs, coxa vara and genu varum or valgum at knee are common deformities. Trivial trauma can cause fractures (often incomplete) in these patients.

Exaggerated lumbar lordosis, protruberant abdomen and visceroptosis are commonly seen.

Rickets often does not manifest clinically in severely malnourished children as the latter often are dwarfed and not growing. However, marked rachitic changes apear in these children with the correction of malnutrition and resumption of growth.

X-rays show widening of physes, small epiphysis alongwith irregularity, fraying, and cupping of epiphyseal end of metaphysis. Flaring (trumpeting) of the metaphyses and rarefaction of bone are also seen. Coarsening of trabeculae is often seen. The deformities are readily appreciated on x-rays. The patients on treatment show a dense white line at the epiphyseo-metaphyseal junction suggesting newly calcified cartilage.

The X-ray features of rickets are shown in Fig. 5.4a-c.

Biochemical Investigations show low/normal calcium and low phosphates (effects of PTH), increased PTH and low levels of vitamin D. Serum

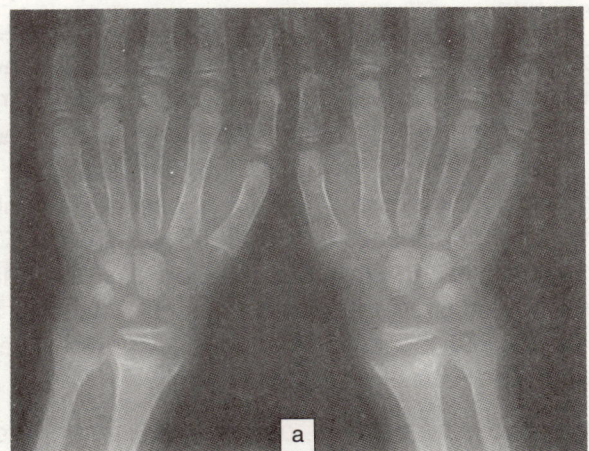

Fig. 5.4a. Florid rickets seen in the lower end of radius and ulna

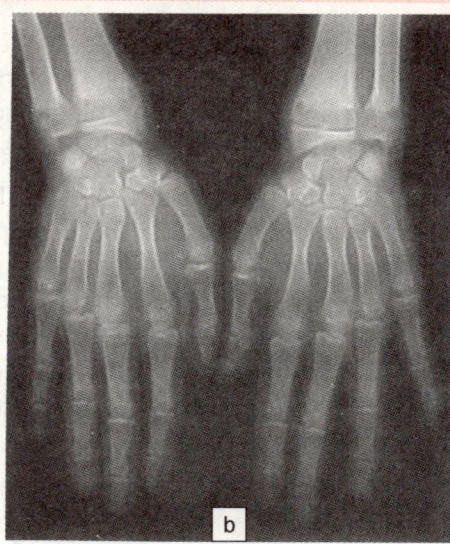

Fig. 5.4b. Healing rickets. Note the appearance of white line and blunting of radiological abnormality

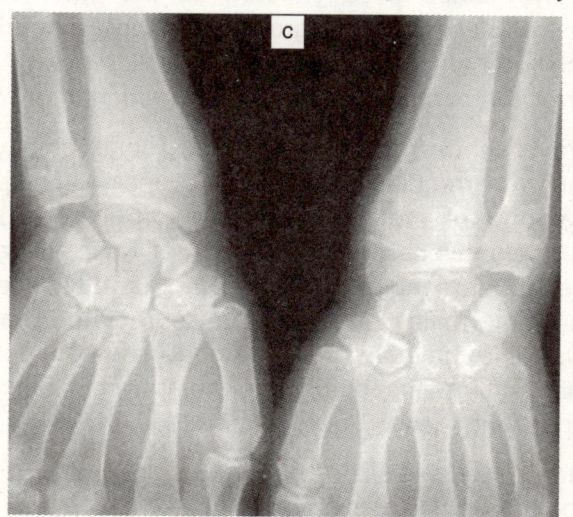

Fig. 5.4c. Healed rickets

alkaline phosphatase is raised. Urinary calcium is reduced while urinary phosphate excretion is increased.

Management of rickets includes oral or IM administration of 6,00,000 IU (or 15000 μg) of vitamin D. If radiological evidence of healing is not seen on x-rays after 3–4 weeks, the (single) dose is repeated. Alternatively, vitamin D can be administered in the doses of 2000–5000 IU (or 50–125μg) of vitamin D daily for 4 weeks. If the child does not respond after two doses of 6,00,000 IU of vitamin D, the child is diagnosed as resistant rickets and investigated accordingly.

Corrective surgery for deformities, when indicated, should be undertaken only after the active disease is controlled.

Gluten sensitive enteropathy induced Rickets

Gluten sensitive enteropathy or Coeliac sprue occurs in infancy and childhood. It is caused by sensitivity to gluten resulting in malabsorption. Disease characteristically starts from the time of weaning. Children have anorexia, irritability and diarrhoea with pale, frothy, foul smelling, bulky stools which stick to the pan and are difficult to flush. Abdomen is distended and there is severe wasting of muscles and subcutaneous tissues. Various deficiency states may arise due to malabsorption such as anaemia, growth retardation and rickets.

Rickets in coeliac sprue is caused by loss of dietary fats and vitamin D (which is fat soluble) in stools due to malabsorption. Excessive unabsorbed fatty acids precipitate the calcium and the latter is also lost in stool.

Radiological features of rickets due to coeliac disease are similar to nutritional rickets.

Biochemical investigations show low levels of serum calcium and low/normal serum phosphate. Excessive fat can be demonstrated in stool examination in these cases. Jejunal biopsy reveals characteristic villous atrophy which improves on withdrawl of wheat from the diet and recurs when wheat is reintroduced in the diet.

Management consists of exclusion of all cereals containing gluten (wheat, barley, oats, rye) from the meal and nutritional supplements including vitamin D and calcium.

Familial Hypophosphataemic Vitamin D Resistant Rickets (FHVDRR) (Phosphate Diabetes)

FHVDRR is X-linked dominant disorder that is a result of *impaired renal tubular reabsorption of phosphate.* Affected patients have a normal glomerular filtration rate (GFR) and impaired vitamin D3 response to usual doses of vitamin D3 . The disease manifests later than nutritional rickets, at about 2 years of age. The clinical and radiological picture of this form of rickets is similar to nutritional rickets though more severe.

Biochemical investigations reveal low serum phosphate, low or normal serum calcium and raised alkaline phosphatase. 24 hours urine examination reveals markedly increased phosphate excretion. Renal function tests are normal.

Management consists of phosphate replacement (1-4 grams daily) alongwith vitamin D3. However, large doses of vit. D3 are often required in these patients and careful vigil should be maintained to diagnose over dosage/toxicity early. Children given excessive amounts of vitamin D develop a toxic syndrome characterized by anorexia, growth failure, constipation, polyuria, polydipsia, soft tissue calcification, elevated serum levels of calcium and eventually renal failure.

The availability of calcitriol and its analogs has facilitated the treatment in these cases as lower doses are required, they are efficacious and toxic symptoms regress quickly once drug is discontinued.

The vitamin D should not be administered to non ambulant patients and should be discontinued 4 to 6 weeks before corrective surgery since after the surgery the patient is likely to be immobilised in a P.O.P. splint.

Treatment with phosphates and vitamin D should be continued till the completion of the growth.

Hypophosphataemic vitamin D resistant rickets may rarely be associated with aminoaciduria (Fanconi's syndrome), culminating in a similar form of rickets with an earlier age of presentation. Treatment is similar to FHVDRR with Vitamin D and neutral phosphates. Other forms include FHVDRR with glucosuria and amino aciduria and late onset Vitamin D Resistant Rickets

Vitamin D dependent Rickets type I (VDDR I)

VDDR I is a rare autosomal recessive disorder that may represent a defect in 1-hydroxylation of vitamin D3 in the kidney due to deficiency of enzyme 25 (OH) vitamin D-1 alpha hydroxylase (Type I). The disease is characterised by low levels of and/or defective 1,25 (OH)$_2$ vitamin D3. The disease features are similar to those of vitamin D-deficiency rickets, except that they may be worse. High levels of Vitamin D are required to treat this form of rickets (20,000–1,00,000 units per day followed by maintenance doses of vitamin D3 analogue).

Vitamin D Dependent Rickets Type II (VDDR II)

VDDR II results from enteric end–organ insensitivity to 1,25–dihydroxy–vitamin D and is probably caused by an abnormality in the 1,25(OH)$_2$ Vitamin D nuclear receptor. Renal conversion of Vitamin D occurs normally. The disease responds to exogenous administration of high doses of Vitamin D (10,000–50,000 units/day) or physiologic doses of synthetic Vitamin D analogues.

Rickets due to Renal Tubular Acidosis

Renal Tubular Acidosis may be acquired in many systemic diseases or may be genetic. Disease results from the loss of fixed base from the distal renal tubules with resulting acidosis. Acidic environment leaches the calcium from the bones and rickets results. The disorder is treated by administration of alkaline solutions to correct systemic acidosis. Renal tubular acidosis may be associated with other renal tubular defects such as

(a) Debre De Toni Fanconi syndrome where phosphates, amino acids and glucose are not reabsorbed through renal tubules,

(b) Lignac Fanconi syndrome where cystinosis (deposition of cystine crystals in the soft tissues) occurs in addition to Debre De Toni Fanconi Syndrome

(c) Lowe's Syndrome–Oculocerebrorenal syndrome characterised by mental retardation, cataracts and glaucoma; and,

(d) Superglycine syndrome, which is a type of Lowe's syndrome along with glycinuria and muscle weakness. Patients with RTA of genetic origin present with severe dehydration due to hyperchloremic, hypokalemic, hyponatremic metabolic acidosis and have poor long term survival rate.

Renal Osteodystrophy

Renal osteodystrophy is classically described as a syndrome complex of osteomalacia, osteoporosis, osteitis fibrosa cystica, osteosclerosis and metastatic calcification owing to chronic end stage glomerular pathology.

Chronic Renal Failure (CRF) leads to an inability to excrete phosphate. Retention of phosphates lowers the serum calcium as a compensatory phenomenon (as the product of serum calcium and phosphate levels in blood remains below 40). The parathyroids are stimulated (secondary hyperparathyroidism) and mobilise calcium from the skeleton but are unable to lower serum phosphate levels due to impaired renal function. In addition, kidney is unable to form $1,25(OH)_2D3$ due to advanced damage. Combination of these factors leads to renal osteodystrophy which is commonly associated with long term hemodialysis. Aluminium toxicity with deposition of aluminium in bone contributes to the development of renal osteodystrophy. This occurs following use of aluminium gels for the treatment of hyperphosphatemia.

Clinically the disease occurs later than nutritional rickets, in children around 5–10 years old. The patients are dwarfed with marked skeletal deformities. However, classical manifestations of nutritional rickets may be conspicuously lacking. The symptoms of end stage renal disease complicate the clinical picture.

The causes of bony changes in renal osteodystrophy are as follows:

1. Osteomalacia/Osteitis fibrosa cystica occurs due to
   (a) hyperphosphatemia
   (b) azotemia and uremia (end organ resistance to vitamin D3)
   (c) decreased synthesis of $1,25(OH)_2$ vitamin D3
   (d) Aluminium toxicity

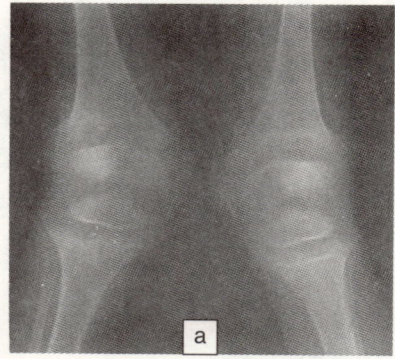

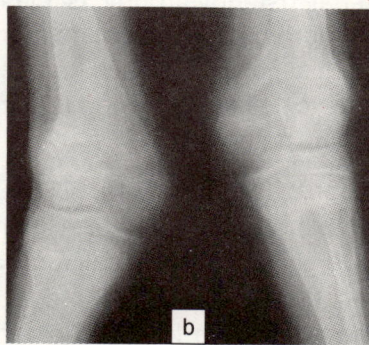

Fig. 5.5a,b. Renal rickets

(e) Secondary hyperparathyroidism

2. Osteosclerosis/Metastatic calcification occurs also
   (a) Treatment related-excessive vitamin D3
   (b) Sudden correction of the deficit
   (c) Sudden changes in pH

X-rays show combined features of rickets (widening of physis, fraying of physeal end of metaphysis) (Fig. 5.5a,b) and hyperparathyroidism (loss of lamina dura of teeth, subperiosteal resorption of bone from phalanges and metacarpals and coarsening of trabeculae). Radiographs of the spine may show rugger jersey spine (Fig. 5.5c,d). Metastatic calcification presents as lead pipe calcification along blood vessels and as calcific deposits at various soft

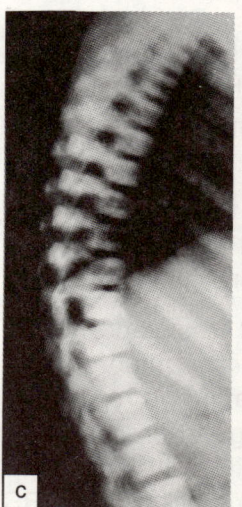
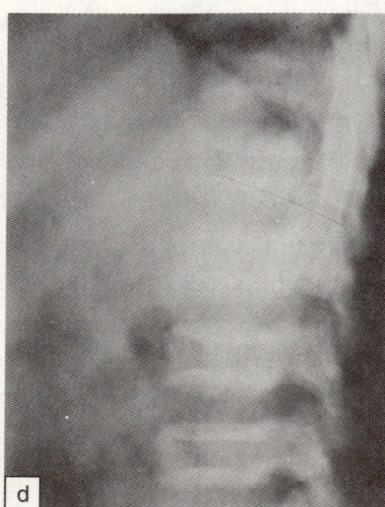

Fig. 5.5c,d. Radiographs of spine in renal osteodystrophy (Rugger Jersey spine)

tissue sites. Clinical and radiological abnormalities in renal osteodystrophy are shown in Fig.5.6.

Biochemical Investigations show a decreased or normal serum calcium, raised serum phosphates, raised serum alkaline phosphatase and reduced urinary excretion of calcium and phosphates. There is, in addition, evidence of impaired renal function manifested as raised blood urea and creatinine and abnormal GFR.

Management consists of treatment of underlying renal disorder. High doses of vitamin D (100,000–500,000 IU daily) alongwith supplemental calcium can control bone changes. Calcitriol which does not need to undergo hydroxylation in kidney is the most appropriate form of vitamin D therapy.

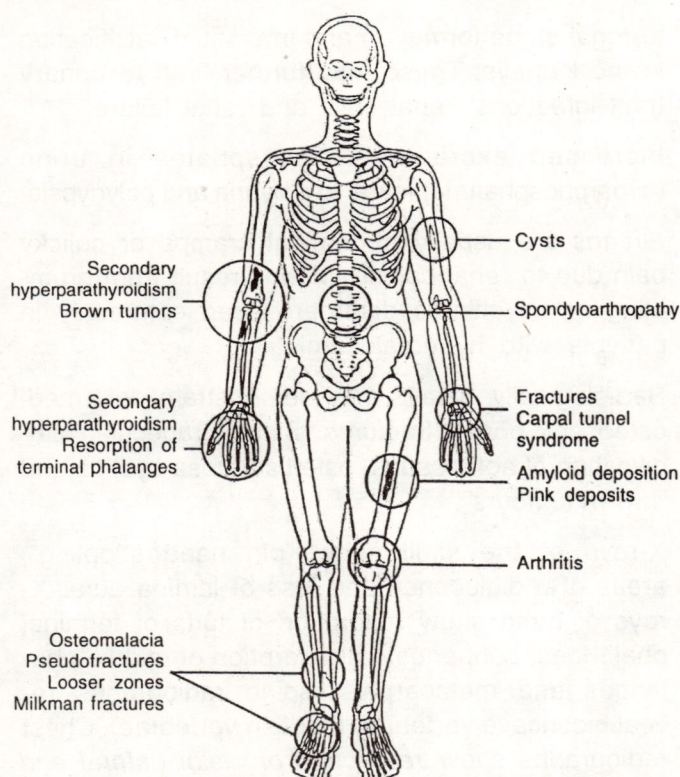

Fig. 5.6. Clinical and roentgenographic abnormalities in renal related bone disease

Labels on figure:
- Cysts
- Secondary hyperparathyroidism Brown tumors
- Spondyloarthropathy
- Fractures Carpal tunnel syndrome
- Secondary hyperparathyroidism Resorption of terminal phalanges
- Amyloid deposition Pink deposits
- Arthritis
- Osteomalacia Pseudofractures Looser zones Milkman fractures

are low and increased urinary phosphoethanolamine is diagnostic.

Hypophosphatasia

Hypophosphatasia is an autosomal recessive disorder caused by low levels of alkaline phosphatase which is required for the synthesis of inorganic phosphate, important in bone matrix formation. Features are similar to those of rickets and treatment may include phosphate therapy. Serum and leucocyte alkaline phosphatase levels

Osteomalacia

The underlying mechanism for both rickets and osteomalacia is the same i.e. failure to mineralise bony matrix, resulting in the presence of unmineralised osteoid about the bony trabeculae. The lack of mineral can be due to nutritional deficiency (vitamin D deficient diet), lack of exposure to sunlight, malabsorption, renal disease or due to anticonvulsant therapy. If this mechanism impacts the skeleton prior to the physeal closure, it results in rickets. If this process occurs after physeal closure, the disease that results is osteomalacia. Naturally, the longitudinal growth of the bones is unaffected. The bones tend to be soft and can bow under the load. In addition, the area of unmineralised osteoid presents as radiographic lucent areas in the bone called *Looser's zones.*

Clinically, these patients present with muscular weakness, generalised bone pains and tenderness. Waddling gait is common due to muscle weakness (hip abductors) along with coxa vara. Femoral neck fractures are common in patients with osteomalacia.

Radiologically, there is generalised demineralization of bone with loss of trabeculae. Looser's zones (microscopic stress fractures) are commonly seen in femoral neck, axillary border of scapula, ribs and pelvis and are often bilateral (Fig. 5.7, Fig. 5.8a,b). Spine may show deformi-

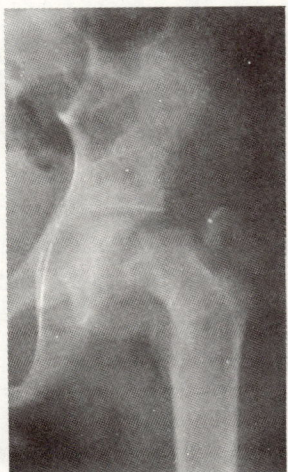

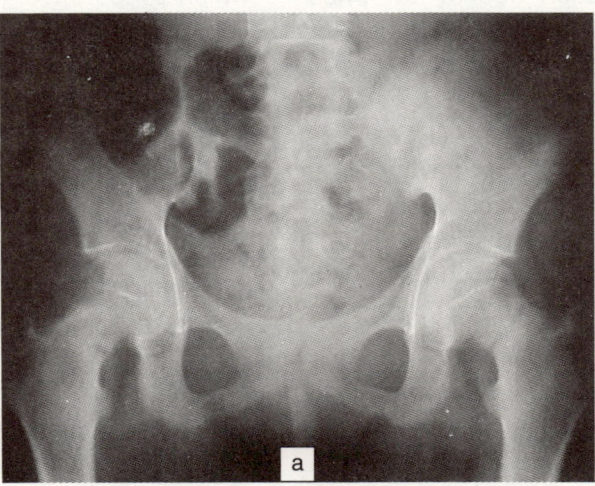

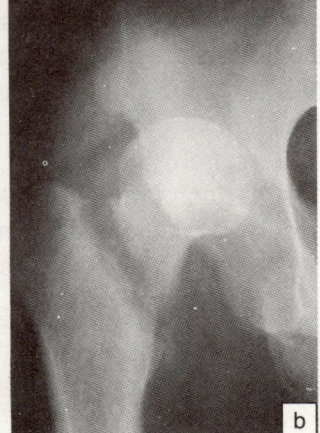

Fig. 5.7. Osteomalacia with pathological subcapital fracture neck of femur

Fig. 5.8a. Osteomalacia with bilateral Looser's zones in the neck of femur
Fig. 5.8b. Osteomalacia with pathologic fracture neck of femur with posterior dislocation of the hip

ties, especially kyphosis and scoliosis and the soft vertebral bodies may be compressed by nucleus pulposus on either side resulting in *biconcave (codfish) vertebrae.*

Pelvis X-rays may show trefoil pelvis and bilateral coxa vara.

Biochemical investigations reveal low or normal serum calcium and low serum phosphate levels. Serum alkaline phosphatase is markedly raised.

Biopsy (transiliac) is required for diagnosis and histological examination shows widened osteoid seams.

Management consists of administration of vitamin D (5000–10,000 IU daily) along with calcium supplements. Fracture neck of femur needs appropriate treatment once the disease heals.

Women with deformed (trefoil) pelvis may need caesarian section for delivery due to feto-pelvic-disproportion.

Primary Hyperparathyroidism

Primary hyperparathyroidism is a disease state characterised by an excess amount of parathyroid hormone (PTH) as a result of a parathyroid adenoma. PTH stimulates osteoclastic activity, causing an intense resorption of bone with consequent hypercalcaemia.

The cavities resulting from bone resorption fill with vascular fibrous tissue (poor repair attempts due to failure of mineralization due to low phosphate levels), resulting in the classic *osteitis fibrosa cystica.* As the cavities coalesce they form a single large cyst called a *"brown tumor"* because of the hemosiderin staining within. Clinical and radiological changes result from this cavitation as well as from the erosive changes occuring under the periosteum. Clinically, the disease usually occurs in middle aged females and is characterised by symptoms of bones, stones, abdominal groans and (psychiatric) moans.

Bony symptoms consist of marked bony pains and tenderness. Frequent fractures and bony deformities are common.

Renal symptoms are commonly seen. Hypercalcaemia leads to hypercalciuria and leads to renal stone formation and interstitial calcification in the kidneys. These may further lead to urinary tract infections, renal colic and renal failure.

Increased excretion of phosphates in urine (hyperphosphaturia) leads to polyuria and polydypsia.

Groans are usually abdominal cramps or colicky pain due to renal calculi. *Moans* result from grumbling or psychiatric disorders seen commonly in patients with hypercalcaemia.

Radiologically, X-rays may demonstrate deformed, osteopenic bones, fractures, shabby trabeculae, calcification of soft tissues, osteitis fibrosa cystica and "brown tumours".

X-rays of the skull show "pin head stippling", areas of radiolucency and loss of lamina dura. X-rays of hand show resorption of tufts of terminal phalanges, subperiosteal resorption of middle phalanges and metacarpals; spine radiographs reveal biconcave vertebrae (codfish vertebrae). Chest radiographs show *resorption of distal (lateral end of) clavicles.* Plain X-rays (KUB) of abdomen may show renal stones.

Biochemical investigations reveal increased serum calcium, increased serum PTH, increased urinary phosphate and decreased serum phosphate.

Histologic changes include osteoblasts and osteoclasts active on both sides of trabeculae, areas of destruction, and wide osteoid seams.

Management consists of surgical parathyroidectomy, which is curative. Prophylactic or definitive fixation of bones is often required for impending or existing fractures respectively. The fractures, when adequately fixed heal reasonably well once parathyroidectomy is done.

Other causes of Hypercalcaemia, in addition to primary hyperparathyroidism, are malignancy (most common), Addison's disease, steroid administration, milk alkali syndrome, hyperthyroidism, vitamin D intoxication and sarcoidosis.

Hypocalcemia

Low plasma calcium can result from low PTH or vitamin D3. Hypocalcemia leads to increased neuromuscular irritability (tetany, seizures, Chvostek's sign), cataracts, fungal infections of nails and ECG abnormalities (prolonged QT interval).

Primary Hypoparathyroidism

Reduced PTH levels cause diminished plasma calcium and increased plasma phosphates. Common clinical findings are blotchy skin due to pigment loss (vitiligo), hair loss and fungal infections of the nails. Skull X-ray may show basal ganglion calcification.

Pseudohypoparathyroidism (PHP)

Pseudohypoparathyroidism is a rare genetic disorder that causes lack of effect of PTH at the target cells. PTH level is normal or even high but PTH action at cellular level is blocked by an abnormality at the receptor, the cAMP system, or by a lack of required cofactors (e.g. Mg^{2+}). Albright hereditary osteodystrophy, a form of PHP is associated with short first, fourth and fifth metacarpals and metatarsals, brachydactyly, exostoses, obesity and diminished intelligence. The serum calcium levels are low while phosphate is high. There may be associated hypothyroidism, diabetes melliltus and gonadal dysgenesis.

PSEUDOPSEUDO HYPOPARATHYROIDISM Rarely the somatic features of pseudohypoparathyroidism may be found in patients with normal plasma levels of calcium and phosphate. This condition is termed as pseudopseudo hypoparathyroidism PTH levels may be normal or slightly raised. It is interesting to note that some of these patrents may develop cataracts even though the serum calcium is essentially normal.

Osteoporosis

Osteoporosis is defined as "microstructural deterioration of skeletal architecture leading to increased fragility and propensity to fracture". WHO definition of Osteoporosis is bone mass more than 2.5 standard deviations (SD) less than the peak bone mass. It is prudent to mention here that according to WHO upto 1 SD loss from peak bone mass may be normal while 1 to 2.5 SD reduction in bone mass is called osteopenia.

Osteoporosis is a quantitative, not qualitative (as osteomalacia) defect in bone. Parallel loss of minerals and matrix occurs, so their ratio remains normal. There is predominance of bone resorption over bone formation. Common causes of osteoporosis are shown in Table 5.2.

Table 5.2. Causes of osteoporosis

Primary	Involutional (post menopausal-I or senile-II)
	Idiopathic (juvenile or adult)
Secondary	Endocrine
	Hypogonadism
	Cushing's
	Hyperparathyroidism
	Hyperthyroidism
	Diabetes Mellitus
	Growth Hormone deficiency
	Nutritional
	Calcium deficiency
	Protein deficiency
	Vitamin C deficiency
	Intestinal malabsorption
	Drugs
	Heparin
	Corticosteroids
	anticonvulsants
	Ethanol
	Methotrexate
	Genetic
	Osteogenesis imperfecta
	Homocystinuria
	Miscellaneous
	Rheumatoid Arthritis
	Immobilisation
	Malignancy (e.g. Multiple Myeloma)
	Chronic liver disease
	Cigarette smoking

Risk Factors

Numerous aetiologies of osteoporosis have been identified but clinically most significant is the postmenopausal type. Sedentary, thin Caucasian women of north European descent, particularly smokers, heavy drinkers, and patients on phenytoin and heparin, patients on low calcium and low vitamin D diets who breast fed their infants are at greatest risk. Premature surgical menopause is an important risk factor. Cancellous bone is markedly affected.

Clinical features include kyphosis and fractures of vertebral bodies (vertebral fractures are commonest fractures in osteoporosis) especially compression fractures of D11–L1, hip fractures, distal radius fractures and fractures of surgical neck of humerus. In addition to pathological fracture, there is frequently a loss of height as a result of the cumulative effects of multiple vertebral fractures as well as progressive development of a kyphotic deformity in the thoracic spine, which is referred to as a *"Dowager's hump"*.

Patients present with a history of pain and/or repeated fractures though at times they may be asymptomatic. Occasionally they complain of early satiety because of abdominal compression resulting from loss of height of vertebral column, and occasionally, they complain of shortness of breath because of increasing kyphosis in the dorsal region.

On examination, typically one finds the prominent Dwager's hump, a barrel chest, a protuberant abdomen, and generalised bone pain with percussion tenderness.

Two types of osteoporosis have been characterized. Type I (post-menopausal) and type II (Age–related).

Type I osteoporosis (Postmenopausal): Affects females between 50–75 years, (6:1, F:M), affects mainly trabecular bone and vertebral (crush) and distal radius fractures are common.

The cause here is mainly increased osteoclastic activity seen after menopause in females.

Type II (senile) osteoporosis is seen in both sexes over 75 years of age, (2:1, F:M), affects both trabecular and cortical bone, and vertebral and hip fractures are common. The cause here is mainly a reduction is osteoblastic activity with age.

Radiologically, findings are decreased bone density, loss of bony trabeculae, thinning of cortices and pathological fractures (Fig. 5.9a,b).

Hematological and biochemical investigations are within normal limits and serve to rule out hyperthyroidism, hyperparathyroidism, Cushing syndrome, hematologic disorders and malignancy.

Histopathological examination (after tetracycline labelling) reveals marked thinning of the bony trabeculae, decreased size of osteons and in-

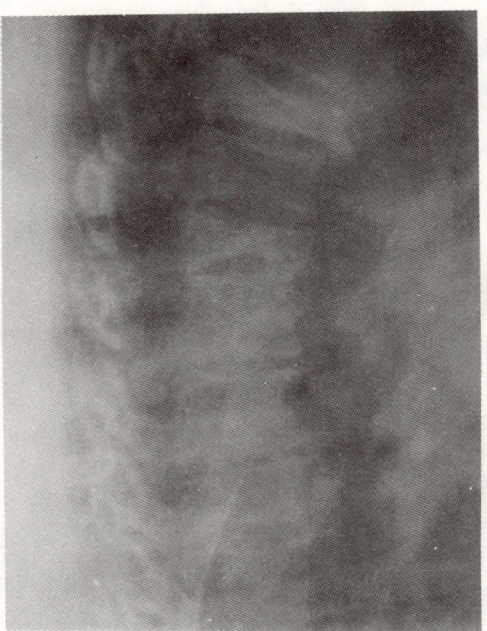

Fig. 5.9a. Osteoporosis with insufficiency fractures of multiple vertebral bodies

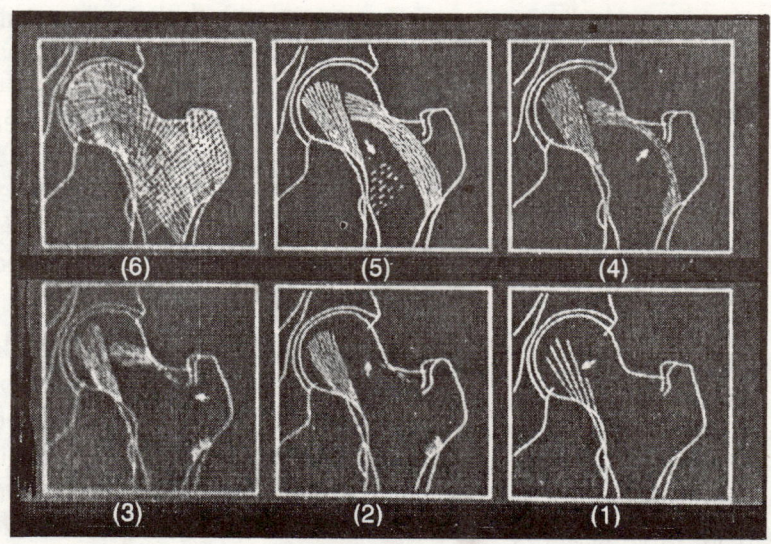

Fig. 5.9b. Singh's Index showing trabecular pattern of proximal femur in progressively increasing severity of osteoporosis

creased porosity of bone with enlarged haversian and marrow spaces.

Bone Mineral Density measurements

One of the most difficult problems in the past has been bone mineral density (BMD) measurement.

Plain radiographs are usually not helpful unless 30–50% bone loss has been present. Special studies now available for work–up of osteoporosis include single photon (appendicular) and double photon (axial) absorptiometry, quantitative computerised tomography (qCT), and Dual energy X-ray absorptiometry (DEXA). DEXA is most accurate with less radiation (equivalent to one chest x-ray).

Management consists of advising physical activity especially weight bearing exercises, calcium supplements (more effective in age related–type II osteoporosis), vitamin D supplements and Hormone Replacement Therapy (HRT) for type I (postmenopausal) osteoporosis. HRT gives best results when started early after menopause. The present recommendation is to continue HRT for 5 years after menopause as longer use may be associated with risk of malignancy. Fluorides, which inhibit bone resorption, increase the cancellous bone mass but make bones more brittle and are associated with high incidence of bone pains and hip fractures. Their use has been discarded. SERM (Selective Estrogen Receptor Modulators) such as Raloxifene can be started two years after menopause and continued for sustained benefits in the form of improved BMD.

Intramuscular/subcutaneous or intranasal calcitonin, di-phosphonates (to block osteoclastic activity) and tamoxifen are other agents often used in the treatment of osteoporosis. Salmon calcitonin has the drawback of tachyphylaxis.

Prevention

The best prophylaxis for patients at risk of developing osteoporosis comprises of

a) diet with adequate calcium intake

b) weight bearing exercises programme, and

c) estrogen therapy evaluation at menopause.

Osteoporosis and Osteomalacia are compared in Table 5.3.

Table 5.3. Comparison of Osteoporosis and Osteomalacia

	Osteoporosis	Osteomalacia
Definition	• Bone mass decreased • Mineralization normal • Bones are brittle	• Variable bone mass • Mineralization reduced • Bones are soft
Age at onset	• Elderly, postmenopausal	• Any age
Aetiology	• Endocrine abnormality • Age • Idiopathic • Inactivity (disuse) • Alcoholism	• Vitamin D deficiency • Abnormality of vitamin D metabolism • Hypophosphatemic syndromes • Hypophosphatasia • Renal tubular acidosis • Calcium deficiency
Symptoms	• Pain at fracture site	• Generalised bone pains
Signs	• Tenderness at fracture site	• Tenderness at fracture site along with generalised tenderness
Radiographic features	• Axial predominance (vertebral crush)	• Appendicular predominance (often symmetric pseudo or true fracture)
Laboratory investigations	• S. Ca/PO$_4^{3-}$ normal • Alkaline phosphatase is normal • Ca^{++} × PO$_4^{3-}$: >30 • Tetracyline labelling-Normal • Urine Ca^{++} normal or high	• S. Ca/PO$_4^{3-}$ normal/low • Alkaline phosphatase is raised • Ca^{++} × PO$_4^{3-}$: <30 • Tetracyline labelling-Abnormal • Urine Ca^{++} normal or low

Scurvy

Scurvy is caused by deficiency of Vitamin C (ascorbic acid). Deficiency of Vitamin C leads to defective collagen growth and repair and impaired intracellular hydroxylation of collagen peptides (reduced activity of lysyl hydroxylase). This leads to scanty and defective osteoid formation.

Clinical features

A rare disease nowadays, scurvy is usually seen in infants 6 to 18 months old who are fed only on boiled milk. Prolonged vitamin C deficiency is required for the disease to develop. Clinical features include fatigue, ecchymosis, joint effusion and iron deficiency. Child is febrile, pale and restless. Gum bleeding and swelling is common. Pain in limbs results in inability to move them ("pseudo paralysis"). Wound healing is delayed. Scorbutic rosary is caused by epiphyseal slips of costal cartilages (differs from rachitic rosary in that it is sharp and angular).

Radiological examination reveals generalised osteopenia, thin cortices and trabeculae, metaphyseal clefts (corner sign) and subperiosteal haemorrhages. Epiphyses appear ringed and separate easily. Fractures are common. Radiological features of scurvy are given in Table 5.4.

Biochemical investigations are within normal limits. Histopathological examination reveals replacement of primary trabeculae with granulation tissue; there are areas of heamorrhage. Physis shows widening of zone of provisional calcification.

Management consists of daily administration of

Table 5.4. Radiologic features of scurvy

- Corner sign
- Pelkan's spur
- White line of Fraenkel
- Wimberger's phenomenon
- Generalised osteopenia
- Thinning of cortices
- Epiphyseal slip
- Widening of growth plate

1–2 gm of vitamin C. Medical treatment alleviates pain and tenderness. Immobilisation and / or open reduction may be needed for fractures and epiphyseal separations.

Bone Tumors

- *General Considerations*
- *Staging of Bone Tumors*
- *Evaluation of Bone Tumors*
- *Biopsy of the Bone Tumor*
- *Surgical Procedures (Types of resection)*
- *Diagnosis & Treatment of Bone Tumors*
- *Benign Osseous Tumors*
  Osteoma
  Osteoid Osteoma
  Osteoblastoma
- *Malignant Osseous Tumors*
  Osteosarcoma
- *Benign Chondroid Lesions*
  Osteochondroma
  Enchondroma
  Chondroblastoma (Codman's Tumor)
  Chondromyxoid Fibroma
- *Malignant Chondroid Tumors*
  Chondrosarcoma
- *Benign Fibrous Tumors of Bone*

- *Fibrous Cortical Defect/Non Ossifying Fibroma/ Metaphyseal Fibrous Defect.*
  Desmoplastic Fibroma
- *Malignant Fibrous Lesions*
  Fibrosarcoma
  Malignant Fibrous Histiocytoma (MFH)
- *Tumors of Unknown Origin*
  Giant Cell Tumors of Bone
  Ewing's Tumor
  Adamantinoma
- *Hematopoietic Tumors*
- *Plasma Cell Tumors*
  Multiple Myeloma
  Plasmacytoma (Solitary Myeloma)
  Osteosclerotic Myeloma
- *Metastatic Bone Disease*
- *Tumor like Conditions*
  Simple (Unicameral) Bone Cyst
  Aneurysmal Bone Cyst (ABC)
  Histiocytosis X

General Considerations

Tumors of the musculo-skeletal system are rare as compared to tumors of the breast, uterus or lung. Metastatic tumors to bone, however, are quite common especially among the elderly.

Primary bone tumors can be broadly divided into three types: malignant bone tumors (sarcomas), benign bone tumors, and lesions that simulate bone tumors (reactive and miscellaneous conditions). Sarcomas are malignant neoplasms of connective tissue (mesenchymal) origin. Sarcomas exhibit rapid growth in a centripetal fashion and invade adjacent soft tissues after destroying the overlying cortex. Sarcomas primarily metastasise via the hematogenous route, most commonly to the lungs. Benign bone tumors usually have limited growth potential but may sometimes be large and destructive. Bone tumor simulators are the conditions occurring in bone but which are not true neoplasms (e.g. osteomyelitis, aneurysmal bone cyst, bone islands and others).

Commonest classification of the bone tumors is based on the cell type and is shown in Table 6.1

Staging of Bone Tumors

Staging systems are useful for evaluation, treatment and predicting prognosis. The staging system

Table 6.1. Classification of primary bone tumors (after Lichtenstein)

Histology type	Benign	Malignant
Hematopoietic		Myeloma
		Lymphoma
Chondrogenic	Osteochondroma	Primary chondrosarcoma
	Chondroma	Secondary chondrosarcoma
	Chondroblastoma	Clear cell chondrosarcoma
	Chondromyxoid fibroma	
Osteogenic	Osteoid osteoma	Osteosarcoma
	Benign osteoblastoma	Parosteal osteosarcoma
		Periosteal osteosarcoma
Unknown origin	Giant cell tumour	Ewing's tumours
	(Fibrous) histiocytoma	Malignant Giant cell tumour
		Adamantinoma
Fibrogenic	Fibroma	Fibrosarcoma
	Desmoplastic fibroma	Malignant fibrous histiocytoma
Notochordal		Chordoma
Vascular	Hemangioma	Hemagioendothelioma
		Hemangiopericytoma
Lipogenic	Lipoma	
Neurogenic	Neurilemmoma	

devised by the Musculoskeletal Tumor Society (also known as Enneking System) is most popular and useful for musculoskeletal lesions. For malignant lesions the system is based on knowing the histologic grade of the lesion (low or high), the anatomic features (Intra or extra compartmental) and the absence (M0) or presence of metastases (M1).

1. **Grade** Grading of tumors is done histologically and is based on degree of anaplasia (loss of structural differentiation, pleomorphism and nuclear hyperchromasia).

Most malignant lesions are high-grade (G2) with over 25% chances of distant metastases. Low-grade malignant (G1) lesions are less common and have less than 25% chances of distant metastases. The typical grading of common bone and soft tissue tumors is shown in Table 6.2.

Table 6.2. Typical low and high grade musculo-skeletal tumors

Low Grade (G1)	High Grade (G2)
Bone	
Parosteal osteosarcoma	Intramedullary osteosarcoma
Primary chondrosarcoma	Post-radiation osteosarcoma
Secondary chodrosarcoma	Paget's sarcoma
Hemangioendothelioma	Fibrosarcoma
Adamantinoma	Malignant fibrous histiocytoma
Soft Tissue	
Myxoid liposarcoma	Malignant fibrous histiocytoma
lipoma-like liposarcoma	Pleomorphic liposarcoma
Angiomatoid malignant	Synovial sarcoma
fibrous histiocytoma	Rhabdomyosarcoma
	Alveolar cell sarcoma

2. **Tumor location** Whether the tumor is confined within the compartment (bone) (intra-compartmental, or T1) or the tumor is extending beyond the confines of bone (extra-compartmental, or T2) can be established by plain radiographs and special studies such as CT and MRI scans.

3. **Metastases** Chest radiographs, CT scan of chest, and a technetium bone scan can exclude the distant spread of the tumor.

Using these parameters, six distinct stages have been devised in the Enneking system (Table 6.3).

Table 6.3. Enneking System of Classification

Stage	GTM	Description
I-A	G1	Low Grade
	T1	Intra compartmental
	M0	No metastases
I-B	G1	Low Grade
	T2	Extra compartmental
	M0	No metastases
II-A	G2	High Grade
	T1	Intra compartmental
	M0	No metastases
II-B	G2	High grade
	T2	Extra compartmental
	M0	No Metastases
III-A	G1 or 2	Any Grade
	T1	Intra compartmental
	M1	With metastases
III-B	G1 or 2	Any Grade
	T2	Extra compartmental
	M1	With metastases

Evaluation of Bone Tumors

1. Clinical Presentation Most tumors cause pain. The pain is typically deep seated and dull. It usually progresses in intensity and becomes constant.

Swelling and local tenderness can be other presenting symptoms. Occasionally, the lesion is discovered accidentally during radiological examination or may present as a pathological fracture.

2. Physical Examination Affected site is inspected for soft tissue swelling, condition of the overlying skin, adenopathy and margins. Rapid growth, warmth, tenderness and ill-defined edge suggest malignancy. A per rectal examination may diagnose a sacral chordoma, which may not otherwise be well delineated on plain x-ray and may be missed. When metastatic disease is suspected, abdomen, breast, prostate and thyroid should be examined as relevant.

3. Radiography Plain radiographs in two planes are the most essential initial radiographic investigations and should be performed even on patients with only a soft tissue mass. Additional views may be obtained to rule out referred pain (as knee pain arising out of a hip lesion) or evaluate a particular area not well visualised on routine films. Skeletal survey should be done in cases of multiple myeloma or suspected metastatic disease.

Sophisticated imaging studies such as Technetium bone scan or MRI can be undertaken to search for occult lesions, especially metastatic lesions. Chest radiographs are routinely taken when a malignant lesion is suspected. Enneking has outlined four basic characters of bone lesions that should be evaluated on plain radiograph:

a) *Location of the lesion*

Certain lesions have a predilection for a certain bone or a particular location e.g. chondroblastoma and giant cell tumors occur in epiphysis of long bones while osteogenic sarcoma occurs commonly in distal femur or proximal tibial metaphysis. Ewing's tumor is common in diaphysis of long bones.

Parosteal osteosarcoma abuts the outer cortex of the bone while classical osteosarcoma arises from an intramedullary location.

b) *Effect of the lesion on the bone*

Effect of the lesion on bone may result in a characteristic pattern of bone destruction with a particular type of zone of transition between the lesion and the normal bone.

i) Geographic bone destruction presents with a clear zone of transition between the lesion and the surrounding normal bone. This pattern implies slow rates of growth of the tumor. (eg. simple bone cyst, Non ossifying fibroma) (Fig. 6.1).

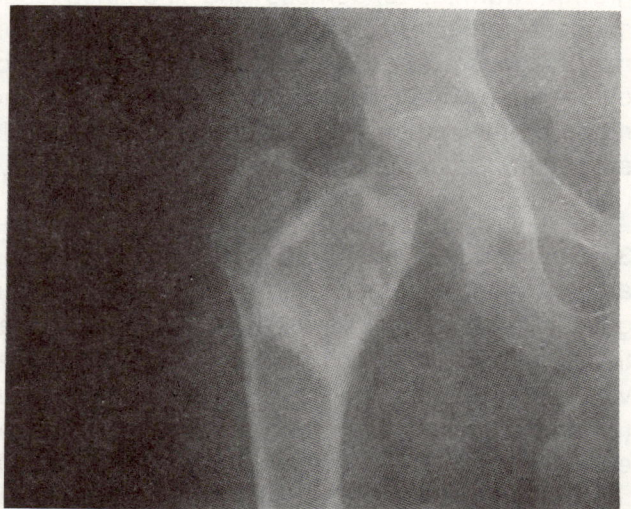

Fig. 6.1. Geographic pattern of bone destruction

ii) Moth-eaten destruction presents with poorly defined zone of transition and usually signals aggressive bone destruction. This pattern of destruction is seen with malignant tumors (such as osteogeonic sarcoma) or chronic osteomyelitis. Lesions with this pattern have intermediate rates of growth.

iii) Permeative pattern presents without any appreciable zone of transition. Permeative pattern is associated with aggressive round cell tumors or acute osteomyelitis. This pattern implies rapid rates of growth.

Apart from the distinctive destruction pattern, other effects of lesion on the bone can be appreciated. High-grade malignant lesions generally spread rapidly through the medullary canal and the cortical bone destruction occurs early. A sizeable soft tissue mass may be associated. Low-grade tumors tend to spread slowly but may also destroy bone and extend to soft tissues.

c) *Response of the bone to the lesion*

Response of the bone to the lesion gives an indication about the lesion. With high grade lesion, host bone has little time to contain the process. Rapid destruction of the cortex occurs early in the disease.

In contrast, in low grade tumors, the host bone

can often contain the lesion with endosteal sclerosis or periosteal bone. In benign lesions, there is often a thick periosteal response.

d) *Any characteristic within the lesion to suggest a specific diagnosis* It is helpful to look for characteristics of the matrix if the lesion produces a matrix. There can be calcification (mineralization of cartilage), ossification (bone formation) or a ground-glass appearance.

In addition it is useful to know the age of the patient as certain lesions involve patients of a particular age group (Table 6.4).

Table 6.4. Common age distribution of various bone tumors

Age	Bone Tumors
Birth–5 years	Metastatic neuroblastoma Metastatic rhabdomyosarcoma
10–20 years	Osteosarcoma Chondroblastoma Ewing's tumour
20–40 years	Giant cell tumour Chondrosarcoma Adamantinoma
40–80 years	Metastatic bone disease Myeloma Lymphoma Paget's sarcoma Post radiation sarcoma

Number of lesions seen in the bone (polyostotic or monostotic) is another important finding on radiography. Diseases such as metastatic lesions, multiple myeloma, lymphoma, fibrous dysplasia and Paget's disease etc. may present with multiple lesions.

Biopsy of the bone tumor

The biopsy of a bone tumor can be of various types:

Needle biopsy is simplest and quick but material retrieved is often inadequate to make accurate diagnosis. A core biopsy can provide greater amount of tissue.

Incisional biopsy removes a piece of tumor for

microscopic study. The problem with incisional biopsy is that it tends to contaminate the surrounding tissues with tumor cells and may compromise definitive treatment.

Excisional biopsy attempts to remove the entire tumor and is often undertaken for malignant tumors involving expendable bones such as fibula, rib etc. or for benign lesions.

Principles of biopsy of bone tumor

Following principles must be adhered to when taking open biopsy from a bone tumor:

1. A *specialised approach* should be used keeping in mind the definitive surgical resection. If the lesion proves to be malignant, the entire biopsy tract must be removed along with the underlying tumor. Longitudinal incision should be used as opposed to horizontal; only a single compartment should be contaminated; muscle splitting approach is better than intermuscular approach; and neurovascular structures should be avoided (neurovascular structures should not be exposed to avoid seeding with tumor cells).

2. *Meticulous hemostasis* should be secured to avoid hematoma formation and subcutaneous haemorrhage. Approaches through the muscle are better as the muscle can be closed tightly. If tourniquet is used, it must be released before closure to obtain adequate hemostasis. If tourniquet is used, exsanguination is contraindicated to avoid spread of tumor cells into systemic circulation avoid spread of tumor cells into systemic circulation.

3. If hemostasis cannot be achieved, a small *drain* should be brought out through the surgical incision to prevent hematoma formation.

4. Biopsy should always be taken from the margin of the tumor, from the *junction* between normal bone and the lesion. Biopsies taken from the main bulk or centre of the lesion often show only necrotic tissue. Whenever possible, the soft tissue component must also be sampled.

5. *Cultures* should always be taken when taking biopsy to rule out unsuspected osteomyelitis.

6. A frozen section must be performed to ensure that adequate and representative tissue has been obtained.

Lastly, clinical history and radiographs should be reviewed with the pathologist prior to biopsy. Interpreting histologic sections may be difficult at times without review of these studies.

Surgical Procedures for bone tumors are graded according to the system of the Musculoskeletal Tumor Society. Types of resection described are :

1. *Intralesional* Plane of dissection goes through the tumor.

2. *Marginal* Goes through the reactive zone (inflammatory cells) of the tumor.

3. *Wide* Takes a cuff of surrounding normal tissue with the tumor.

4. *Radical* Entire tumor and its compartment(s) that the tumor lies within are removed.

Diagnosis & Treatment of Bone Tumors

Benign Osseous Tumors

1. *Osteoma*

Osteomas are benign slow-growing radiodense lesions characterised pathologically by predominantly mature lamellar bone. These are tumor-like lesions rather than true tumors. Osteomas may be composed of spongy bone (cancellous osteoma) or hard compact bone (ivory osteoma).

Osteomas may particularly affect the skull and facial bones especially the mandible and frontal and ethmoid sinuses. Dome shaped ivory-like excrescences on the inner or outer surface of the calvarium or protruding into the orbit or paranasal sinuses are typical. Clinically, these may present as a painless mass. Sinusitis, headache, pain and loss of smell may sometimes be presenting symptoms. In the frontoethmoid sinuses, large growths may erode the dura. Orbital lesions may produce exophthalmos, double vision and even impairment of vision. Multiple osteomas in association with colonic intestinal polyps are seen in Gardner's syndrome.

Radiologically, a dense or oval shaped mass is noted contiguous with the cortical surface of the bone. The surface is smooth or lobulated. The underlying cortex of the host bone may be slightly thickened.

Treatment consists of excision of the tumor.

2. *Osteoid Osteoma*

Osteoid Osteoma is the most common benign osteoid forming tumor. It characteristically produces pain in young patients (ages 5-30 years most commonly). Pain, often most severe at night, and relieved by aspirin, increases with time. The pain may be referred to an adjacent joint. When intracapsular, the lesion may mimic arthritis. In the spine, it may cause scoliosis, disk problems and neurologic symptoms. Half of the cases involve the lower extremity with upper portion of former being the most common location.

The explanation of pain in osteoid osteoma has received some attention. High concentrations of prostaglandins (E_2, I_2 and F_1 alpha) have been found in the nidus of the lesion and this explains why the prostaglandin inhibitors are beneficial therapeutic agents.

Osteoid Osteoma has a classic roentgenographic appearance (Fig. 6.2). Central lytic nidus measuring up to 10mm is surrounded by sclerotic cortical bone especially in the common cortical lesion. The more centrally located lesions in metaphyseal bone do not elicit much sclerosis and are difficult to diagnose.

The two most important imaging studies for this tumor are the bone isotope scan (shows "target" lesion) and CT scan.

Histologically the nidus shows aggressive but benign woven bone formation, with large number of osteoblasts and osteoclasts in a vascular fibrous stroma.

Treatment consists of complete removal of the nidus or curettage of the nidus. Surrounding sclerotic bone does not need to be removed. Use of preoperative radioisotope labelling and intra-operative image intensifier (fluoroscopy) examination ensures complete removal of the nidus.

Spontaneous regression or even complete disappearance of osteoid osteoma is known without any treatment.

Osteoblastoma

Osteoblastoma is a rare, benign bone-producing tumor that is like osteoid osteoma in many ways but can attain a large size and is not self-limited. Osteoblastoma is found in young patients (5-30 years), more commonly in males. The most common location is posterior elements of the spine and sacrum. Pain is always present, as is tenderness. Pain usually increases with movements and is often radicular. Scoliosis is often seen.

Radiographically, the osteoblastoma has a more lytic and destructive appearance than the osteoid osteoma. Its nidus is greater than 2 centimetres and has less sclerotic reactive bone at the periphery and may take on the appearance of aneurysmal bone cyst.

In general, a lesion greater than 2.5 centimetres is categorised as osteoblastoma whereas the osteoid osteoma remains smaller than 2.5 centimetres.

Histologically, the nidus of osteoblastoma is similar to that of osteoid osteoma and shows excessive osteoblastic activity and osteoid formation with numerous giant cells in a vascular fibrous stroma.

Treatment consists of curettage (with or without bone grafting). Complete resection should be done whenever the lesion is surgically accessible. Radiotherapy is rarely indicated; it may be necessary for large lesions in difficult areas such as spine and pelvis.

Malignant Osseous Tumors

Osteosarcoma

Osteosarcoma is one of the most common pri-

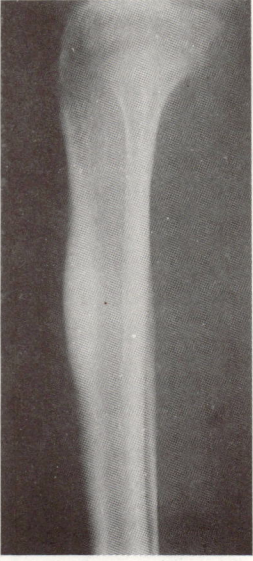

Fig. 6.2.   Osteoid osteoma of the tibia. Note the nidus in the centre of the lesion

mary malignant tumors of the adolescence (second only to multiple myeloma in overall incidence). It is a highly malignant tumor, which, by definition, produces neoplastic osteoid or bone or both. The osteosarcoma can be classified into various types as shown in Table 6.5.

Types of Osteosarcoma

1. Classic/Conventional

Osteosarcoma characteristically arises in the metaphysis of the long bones and grows circumferentially through the cortex into the soft tissues raising the periosteum. Nearly half the lesions are seen about the knee joint. Distal femur is the most common site followed by proximal tibia and then proximal humerus.

Table 6.5 . Classification of Osteosarcoma

I. Primary Osteosarcoma
  1. Conventional
        a) Osteoblastic
        b) Chondroblastic
        c) Fibroblastic
        d) Small cell
        e) Telangiectatic
  2. Surface Osteosarcoma
        a) Parosteal Osteosarcoma
        b) Periosteal Osteosarcoma
        c) High grade surface osteosarcoma
II. Secondary Osteosarcoma
        a) Post-irradiation (Ionizing radiation)
        b) Paget's Sarcoma
        c) Solitary/Multiple Osteochondromatosis
        d) Solitary/Multiple Enchondromatosis
        e) Bone Infarction
        f) Chronic Osteomyelitis
        g) Miscellaneous—GCT, Fibrous Dysplasia, Chondroblastoma, Osteoblastoma
III. Rare Osteo-
   sarcomas
        a) Li Fraumeni Syndrome (p53 mutation : in association with Retinoblastoma)
        b) Osteosarcoma of the Jaw
        c) Multicentric Osteosarcoma

Osteogenic sarcoma characteristically occurs at the adolescent growth spurt, with the peak age of occurrence between 10 and 20 years of age. Osteogenic sarcoma typically presents with pain, which is often mild and intermittent initially, but more continuous later. Patients may present with a pathologic fracture. In general patients are symptomatic for several weeks before diagnosis. A mass near a major joint may often be palpable at the time of diagnosis. Dilated veins are commonly seen in overlying skin (Fig. 6.3).

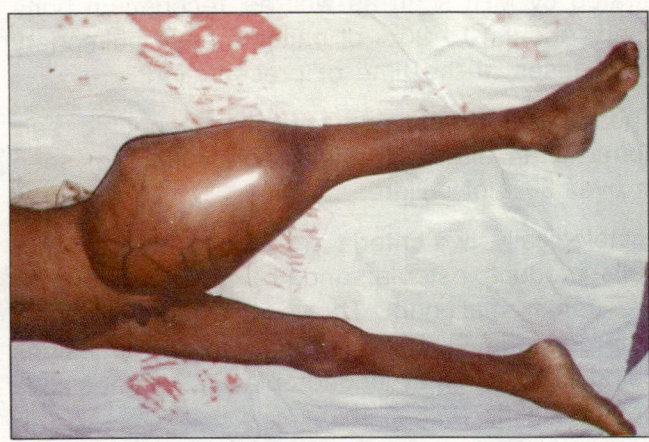

Fig. 6.3. Osteosarcoma left thigh. Note the dilated veins on surface

Radiographic findings include a moth eaten appearance of bony cortical destruction and spread of tumor into the soft tissues with characteristic ossification and periosteal reaction in a "sunburst" pattern and a "Codman's triangle" (triangle created by the raised periosteum) (Fig. 6.4a).

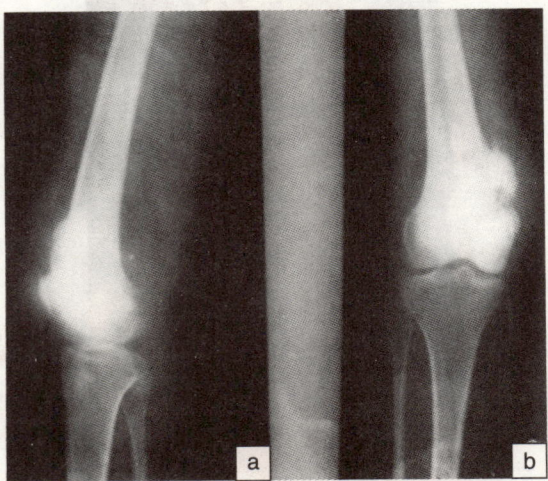

Fig. 6.4a,b. Osteogenic sarcoma of distal femur. Note the cortical destruction, Codman Triangle and Sunburst appearance

The tumor is limited by growth plate, which resists invasion. Though blastic types predominate, mixed lesions with patchy lysis and sclerosis admixed may be seen. Telengiectatic osteosarcomas are lytic.

CT and MRI scans are helpful in demonstrating soft tissue component, involvement of neurovascular structures or joint penetration. MRI also defines involvement of cancellous and medullary bone. The "skip lesions", seen in the marrow cavity of the bone in less than 3% cases, can be demonstrated by MRI scan as well as Technetium bone scan. About 10 - 20% of patients have pulmonary metastases at the time of presentation.

The laboratory hallmark of an osteogenic sarcoma is an elevated alkaline phosphatase, seen in over 50% of children.

Histologically, two criteria are utilised: a) the tumor cells produce osteoid; and, b) the stromal cells are frankly malignant. The lesions may be highly heterogenous in appearance, with some lesions being predominantly chondroblastic, osteoblastic or fibroblastic (Fig. 6.4b,c).

Treatment for osteosarcoma must be aggressive. Amputation is often required, especially if there has been delay in diagnosis, inappropriate surgery or a pathological fracture.

Use of multi-modality therapy in conjunction with improved imaging techniques to detect pulmonary metastases has improved the outlook considerably. Before the advent of adjuvant multi drug chemotherapy, 80% of patients died of pulmonary metastases after high amputation. The prognosis for 5 years survival has risen to about 75% at the present date with the use of combination chemotherapy and surgical treatment. The drugs commonly used today include high dose methotrexate, doxorubicin, cisplatinum and ifosfamide. Neoadjuvant chemotherapy effectively destroys malignant cells and in many patients there is total necrosis of tumor. Neoadjuvant chemotherapy refers to the use of chemotherapeutic agents for a minimum of three cycles preoperatively. The use of these agents prior to surgery decreases the tumor bulk, destroys micrometastases and thus improves survival by minimising the chances of distant metastases. It also helps in achieving better local control of the disease. Another advantage is that histopathologic examination of the excised tumor specimen and evaluation of percentage tumor necrosis can assess the response to chemotherapy. Response to preoperative chemotherapy has prognostic value when more than 90% of the tumor cells show necrosis. In these cases prognosis for a 5-year cure is about 85–90%. Limb salvage surgery is now possible with 8–12 weeks of neoadjuvant chemotherapy, surgical (wide) excision of the tumor and postopera-

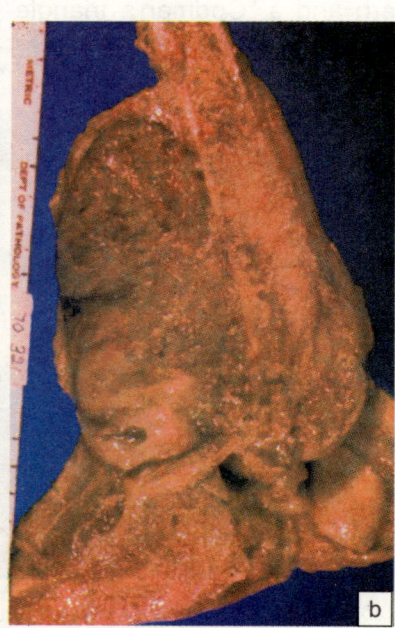

Fig. 6.4b. Gross pathology specimen of Osteosarcoma

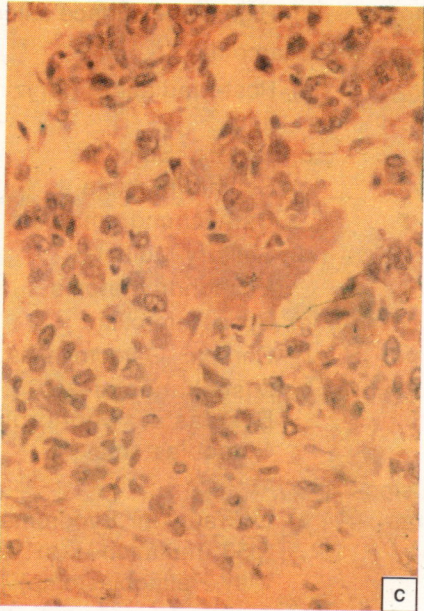

Fig. 6.4c. Histopathologic appearance of Osteosarcoma. Note the osteoid formation by the tumor cells

tive chemotherapy for 6-12 months. Allograft or prosthetic reconstruction is often required for limb salvage surgery. Relative contraindications to limb salvage surgery are pathological fracture, involvement of neurovascular bundle, inappropriate biopsy site, infection, immature skeletal age and extensive muscle involvement.

Pulmonary metastases are no more considered fatal in osteosarcoma. Preoperative chemotherapy followed by surgical removal (lobectomy or wedge resection) is used to ablate pulmonary disease.

2. Parosteal (Juxtacortical) Osteosarcoma

This low-grade osteosarcoma occurs on the surface of metaphysis of long bones. It is slow growing and is often underdiagnosed on biopsy. It accounts for only 4% of all osteosarcomas.

Parosteal osteosarcoma has many features distinct from classical osteosarcoma such as female preponderance (1.4:1), older age group (95% occur between 15–40 years), a higher prevalence of location around the knee (71% occur at knee) and slow rate of growth.

Distal femur, especially its posterior aspect is the most common site. Tumor may be asymptomatic initially or may present as slowly growing painless mass, most commonly in the popliteal fossa. Pain and swelling occur late in the course of disease.

Radiographic examination reveals a radiodense mass at the surface of the bone. Tumor may encircle the bone before invading it, creating a characteristic radiolucent line ("cleft") between the tumor and cortical bone. Significantly, obliteration of this cleft implies invasion of the medullary canal (25% cases) and the prognosis changes to that of classic intramedullary osteosarcoma. CT scan and MRI can also help in ascertaining the cortical invasion. CT scan can also help in differentiating parosteal osteosarcoma from a sessile osteochondroma. The latter typically shows continuity of cortex and medullary cavity of the lesion with the cortex and medullary cavity of the parent bone while no such continuity is seen in parosteal osteosarcoma.

Histological examination reveals extremely well differentiated osteoblasts with very few mitotic figures. Trabeculae are regularly arranged. However, rarely this low-grade tumor can dedifferenti-

ate into a high grade sarcoma with poor prognosis. Histologically the differential diagnosis is myositis ossificans in which there is characteristic zone phenomenon (more activity towards the centre) unlike osteosarcoma which shows central necrosis.

Parosteal osteosarcoma being a low-grade tumor does not respond well to either chemotherapy or radiation therapy. The clinical course is that of slow progression. Metastases are rare, occur by hematogenous route and may present more than 5 years after excision of the tumor. Incomplete excision always leads to recurrences.

Treatment of choice is wide excision including cortex of the underlying bone. Overall survival is approximately 80%. Recurrences are rare after wide excision, but may occur as long as a decade after surgery.

3. Periosteal Osteosarcoma

Periosteal osteosarcoma occurs on the surface of bone and is predominantly chondroblastic. Periosteal osteosarcomas occur almost always in the lower extremity and involve the diaphysis of femur or tibia. It occurs most frequently in children and is slightly more common in females. Pain or swelling over the involved bone is the most common presentation.

The radiographic examination reveals a mixed radiodense/radiolucent lesion on the diaphysis of the bone with irregular bone contour. Radiodensities reflecting matrix mineralization are usually seen alongwith periosteal reaction and thickened cortical bone. Linear intralesional mineralization lines ("sunburst type") perpendicular to the long axis of the affected bone are characteristic.

Histologically the microscopic pattern resembles neoplastic cartilage similar to that of a surface chondrosarcoma seen in older patients. Neoplastic osteoid formation, however, suggests the diagnosis of periosteal osteosarcoma.

Prognosis wise, Periosteal osteosarcoma is intermediate between parosteal osteosarcoma (very low grade) and high grade intramedullary osteosarcoma. Death occurs in 20–40% patients. Surgical treatment is wide excision and usually a limb-sparing procedure. Chemotherapy is rarely required.

4. Secondary Osteosarcoma

Osteogenic sarcoma can arise from a wide range of benign diseases (Table 6.5) and usually occurs at a later age (Fig. 6.5).

Table 6.5. Secondary osteosarcomas

Underlying bone disease
    Paget's Disease
    Radiation injury
    Bone infarction
    Chronic osteomyelitis

Malignant transformation in benign tumours
    Solitary osteochondroma
    Solitary enchondroma
    Multiple Hereditary exostoses
    Enchondromatosis

Miscellaneous
    Giant cell tumour
    Fibrous Dysplasia
    Chondroblastoma
    Osteoblastoma

The classic example of secondary osteosarcoma is that arising in the presence of Paget's disease. Pagetic sarcoma is the commonest osteosarcoma in old age and comprises 3% of all osteosarcomas. The most common location is humerus, followed by the pelvis and femur.

The prognosis for patients with pagetic osteosarcoma is extremely poor and chemotherapy is usually not preferred in view of advanced age of the patients.

Benign Chondroid Lesions

1. Osteochondroma

Osteochondroma is a benign cartilage capped protuberance of bone growing outward from the surface of a normal bone. The lesion is contiguous with underlying cortical trabecular bone and marrow. The lesion can be pedunculated or sessile. Sessile lesions are more likely to be multiple and are more prone to malignant transformation. The cartilage in the cap undergoes endochondral ossification. Thus the lesions continue to grow with growth, away from the metaphysis (from where they originate), and stop growing at skeletal maturity with ossification of cartilage cap. Continued growth beyond this time may suggest malignant degeneration.

Osteochondroma is a developmental or hamartomatous process, which arises from a defect in the metaphyseal side of growth plate.

Osteochondromas arise most commonly from metaphysis of the distal femur (>50%) (Fig. 6.6a-c). Other sites are proximal humerus and proximal tibia. Clinically, osteochondromas are usually asymptomatic. When detected, osteochondroma may present as long-standing mass, sometimes

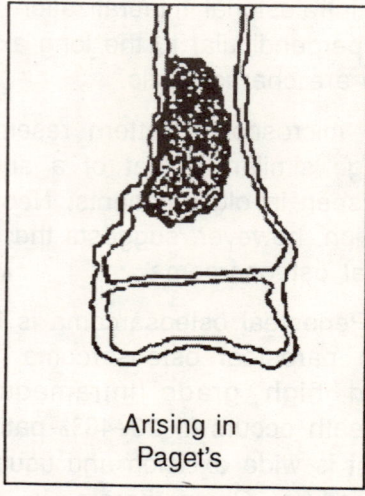

Arising in Paget's

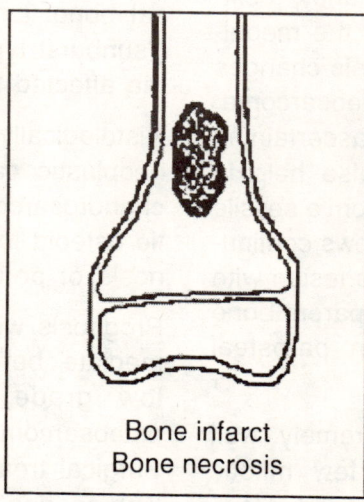

Bone infarct
Bone necrosis

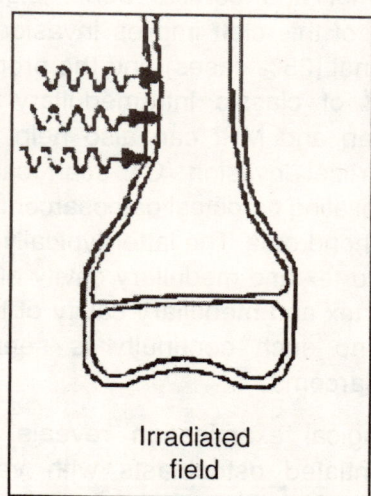

Irradiated field

Fig. 6.5.   Secondary Osteosarcoma

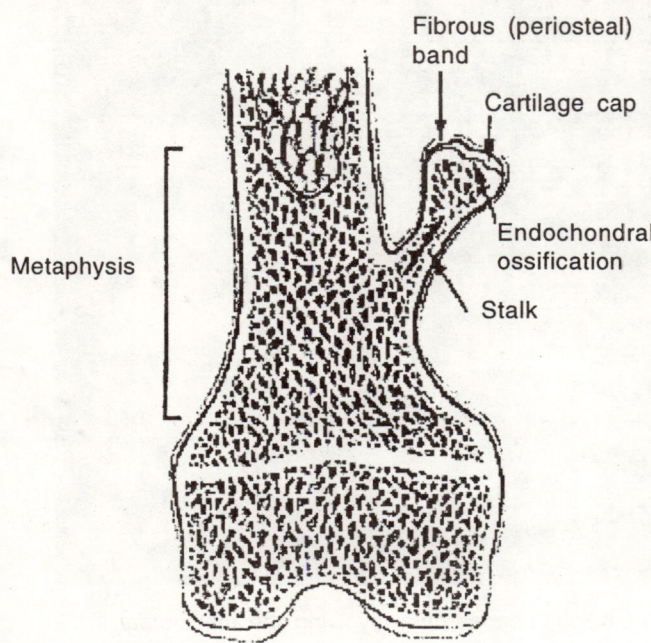

Fig. 6.6a. Schematic diagram of an osteochondroma

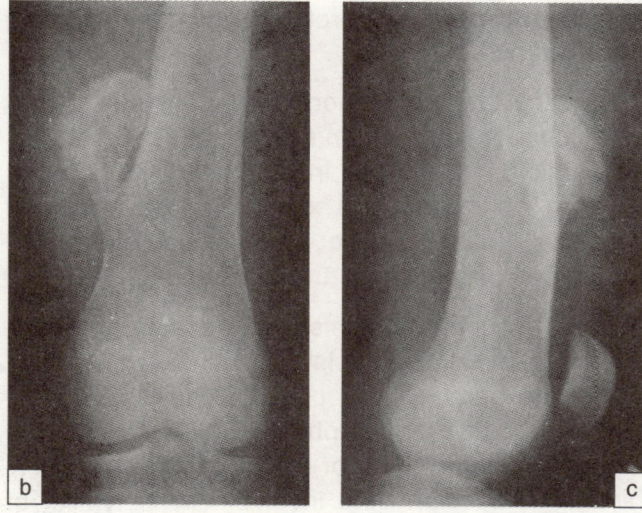

Fig. 6.6b,c.   Pedunculated osteochondroma arising from the distal femur. Note the growth of osteochondroma away from the adjacent joint.

painful, in male adolescents. Patients may experience pain secondary to inflamed bursa over the lesion, muscle irritation, and impingement of nerve, fracture of the stalk or malignant transformation. Osteochondromas can also cause aneurysms, fractures of the bone or formation of osteocartilaginous loose bodies following fracture. Occasionally some lesions may attain large sizes and cause mechanical restriction of joint motion.

Radiographically, the lesion appears as radiodense, pedunculated or sessile lesion (Fig. 6.7a-c) extending into soft tissues, pointing away from the nearest joint.

CT scan can establish cortical and medullary continuity between the lesion and the host bone. This is an important differentiating feature from periosteal or juxta-cortical chondromas and parosteal osteosarcomas which have an interface with cortical bone.

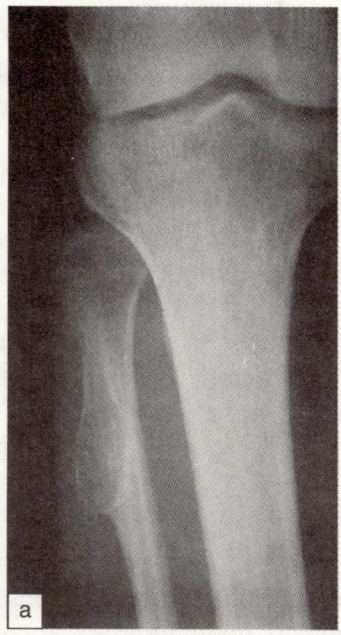

Fig. 6.7a. Sessile osteochondroma arising from the proximal fibula

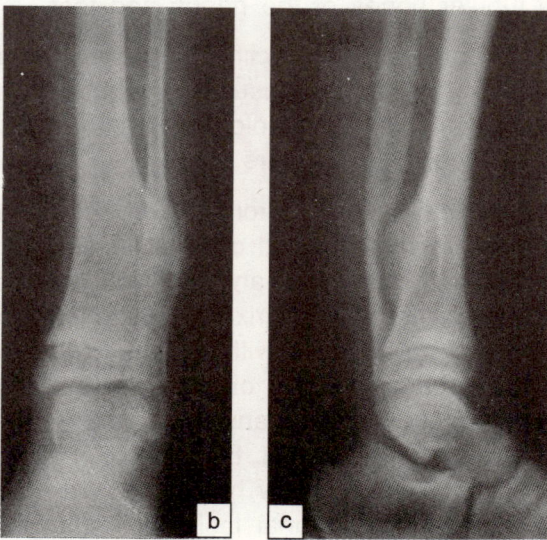

Fig. 6.7b,c.   Sessile osteochondroma arising from the distal tibia. Note the pressure effect on the fibula

Histology reveals normal bone with (hyaline) cartilaginous cap.

When asymptomatic, these lesions are treated with observation only. Surgery is indicated for pressure on neurovascular structures, unsightly deformity, impairment of articular function and motion, development of painful bursa or for suspected or established malignant transformation. Surgery involves excision of lesion at its base along with covering periosteum (so called extraperiosteal excision) and the cartilage cap.

Conversion of solitary osteochondroma to chondrosarcoma (usually) or osteosarcoma (rarely) occurs only during adulthood. The overall rate of malignant transformation for solitary lesions is less than one percent. The rate of malignant degeneration in multiple hereditary exostoses is 10–20% especially in the larger, more proximal lesions. Other problems with multiple osteochondromas include growth disturbances, such as angular deformity or limb length discrepancy; secondary impingement on nerves, vessels and tendons; spinal cord compression or pleural irritation.

2. Enchondroma

Enchondroma is accumulation of cartilage rests within the bone. Enchondromas constitute about 12% of all benign bone tumors. Enchondroma is the commonest benign neoplasm of the bone. In 50% of the cases an enchondroma is found in the small tubular bones of the hands and feet.

Enchondromas may be clinically asymptomatic. When symptomatic, they usually present with pain or swelling or even pathological fracture in patients between 10–30 years of age.

Radiographically, enchondromas are well-defined, sharply demarcated, round or oval lesions, which are lobulated with thin and sclerotic borders. Mineralization of the matrix in these lesions is variable and calcification within them can be flocculent, punctate, speckled or ring like. In case of an enchondroma of the hand, the lesion may be expansile with thinning of the cortex (Fig. 6.8). Bone scans typically show hot spots and lead to the discovery of additional lesions. Histologically, enchondromas appear as lobulated islands of benign cartilage surrounded by calcifying tissue and bone.

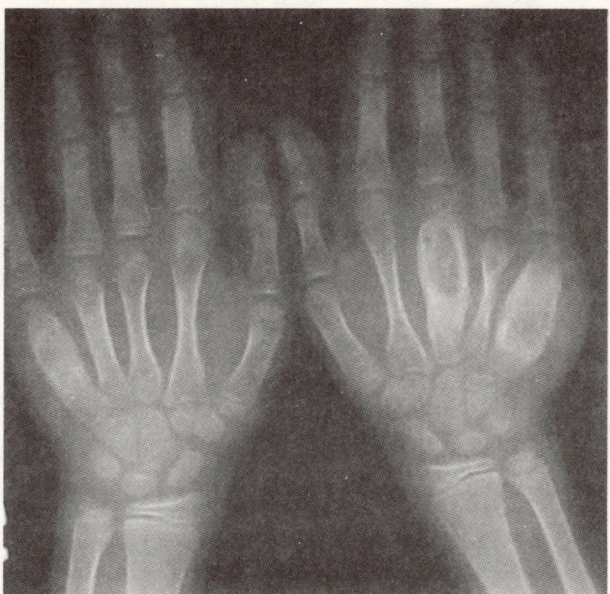

Fig. 6.8. Enchondroma involving the metacarpals.

Asymptomatic solitary enchondroma of the hand or foot needs no treatment. If the patient has a pathologic fracture, it is best to allow the fracture to heal and perform curettage and bone grafting subsequently.

A large solitary osteochondroma converts to low-grade chondrosarcoma in fewer than 5% of cases. Conversion takes place in adulthood. Pain in the absence of trauma and x-ray showing extension into soft tissues in the older patient is highly suggestive of malignant transformation.

Multiple enchondromatosis or *Ollier's disease* is a rare nonfamilial dysplasia typically seen on one half of the body. Ollier's disease shows extensive involvement of the metaphyseal areas resulting in bowing and shortening of the long bones. Cortical thinning and epiphyseal involvement is typical of Ollier's disease. In 25% of patients with Ollier's disease, a secondary chondrosarcoma develops subsequently. Lesions of proximal femur and pelvis are particularly high risk.

Mafucci's syndrome is characterised by the presence of multiple enchondromas along with hemangiomas.

3. Chondroblastoma (*Codman's Tumor*) is a benign cartilaginous lesion of the epiphysis or apophysis in adolescents. Patients are between the ages of 10 and 20 years in 90% of the cases. The lesion occurs most commonly in the lower extremity (three fourth cases), especially around the knee. Upper end of the humerus is the next most common site. Triradiate cartilage of pelvis is also a common location. Males are more commonly affected than females (2.5:1).

Clinically, the patients usually have pain, often localised to the adjacent joint, which is tender on palpation. Limping, muscle wasting and restriction of movements may occur in a lesion located close to the knee joint. Effusion and signs of inflammatory arthritis may also be noted in the knee joint. The lesion may occur in the presence of open, closing or closed growth plate.

Radiological examination demonstrates a well-circumscribed, ovoid, lytic lesion present eccentrically in the epiphysis, often extending to metaphysis (Fig. 6.9a-c). Lesion has a thin, sclerotic margin. Lytic lesion shows central stippled or flocculent calcification occurring in chondroid portion of the tumor. Bone scans are hot in chondroblastoma.

Histologically, the chondroblastoma resembles giant cell tumor with numerous macrophages seen usually in areas of hemorrhage.

The stromal cells are polyhedral which are consistent histogenetically with chondroblasts. Calcification in a lacy network ("Chicken - wire" calcification) is seen around these stromal cells.

Treatment for chondroblastoma consists of curettage and bone grafting. Recurrences can occur in about 15% cases after curettage. In such patients, repeat curettage is often successful.

The spontaneous conversion of chondroblastoma to a malignant tumor is extremely rare. Malignant degeneration can occur following radiation treatment. Chondroblastoma, though benign, can rarely metastasise to lung just like giant cell tumor (in 2% cases). The prognosis in the metastatic disease, however, is excellent.

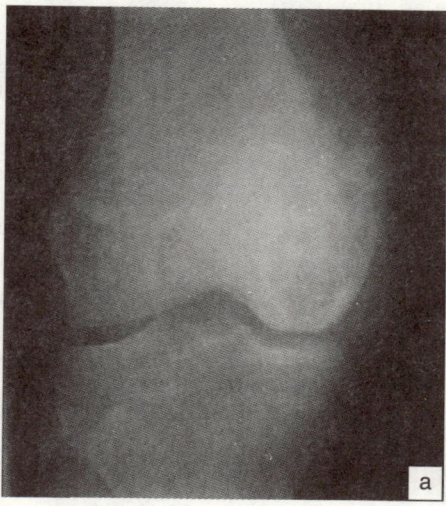

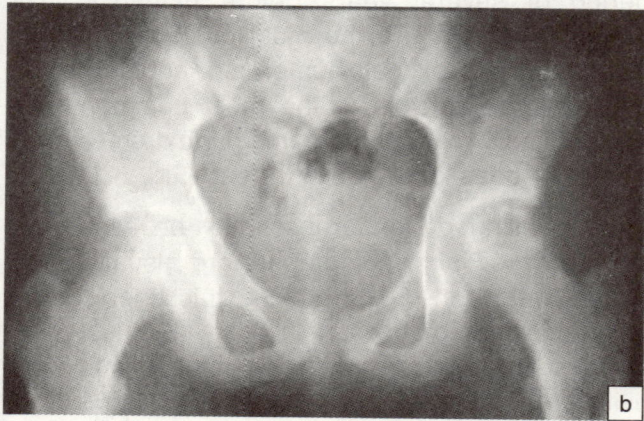

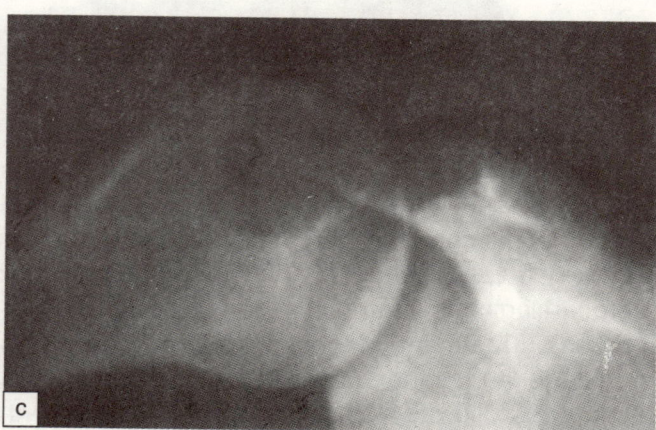

Fig. 6.9a-c.   Chondroblastoma (a) distal femur (b) left femoral head and (c) humeral head. Note the epiphyseometaphyseal location of the tumor with involvement of the growth plate

4. Chondromyxoid Fibroma

Chondromyxoid fibroma is a rare benign cartilage tumor containing variable amounts of chondroid, fibromatoid and myxoid elements. Most patients are seen in the second and third decades of life, 80% before 40 years of age. Men are more commonly affected than women. The lesion tends to involve long bone of lower limb (up to 70% cases) especially proximal tibia followed in frequency by distal femur and the first ray of the foot.

Pain is the most common symptom. Local swelling in small bones is common. Tenderness is often present.

Radiographs show an expansile, lobulated, lytic tumor with sharp sclerotic margins and a pseudoloculated pattern resembling bone cyst (Fig. 6.10). Lesion is eccentrically located in metaphysis and often erodes the cortex. None or faint mineralization may be noted within the lesion. Bone scans are hot.

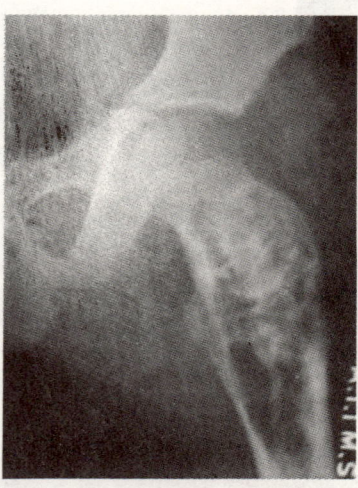

Fig. 6.10. Chondromyxoid fibroma of the proximal femur

Histologically, the lesion shows a mixture of fibrous, myxomatous and chondroid tissue. Giant cells are also seen. The tumor grows in lobules and often there is condensation of cells at the periphery of the lobules. Production of either chondroid or fibrocartilaginous matrix is seen in variable proportions. Treatment of chondromyxoid fibroma is curettage and bone grafting. Recurrence rate is about 25% following this procedure. Ideal treatment, when feasible, is enbloc resection. Conversion to chondrosarcoma is extremely rare.

Malignant Chondroid Tumors

Chondrosarcoma

Chondrosarcoma is a malignant tumor of cartilage that can occur in any bone preformed in cartilage. Patients with multiple benign cartilage lesions run the risk of eventually developing malignant change, particularly in the pelvis, proximal femur or humerus. The patients are, thus, in middle life or older for these secondary tumors. Primary chondrosarcoma may occur during the third or fourth decade of life. Classification of chondrosarcoma is given in Table 6.6.

Table 6.6. Classification of Chondrosarcoma

1. Conventional Chondrosarcoma
     Borderline
     Low-grade
     High-grade

2. Secondary Chondrosarcoma
     Solitary / Multiple exostosis
     Solitary / Multiple enchondromatosis

3. Peripheral Chondrosarcoma

4. Dedifferentiated Chondrosarcoma

5. Miscellaneous
     Mesenchymal Chondrosarcoma
     Chondrosarcoma of small bones
     Synovial Chondrosarcoma

The typical primary chondrosarcoma is a low-grade tumor seen in adults between 30 and 60 years of age. Men are more commonly affected. Minimal symptoms of pain may occur over a period of several years before diagnosis. The pelvis and femur are the most common locations followed by proximal humerus, shoulder girdle and ribs. Metaphysis is the most common location. Primary chondrosarcoma is extremely rare in small bones of hands and feet (Fig. 6.11a).

Pain, swelling or tenderness may be associated complaints. Plain radiographs are usually diagnostic with bone destruction, thickened cortex and flocculent matrix calcification (Fig. 6.11b-d). Bone scans are hot indicating mineralization activity.

Histologically, chondrosarcomas are usually cellular but degree of cellularity varies in different

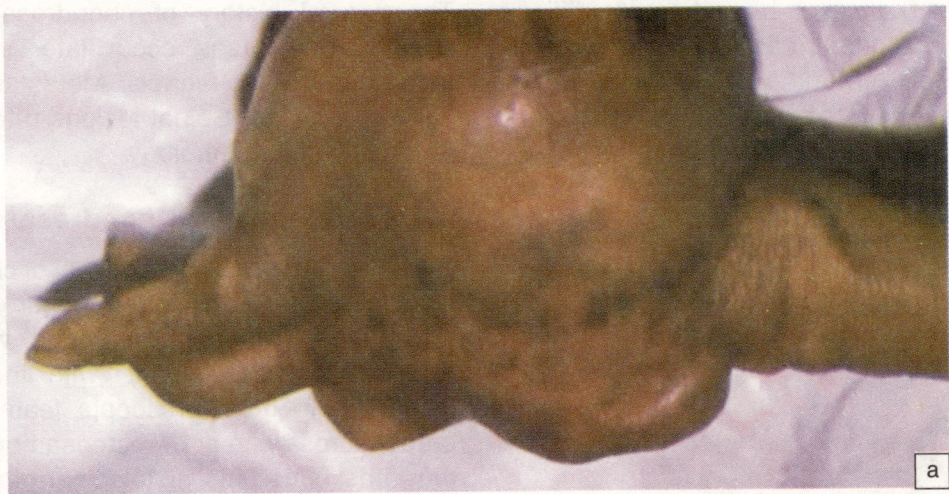

Fig. 6.11a.   Chondrosarcoma arising from the palm

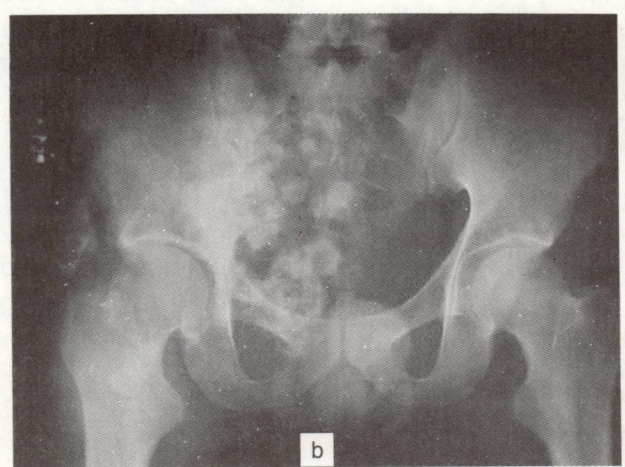

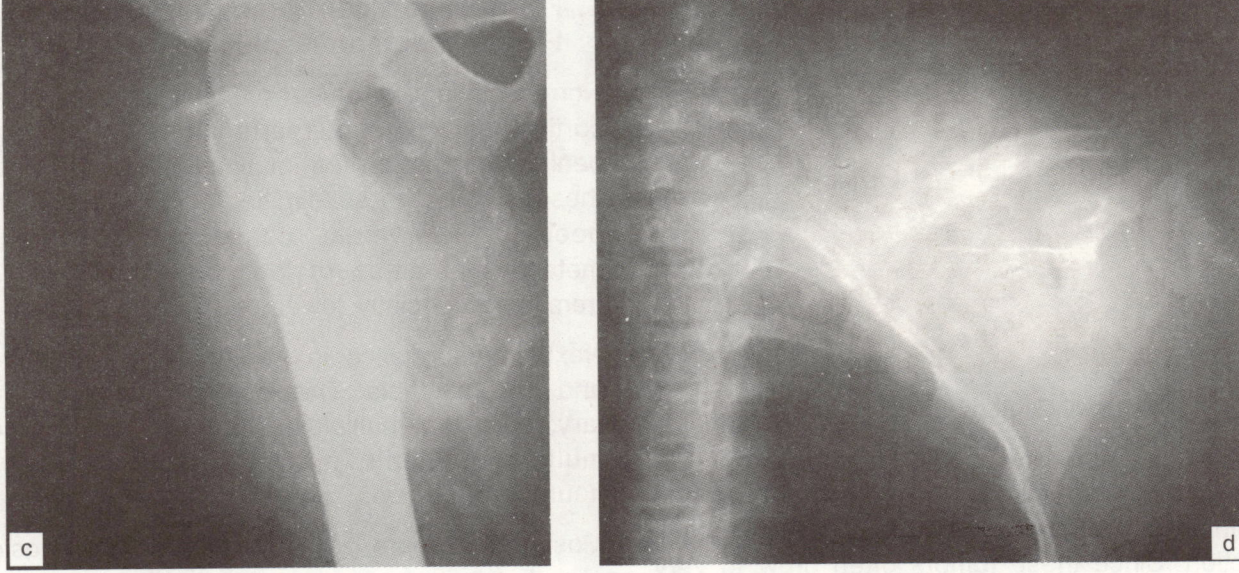

Fig. 6.11b-d. Radiologic features of chondrosarcoma arising from (b) Pelvis, (c) Proximal femur and (d) Scapula. Note the bony destruction and flocculent matrix calcification.

fields (Fig. 6.11e,f). It may be extremely difficult to differentiate malignant cartilage only on the basis of histologic criteria. The clinical, radiographic and histologic features of a particular lesion must be considered together to avoid incorrect diagnosis.

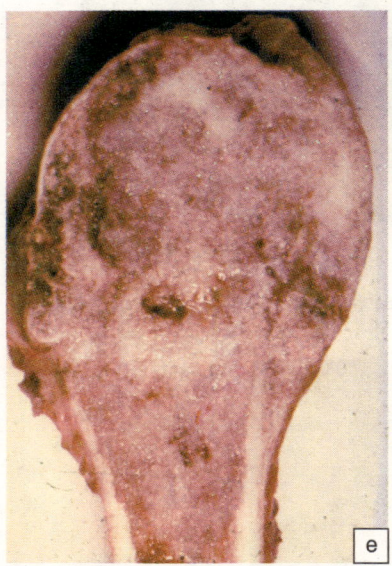

Fig. 6.11e. Gross pathologic specimen of chondrosarcoma

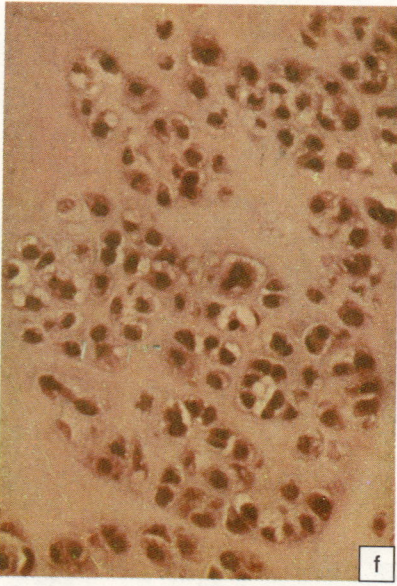

Fig. 6.11f. Histopathology of chondrosarcoma

Most (almost 90%) of chondrosarcomas are low grade and do not respond to chemotherapy and radiotherapy. Treatment consists of wide surgical resection. Since these tumors often grow to very large size before the patient presents for treatment, amputation often is the only choice.

The natural history of chondrosarcoma is slow growth. Metastases occur late and are usually through venous channels. Metastases usually occur to the lungs. Spinal lesions often cause death by local tumor pathology.

2. Dedifferentiated Chondrosarcoma

This is the most malignant variety of chondrosarcoma. It accounts for 10% of all chondrosarcomas. It is most likely a second mutation within the pre-existing chondrosarcoma, with the second sarcoma taking on microscopic features of a high-grade fibrosarcoma or osteosarcoma. The tumor thus has bimorphic histological picture.

Dedifferentiated chondrosarcoma occurs in older patients, usually between the age of 50–70 years. The clinical pictures and site of involvement are similar to that of low grade chondrosarcoma.

Radiographic picture is also dimorphic. Most commonly the radiographs show a typical chondrosarcoma with a superimposed highly destructive area.

Treatment is wide resection with reconstruction using allografts and/or modular tumor prostheses. Adjuvant multi-agent chemotherapy is used in the patients who are not very old.

The prognosis is poor and the long-term survival is less than 10%. Patients usually die of metastases.

Benign Fibrous Tumors of Bone

1. Fibrous Cortical Defect/Non Ossifying Fibroma/Metaphyseal Fibrous Defect

Non ossifying fibromas or their smaller fibrous cortical defect counterparts are the commonest benign lesions of the skeletal system. Most of these lesions are self-limiting and resolve spontaneously. The most common locations are metaphyseal areas of long bones of lower extremities especially lower end of femur.

Next common sites in frequency are distal tibia and proximal tibia. The lesions are usually solitary; however, multiple lesions can occur. These multiple lesions may be associated with neurofibromatosis.

Most patients are asymptomatic and the lesions are discovered accidentally during radiographic examination. Rarely, the lesion becomes large enough to fracture.

Radiographic examination reveals a metaphyseal, eccentric lytic lesion surrounded by a sclerotic rim. The cortex may be thinned and expanded.

Histological examination reveals cellular, fibroblastic connective tissue background with cells arranged in whorled bundles. There are numerous giant cells, lipophages, and variable amounts of hemosiderin pigmentation.

Treatment is not required for asymptomatic lesions. Symptomatic patients with large lesions involving more than 75% of the cortex with imminent fracture require curettage and bone grafting.

2. Desmoplastic Fibroma

These are fibrous lesions of bone with histologic characteristics of the extraosseous desmoid tumors. This is a rare, locally aggressive, benign lesion. This lesion is often difficult to differentiate from desmoids and low-grade fibrosarcomas histologically.

Desmoplastic fibroma occurs in the first three decades of life without any sexual predilection. Commonly involved bones are ilium, long bones and mandible. Lesions are often asymptomatic or only slightly painful and may present with pathological fracture.

Radiographic examination reveals a distinct, lucent, expansile lesion with well-defined margins. Cortical erosion with pathological fracture may be seen.

MRI can help in differentiating intraosseous tumor from normal marrow and is extremely useful in pre-operative planning.

Histologically lesion shows dense, collagenized tissue surrounding uniform appearing, benign fibroblasts. Histology alone at times may be unable to distinguish between desmoplastic fibromas and desmoid, low grade fibrosarcoma, or even fibrous histiocytoma.

Treatment is wide surgical excision. Non resection procedures have high recurrence rates.

Metastases may occur after local recurrences

Malignant Fibrous Lesions

1. Fibrosarcoma

Fibrosarcoma of bone is a malignant, primary, spindle cell sarcoma of bone composed of fibroblasts. Primary fibrosarcoma is a rare lesion accounting for 4 percent of malignant tumors of bone. The common sites are distal femur, proximal tibia, pelvis, proximal femur and proximal humerus in that order. Tumor can occur at any age (15-60 years) but more commonly affects young adults.

Patient often presents with pain and a mass and occasionally may present with a pathological fracture.

Radiographically, the lesion is purely osteolytic, permeative and poorly marginated.

Histologically, fibrosarcomas are characterised by interwoven bundles of spindle cells with narrow tapering nuclei and ill-defined cytoplasmic borders and herringbone pattern. High-grade forms show greater anaplasia of fibroblasts with higher index of mitotic activity and lesser collagen fibre formation as compared to low-grade form.

Treatment consists of wide or radical resection to prevent recurrences. Amputation may be required to control the disease. Adjuvant chemotherapy has to be added for the treatment of high-grade fibrosarcoma in young patients who can tolerate systemic toxicity. Chemotherapy is not effective for low-grade forms. Prognosis for fibrosarcoma is generally poor.

Secondary fibrosarcomas may be seen in association with Paget's disease, irradiation or bone infarction.

2. Malignant Fibrous Histiocytoma (MFH)

Malignant fibrous histiocytoma, though more common in soft tissues, can arise de novo in the skeleton. It runs a clinical course similar to fibrosarcoma. MFH is seen in middle aged and older adults with male preponderance. It most frequently involves the bones around the knee (distal femur, proximal tibia), ilium, humerus and skull. MFH can occur following Paget's disease, bone infarction or irradiation. Patients usually present with pain and swelling.

Radiographs show aggressive permeation of metaphyseal-diaphyseal bone. Lesions are diffuse without any evidence of periosteal response or calcification. CT and MRI are extremely useful for early detection of the tumor, destruction of bone and determination of position of the tumor in relation to adjacent neurovascular structures, which is important for the preoperative planning.

Histological examination shows tumor to be high grade showing highly anaplastic fibroblasts with abundant cytoplasm mixed with malignant histiocytes and a few giant cells in a typical cartwheel or storiform (Greek: storis, meaning matted) growth pattern.

Treatment is aggressive wide resection. Radiation and chemotherapy do not have established benefit.

Overall prognosis for MFH is poor with high rates of local recurrence and metastasis.

Tumors of Unknown Origin

1. Giant Cell Tumors of Bone

Various types of tumors contain giant cells (Giant cell variants) but are not true benign giant cell tumors.

Giant Cell Tumor (GCT) is a distinct clinical-radiological-pathologic entity characterised by lytic expansile lesion in epiphysis or apophysis without any new bone formation occurring in skeletally mature adults 20–40 years old (after closure of epiphysis). Females are more commonly affected. Tumor is found around the knee in about half the cases. The next common locations are distal radius and sacrum (Commonest tumor of sacrum). GCT can occur in hand and foot bones. Such lesions are often multicentric.

Clinically the tumor is usually painful for several months before the diagnosis. Pathologic fracture may sometimes be the presenting feature. Swelling or painful effusion can be a feature due to its proximity to a major joint. Weakness or limitation of range of motion may be other symptoms.

Radiologic examination reveals usually a well-circumscribed, expansile, purely lytic lesion, with pseudotrabeculations, in the epiphysis/epiphyseal-metaphyseal region extending up to the subarticular margin without any periosteal reaction. Lesions have no sclerosis around them. The radiologic picture has been classically described as "soapbubble" appearance (Fig. 6.12d,e). Cortex may be eroded sometimes with extension into the soft tissues. The lesion grows towards the joint surface and frequently abuts the articular cartilage but does not break into the joint. Histological examination reveals proliferating stromal cells with round, oval or even spindle shaped nucleus with multinucleated giant cells scattered evenly throughout the lesion (Fig. 6.12a-c). Mitotic figures may be variable. Light microscopic characteristics are poor at defining the biologic behaviour of the tumor. Enneking classified giant cell tumors into three types based on clinical, radiological and histopathologic appearance viz. Grade A-Latent; Grade B-Active; and, Grade C-Aggressive.

The differential diagnosis most importantly includes chondroblastoma. The latter, however, is much rarer, occurs in younger patients when physis is still open and shows calcification in about 50% cases. Other differentials are enumerated in Table 6.7.

Like chondroblastoma the benign giant cell tumor has a 1–2% chance of metastasising to the lungs. Recurrent tumors have a much higher risk (6%).

The prognosis for survival with pulmonary metastasis is good and some of the tumors may resolve spontaneously. Approximately 90% of giant cell tumors are benign. The benign giant cell tumors can later convert to malignant form. The risk of malignant transformation is much higher following radiation therapy.

Treatment aims to remove the lesion with preser-

Table 6.7. Giant cell variants (Reactive and tumorous conditions showing proliferation of giant cells)

– Non ossifying fibroma	– Chondromyxoid fibroma
– Chondroblastoma	– Osteoblastoma
– Unicameral bone cyst	– Aneurysmal bone cyst
– Osteoid Osteoma	– Giant cell reparative granuloma
– Benign fibrous histiocytoma	– Malignant fibrous histiocytoma.
– Brown tumor of hyperparathyroidism	

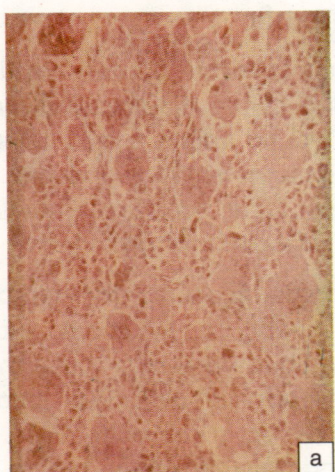

Fig. 6.12a.   Microscopic appearance of Giant cell tumour

vation of the involved joint. Curettage and bone grafting attempts to achieve these ends but has significant recurrence rate. Recurrent tumors are more aggressive in their biologic behaviour. Most surgeons presently elect curettage followed by adjuvant phenol, hydrogen peroxide, or liquid nitrogen (cryotherapy) to destroy remaining cells in the walls of tumor cavity. Bone defect is subsesquently filled with bone cement with or without additional steinmann pins to support subchondral bone and prevent collapse. This treatment gives local control in 80–90% cases. When lesions are extensive, resection arthrodesis, allograft reconstruction or custom made pros-

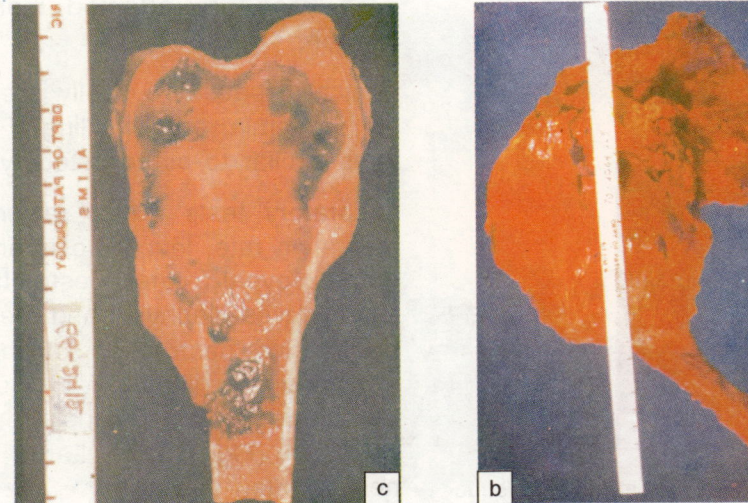

Fig. 6.12b,c. Gross pathology specimen of giant cell tumor

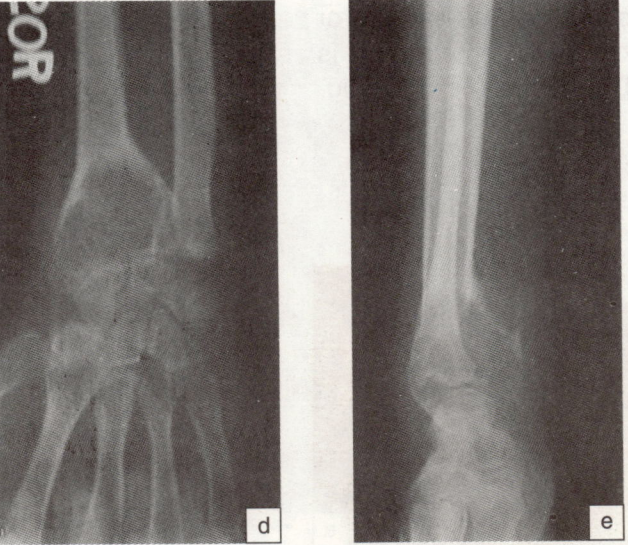

Fig. 6.12d,e. Giant cell tumor arising from the lower end of radius

thetic replacement are other alternatives. The GCTs of lower end of the radius (12% cases) present a special problem. The treatment options in these cases include curettage and bone grafting for small lesions, excision with centralisation of ulna and, excision and reconstruction with upper end of contralateral fibula (Fig. 6.12d-f).

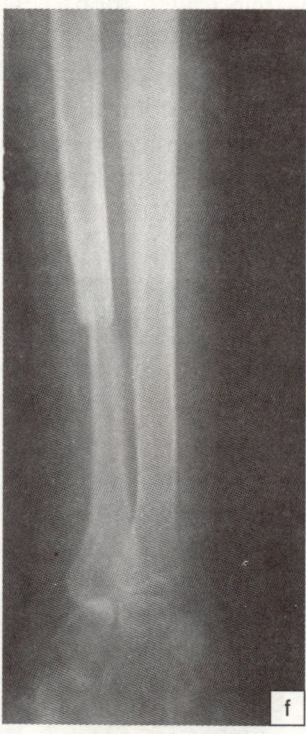

Fig. 6.12f.   X-ray following tumor excision and reconstruction with proximal fibula

In surgically inaccessible sites such as sacrum or spine, radiotherapy is considered though it is associated with increased risk of causing malignant change.

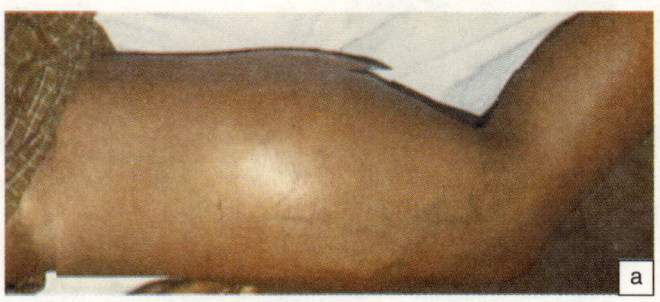

Fig. 6.13a.   Clinical appearance of Ewing's Sarcoma

2. Ewing's Tumor

Ewing's sarcoma is a primary malignant bone tumor, growing in the diaphysis of long bones in children and young adults and is composed histologically of uniform small round cells with indistinct cytoplasm, fine nuclear chromatin, indistinct nucleoli and cytoplasmic glycogen.

Ewing's sarcoma accounts for approximately 5–10% of malignant bone tumors and commonly affects femur, tibia, humerus, fibula and flat bones (pelvis, ribs, and scapula). Two third cases are found in pelvis or lower extremities. Majority of cases occurs between 5–15 years of age. In patients younger than 5 years of age, metastatic neuroblastoma and leukaemia should be considered. Men are affected more commonly than women.

Clinically, patients usually present with pain, fever, anaemia, and swelling (Fig. 6.13a) – symptoms similar to acute osteomyelitis.

Laboratory tests reveal raised erythrocyte sedimentation rate, leucocytosis and anaemia. Radiographs reveal a large destructive lesion that usually involves diaphysis and metaphysis. Extensive permeative destruction of the cortex is seen. Periosteum is lifted off in multiple layers giving the characteristic onionskin, multilaminated appearance (Fig. 6.13b). Large soft tissue component is often seen.

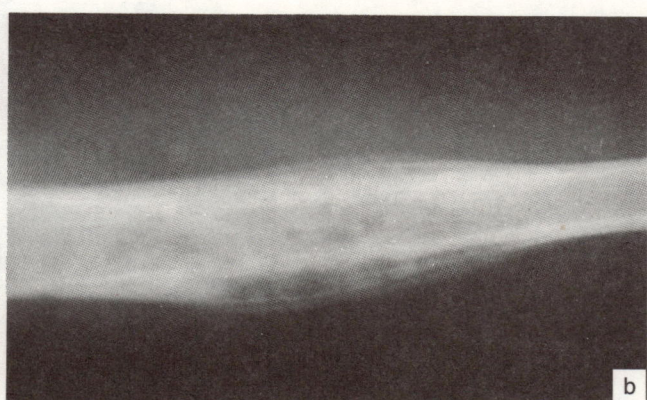

Fig 6.13b.   X-ray appearance of Ewing's Sarcoma. Note the onion peel periosteal reaction

Histologically, tumor consists of sheets of uniform round cells containing glycogen in cytoplasm

(Fig. 6.13c). Pseudorosette formation is seen as a result of central necrosis in a small clump of tumor cells. Central tumor necrosis is quite common in Ewing's tumor leading to liquefaction, which can appear like pus. Special staining with HBA-71, which recognizes a product of the MIC-2 gene, has been suggested to be specific for Ewing's sarcoma and neurectodermal tumors.

Combined with radiographic appearance and the presence of fever, the tumor can often be misdiagnosed as infection. Ewing's sarcoma is associated with chromosomal translocation (11, 22). The tumor markers include neuron specific enolase and myeloperoxidase.

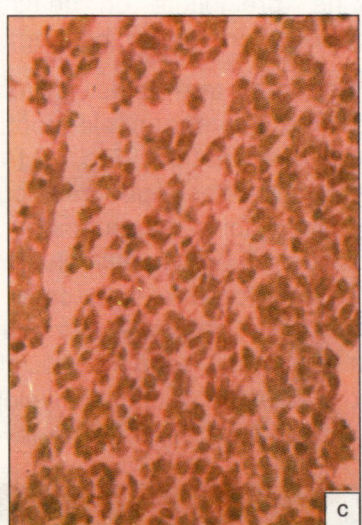

Fig. 6.13c. Histopathologic appearance of Ewing's Sarcoma. Note the sheets of round cells with attempts at pseudorosette formation

Treatment consists of chemotherapy and radiotherapy and surgical ablation, when possible (e.g. in expendable bones such as fibula, clavicle, scapula). Radiotherapy provides excellent local control but chemotherapy is required to control occult micrometastases, which are believed to be present in 80% of cases at the time of presentation. Long term survival with multimodality treatment may be 60–70%.

Prognostic factors in Ewing's Tumor include location (with patients who have pelvic, sacral or spinal involvement doing worse), extensive destruction and unhealed pathologic fracture.

Ewing's sarcoma is the most common source of brain metastases in children with solid tumors.

More than one bone involvement or skip metastases in the bone are seen in less than 5% cases.

3. Adamantinoma

Adamantinoma is a rare, slow growing malignant tumor of the bone occurring in second and third decades of life and composed of epithelial like islands of cells. Adamantinomas comprise 0.33% of all malignant bone tumors. Males and females are equally affected. Approximately 90% lesions occur in tibia and about 5% in fibula. Tumors are usually diaphyseal in location and frequently start in the anterior cortex. Most patients are young adults and present with pain of several months' or years' duration. These lesions are distinct from adamantinoma/ameloblastoma of the jaw.

Radiographs reveal a well demarcated lytic or mixed lytic and sclerotic loculated lesion involving diaphysis and bulging the anterior cortex. There may be multicentricity or involvement of ipsilateral tibia as well as fibula so physician should look for multiple sites.

Histological examination reveals epithelial or angioid tissue growing in a fibrous stroma. Presence of S-100 and cytokeratin on special staining confirms the epithelial origin of the tumor. The histological differential is from osteofibrous dysplasia.

Treatment is wide resection of involved segment of diaphysis followed by allograft reconstruction or bone transport using external fixators.

The lesion metastasises occasionally to regional lymph nodes and the lung. Metastases may occur early or after multiple attempts at local control. Even if pulmonary metastases occur, they can be resected with good expectation of survival.

Hematopoietic Tumors

Plasma Cell Tumors

1. Multiple Myeloma

Multiple myeloma is the commonest primary bone tumor and accounts for 45% of all malignant bone tumors. Classically it is a malignant tumor of plasma cells associated with widespread intraosseous proliferation of the plasma cells resulting in destruction of bone and lytic lesions throughout the skeleton. Tumor commonly occurs in patients between 50 and 80 years of age. Males are more commonly affected (M: F=2:1). Patients usually present with bone pain in spine and ribs or pathologic fracture (fracture of the sternum is considered pathognomonic by some). Constitutional symptoms such as fever, weakness, weight loss and anaemia with resultant fatigue are commonly associated. Symptoms may be related to complications such as renal insufficiency ("myeloma kidney" caused by protein plugging of renal tubules and renal failure), hypercalcaemia and amyloidosis.

Radiographically, myelomas are characterised by discrete, punched out lesions at multiple sites (Fig. 6.14a,b). Diffuse osteoporosis with vertebral compression fracture may be prominent feature. Lesions are always purely lytic without new bone formation and do not show uptake on bone scanning. Vertebral lesions may be associated with soft tissue extension causing difficulty in differentiation from tuberculosis of the spine. *Intravenous Pyelography (IVP) is contraindicated.*

Laboratory investigations reveal anaemia, raised erythrocyte sedimentation rate (often in excess of 100/1st hour), hyperproteinemia with reversal of albumin/globulin ratio and hypercalcaemia. Serum creatinine is raised in about 50% patients. Serum alkaline phosphatase is usually normal. Urine examination reveals the presence of Bence-Jones proteins (precipitate on heating urine to 50°C and dissolve on further heating).

The two most important tests for diagnosis of multiple myeloma are serum electrophoresis and bone marrow examination (Fig. 6.14c). Serum (as well as Urine) electrophoresis confirms the presence of monoclonal gammopathy i.e. monoclonal production of one heavy chain (IgM, IgG, IgA or others) and/or one light chain (kappa or lambda) in any combination. Tumors with IgG and kappa chain are most frequent. α_2 microglobulin is the tumor marker for multiple myeloma and its levels are markedly raised. The investigations

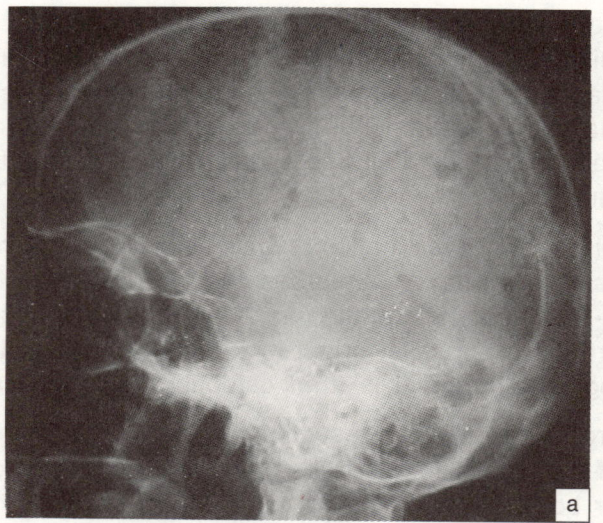

Fig. 6.14a. Multiple Myeloma with punched out lesion in the skull

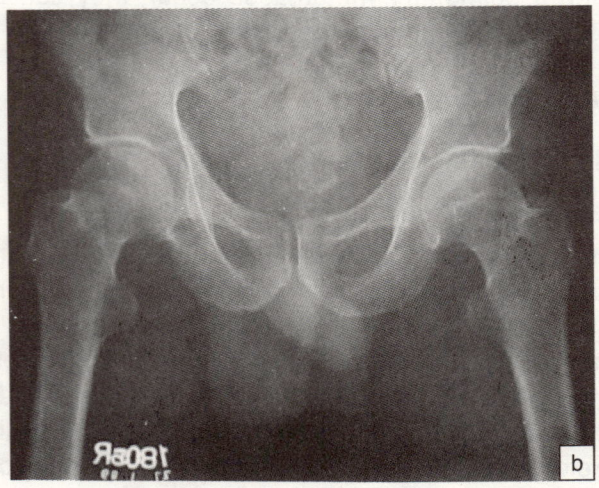

Fig. 6.14b. Multiple Myeloma with lytic lesions in pelvis

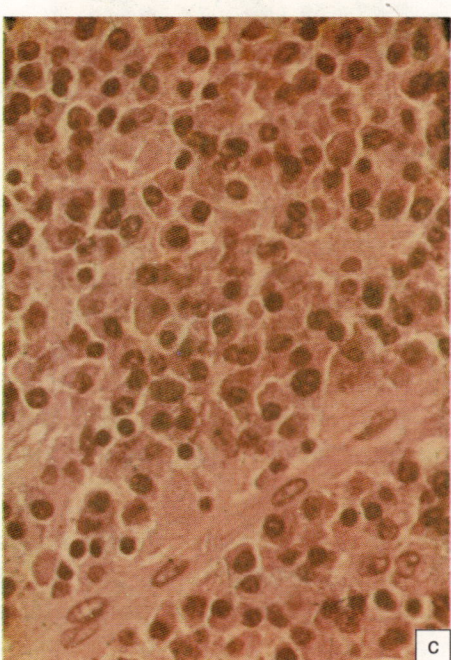

Fig. 6.14c. Microscopic picture of multiple myeloma. Note the sheets of plasma cells having eccentric nucleus and cart-wheel chromatin

commonly performed for multiple myeloma are given in Table 6.8.

Table 6.8. Investigations for Multiple Myeloma

Serum Calcium	High or Normal
Serum Phosphate	Normal
Serum Alkaline Phosphatase	Normal (raised only if pathological fracture)
Serum α_2 microglobulin	Increased (Tumor Marker)
Urinary Bence Jones Proteins	Positive only in 30% patients
Serum Protein Electrophoresis (M Spike)	Positive (Highly Specific) Ig G- 60% Ig A- 25% Others- 15%
Bone Marrow Examination	5%–100% Plasma cells

Histopathological examination of bone marrow biopsy or aspiration specimen shows sheets of plasma cells. Plasma cells have eccentric nucleus with stippled chromatin along its rim in "cartwheel" appearance and abundant cytoplasm. There is perinuclear clear zone (halo). Treatment consists mainly of chemotherapy with Melphalan and cortisone. Local treatment is similar to metastatic disease. Surgical stabilisation with irradiation is used for impending fractures (Prophylactically) and complete fractures (definitive treatment). Intralesional debridement followed by cemented nail or prosthetic devices is done. After surgery, the entire bone is irradiated with 5500 cGy.

Multiple myeloma has extremely poor prognosis along its natural course. Prognosis also depends on the stage of the disease. With the availability of chemotherapy, the average survival time has improved to 2-4 years.

2. Plasmacytoma (Solitary Myeloma)

Plasmacytoma is a solitary tumor identical otherwise to myeloma but with a more favourable prognosis. Solitary plasmacytoma is diagnosed when a solitary lesion is diagnosed on the skeletal survey. Tumor contains plasma cells on histologic examination and the results of serum electrophoresis, bone marrow examination and urine examination are normal. The histologic and radiographic features of plasmacytoma are same as multiple myeloma.

Solitary plasmacytomas constitute less than 10% of the myeloma. It is a low-grade lesion, which involves a younger age group, and the sex distribution is equal. However, in about 30% of patients, systemic evidence of multiple myeloma develops if they are followed for 20 years.

Treatment is wide resection if possible. If surgical excision is not warranted intralesional debridement and reconstruction followed by radiation therapy is treatment of choice. Intensive radiotherapy achieves local eradication in almost all patients.

3. Osteosclerotic Myeloma is a rare variant characterised by sclerotic or mixed sclerotic / lytic lesions involving spine, pelvis and ribs and amyloidosis leading to chronic inflammatory demyelinating polyneuropathy. Patients may have *POEMS* syndrome (polyneuropathy, organomegaly, endocrinopathy, 'M' protein and skin changes). Alkaline phosphatase may be raised in serum in these cases and recently, increased levels of osteocalcin (bone gla protein), the major non-collagenous bone protein have been linked to osteosclerotic variant.

Radiotherapy is the primary modality of treatment but neurologic changes may not improve with treatment.

Metastatic Bone Disease

Metastatic cancer to the skeleton is the most common malignant tumor affecting bone. The bone is the third most common site after the lung and liver. When a destructive lesion is seen in a patient over 40 years of age, metastases must be considered a differential. The carcinomas of breast, prostate, lung, thyroid and kidney account for 80% of bone metastases.

The most common locations are pelvis, vertebral bodies, ribs and proximal limb girdles. Metastases are rare distal to elbows or knees. Metastases to hand are seen in lung cancers. Metastases have a predilection for red marrow; therefore, metastases in children occur in long-bones while axial skeleton is commonly involved in adults (due to Batson's venous plexus). The most commonly affected part of skeleton is spine. In general lumbar and sacral vertebrae are commonly affected by prostate cancer while breast and lung cancer prefer thoracic vertebrae.

Clinically the metastatic disease is associated with considerable morbidity. Pain, pathologic fracture and spinal compression syndromes are most common. Hypercalcemia and marrow replacement may be responsible for other symptoms. Pulsating tumors are seen with hypernephroma, multiple myeloma and thyroid carcinomas. The radiographic examination reveals lesions that may be lytic, sclerotic (prostate carcinoma, breast carcinoma, lymphoma) or mixed (Fig. 6.15). Blastic/ sclerotic lesions are often painless and have lower incidence of pathological fractures.

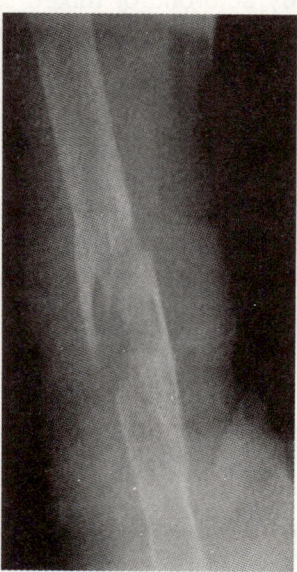

Fig 6.15. X-Ray showing pathologic fracture of shaft of femur

Laboratory examination reveals non specific findings. Alkaline phosphate is elevated in slightly over 50% cases. SGOT, LDH and uric acid levels are usually higher than normal. Those with prostate cancer may show raised serum acid phosphatase levels and serum Prostate Specific Antigen (PSA) levels.

Radiological investigations recommended for evaluation of single metastatic lesion of unknown origin is shown in Table 6.9. Complete blood counts including ESR, serum chemistry including liver function tests and urine and blood electrophoresis are other useful screening investigations.

Even with best investigating modalities, the site of

Table 6.9. Radiological evaluation of a single metastatic lesion of unknown origin

Plain X-rays in two planes of affected area

Technetium bone scan – to detect multiplicity of lesions and to look for more accessible site(s) for biopsy.

Radiographic studies to search for occult neoplasm

Chest x-ray

CT of chest: for occult lung cancer or associated metastatic disease in lungs

Ultrasound and/or CT of abdomen: To detect GIT malignancy, Renal cell carcinoma or lymphoma.

primary malignancy can be found only in less than 30% cases.

Treatment of metastatic bone disease aims to control pain and maintain independence and ambulation of the patient. Prophylactic internal fixation should be undertaken when more than 50% diaphyseal cortex is destroyed, when there is permeative destruction of the subtrochanteric femoral region, and, when there is persistent pain following irradiation. Intramedullary fixation/ prosthetic fixation with cementing followed by radiotherapy is the mainstay of pain alleviation. Radioactive strontium or phosphorus is also effective in relieving bone pains. The primary, when detected, should be treated according to the stage and recommended protocols.

Tumor like Conditions

1. Simple (Unicameral) Bone Cyst

is the most common cystic condition and the most frequent cause of pathological fracture in children. The lesion occurs most commonly in patients between 5 and 15 years of age and occurs most commonly in the proximal humerus. The lesion is characterised by cystic, symmetric expansion with thinning of involved cortices. Patients are asymptomatic till accidental discovery on x-rays or pathological fracture.

Radiographs show central expansile lytic area. The longitudinal extent of the lesion is more than the horizontal extent (Fig. 6.16). The lesion often appears trabeculated. Often, there is a bony fragment in the dependent part of cyst ("fallen fragment" or "fallen leaf" sign). With age, the lesion tends to move away from the physis. A

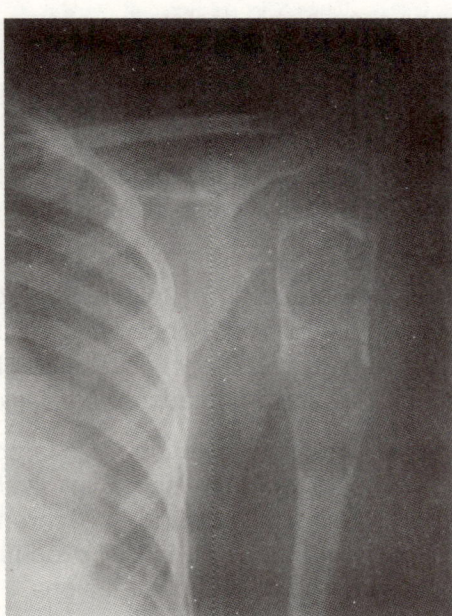

Fig. 6.16. Simple bone cyst involving the proximal humerus

bone cyst is called "active" when it is still attached to physis and inactive when it separates from the physis.

Histologically, the cyst has a thin fibrous lining, which contains giant cells, hemosiderin pigment and a few chronic inflammatory cells.

Treatment of simple bone cyst consists of aspiration followed by methyl prednisolone acetate (DEPO-MEDROL®) injection. Recalcitrant lesions are treated with curettage and bone grafting. Simple bone cysts may spontaneously resolve following a pathologic fracture.

2. Aneurysmal Bone Cyst (ABC)

ABC is a painful hemorrhagic reactive lesion that may be aggressive in its ability to destroy normal bone and extend into soft tissues. The lesion may arise in bone primarily or can occur secondarily in pre-existing lesions such as giant cell tumor, chondroblastoma, chondromyxoid fibroma, fibrous dysplasia or even osteosarcoma.

Three fourth of patients with ABC are less than 20 years old. ABC is usually subperiosteal in origin and seen in metaphysis. The femur is the most frequently affected site followed by tibia, pelvis and spine (esp. posterior elements). Patients present with swelling and pain of prolonged duration. Pathological fractures may occur. Radiographs demonstrate eccentric, lytic, expansile

area of destruction in the metaphysis with a thin rim of periosteal (reactive) new bone surrounding the lesion (Fig. 6.17).

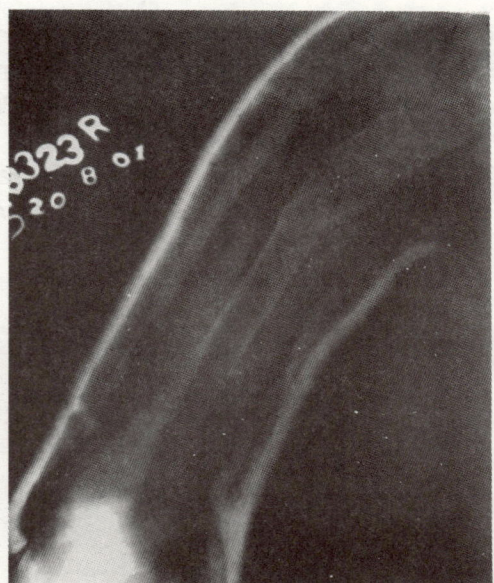

Fig. 6.17. Aneurysmal bone cyst of proximal humerus with pathological fracture.

Histologically the lesion shows cavernous blood filled spaces without an endothelial lining. There are thin strands of bone present in the fibrous tissue of the septae. Benign giant cells may be found in abundance. Carefully placed multiple biopsies should be taken to rule out the presence of other malignant neoplastic process.

Treatment is curettage and bone grafting. Radiation therapy can be employed for inaccessible sites such as spine. The radiation therapy, however, can convert this lesion into a sarcoma. Repeated embolization has been described for extremely large lesions to reduce hemorrhagic expansion.

Spontaneous resolution has been described in untreated ABC over 2-3 years. Surgical treatment or radiotherapy can hasten this process.

3) **Fibrous dysplasia**, 4) **Paget's Disease**, 5) **Neurofibromatosis**, and 6) **Gaucher's disease** have been described elsewhere.

Histiocytosis X

Histiocytosis X is a disease of the reticulo-endothelial system characterised by granulomatous lesions with histiocytic proliferation. The disease may manifest in a range from *eosinophilic granu-*

loma (usually involves a single bone and is self limiting), through *Hand-Schuller-Christian disease* (Disease of intermediate severity) to *Letterer-Siewe disease* (fulminant lethal form).

Eosinophilic granuloma is the most common form. It commonly occurs in adolescents. It commonly involves single and rarely multiple bones. Patients present with pain and swelling. Skull, spine (Fig. 6.18a,b), pelvis, ribs and long bones are the sites of predilection. Extra skeletal involvement does not occur.

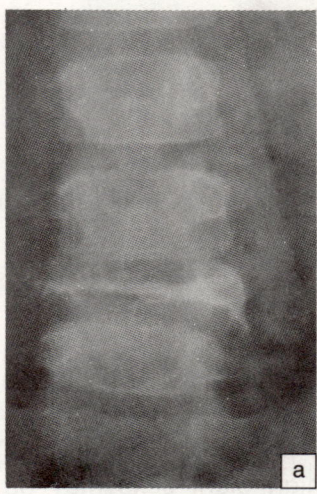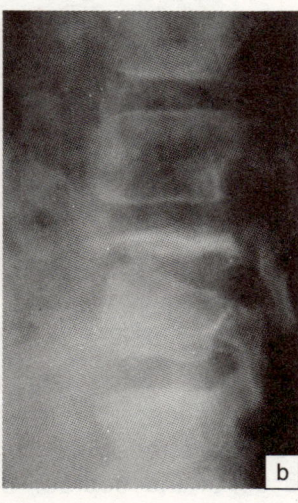

Fig.6.18a,b. X-rays showing Eosinophilic granuloma (Vertebra plana). Note maintenance of disc space.

Radiographs show highly destructive, often-expansile lesion with a well-defined margin. Cortex may be destroyed and soft tissue extension may occur.

Histologically, examination reveals proliferating histiocytes with indented nucleus and eosinophilic cytoplasm. Birbeck granules are seen in the cytoplasm.

Eosinophilic granuloma is a self-limiting condition and can often be kept under observation. Curettage and bone grafting can treat accessible lesions. Radiotherapy is used for inaccessible lesions.

Hand-Schuller-Christian disease is characterised by bone lesions as well as visceral involvement. It begins at 2–3 years of age and is a chronic form of histiocytosis with classic triad of exophthalmos, diabetes insipidus and lytic skull lesions.

Treatment consists of corticosteroid administration and radiation therapy for the skeletal lesions. Letterer Siewe is acute and generalised form of disease which occurs in infants. It has bone lesions similar to eosinophilic granuloma along with severe widespread visceral involvement characterised by lymphadenopathy, hepatosplenomegaly and pancytopenia. The disease is invariably fatal and no effective treatment is available. Antibiotics, chemotherapy, radiotherapy and corticosteroid can be used judiciously to provide symptomatic relief.

CHAPTER 7

Disorders of the Peripheral Nerves

Peripheral Nerve: Structure and Function

The peripheral nerve is composed of nerve fibres, blood vessels, and connective tissue.

An outermost epineural sheath encloses fascicles with the surrounding alveolar tissue called epineurium. Fascicles are nerve bundles covered with connective tissue called perineurium. These nerve bundles are in fact groups of axons coated with the fibrous tissue called endoneurium (Fig. 7.1). Nerve fibres or axons vary in diameter from 2 to 25 µm.

Three types of nerve fibres are known (Table 7.1).

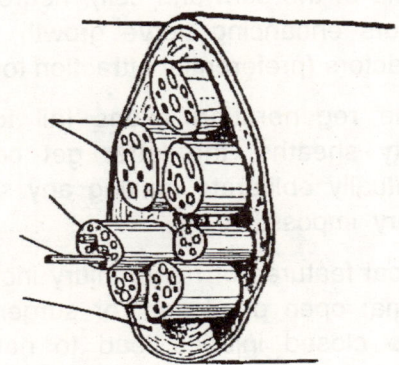

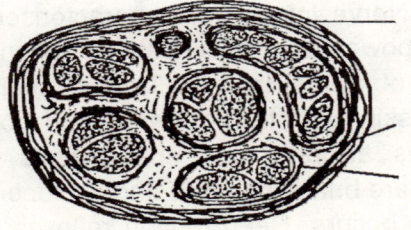

Fig. 7.1. Cut section of a peripheral nerve

Table 7.1. Types of nerve fibre

Characteristic	Type		
	A	B	C
Diameter (µm)	10–20	<3	<1.3
Myelination	Heavy	Inter-mediate	None
Speed	Fast	Medium	Slow
Conduction velocity	12–120m/s	3–15m/s	0.5–2m/s
Function	Touch, Pressure, Proprio-ception	Pregan-glionic auto-nomic	Postgan-glionic auto-nomic
Somatic	Motor	pain, touch	

Type A fibres are classically the fibres conducting the touch sensation; while type C (unmyelinated, slow conducting) fibres are associated with pain transmission. Type B fibres are found in the Autonomic Nervous System. Myelinated fibres have one schwann cell per axon while unmyelinated fibres can have one schwann cell for many axons.

Resting potential of the neuron is - 50 to - 80 mV, with the inside of the cell being negative relative to the external environment.

Nerve action potential transmits electrical potentials to other neurons or the muscle and results from an increase in cell membrane permeability to Na$^+$ in response to a stimulus.

Conduction in the myelinated fibres is rapid and is facilitated by gaps in between the schwann cells known as *nodes of Ranvier*. This type of conduction, jumping from one node to other, is called *saltatory conduction.*

Blood supply to a peripheral nerve is intrinsic as well as extrinsic. Extrinsic vessels run in loose connective tissue surrounding the nerve trunk (mesoneurium) while intrinsic blood supply is via the vascular plexuses in the epineurium, perineurium and endoneurium with extensive communication between the three plexuses.

Nerve Injury

Nerve injury has been classified by Seddon into three types:

1. **Neuropraxia** is a reversible conduction block, which occurs without any anatomical damage to the nerve. Neuropraxia is caused usually by nerve compression leading to local ischaemia. Tinel's sign is absent. Prognosis for recovery is good. Recovery does not follow any definite pattern. Recovery may occur within a few hours to a few days. Expectant treatment is adequate.

2. **Axonotmesis** is a more severe injury. The nerve fibres are interrupted within their sheaths but endoneurium remains intact. Spontaneous regeneration of axons occurs and prognosis for recovery is fair.

3. **Neurotmesis** is the most severe injury. Complete transection of nerve (including axons and endoneurium) occurs and the prognosis for recovery is poor.

Traction injury is a very severe form of injury which is essentially neurotmesis along with ischaemic changes resulting from injury to vessels. The damage may extend to extensive area with very poor prognosis for recovery. 8% elongation diminishes microcirculation while 15% elongation disrupts the axons.

Sunderland classified nerve injuries into five types. Type I to type V indicate increasing severity of injury (Table 7.2).

Biological Response to nerve injury

Peripheral nerve injury leads to the death of distal axon. The Wallerian degeneration of myelin is seen in distal axon as well as proximally to the node of Ranvier just proximal to the site of injury. Proximal axonal budding occurs after a delay of one month and if these newly grown axons enter the schwann sheaths, they continue to grow at the rate of 1mm/day (In children, the rate of regeneration can be as fast as 3–5mm/day). The proliferating axoplasms at the proximal end along with fibrous tissues form neuroma while the proliferating schwann cells at the distal stump along with fibrous tissue form the glioma.

Nerve regeneration is influenced by contact guidance (regenerating cell is attracted to the basal lamina of the schwann cell), neurotrophic factors (factors enhancing nerve growth) and neurotropic factors (preferential attraction towards nerves).

If the regenerating axons fail to enter distal empty sheaths, the latter get constricted and eventually obliterate making any subsequent recovery impossible.

Clinical features of nerve injury include history of trauma; open or closed, or surgery (iatrogenic). While closed injuries lead to neuropraxia, the open injuries are likely to be more severe, often neurotmesis. Nerve injuries are characterised by loss of motor power, and/ or sensations depending on the type of nerve injured. Trophic changes occur in the skin, soft tissues, nails and bones. Skin becomes atrophic and shiny, digits look tapered, nails are brittle; hair loss and osteoporosis of bones also occurs. Deep tendon reflexes may be diminished or absent. Painful neuromas form

Table 7.2. Nerve injury classification

Sunderland classification	Salient features		Seddon's classification
First Degree	-	Physiologic conduction block at the level of injury to the axon	
	-	No Wallerian degeneration	
	-	Recovery is spontaneous	
	-	Motor loss > Sensory loss	
	-	Prognosis good	
			Neuropraxia
Second Degree	-	Disruption of the axon present, endoneurium intact	
	-	Wallerian degeneration occurs	
	-	Recovery may occur	
	-	Neurologic deficit complete	
	-	Advancing Tinel's sign present	
	-	Prognosis is good	
			Axonotmesis
Third Degree	-	Disruption of axons and endoneurium (Perineurium intact)	
	-	Wallerian degeneration present	
	-	Recovery doubtful	
	-	Marked neurologic loss	
	-	Tinel's sign present	
	-	Complete recovery never seen	
Fourth Degree	-	Disruption of axon, endoneurium and part of perineurium	
	-	Wallerian degeneration severe	
	-	Retrograde degeneration-leading to neuronal death	
	-	Healing by scar tissue	
	-	No advancing Tinel's sign	
	-	Prognosis poor without surgery	
Fifth Degree	-	Nerve is completely transected	
	-	Chances of recovery remote	
			Neurotmesis

and may be exquisitely tender to touch. "*Stingers*" (or "*Burners*") are seen in football players and are due to neuropraxia from stretch injury to brachial plexus. Sympathetically Mediated Pain (SMP) or causalgia or Reflex Sympathetic Dystrophy commonly occurs after injury to some nerves e.g. infrapatellar branch of saphenous nerve at the knee. Tinel sign helps to localise the site up to which axonal regeneration has advanced. Percussion or placing a tuning fork on the course of nerve, proceeding proximally from distally indicates the extent of regeneration as the most distal area where the patient experiences tingling in the supply of that nerve with above mentioned manoeuvre. Tinel's sign progressing from proximal to distal (i.e. better elicited distally) indicates good recovery. Tinel's sign present only at the site of nerve injury implies neuroma formation.

Electrical Diagnostic Studies can help diagnose compression, transection or recovery of a nerve lesion and are often used to prognosticate or decide about the timing of intervention after the nerve injury.

1. Nerve conduction studies

Nerve conduction studies are used to measure nerve conduction velocity and latency and are most useful to diagnose nerve compression (increased latency and reduced velocity across the site of compression) and transection of the nerve. They can also be useful to distinguish nerve root lesions such as radiculopathy following prolapsed intervertebral disc from the peripheral nerve lesions. Measurement of sensory nerve conduction is more reliable than motor nerve conduction.

2. Erb's Reaction of Degeneration

Up to two weeks after injury, the muscle supplied by the injured nerve continues to respond (i.e. contract) to faradic current which stimulates the muscle via the distal nerve and motor end plate. However, after two weeks the muscle stops responding to faradic current and responds only to galvanic current which stimulates the muscle fibres directly. This sequence of events occurring after nerve injury is called Erb's reaction of degeneration.

3. Strength Duration curve

It is a test devised to measure excitability of muscle to electrical stimuli of progressively shorter duration. Two terms are defined in relation to this test.

a) *Rheobase* is that minimum amount of current which, subjected to the muscle for indefinite period, will provide a minimal muscle contraction.

b) *Chronaxie* is twice the rheobase.

The test is based on the observation that in a normal muscle, except for currents of very short duration (where higher voltage is required), the same amplitude of the current produces muscle contraction at nearly all durations of current. In denervated muscles, however, much higher voltages are required, as the pulse duration is reduced, to produce minimal contraction.

Strength duration curve is a very reliable indicator of denervation and begins to rise within a few days after denervation. Strength duration curve shows a shift to the right with denervation. Subsequent reinnervation is evident by shift of the curve to the left towards the normal curve pattern.

A normal S.D. curve at the end of one week suggests that the nerve lesion is neuropraxia.

The normal, denervation and partial innervation patterns on a strength duration curve are shown in Fig. 7.2.

4. Electromyography (EMG)

Electrical activity of contracting muscle can be

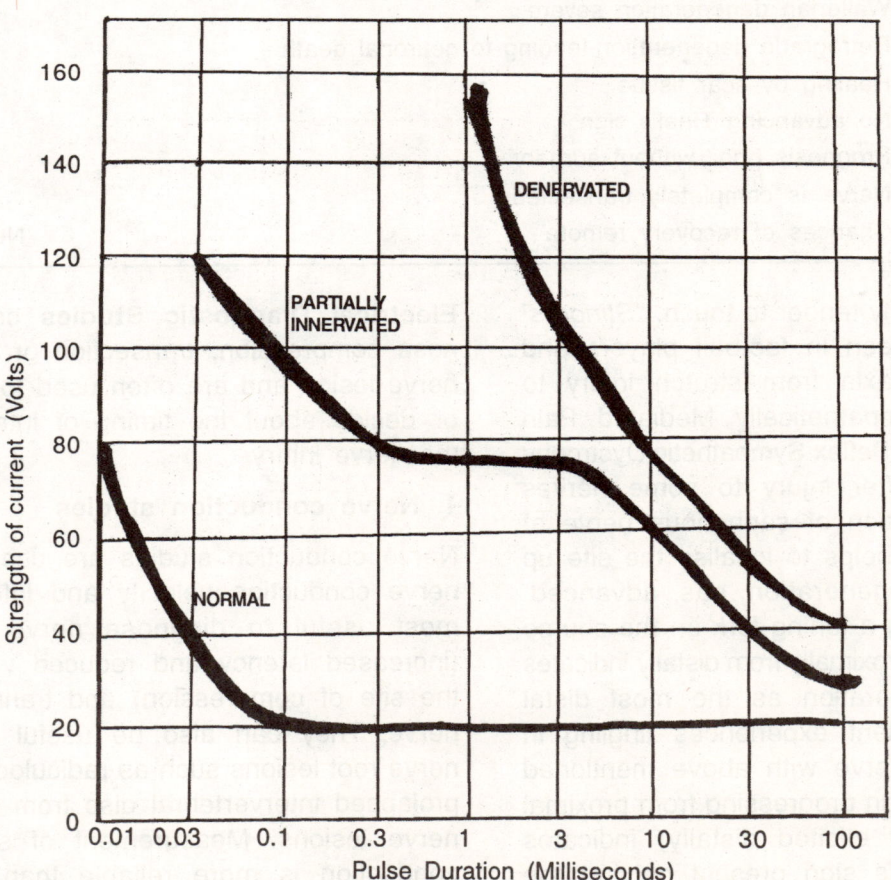

Fig. 7.2. Strength Duration curves showing denervated, partially innervated and normal patterns

picked up and recorded by special muscle electrodes. This test, called electromyography (EMG), shows abnormality within 2–3 weeks of denervation. EMG pattern in denervated muscles shows fibrillation potentials which are biphasic, low voltage potentials of short duration. Recovering muscles show complex polyphasic waves, voluntary action potentials and interference pattern of the normal muscle. EMG can be used to differentiate the spinal (segmental) lesions from the peripheral nerve lesions depending on which myotomes are involved.

Treatment of Injury

General treatment consists of prevention of injury, splintage, and passive physiotherapy to avoid stiffness and muscle stimulation by (galvanic) electric currents to avoid wasting.

Expectant treatment is required when neuropraxia is suspected. Closed nerve injuries associated with the closed fractures are best treated expectantly. Only when the nerve shows no signs of recovery at the end of 6 weeks following injury should the electrical studies be undertaken to plan further treatment.

Types of Nerve Repair

1. *Direct muscular neurotization* implies embedding the proximal stump of the cut nerve directly into the muscle. This method is rarely used.

2. *Neurotization* is often used in brachial plexus injuries in cases with root avulsions when there is practically no proximal stump. The intercostal nerves are transected and anastomosed to the distal stump of the cut nerve.

3. *Epineural repair* is done by apposing the nerve ends and suturing the circumferential epineurium. Correct orientation of the nerve ends is extremely important for optimum regeneration. Malalignment of the nerve ends will result in sensory axons growing into motor axon sheaths of distal nerve end and vice versa.

4. *Group Fascicular repair* is done by apposing the respective groups of fascicles and suturing their circumferential perineurium. Theoretically, this type of repair ensures better coaptation of fascicles with better regeneration. However, expensive microscope and microsurgical instruments as well as expertise is required to perform this type of repair.

Timing of Nerve Repair

Primary repair Repair immediately after injury is done in cases where wound exploration is anyway being done or associated fractures or injuries to other structures need to be repaired. However, the local wound bed must be healthy for successful outcome otherwise cut nerve ends are just tagged to soft tissues with marking sutures to avoid retraction and enable easy identification at the time of subsequent repair.

Delayed Primary repair A repair done after 2 weeks of injury is called delayed primary repair. The nerve ends at this time are easy to handle as the epineurium becomes thick and fibrosed (unlike after acute injury when it is friable, tears easily and does not hold sutures well). The local wound heals by this time and host bed becomes favourable with minimal risk of infection. Delayed primary repair is also done when the patient has to be referred elsewhere for lack of adequate facilities and/or expertise.

Secondary Repair Late repair is done when the local conditions are not conducive (such as presence of infected wound), the required expertise is not available or the surgery is not possible earlier because of poor general condition of the patient. The neuroma and gliomas are well formed by this time and their excision, along with retraction of cut nerve ends often leaves a gap in the nerves.

The gap in the nerve ends can be overcome partly by positioning of neighbouring joints (e.g. extension at hip and flexion at knee for the sciatic nerve, flexion at elbow and wrist for median nerve), transposition of nerve (e.g. anterior transposition of the ulnar nerve), sacrifice of (articular) branches and mobilisation of nerves, neurotization, nerve grafting or by shortening of bones. Sural, saphenous and medial cutaneous nerve of the forearm are some of the examples of donor nerves for nerve grafting.

Nerve grafting, wherever possible, should be preferred to end to end anastomosis of a nerve under tension across a gap. The latter has been shown to compromise microcirculation to the nerve and incite severe intraneural scarring which constricts the regenerating axons.

Factors affecting results after nerve repair

1. *Type of injury* The more proximal the injury, the worse is the recovery after the nerve repair.

2. *Type of nerve* Purely sensory or motor nerves recover better than mixed nerve. Radial nerve repair shows consistently better results than ulnar or median nerve.

3. *Timing of repair* Early repairs give better results. If the repair is delayed by more than a few months, the end organs may start degenerating and compromise the result. Generally, ulnar and median nerve repairs seldom give good results if done one year after the injury whereas radial nerve can be repaired up to 18 months after injury with satisfactory outcome. This period is often referred to as the critical period, which varies for different nerves.

4. *Size of the gap* between nerve ends/Tension at the suture line The more the gap between the nerve ends, the poorer is the quality of recovery after nerve repair. The greater the tension at the suture line, worse is the nerve regeneration.

5. *The condition of the host bed* Extensive scarring or infection of the host bed precludes satisfactory recovery after the nerve repair.

6. *Vascularity of the nerves* Extensive stripping of the nerves from their bed to mobilise them deprives them of their vascularity and mars the results after nerve repair.

Reconstruction after Failed Nerve Regeneration

Several salvage procedures are available to obtain optimum function and to reduce disability following the failure of nerve to regenerate after repair. These procedures include muscle transfer (e.g. Trapezius transfer for deltoid paralysis), tendon transfers (e.g. for foot drop), capsulodesis (e.g. Zancolli's procedure for ulnar n. palsy), arthrodesis (e.g. for flail foot or abductor paralysis of shoulder) or even amputation (for an anaesthetic and useless limb after high sciatic nerve palsy).

Regional Nerve injuries

1. Brachial Plexus Injuries The brachial plexus injuries can occur during birth or during the adulthood. The formation of the brachial plexus is given in Fig. 7.3. Leffert classification of brachial plexus injuries is shown in Table 7.3.

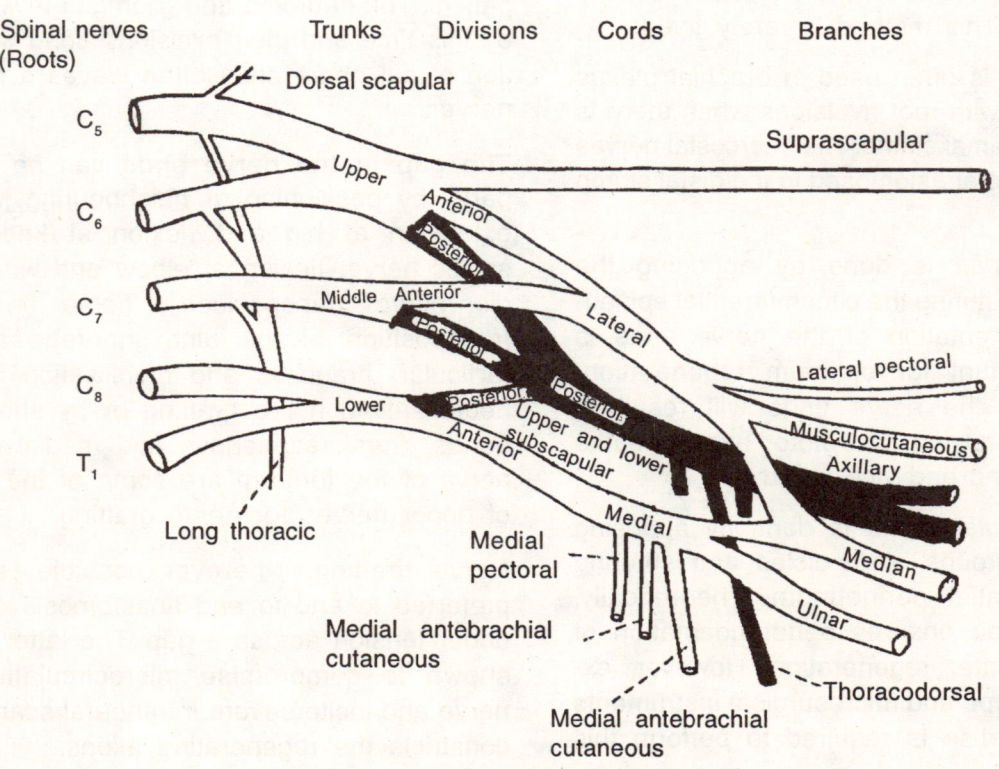

Fig. 7.3. Formation of the brachial plexus

Table 7.3. Leffert classification of Brachial Plexus Injuries

1. Open injuries of the brachial plexus
2. Closed (traction) injuries of the brachial plexus
   a) Supraclavicular injuries
      i) Supraganglionic
      ii) Infraganglionic
   b) Infraclavicular injuries
   c) Post anaesthetic palsy
3. Radiation injury to the brachial plexus
4. Obstetric palsy

(a) Brachial Plexus Injuries at Birth

Brachial plexus injuries occur during difficult deliveries because of the stretch most commonly caused by an increase in the angle between the neck and the shoulder due to forcible lateral flexion of the head to the opposite side.

Erb's Palsy occurs when the fifth and the sixth cervical nerve roots or their derivatives are involved. These patients have paralysis of abductors and external rotators of the shoulder and the flexors of the elbow. The classical attitude of the arms is one of adduction and internal rotation at shoulder and extension at the elbow giving typical *"policeman accepting tip"* appearance. Fingers and wrist have normal function. Usually the prognosis is good and full recovery can be expected. Prevention of contractures by splintage and passive stretching is the mainstay of treatment. Untreated cases tend to develop adduction and internal rotation deformity at the shoulder. Treatment of the neglected cases aims at correction of these deformities by release/lengthening of the subscapularis followed by mobilisation using stretching.

Klumpke's Palsy occurs when eighth cervical and the first dorsal nerve roots are affected. These patients have the paralysis of flexors of the wrist and fingers and intrinsic muscles of hand. The classical attitude is of the extension at the wrist and clawing of the fingers. Shoulder and elbow have normal function. Horner's syndrome may complicate the clinical picture when cervical sympathetic fibres are also damaged. The prognosis for recovery in this type of paralysis is not good and the recovery is only partial in most cases. Splintage and passive stretching are important while waiting for recovery. Tendon transfers may be required for residual disabilities.

Complete paralysis of the entire arm involving all components of the brachial plexus may occur rarely and the prognosis in these cases is extremely poor.

(b) Brachial Plexus Injuries in Adulthood

Brachial plexus injuries in adult occur commonly during motor vehicular accidents, gunshot injuries and by penetrating wounds to the neck. The injuries may vary in severity and often are associated with skeletal injuries such as fracture of the clavicle or humerus or dislocation of the shoulder joint. Fractures of transverse process of cervical vertebra may be present. It is important to differentiate between preganglionic (nerve root avulsion or injury) and postganglionic lesions as the prognosis is poor in the former.

In general, presence of Horner's syndrome, paralysis of rhomboids and serratus anterior, preservation of triple reaction, demonstration of pseudomeningocele on myelography and dural ectasia on MRI suggest pre-ganglionic lesions.

The surgical treatment of brachial plexus injuries is being undertaken increasingly and progressively better results are being reported. Direct repair of transected neural tissue or rarely neurotization is required during exploration. The associated skeletal injuries should be treated on their merits.

2. Axillary Nerve (C_5, C_6)

Axillary nerve is damaged following shoulder dislocation, fracture of surgical neck of humerus or during surgery on the shoulder (When operating on rotator cuff it is important that the split in the deltoid should not extend more than 5 cm distal to the angle of acromion to avoid injury to the axillary nerve).

Clinically the patient has paralysis of abduction and sensory loss over the *"regimental badge"* area.

The treatment is expectant as most cases recover with time. If the recovery does not occur, the abduction can be restored by the trapezius muscle transfer or the shoulder arthrodesis when the scapulothoracic muscles can abduct the stabilised shoulder at the scapulothoracic joint.

3. Radial Nerve (C_6, C_7, C_8, T_1)

Radial nerve can be injured in the axilla, in the spiral groove of the humerus or at the elbow (where its posterior interosseous branch is commonly injured).

Injury to the radial nerve in the axilla results from the pressure due to crutch ("crutch" palsy) or the back of the chair (*"Saturday night palsy"*) or because of penetrating injuries or gunshots. All the muscles acting at elbow, wrist and fingers supplied by the radial nerve are paralysed. Thus, triceps is paralysed; there is wrist drop and inability to extend metacarpophalangeal joints of fingers and metacarpophalangeal and interphalangeal joints of the thumb. In addition, there is sensory loss in the autonomous area of radial nerve supply on the dorsum of the first web space.

Radial nerve injury in **Spiral groove** results from the fractures of the humerus at this level. All the features enumerated above are present except that innervation to part of the triceps (long head) escapes injury.

Radial nerve injury at the **elbow** usually involves posterior interosseous nerve (wholly motor branch of radial nerve). The injury at this level is caused by radial head dislocations (e.g. in Monteggia # dislocation), during surgical procedures (e.g. radial head excision) or penetrating or gunshot wounds. There is no sensory loss and some power of wrist extension is preserved as extensor carpi radialis longus muscle escapes injury. Also preserved is the power of brachioradialis muscle, which can be tested by asking patient to flex the elbow against resistance with forearm in mid prone position.

Injury to superficial radial nerve (wholly sensory branch of radial nerve) occurs during surgical exposure of mid and distal forearm and by the penetrating injuries.

Treatment of the radial nerve palsy depends on the site and the type of the lesion. Closed lesions are best managed by expectant treatment. When indicated (e.g. open injuries, radial nerve palsy appearing for the first time after closed manipulation, inability to show signs of recovery after 6–8 weeks), nerve injuries proximal to the elbow can be explored and repaired and good results can be expected. Radial nerve is almost purely motor and repairs done even 18 months after the injury have been known to result in complete recovery. Radial nerve lesions distal to elbow are difficult to repair as the posterior interosseous nerve is deep seated and gaps in the nerve are difficult to overcome due to limited possible mobilisation of the nerve. The sensory branch, if injured, leads to minimal disability and is usually ignored.

If the nerve cannot be repaired for some reason or does not recover after repair, tendon transfer can be undertaken to restore function. Modified "Jones' transfer", the most commonly performed procedure for radial nerve palsy, is depicted in Table 7.4.

4. Median Nerve ($C_{6,7,8}$, T_1)

Median nerve is rarely injured in forearm due to its deep situation except in cases of volkmann's ischaemic contracture. Direct injury to the nerve occurs most commonly at the wrist and at the elbow.

Median nerve is injured at the wrist commonly due to lacerations or penetrating wounds or due to skeletal injuries such as the fractures of the distal radius or dislocation of the lunate. The injury at this level results in the sensory loss over the lateral three and half digits and the corresponding area of the palm anteriorly and distal two thirds of the same digits on the posterior aspect. Trophic changes occur in these digits.

The motor paralysis involves thenar muscles

Table 7.4. Modified Jones' transfer for radial nerve palsy

Motor	Recipient	Function
Pronator teres	Extensor carpi radialis brevis	Wrist extension
Flexor carpi ulnaris	Extensor digitorum	MCP joints extension
Palmaris longus	Re-routed extensor pollicis longus	Extension and abduction of thumb

though the nerve supply to the flexor pollicis brevis and opponens pollicis is variable and these muscles may not always be paralysed. Thenar eminence appears wasted. *"Ape thumb"* may be seen. The paralysis of abductor pollicis brevis can be tested by active abduction of thumb against resistance or by asking the patient to abduct the thumb and touch examiner's pen (*Pen Test*). The injury at the elbow level occurs due to penetrating injuries or by skeletal trauma such as elbow dislocation or supracondylar fracture of the humerus or due to iatrogenic causes as due to injury by kirschner wires passed to stabilise the supracondylar fracture of the humerus. The sensory loss in these cases is similar to a more distal injury.

The muscles paralysed include flexor digitorum superficialis and the lateral half of flexor digitorum profundus, flexor carpi radialis, palmaris longus and flexor pollicis longus. Since the index finger loses both its flexors a *"pointing index"* is seen.

Interestingly, the closed injuries to median nerve at the elbow often involve only the anterior interosseous nerve component (much the same way as only the lateral popliteal nerve component is injured in sciatic nerve injury). Consequently one may see paralysis of flexor pollicis longus, flexor digitorum profundus and pronator quadratus only.

Treatment of median nerve injury is important because it supplies sensations to a very important area of hand concerned with grasping objects. Nerve should be explored and repaired when neurotmesis is expected or the nerve is not showing any signs of recovery on waiting. Useful recovery can be expected after repair. Opponensplasty can be done for residual opponens paralysis.

5. Ulnar Nerve (C_8, T_1)

Ulnar nerve is commonly injured at the wrist or elbow.

At the **wrist** the nerve is commonly injured due to cut injuries. The injury at the level of wrist results in sensory loss over ulnar one and a half fingers and corresponding area of the palm. Trophic changes commonly occur in these fingers and medial part of the palm.

The muscles paralysed include hypothenar muscles,

adductor pollicis, interossei and medial two lumbricals. Clinically, this is evident by clawing (hyperextension at the metacarpophalangeal joints (due to unopposed action of EDL and flexion at the interphalangeal joints due to unopposed action of long flexors of the little and ring fingers).

This deformity is known as *"intrinsic minus"* deformity. There is wasting of interossei seen as appearance of hollows between metacarpals on the dorsum of hand. Wasting of the first dorsal interosseous is particularly conspicuous. The transverse metacarpal arch is lost and there is hyperextension of the MCP joint of the thumb.

Adductor pollicis is tested by *"Froment Sign"* implying that when patient is asked to hold lightly onto a piece of paper between his index finger and thumb, interphalangeal joint of thumb gets flexed due to compensatory over-activity of flexor pollicis longus (as the thumb itself is incapable of adequate adduction due to weak adductor pollicis).

A card held between the fingers can be easily removed due to weak interossei (*Card Test*).

"Igawa Test" also tests interossei by asking patient to adduct and abduct fingers in a horizontal plane.

The injury to ulnar nerve at the elbow occurs commonly following skeletal trauma such as fractures of medial epicondyle, elbow dislocation, fractures of the supracondylar region of the humerus or tardy ulnar palsy following a longstanding cubitus valgus deformity.

The sensory loss in these cases is similar to a more distal injury. The additional muscles paralysed include flexor carpi ulnaris and flexor digitorum profundus (medial half). Since FDP is paralysed, it does not aggravate the clawing deformity. The clawing deformity seen with proximal lesion, therefore, is less severe than that seen with more distal lesion – this is called *"Ulnar Paradox"*.

The signs of ulnar nerve palsy are shown in Table 7.5.

Treatment of ulnar nerve injury comprises of exploration and repair. Delay compromises the degree and quality of recovery. In cases of tardy ulnar nerve palsy, only anterior transposition of the nerve is sufficient. If the median nerve is intact, useful hand function is preserved (except

Table 7.5. Signs of ulnar nerve palsy

Clawing of ring and little fingers	Duchenne's Sign
Correction of clawing by stabilising the MCP joint in flexion passively	Bouvier-Beevor Sign
Inability to abduct the ring finger	Pitres-Testud Sign
Hyperextension of MCP joint of thumb	Jeanne's Sign
Loss of transverse metacarpal arch	Masse's Sign
Loss of thumb adduction (key pinch)	Froment's Sign; Bunnel's 'O' Sign
Inability to adduct the little finger	Wartenberg Sign
Loss of sensibility on the volar aspect of ulnar one and a half fingers	
Inability to flex the DIP joint of the ring and little fingers	Pollock's Sign♣
Partial loss of wrist flexion♣	
Loss of sensations over dorsoulnar aspect of the palm and dorsal side of little finger♣	

♣ Implies the sign seen only in high ulnar nerve palsy

fine movements as ulnar nerve is the *Musician's Nerve*) even if ulnar nerve does not recover. A plethora of treatment options are available to treat clawing of the fingers (including Zancolli's capsuloplasty, Dermadesis, tendon transfers etc) and loss of adduction of the thumb (tendon transfers).

6. Sciatic Nerve ($L_{4,5}$, $S_{1,2}$)

Sciatic nerve is formed by the anterior and posterior divisions of the ventral primary rami of L_4–S_2 nerve roots from the lumbosacral plexus (Fig. 7.4). Sciatic nerve is injured following skeletal trauma such as posterior dislocation of the hip, during surgery (for pelvis fractures or during posterior approach for hip surgery), gunshot or penetrating injury.

Sensory loss following sciatic nerve injury occurs over the entire limb distal to the knee. The muscles paralysed are hamstrings and all the muscles distal to the knee. Incomplete lesions of sciatic nerve often involve only common peroneal component of the nerve.

Treatment of sciatic nerve injury is exploration and repair. The results of the nerve repair are poor and often the common peroneal component does not recover. If sensations recover the patient is spared the agony of recurrent trophic ulcers with osteomyelitis of the foot bones and can be given a caliper for motor paralysis. How-

ever, if the sensations do not recover the patient may eventually need below knee amputation.

7. Common Peroneal Nerve ($L_{4,5}$, $S_{1,2}$)

Common peroneal nerve is most commonly injured by compression or stretching. Compression occurs most commonly at the neck of fibula where the nerve winds around to enter the leg through the peroneus longus muscle. Compression occurs due to tight plaster, tight bandage or by direct pressure on fibular neck when the extremity is externally rotated in an unconscious patient.

Stretching occurs when the knee is forcefully adducted following trauma or while correcting genu valgum deformity, skin traction or during correction of knee flexion deformity.

Direct injury to the nerve occurs by impalement of nerve by steinmann pin passed for upper tibial skeletal traction, following fracture of the neck of fibula or by cut injuries.

Clinically, the sensory loss extends over anterior and lateral half of the leg and dorsum of the foot and toes. The muscles paralysed are those of the anterior and the peroneal compartments. *"Foot drop"* and equino-varus deformity result.

Treatment consists of exploration and repair of the nerve if transection is suspected. The prognosis for recovery is poor. If the recovery does not occur, tibialis posterior transfer (either subcu-

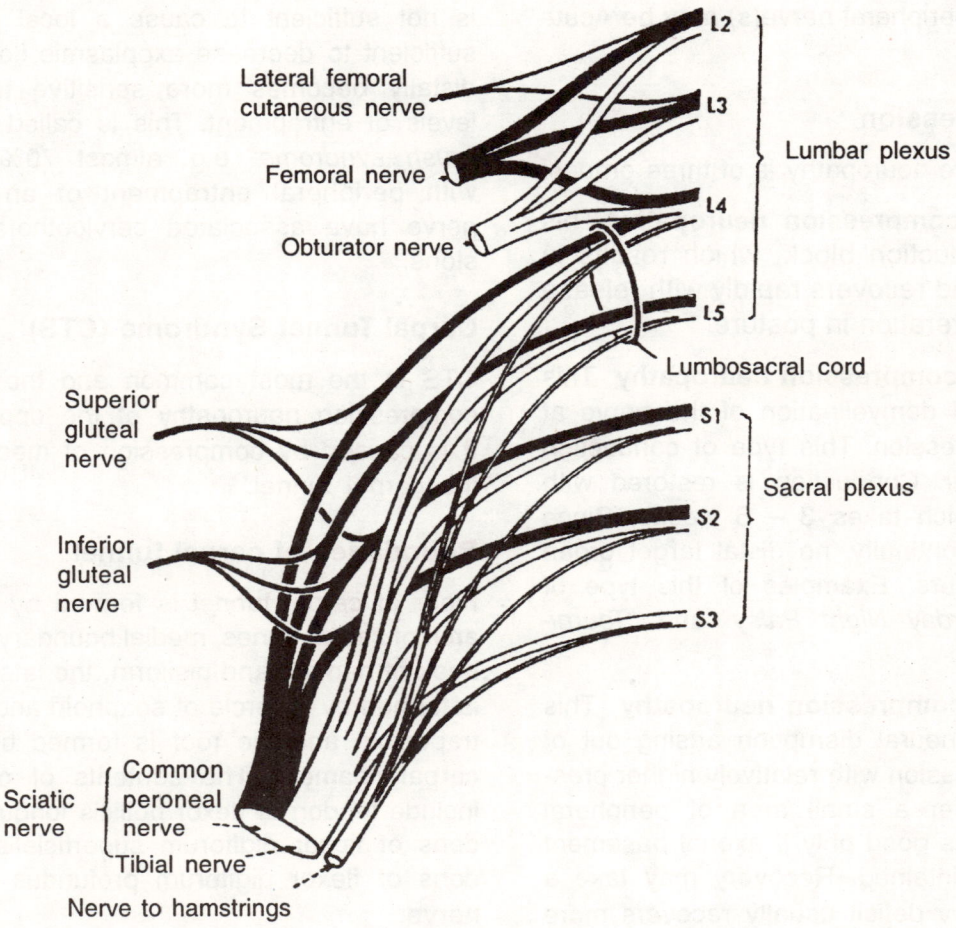

Fig. 7.4. Formation of Lumbosacral plexus

Labels in figure: Lateral femoral cutaneous nerve, Femoral nerve, Obturator nerve, Superior gluteal nerve, Inferior gluteal nerve, Sciatic nerve, Common peroneal nerve, Tibial nerve, Nerve to hamstrings, L2, L3, L4, L5, Lumbar plexus, Lumbosacral cord, S1, S2, S3, Sacral plexus

taneously or across the interosseous membrane) to dorsum of foot can be done to treat foot drop. However, often the transfer acts only as tenodesis and results are not very good. The patient has to wear below knee caliper for foot drop.

The surgical intervention is of no use in traction injury and tendon transfer or below knee caliper is required.

8. Posterior Tibial Nerve (Medial Popliteal Nerve) ($L_{4,5}$, $S_{1,2,3}$)

Posterior tibial nerve is injured by penetrating injuries or gunshot wounds. Clinically, the sensory loss extends to sole and distal calf. Trophic ulcers on the sole are common. The paralysed muscles include gastrocnemius, soleus, flexors of toes and intrinsic muscles. The calf is wasted and the gait is peg like due to paralysis of triceps surae. The toes get clawed due to the unopposed action of toe extensors, which are supplied by the common peroneal nerve.

Treatment consists of exploration and repair of the nerve. The prognosis for recovery is not good and the patient often needs below knee caliper. Recurrent trophic ulcers remain the main cause of morbidity and may necessitate below knee amputation.

Peripheral Compression Neuropathies

Compression neuropathies commonly occur when nerves are located superficially with minimal surrounding connective tissue, either close to bone or in a fibro-osseous tunnel. Nerve fibres with large closely packed fascicles and little epineural tissue are more susceptible to compression. Some systemic conditions increase the susceptibility to peripheral compressive neuropathies. The examples of these conditions are pregnancy, acromegaly, diabetes, systemic lupus erythematosus, myxedema, chronic renal failure, Rheumatoid arthritis, vitamin B6 deficiency and chronic demyelinating inflammatory polyneuropathy.

Compression of peripheral nerve(s) may be Acute or Chronic.

1. Acute Compression

Acute compressive neuropathy is of three grades:

a) Neuropraxic compression neuropathy This is transient conduction block, which results in paraesthesiae and recovers rapidly with release of pressure or alteration in posture.

b) Axonotmesic compression neuropathy This results from focal demyelination of the nerve at the site of compression. This type of conduction block lasts longer. Conduction is restored with remyelination, which takes 3 – 6 weeks. Since there is axonal continuity, no distal target organ degeneration occurs. Examples of this type of lesion are *"Saturday Night Palsy"* and *"Tourniquet Palsy"*.

c) Neurotmesic compression neuropathy This results from intraneural disruption arising out of prolonged compression with relatively higher pressures exerted over a small area of peripheral nerve. Recovery is good only if axonal basement membrane is maintained. Recovery may take a long time. Sensory deficit usually recovers more rapidly than motor deficit.

Tourniquet palsies can be avoided by tying the tourniquet over the portion with greater soft tissues; cotton padding should always be applied beneath the tourniquet. Tourniquet pressure should not be more 50 mm above the systolic pressure for the upper limb and more than twice above the systolic pressure for the lower limb; the pressure of tourniquet should be periodically checked and the tourniquet time should not exceed two hours in the lower limb and one hour in the upper limb.

2. Chronic compression neuropathies are caused by peripheral nerve entrapment. Myelinated fibres are more susceptible than unmyelinated. Demyelination due to compression is responsible for decreased conduction velocity. In addition, vascular factors (due to reduction of blood flow by compression) result in reduced efficacy of axon transport system, Na^+ / K^+ membrane pump and maintenance of axonal cell membrane.

It has been shown that when compressive force is not sufficient to cause a local injury but is sufficient to decrease axoplasmic flow, the nerve distally becomes more sensitive to subclinical levels of entrapment. This is called *"The double crush syndrome"* e.g. almost 70% of patients with peripheral entrapment of an upper limb nerve have associated cervicothoracic root lesions.

Carpal Tunnel Syndrome (CTS)

CTS is the most common and the best known compression neuropathy of the upper extremity. It is caused by compression of median nerve in the carpal tunnel.

Boundaries of carpal tunnel

Floor of carpal tunnel is formed by the concave arch of carpal bones, medial boundary is formed by hook of hamate and pisiform, the lateral boundary is formed by tubercle of scaphoid and the ridge of trapezium and the roof is formed by transverse carpal ligament. The contents of carpal tunnel include tendon of flexor pollicis longus, (four) tendons of flexor digitorum superficialis, (four) tendons of flexor digitorum profundus and median nerve.

The causes/risk factors for CTS are enumerated in Table 7.6.

Clinically, the patients have history of pain and paraesthesiae in thumb, index and middle fingers. Pain classically becomes severe at night and causes interruption of sleep; the pain may also aggravate with repetitive use. CTS may often be bilateral.

Table 7.6. Causes/Risk factors for Carpal Tunnel Syndrome

Intrinsic Factors	Other factors
Female sex	Ganglion in the wrist
Pregnancy	Anomalous tendons and muscles
Rheumatoid Arthritis	Osteoarthritis of carpal bones
Diabetes Mellitus	Infection
Myxedema	Haemorrhage in tunnel
Acromegaly	Occupational exposure to vibration
Hemodialysis	
Amyloidosis	

Examination reveals wasting of thenar eminence and loss of thumb abduction (*"Simian Hand"*) in severe cases. Sensory hypoesthesia may involve the first three digits. Vibratory test is more sensitive as compared to pinprick and two-point discrimination. Trophic changes may occur in involved digits.

Diagnosis

A) Provocative Tests include i) positive Tinel's sign at the wrist; ii) Phalen's test; iii) Tourniquet test; iv) Flick test, and v) Tethered median nerve stress test.

Phalen's Test Maximal wrist flexion for one minute produces numbness or paraesthesiae.

Tourniquet test Occlusion of blood flow by pneumatic cuff leads to paraesthesiae in the median nerve distribution.

Flick test Patient flicks or shakes the symptomatic hand in an attempt to alleviate symptoms.

Tethered median nerve test Hyperextension at distal interphalangeal joint with wrist supinated produces volar forearm pain.

B) Electrodiagnosis

Electrical studies reveal focal slowing of median nerve conduction at the wrist and increased latency. Electromyography may show fibrillation potentials in the median nerve innervated muscles of the hand. Motor studies are less sensitive than sensory.

C) Carpal Tunnel Injection

In questionable cases, an injection of a steroid preparation can be given into the carpal tunnel. Relief in pain with injection even for a few days gives diagnostic information regarding median nerve compression. Relief with injection indicates good prognosis after surgery.

Treatment

Conservative treatment can be tried in patients with mild to moderate symptoms and in patients where CTS is associated with pregnancy or fluid retention. Anti-inflammatory drugs (NSAIDs) can be given to control pain and inflammation in cases with synovitis while diuretics can ease fluid retention. Steroidal injections given at the level of distal wrist crease in line with little finger and with needle directed at 45 degrees distally and radially can relieve the symptoms. Injection should never be given in the substance of the nerve.

Splints to limit the wrist movements can help in CTS. Splints should be worn for most of the day and the entire night.

Underlying diseases such as hypothyroidism should be treated.

Surgical Treatment

Median nerve decompression has to be undertaken in recalcitrant cases. Transverse carpal ligament is divided to relieve the compression and a small segment excised from it.

Neurolysis and epineurectomy is done in longstanding cases associated with atrophy of thenar muscles and thickened epineurium.

Tenosynovectomy is done when the synovium is hypertrophied and leading to median nerve compression as in rheumatoid arthritis.

Endoscopic Carpal Tunnel Release (ECTR) is now in vogue to release transverse carpal ligament endoscopically as a minimally invasive procedure.

Other Sites of Median Nerve Compresssion are at the shoulder girdle (*Saturday night palsy, honeymoon palsy*), elbow (*Pronator teres syndrome, Compression by ligament of Struthers, Anterior interosseous nerve syndrome*) and palm (entrapment of digital nerves).

Ulnar Nerve Compression

Ulnar nerve compression occurs most commonly at the elbow. Ulnar nerve can be compressed at the following sites around the elbow:

1. From the arcade of Struthers to the area of medial epicondyle – most common site

2. At or just proximal to medial epicondyle

3. The epicondylar or olecranon groove.

4. Between the two heads of flexor carpi ulnaris

Clinically, the compression is characterised by pain in the medial elbow and proximal forearm and sensory disturbance in ring and the little finger. Ring and the little fingers may show clawing.

Electrical studies help in localising the lesion.

Treatment Conservative treatment involves trial of splinting with elbow flexed about 45 degrees. Failure of conservative treatment warrants surgical treatment, which involves decompression in situ, or anterior transposition of the ulnar nerve.

Other Sites of Ulnar Nerve Compression include shoulder and axilla (Saturday night palsy) and at the wrist (in the Guyon's canal or distally).

Chieralgia Paraesthetica is caused by entrapment of superficial radial nerve proximal to wrist.

Tarsal Tunnel Syndrome

It is analogous to the carpal tunnel syndrome. The posterior tibial nerve gets compressed beneath the flexor retinaculum (laciniate ligament). The causes of tarsal tunnel syndrome may be outside the canal (displaced distal tibial, talar and calcaneal fractures, ganglion / tenosynovitis of adjacent tendon sheath or rheumatoid arthritis) or inside the canal (varicosities, neural tumour or perineural fibrosis).

Clinically the patient complains of burning pain in the plantar aspect of the foot and toes. Paraesthesiae are worse at night and may be partly relieved by hanging the foot in dependent position.

Treatment Conservative treatment includes local steroid injection, ankle immobilisation in night splint (for 6–8 weeks), anti inflammatory drugs and wide, cushioned and comfortable shoes.

Recalcitrant cases should be treated by surgical decompression of the nerve involving division of flexor retinaculum.

Anterior Tarsal Tunnel Syndrome is caused by entrapment of the deep peroneal nerve beneath the inferior extensor retinaculum.

Meralgia Paraesthetica is caused by compression of lateral femoral cutaneous nerve (L_2–L_3) beneath the inguinal ligament. Clinically, the patients experience pain, tingling or numbness over the cutaneous distribution of the nerve. The common causes are tight fitting brace or corset, tight belt, pagers, obesity and diabetes mellitus. The symptoms often recover spontaneously. If not, the treatment involves local injection of steroid and local anaesthetic agent 1 inch distal and medial to anterior superior iliac spine. Surgical treatment is rarely required. It consists of decompressing the nerve by dividing the portion of inguinal ligament overlying the nerve.

Leprosy is the commonest cause of peripheral neuropathy in India.

Peripheral nerves are involved by the tuberculoid form of leprosy. Leprosy affects the nerves in superficial locations such as ulnar nerve at elbow, superficial radial nerve, lateral popliteal nerve, greater auricular nerve etc. Musculocutaneous and posterior tibial nerves are least often involved.

Clinically the patients present with hypoesthesia with or without motor dysfunction characteristic of the involved nerve. The affected nerves are thickened on palpation. Involvement of the nerves of lower limb leads to development of severe and resistant trophic ulcers.

Treatment is mainly antileprosy drugs namely dapsone and rifampicin. Good general care of anaesthetic skin and trophic ulcers should be taken. Tendon transfers and /or calipers are often required for functional deficits such as foot drop.

Nerve deficits due to leprosy are treated by multi-drug therapy and corticosteroids.

Sometimes the nerves may be involved acutely in leprosy with formation of nerve abscesses and oedema of nerves leading to acute compressive neuropathy due to compression in fibro-osseous tunnel. Ulnar nerve is most commonly involved. These cases should be taken up for urgent surgical intervention in the form of decompression of nerve and drainage of nerve abscess to contain the damage and prevent irreversible nerve deficit.

Neuromuscular Disorders

- *Poliomyelitis*
- *Cerebral Palsy* (*Little's Disease*)
- *Myelodysplasia* (*Spina Bifida*)
- *Arthrogrypotic Syndromes*
  Arthrogryposis Multiplex Congenita (*Amyoplasia*) (*AMC*)
  Larsen Syndrome
  Multiple Pterygium Syndrome
- *Myopathies* (*Muscular Dystrophies*)
- *Duchenne's* (*Pseudohypertrophic Muscular Dystrophy*)
  Becker's Muscular Dystrophy
  Facioscapulohumeral Muscular Dystrophy
  Limb-Girdle Muscular Dystrophy
- *Hereditary Neuropathies*
  Friedreich's Ataxia
  Charcot-Marie-Tooth (*Peroneal Muscular Atrophy*)
- *Acute Idiopathic Postinfectious Polyneuropathy* (*Gullain Barre Syndrome*)

Poliomyelitis

Poliomyelitis is an acute infectious disease caused by one of the three antigenic types of poliovirus (an enterovirus) that destroys anterior horn cells in the spinal cord and brain stem. The virus enters the body through gastrointestinal and respiratory tract and spreads to central nervous system by the hematogenous route. The hallmark of poliomyelitis is asymmetric muscle weakness with lower motor neuron type of paralysis (areflexia, hypotonia) and normal sensations. Involvement of the nervous system varies from the minimal involvement to complete paralysis, and is proportionate to the number of anterior horn cells damaged. Quadriceps in lower limbs and deltoid in upper limb are the most commonly affected muscles. Tibialis anterior is most commonly paralysed muscle.

Effective nation-wide immunisation programmes (Pulse Polio) have reduced the incidence of poliomyelitis in India.

Classification

Clinical course of poliomyelitis is characterised by four stages:

1. **Acute Poliomyelitis** is an acute illness characterised by sudden onset of paralysis and presence of fever, acute muscle pain and neck rigidity. This acute illness can last up to ten days and varies in severity. Many cases can abort at this stage while others may experience diffuse and severe paralysis.

2. **Subacute Poliomyelitis or convalescent stage** Subacute phase is characterised by recovery of the muscle power by anterior horn cell survival (average 47% of anterior horn cells in spinal cord escape the initial attack), axon sprouting and hypertrophy of the muscles. The maximum recovery occurs in the first 3 to 6 months but the recovery may go on till 18–24 months. The surgical interventions should therefore be delayed for a period of 18–24 months. The recovery is determined by the extent of initial damage thus implying that completely paralysed muscles are less likely to recover than partially paralysed.

3. **Residual Poliomyelitis** Post polio-residual paralysis (PPRP) is the stage 18–24 months after the initial attack when no further recovery is expected and definitive procedures to restore function and provide structural stability can be undertaken.

4. **Post poliomyelitis Syndrome** Post poliomyelitis syndrome occurs in adults who had acute

poliomyelitis in childhood. These patients start complaining of increased muscle weakness three to four decades after the acute illness. Chronic overuse of muscle leads to deterioration of function in these patients. These patients have a history of the poliomyelitis, a random, asymmetric pattern of muscle weakness and often have additional symptoms such as muscle fatigue, cramps, joint pains, sleep apnea and depression.

Management

1. Acute Poliomyelitis

Patient is advised complete bed rest and given analgesics and moist heat to relieve muscle pains and spasm. Muscle fatigue and administration of intramuscular injections can lead to paralysis and should be avoided. Tonsillectomy in acute stage has been associated with bulbar poliomyelitis. Involvement of shoulder muscles (progressive paralysis of deltoid) may herald the onset of respiratory paralysis by involvement of intercostal and diaphragmatic muscles. Mechanical support of ventilation should be instituted at the earliest sign of respiratory compromise. Similarly, weakness of anterior neck muscles, difficulty in swallowing, paralysis of facial muscles or nasal intonation of voice may point towards the onset of bulbar paralysis.

Acute phase contractures in fascial structures may occur in the acute phase. Splinting to prevent deformity and regular range of motion exercises several times a day to prevent stiffness are instituted.

2. Subacute Poliomyelitis

Treatment of subacute poliomyelitis consists of maximising function, restoration of joint motion and prevention of deformities. Regular physiotherapy is instituted to achieve hypertrophy of the functioning muscle fibres. Splints and braces are used to maintain joint position and supplement function.

3. Residual Paralysis

Orthopaedic surgery is commonly performed at this stage to restore function and provide structural stability. It is particularly important to prevent skeletal deformities arising out of muscle imbalance in the growing children. The correction of the deformities should be performed carefully

to avoid causing the fractures in the osteoporotic bones (Fig. 8.1a,b). Physiotherapy aims to improve function in the undamaged muscles, educate patient to use all the available muscles for useful function and prevent contractures.

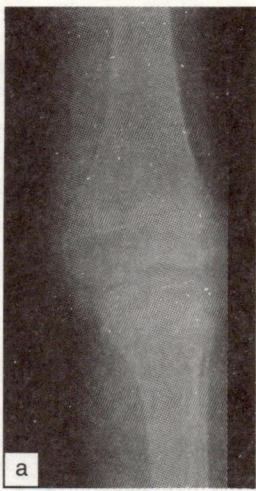

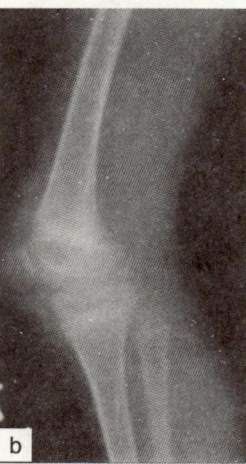

Fig. 8.1a,b. X-rays of a patient with poliomyelitis showing flexion deformity of the knee. Note the cortical thinning and osteopenia.

Orthotic devices can be used judiciously for several purposes:

a) To enable a non-ambulatory patient to walk; e.g. bilateral above knee orthoses can enable a patient to walk with the help of a walker/ bilateral crutches.

b) To protect weak muscles from over stretching; e.g. an inside iron and an outside T-strap with below knee caliper prescribed in evertor deficient foot prevents over stretching of peroneii.

c) To augment and / supplement the function of a weak muscle; e.g.

- a floor reaction orthosis (F.R.O.) can help a patient with weak quadriceps muscles to walk better by supplementing action of knee extensors.

- a dorsiflexor assist spring in a below knee caliper substitutes the function of paralysed ankle dorsiflexors.

d) To control a deformity; e.g. spinal brace can control paralytic scoliosis and collapsing paralysed spine can be effectively supported.

e) To prevent occurrence of deformity.

Surgical Treatment in poliomyelitis has following aims:

a) A patient who is not ambulant should be made ambulant

b) A patient who is ambulant with an above knee caliper should be made to ambulate with a below knee caliper. A smaller caliper makes ambulation easier, is light and cosmetically more acceptable.

c) A patient who is ambulant with a below knee caliper should be made ambulant without the caliper.

d) Correction of deformities which prevent fitting calipers/braces. This can be achieved by fasciotomy, tenotomy, Z-lengthening of tendon(s), osteotomy and arthrodesis.

e) Stabilisation of joints which are flail or which have severe muscle imbalance around them. The functioning muscles in the latter case can be used to provide motor function at other joints. This is usually achieved by arthrodesis.

f) To achieve equalisation of limb lengths when the paralysed limb is significantly shorter than the normal limb.

g) Reduction and stabilisation of unstable joint such as the hip dislocated due to paralysis. This can be achieved by muscle transfers and /or bony operations.

h) Stabilisation of spine when collapsing spine is causing symptoms and prevents wheelchair mobilisation in case of severe paralysis.

4. Postpoliomyelitis Syndrome

Treatment in these cases aims to preserve muscle strength and prevent further weakness. Life-style modification to prevent chronic overuse, limited exercises program incorporating periods of rest and orthotic support to limbs are useful measures in the management.

Cerebral Palsy (Little Disease)

Cerebral Palsy (CP) is a non-progressive and non hereditary disorder with onset before 2 years of age resulting from injury to the immature brain. The onset may be prenatal, perinatal or postnatal. An exact cause is not always known but etiological factors include prematurity (most common), perinatal infections (TORCH), anoxic injuries, cerebral trauma, meningitis and neonatal jaundice.

Cerebral palsy is an upper motor neuron disease with a mixture of muscle weakness and spasticity. Initially, the spastic muscles cause dynamic deformity at joints. Persistent spasticity leads to shortening of muscles, joint contractures, subluxation or dislocation of joints and bony deformities. Intelligence is often impaired in these cases.

Types of Movement Disorders in CP

1. *Spasticity* is characterised by increased muscle tone and hyperreflexia with slow restricted movements because of simultaneous contraction of agonist and antagonist muscles.

   This is the most common pattern and results from lesion in cerebral cortex. Characteristic deformities include adduction and internal rotation at the shoulder, pronation of forearm, flexion at wrist, flexion at knee, equinus at ankle etc. This form of CP is most amenable to operative intervention.

2. *Athetosis* is characterised by a constant succession of slow, writhing involuntary movements. These movements are aggravated during voluntary actions or by attempts to control them. This pattern is caused by lesion in basal ganglion. This form is very difficult to treat and not amenable to surgical correction.

3. *Ataxia* is characterised by poor co-ordination of muscles for voluntary activity. These patients have an unbalanced, wide-based gait. This form is caused by a lesion in cerebellum and is also less amenable to orthopaedic treatment.

4. *Mixed disorders* typically involve a combination of spasticity and athetosis.

Topographic Classification of CP

1. *Monoplegia* Single limb involvement, usually spastic. It is relatively rare.

2. *Hemiplegia* Spasticity of ipsilateral upper and lower extremities.

3. *Paraplegia* Neurological deficit involves only lower limbs. However, it is rare and existence of other spinal cord lesions must be ruled out.

4. *Diplegia* Most common type. Spasticity pattern. Lower limbs are more involved than upper limbs. Speech and intelligence are usually normal or slightly impaired. Esotropia and visual perception problems are common.

5. *Total body involvement* has involvement of all four limbs (Quadriplegia), head and trunk. Sensory deficits are typical. Mental retardation is common. These patients are usually non-ambulators.

Evaluation of the CP patient

Assessment of a patient with CP is based on thorough birth and development history and physical examination. Proper assessment of IQ should be made to predict the degree of physical dependence and ability to carry out activities of daily living. Locomotor profile is based on the persistence of primitive reflexes. Commonly tested reflexes include the Moro startle reflex (disappears by age of 6 months) and the parachute reflex (normally appears by 12 months of age). Persistence of primitive reflexes suggests that the child will be a non-ambulator.

Gait disorders are the most common problem seen by the orthopaedists. Diplegics have crouched gait, toe walking and knee flexion deformity while, hemiplegics usually present with toe walking only. Scissoring gait is seen commonly in spastic cerebral palsy (Fig. 8.2). Use of three dimensional computerised gait analysis with dynamic EMG and force plate studies enable a more scientific preoperative decision making and individualised treatment plan for patients with CP. Continuously active muscles, when identified can be lengthened or transferred out of phase.

Hip dislocation and subluxation is quite common in CP (Fig. 8.3).

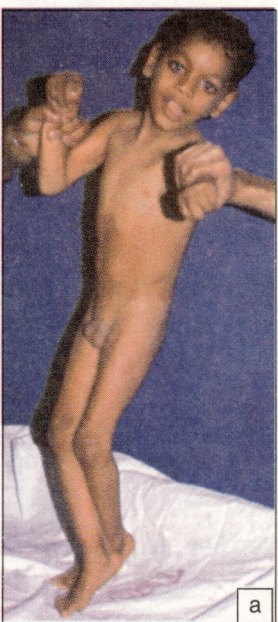 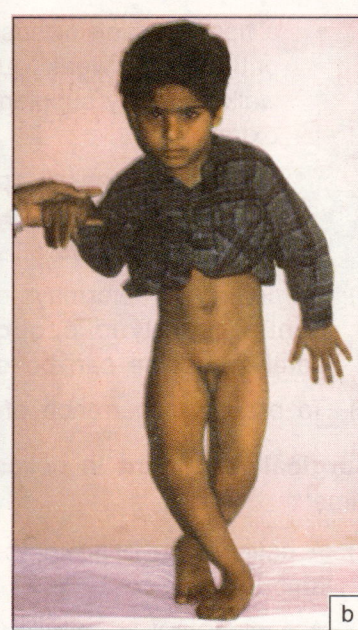

Fig. 8.2a,b. Scissoring gait seen in spastic cerebral palsy

Windswept hips deformity, characterized by abduction of one hip and the adduction of contralateral hip is also commonly seen.

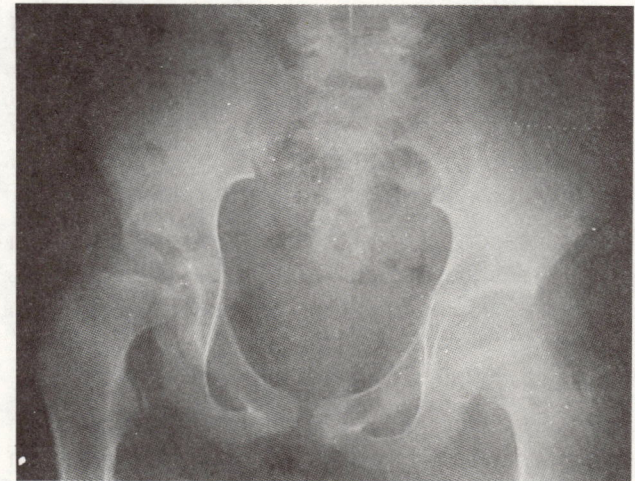

Fig. 8.3. X-rays of a patient with cerebral palsy showing subluxated right hip.

Bilateral coxa valga may be seen (Fig. 8.4).

Knee abnormalities include flexion contractures and decreased range of motion.

Foot and ankle abnormalities are common in CP. Gait and dynamic EMG evaluation is helpful. Equino-valgus caused by contracted tendo achilles and spastic peroneii is more common in spastic diplegia. Equinovarus in more common in spastic

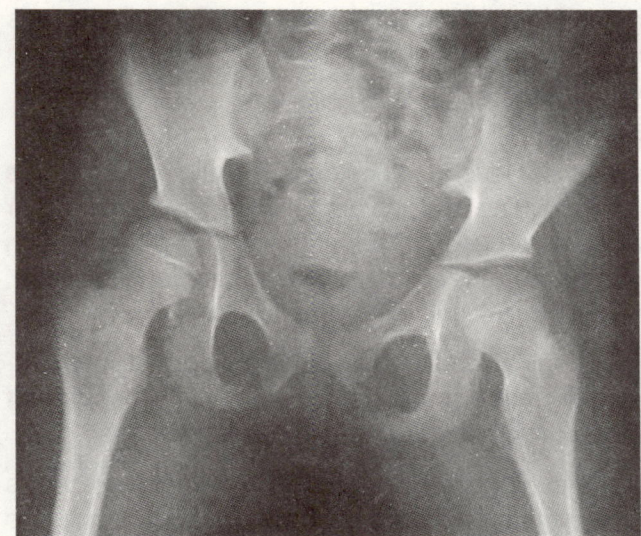

Fig. 8.4. Cerebral Palsy with bilateral coxa valga

hemiplegia and is caused by over action of tibialis anterior or posterior tendon (or both). Weight bearing in the presence of tight tendo achilles causes break in the midfoot giving rise to rocker bottom foot type of deformity (Fig. 8.4a).

Spinal disorders most commonly involve scoliosis, which may be very severe, making wheel chair sitting difficult. Kyphosis is also commonly seen.

Treatment

Specific goals must be set for the patient of CP

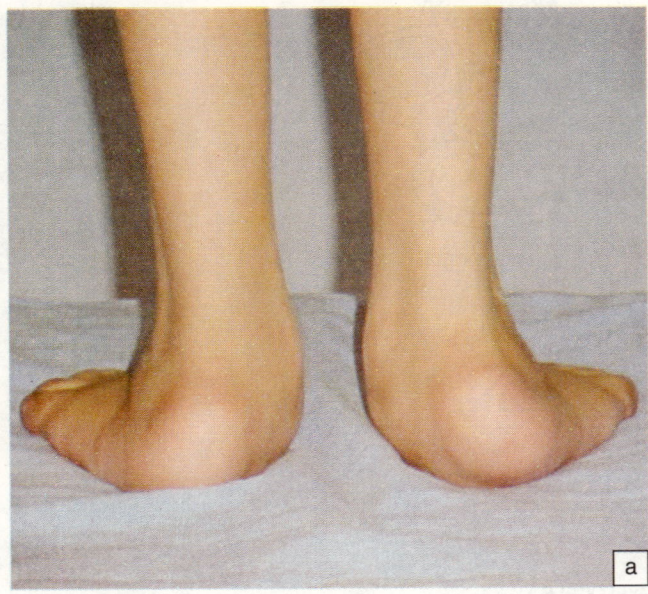

Fig. 8.4a. Equinovalgus deformity of both feet in a child with CP

before starting treatment. The treatment needs multidisciplinary approach involving paediatricians, orthopaedists, neurologist, physiotherapist, speech therapist and vocational counsellor. Physiotherapy and splintage are used to control joint deformities.

Orthopaedic treatment in CP aims to improve ambulation by releasing muscles or joint or improve sitting position in wheelchair. Surgery may be needed for indications such as toilet care and personal hygiene (e.g. surgery to release severe adduction contractures of both hips in a severely affected CP patient). Surgery is also performed on ambulatory patients to keep hips reduced (and avoid painful arthritis) and to stabilise the spine in scoliosis to improve and maintain sitting position.

Surgery to improve function is considered in child over 3 years of age with spastic CP and voluntary motor control. The only exception to this rule is an impending dislocation of hip in a child with CP where adductor and psoas release in done early.

Selective dorsal root rhizotomy, neurectomies and intramuscular botulinum toxin injections are used to control muscle spasticity. Deformities are corrected by lengthening of contracted muscles by myotomy, tenotomy or aponeurotomy (e.g. tendo achilles, adductors of hips, hamstring muscles). Tendon transfers are done to correct muscle imbalance e.g. distal transfer of rectus femoris muscle to semitendinosus or gracilis improves knee flexion.

Hip subluxation is treated in young children by adductor and / or psoas release while in older children bony reconstruction in the form of varus derotation osteotomy, femoral shortening and Salter, Dega, Ganz, triple or Chiari osteotomy is required.

Treatment of scoliosis is tailored to the needs of the patient. Small curves without functional deficit or large curves in severely involved patients are only kept under observation. Severe curves in ambulatory patients or curves associated with pelvic obliquity are treated with posterior and/or anterior fusion with or without spinal instrumentation.

Myelodysplasia (Spina bifida)

Myelodysplasia is a disorder of spinal cord development, neural tube closure, or a rupture of the developing cord, most commonly caused by hydrocephalus. Although the exact cause is not known, there is a significant hereditary component.

In its mildest form, this spinal dysraphism consists of *spinal bifida occulta* (defect in vertebral arch with confined cord and meninges). The other varieties are shown in Fig. 8.5a.

Meningocele Defect with bulging sac without protrusion of neural elements through the defect.

Myelomeningocele Spina bifida with protrusion of the sac with neural elements. Spinal cord is dysplastic. The defect is commonly associated with hydrocephalus and congenital scoliosis. The defect must be surgically closed in the first few days of life.

Rachischisis Neural elements are exposed on the surface without any covering with spinal cord's canal open. Children are still born or die soon after birth.

Spina bifida occulta occurs commonly at L5, S1, or cervical level. The lesion is mostly asymptomatic and is discovered incidentally on x-rays taken for unrelated reason. The skin overlying the lesion may be normal or may show a dimple (Fig. 8.5b), nevus, tuft of hair or a lipoma.

Neurological deficit may arise in a small percentage of these patients in later life because of tethered spinal cord, which needs release.

Myelomeningocele can occur at any level but is seen commonly between D_{12} and S_2. Since the neural tissue fails to form properly, these patients are paraplegic and insensate below the level of dysraphism. Hydrocephalus develops rapidly soon after birth. Muscle imbalance and intrauterine

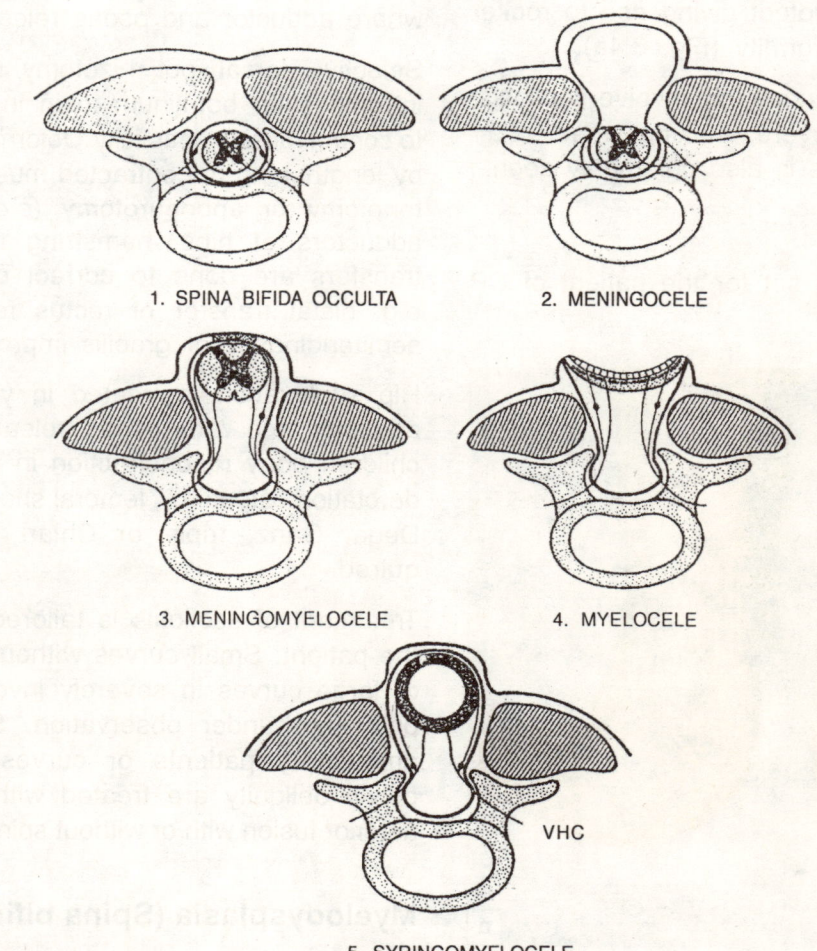

1. SPINA BIFIDA OCCULTA   2. MENINGOCELE

3. MENINGOMYELOCELE   4. MYELOCELE

VHC

5. SYRINGOMYELOCELE

Fig. 8.5a. Different types of spina bifida

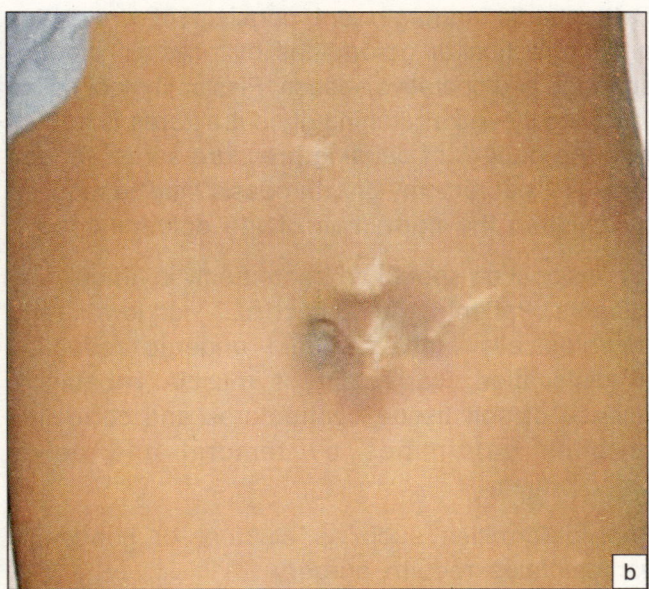

Fig. 8.5b. Dimpling of the skin and scar of previous surgery in a patient with myelomeningocele.

positioning frequently lead to hip dislocations, knee hyperextension and club feet (Fig. 8.6).

Scoliosis, torsional deformities of legs, contractures and congenital vertical tali are also noted often at birth. Bladder and bowel paralysis is common. Function in a child with myelodysplasia is related to the level of the defect and associated congenital abnormalities. The higher the level of defect, the poorer is the function and hence, prognosis. A child with an S_1 level (i.e. the last functioning level is S_1) will have only minimal motor involvement and will be able to walk whereas a patient with function proximal to L_4 will require wheelchair (L_4 is the key level because quadriceps can function and allow community ambulation). The combination of deformities is typical for various levels due to different combinations of paralysed and spared motor units. e.g.

- Hip dislocation is most common at L_3/L_4 level.

- L_4 level patients present with rigid clubfoot due to functioning tibialis anterior and posterior muscles and paralysed peroneii.

- The lesion at L_5, however, leads to calcaneovalgus because of the unopposed action of dorsiflexors and peroneii while tendo-achilles is paralysed.

Sudden changes in neurological status, (spasticity or new neurological deficit or sudden changes in function such as rapid increase in scoliotic curve or late hip dislocation at the lower lumbar level, recurrence or progress of foot deformities) may indicate hydrocephalus (most common), tethered cord or hydromyelia.

Fractures are common in myelodysplasia and may often go unnoticed because of insensate lower extremities. Patients with fractures present with redness, warmth, and swelling of lower extremity. X-rays are needed to confirm the fractures.

The insensate lower extremities in patients with myelodysplasia often lead to foot ulceration (Fig. 8.7), infection and development of neuropathic joints.

Spinal problems in myelodysplasia are due to scoliosis, pelvic obliquity and kyphosis. Hemivertebrae, diastematomyelia and unsegmented bars are commonly associated.

These patients may be allergic to latex possibly due to repeated catheterization with latex rubber catheters. Sensitisation may be severe, leading even to anaphylaxis. Therefore, these patients should be spared any contact with latex products such as gloves, catheters etc.

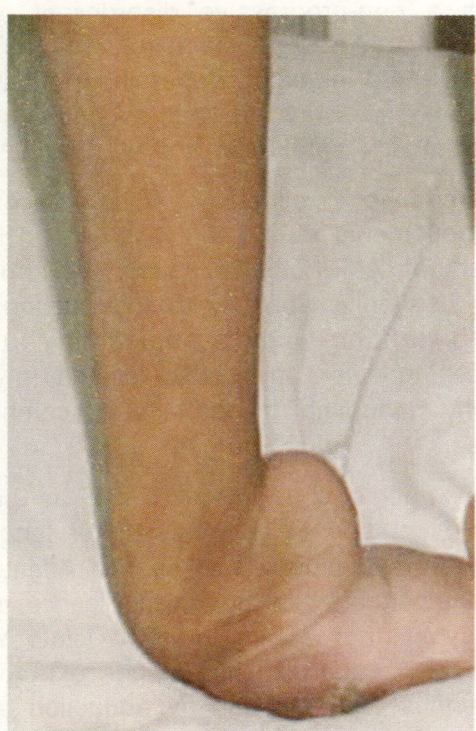

Fig. 8.6. Rigid clubfoot in association with Myelomeningocele

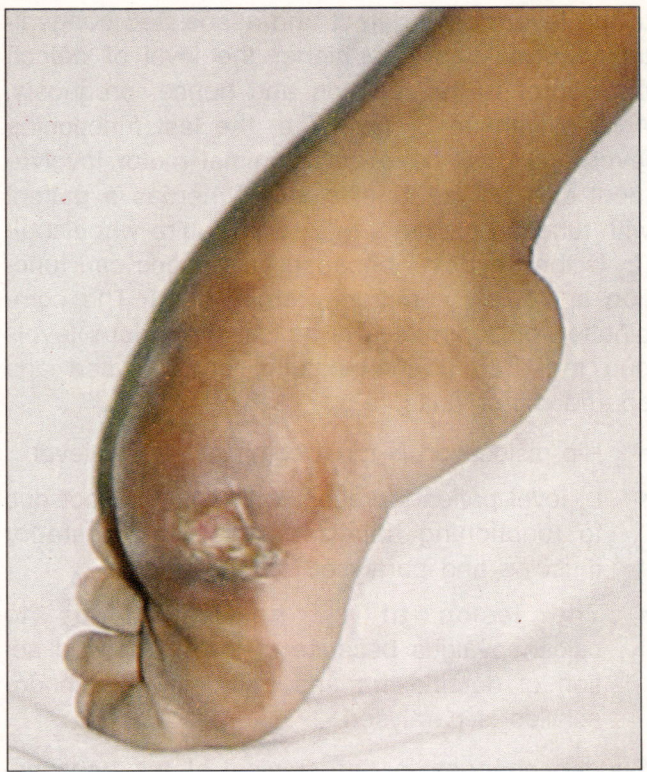

Fig. 8.7. Foot ulceration in a patient with myelodysplasia

Prenatal diagnosis of myelodysplasia is now possible by estimation of amniotic fluid or maternal serum alpha-fetoprotein levels estimated at 16 weeks of gestation. Raised levels of AFP suggest neural tube defect. Ultrasonography is a valuable tool to diagnose severe neural tube defects in-utero.

Treatment

It is important to realise that these children are multiply handicapped and have learning disorders, perceptual problems, hearing and visual impairment and emotional problems. All these problems require a co-ordinated effort by a multidisciplinary team comprised of neurosurgeons, orthopaedists urologist, paediatricians, physiotherapist, social worker, occupational therapist, orthotist and psychologist.

Closure of the defect is an emergency in myelomeningocele and must be done within 48 hours of the birth. Hydrocephalus, if is develops, should be managed on priority. Urologist will be required to tackle the problems of urinary incontinence. Neurosurgeon will be required to tackle the problems arising out of tethered cord.

Orthopaedic management consists of prevention and correction of deformities by physical therapy, splintage and operative release. Plaster immobilisation following closed stretching of contractures is fraught with the danger of causing pressure sores. Tendon transfers, neurectomy or arthrodesis may be required to maintain the correction of the deformity.

Hip dislocation should be treated only in ambulatory patients. Patients with defect at L_4 or lower (and neurologically stable) should undergo reduction of dislocation, correction of muscle imbalance, release of soft tissue contractures and correction of bony deformities by femoral and pelvic osteotomies.

Foot deformities such as clubfoot or congenital vertical talus require surgery.

Scoliosis in myelodysplasia is often refractory to bracing and anterior fusion with or without instrumentation is often required. Fractures in myelodysplasia can be treated conservatively with good results.

Arthrogrypotic Syndromes

1. Arthrogryposis Multiplex Congenita (Amyoplasia) (AMC)

AMC is a non-progressive disorder of multiple aetiology characterised by joint contractures or dislocations, rigid skeletal deformities, shiny skin with decreased wrinkling and subcutaneous tissue and muscle weakness and wasting.

AMC is caused by oligohydramnios or decreased foetal movements during a critical period in limb development. AMC can be caused by neurologic lesions (congenital absence of anterior horn cells, Werdnig-Hoffman spinal muscular atrophy, myelomeningocele), myopathic lesions (myotonic dystrophy, congenital myopathies) or combination of both.

AMC resembles polio in as much as sensory function is preserved and only motor function is lost. DTR are diminished or absent. Affected patients have normal facies, normal intelligence, multiple (often symmetric) contractures of joints without any visceral abnormalities. Upper extremity involvement is characterised by adduction and internal rotation of humerus, elbow extension and wrist flexion with ulnar deviation.

Lower extremity involvement is characterised by dislocation of hip, knee (flexion or extension) contractures and rigid clubfoot deformities.

The spine may have scoliosis. Fractures may be seen in one fourth of patients.

Evaluation of these patients includes neurologic studies, enzyme test and muscle biopsy (at 3–4 months). Microscopic examination reveals fatty degeneration of muscle fibres.

Treatment has to be started early and is prolonged. Passive stretching, serial casting, soft tissue releases and osteotomies may be required for correction of contractures. Aggressive treatment of clubfoot is attempted to enable the child to wear shoe and ambulate. An initial posteromedial soft tissue release is done and is followed by bony procedures if deformity recurs. Knee contractures are corrected before reduction of hip dislocation to maintain reduction.

Dislocated hips are treated with open reduction though bilateral hip dislocations in AMC are best left alone due to poor results after surgery.

2. Larsen Syndrome

Larsen syndrome is similar to AMC but joints are not as rigid as in the latter. Abnormal facies, multiple joint dislocations, scoliosis and cervical kyphosis are associated features.

3. Multiple Pterygium Syndrome is an autosomal recessive disorder characterised by cutaneous flexor surface webs, congenital vertical talus and scoliosis.

Myopathies (Muscular dystrophies)

Myopathies are non-inflammatory inherited disorders with progressive muscle weakness. Several types of muscular dystrophies are described based on their inheritance pattern.

1. Duchenne's (Pseudohypertrophic Muscular Dystrophy)

Duchenne's is sex linked recessive abnormality of young men manifested as clumsy walking, impaired motor skills, calf pseudohypertrophy (Fig. 8.8a) and lumbar lordosis. Examination reveals positive *Gower's Sign* (patient rises by walking the hands up the legs to compensate for gluteus maximus and quadriceps weakness)(Fig. 8.8b). Hip extensors are often the first group of muscles to get involved. Spinal deformity (scoliosis) is commonly associated. Laboratory investigations reveal markedly elevated creatine phosphokinase (CPK) level in serum and absent dystrophin protein on muscle biopsy DNA testing.

Histopathological examination of muscle biopsy reveals foci of necrosis and connective tissue infiltration.

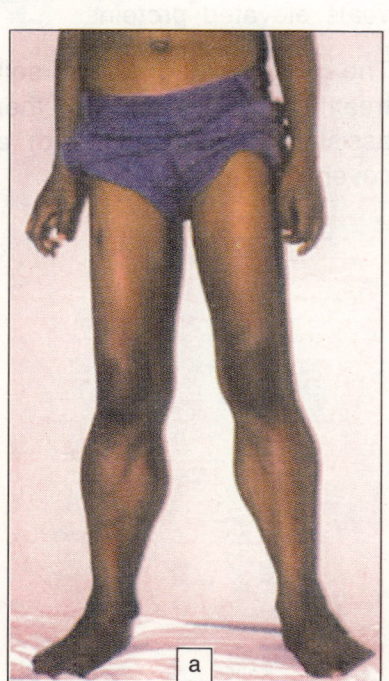 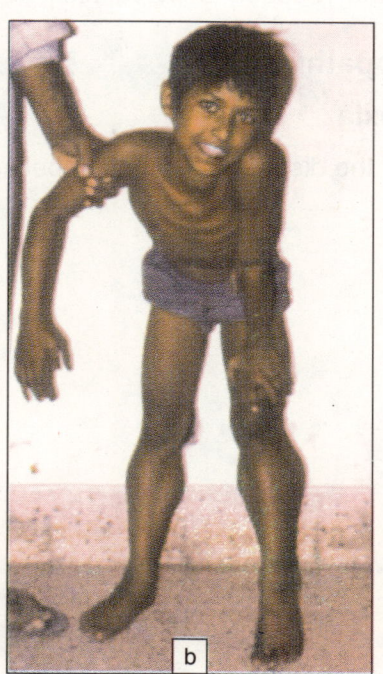

(a)

Fig. 8.8a,b. Duchenne's Muscular Dystrophy. (a) Note the pseudohypertrophy of calf muscles (b) Gower's Sign

Natural history of the disorder is of relentless progression. Patients usually lose independent ambulation by the age of 10 years and are bed-ridden by age 16. Children usually die of cardio-respiratory complications by 20 years of age.

Treatment aims to keep the patients ambulatory as long as possible by use of orthotic devices and release of contractures.

2. Becker's Muscular Dystrophy

Becker's dystrophy is also x-linked recessive (similar to Duchenne's) but is less severe. The patients can live beyond 22 years age without respiratory support. Affected individuals typically have red/green colour blindness. Abnormal dystrophin protein is present on muscle biopsy DNA testing.

3. Facioscapulohumeral Muscular Dystrophy

Autosomal dominant disorder typically seen in patients between the ages of 6 to 20 years. Facial abnormalities, winging of scapulae and normal CPK levels in serum are typical findings.

Scapulothoracic fusion stabilises the winging of scapula.

4. Limb-Girdle Muscular Dystrophy

Autosomal recessive disorder common between the ages of 10 to 30 years with pelvic or shoulder girdle involvement and reduced CPK values.

Hereditary Neuropathies

1. Friedreich's Ataxia

Friedreich's ataxia is the disease of spinocerebellar degeneration with a typical onset before 10 years of age. Affected child presents with staggering, wide-based gait, nystagmus, cardiomyopathy, cavus foot and scoliosis. Disorder involves both motor and sensory defects. Ataxia interferes with ambulation by the age of 30 years and patients die by 40-50 years age.

2. Charcot-Marie-Tooth (Peroneal Muscular Atrophy)

Peroneal muscular atrophy is autosomal dominant motor sensory demyelinating neuropathy (motor more than sensory). Patients present with *"STORK LEGS"*, peroneal weakness, hammer toes and pes cavus. Intrinsic muscle wasting may occur in hands. Nerve conduction studies reveal low nerve conduction velocities with prolonged distal latencies in peroneal, ulnar and median nerves. Treatment consists of correction of foot deformities by soft tissue releases with or without bony procedures.

Acute Idiopathic Postinfectious Polyneuropathy (Gullain Barré Syndrome) is characterised by symmetric ascending motor paresis caused by demyelination following viral infection. Sensations are preserved. Respiratory compromise may occur in severe cases.

Examination of cerebrospinal fluid typically reveals elevated proteins.

The disorder is usually self-limited. Expectant treatment with supportive therapy and ventilatory assistance (when required) are provided till recovery occurs.

CHAPTER 9

Limb Length Discrepancy

Introduction

The problem of limb length discrepancy is common and its importance is unlikely to diminish, despite the fact that the etiologic factors have changed considerably during the past two decades. In India, poliomyelitis remains the most common cause of limb length discrepancy.

Limb length discrepancy can arise either by shortening or overgrowth of one or more bones in the limb. The limb length discrepancy causes significantly more functional impairment in the lower limbs as compared to the upper limbs.

Normal Growth of Long Bone

The appendicular skeleton is preformed in cartilage, which is gradually replaced by bone. The growth occurs by proliferation of cartilage at the growth plate and articular cartilage. This process is called as endochondral ossification.

The growth in the appendicular skeleton is maximum towards the knee (65% of growth of the lower limbs occurs at the knee) and away from the elbow. Femur contributes 54% of the total length of the lower limb (35% from its lower end and 19% from the proximal femoral epiphysis) and the tibia contributes 46% (30% from its upper end and 16% from its lower end). In general, 1 cm of growth per year takes place in distal femur and 0.6 cm in proximal tibia, till skeletal maturity. Lower femoral physis contributes 70% of the total length

of the femur and, upper tibial physis contributes 60% of the total length of the tibia (Fig. 21.14).

Understandably, injuries / diseases occurring in the growth centers about the knee lead to much greater alteration in growth than those occurring away from the knee.

Etiology   A variety of diseases can give rise to the limb length discrepancy.

1. **Congenital and Developmental causes**

   a) Terminal limb deficiencies:

      Paraxial hemimelia

      Proximal focal femoral deficiency

   b) Congenital short femur

   c) Hemiatrophy or Hemihypertrophy

   d) Bowing of tibia

   e) Ollier's disease

   f) Congenital dislocation of hip

   h) Congenital coxa vara

   i) Arthrogryposis multiplex congenita

   j) Arteriovenous fistula

   k) Congenital pseudarthrosis of the tibia

   l) Hemangiomatosis and Neurofibromatosis.

2. **Traumatic**

   a) Causing growth retardation or arrest e.g. Injuries to the physeal plate

129

b) Causing growth acceleration e.g. Fractures of the metaphysis and diaphysis

c) Resulting in shortening e.g. Malunion (excessive overriding or angulation) of fractures

3. **Infection of bone and joint**

a) Causing growth retardation or arrest : Acute osteomyelitis

: Pyarthrosis/septic arthritis

: Chronic osteomyelitis

b) Causing growth acceleration : Chronic osteomyelitis

Note: Any condition causing chronic hyperemia of the growth plate can lead to stimulation of bone overgrowth eg: Meta/diaphyseal fractures, chronic osteomyelitis

4. **Neurogenic** Poliomyelitis, Cerebral palsy, Myelopathy, Myelomenigocele.

5. **Neoplastic**

(a) Tumours or Tumourous conditions producing over growth

   (i) Fibrous dysplasia

   (ii) Osteoid osteoma

   (iii) Hemangiomatosis

   (iv) Neurofibromatosis

(b) *Tumors or Tumorous conditions causing growth retardation*.

   (i) Solitary enchondroma.

   (ii) Solitary bone cyst.

   (iii) Neurofibromatosis.

6. **Miscellaneous** Perthes' disease, Slipped capital femoral epiphysis, Prolonged immobilisation in growing age (May lead to epiphyseal growth arrest).

Limb Length Discrepancy (LLD) and Poliomyelitis

This is the commonest cause of LLD in India. The cause of shortening is two fold:

1. Muscle atrophy is the most significant factor, causing reduced stimulation of normal skeletal growth.

2. The second factor is a peculiar coldness of the limb (Virchow sign), which in some instances seems to produce even further atrophy or lack of growth. This is probably related to some alteration of vasomotor control. This factor explains the variable degrees of shortening seen in various patients who have similar degrees of muscle weakness.

Evaluation of a Patient with Limb Length Discrepancy

A detailed history and examination is mandatory for the evaluation of a patient with limb length discrepancy. An attempt should be made to determine the cause of the limb length discrepancy. The stance and the gait should be observed. A *short limb gait* is characterized by equinus at the ipsilateral ankle, dipping down of the shoulder and the pelvis on the ipsilateral side and the flexion of the knee on the normal side when the affected limb is in the stance phase (cf the *Trendelenberg gait* where the pelvis dips down on the opposite side and the opposite shoulder dips down when the affected limb is in the stance phase). All the joints of the affected extremity should be examined for deformities/dysplasias, range of motion and stability. It is important to localize the site of inequality because it is desirable to keep the segment of the lower limbs as equal as possible so that the knee levels remain nearly the same.

Assessment of the strength and balance of muscles in the shortened limb is important for two reasons. Firstly, it is a questionable practice to lengthen a short limb where above knee brace is already required for ambulation; and, secondly, to elongate a very weak, shortened limb may create a situation where an above knee brace is needed for independent ambulation, whereas prior to surgery a brace was not needed. This occurs because of weakening of existing musculature by elongation or the production of a long lever arm.

Spine should be examined for flexible or structural scoliosis. Pelvic obliquity should be looked for. Neurological examination and assessment of the distal vascular status are mandatory.

An attempt must be made to differentiate between the true and the apparent length.

A true limb length is described between the anterior superior iliac spine and the medial malleolus on the two sides with the pelvis square and the limbs in identical position. Pelvis is said to be square when a line joining the two anterior superior iliac spines is perpendicular to the bed. Relative (apparent) lengthening and shortening can be produced by an abduction deformity of the apparently long limb or an adduction deformity of the apparently short limb respectively. This is basically the result of fixed pelvic obliquity. (In such instances, treatment should be directed towards the correction of pelvic obliquity. Limb shortening or lengthening in such cases is almost always contraindicated).

Limb length discrepancy can be documented by the clinical and radiographic methods. The clinical methods are the block method and the tape method.

Block Method This is an accurate method for evaluating limb length discrepancy. Wooden blocks of varying thickness are used to elevate the shorter limb till the pelvis is squared. The height of these wooden blocks needed reflects the limb length inequality.

Tape Method The pelvis is squared and with both limbs in identical position the distance between the anterior superior iliac spine and the tip of the medial malleolus is measured.

Radiologic assessment includes the assessment of the degree of discrepancy, deformity if any, and skeletal age. Currently, the three most commonly used techniques for the measurement of limb length discrepancy are orthoroentgenogram, scanogram and computerized digital scanograms.

Orthoroentgenogram is the best roentgenographic technique for determining limb length discrepancy. This procedure uses three separate exposures with the beam sequentially centered over the hip, the knee and the ankle joints. The distances between the major joint surfaces are calibrated by a centimeter ruler placed at the same level as that upon which the patient lies. The tube to film distance is standardized, usually to 6 feet.

The advantages of this method are simplicity, minimal radiation and accurate measurement of true limb length. Individual segment length can be measured. The method also allows for evaluation of angular deformity if any.

CT scan Recently, CT scan determination of limb

lengths has been developed. This technique is simple, accurate and visualizes the entire pelvis and lower limb, and the scans are easy to store.

Skeletal Age

It is necessary to determine the skeletal age of the patient in cases of LLD, especially if correction by growth arrest is contemplated. The Greulich-Pyle Atlas is the most highly accepted method of documentation of skeletal age. Standards are based on the stage of development of various primary and secondary ossification centers in the wrist and hand.

Progression of the Discrepancy

Shapiro classified progression of lower limb length inequality into five patterns.

Type 1   Upward slope pattern (Graph 1)

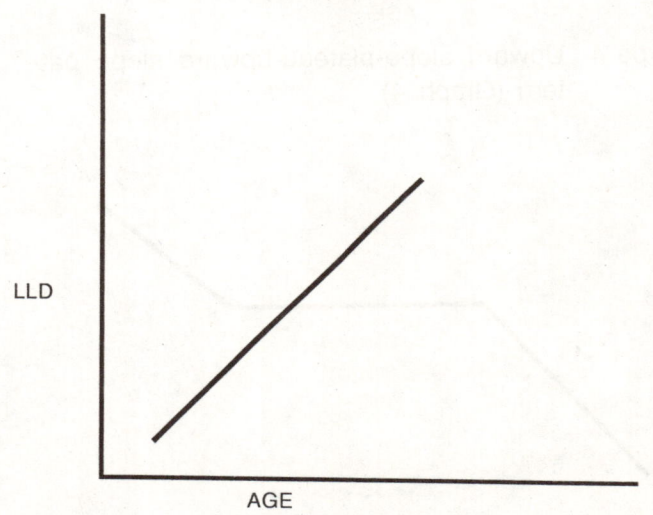

Type 2   Upward slope-Deceleration pattern (Graph 2)

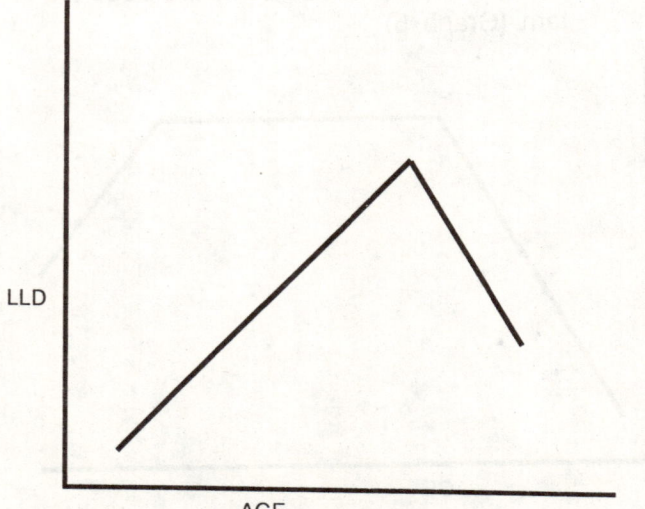

Type 3   Upward slope-Plateau pattern (Graph 3)

        3a Downward slope-plateau pattern

        3b Plateau pattern

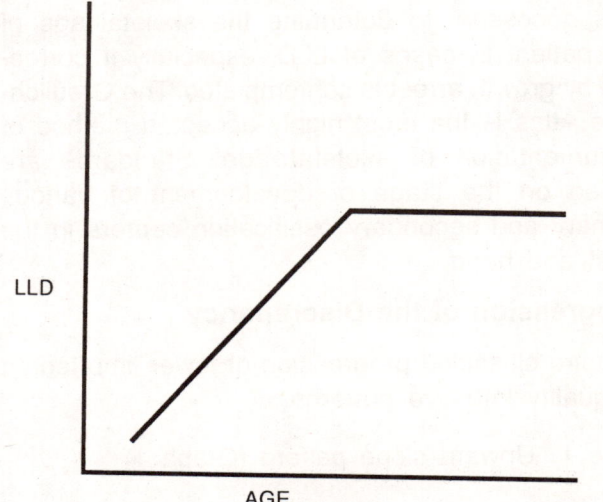

Type 4   Upward slope-plateau-upward slope pattern (Graph 4)

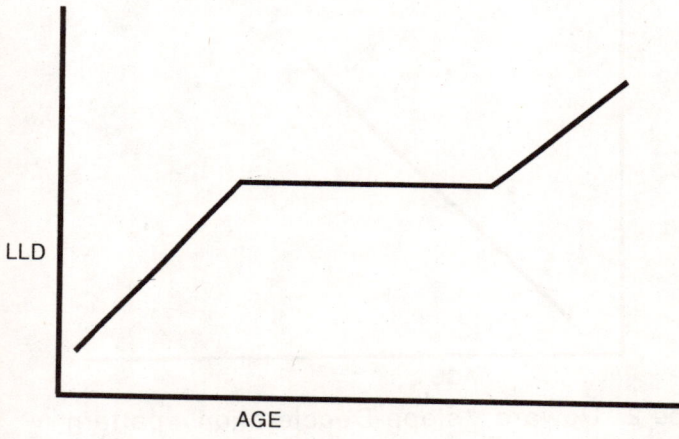

Type 5   Upward slope-plateau-downward slope pattern (Graph 5)

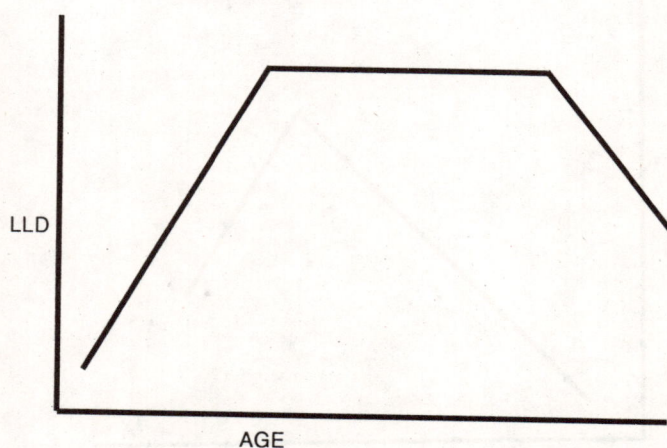

Progression of the discrepancy is important for several reasons. If the LLD is static or relatively so, the best form of equalization treatment can be planned more accurately. If the LLD is progressive, it is very important to document this progression. On rare occasions minor discrepancies may stabilize or correct spontaneously.

Growth Prediction Methods

1. Green and Anderson growth remaining chart.
2. Moseley straight line graph
3. Tupmans formula

1. Green and Anderson method

The growth remaining method uses a chart depicting the amount of additional growth to be expected from a normal proximal tibia and distal femur in different sexes at different skeletal ages. In addition the percentage growth inhibition over a minimum period of 3 months is determined by

$$\frac{(\text{Growth of the normal limb} - \text{growth of involved limb}) \times 100}{\text{Growth of normal limb}}$$

The two are used in conjunction to decide the course of action and optimal timing to pursue that course.

2. Moseleys Method

This is the straight line graph and uses the same determinants as the growth remaining chart. This has the following advantages.

(a) It does not require mathematical calculations
(b) The short and long sides can be compared at a glance, and,
(c) The height of the patient relative to his skeletal age is quickly determined

3. Tupmans formula

This determines the age to perform epiphyseal arrest for correction of LLD.

	Femur	Tibia
Boys	$A=\dfrac{25-(D\div0.7)}{1.69}$	$A=\dfrac{24.5-(D\div0.55)}{1.59}$
Girls	$A=\dfrac{19.4-(D\div0.7)}{1.41}$	$A=\dfrac{17.9-(D\div0.55)}{1.34}$

A=Age of growth arrest
D=Discrepancy

Anticipated Adult Height

This is important for planning the appropriate surgical intervention.

For example, a patient with a predictable ultimate stature of normal or taller than average proportions is more amenable to some sort of shortening procedure, if the discrepancy is not more than 5 cm. Conversely a patient of anticipated short stature will more likely benefit from limb lengthening procedure.

Degree of discrepancy

This is the most significant factor in deciding the appropriate management of limb length discrepancy.

< 2 cm	Customarily accepted and can be treated by non surgical methods.
2–4 cm	Grey area.
4–18 cm	Surgical correction
>18 cm	This degree of inequality is excess of the amount that any combination of procedures can be effectively or predictably used to equalize the discrepancy.

Some form of surgical treatment becomes necessary with a limb length discrepancy greater than 4 cm because:

1. This leads to a very awkward gait with fast walking and running being difficult or impossible.
2. Increased energy expenditure during ambulation.
3. Shoe raises greater than 4 cm are cumbersome and make walking more tedious.
4. This can lead to knee pain and early degenerative changes in lower limb joints.

Treatment of Limb length inequality

Proper management of the problem of limb length inequality depends on three factors.

1. *Assessment of the patient* whether the discrepancy warrants surgical intervention.
2. *Understanding of the various methods* of surgical equalization and application of the most appropriate one for the given case.
3. *Technical aspects of surgical equalization* should be mastered.

The degree of discrepancy is the most significant factor in deciding the appropriate management of limb length discrepancy. Minor limb length discrepancies up to 2 centimeters are common and can be either ignored or treated with a shoe lift. Discrepancies between 2 to 4 centimeters fall in the grey zone. Discrepancies between 4 to 18 centimeters constitute the indication for the limb length equalization.

Factors governing the decision for equalization include etiology, degree of discrepancy, skeletal age, progression of the discrepancy, anticipated adult height, strength and balance of the musculature, status of the foot and ankle, site of inequality (thigh or leg), needs and desires of parents/patient and, the general health factors. Pre-existent deformities in the limb should be corrected after limb lengthening as the latter procedure can lead to the occurrence of secondary deformities, which may need treatment.

Equalization of limb lengths can be achieved either non-surgically or surgically.

Non-surgical Methods

A shoe lift is a simple method of equalizing limb lengths, but children often refuse to wear it. The indications of shoe lift are difficult to define. If ambulation is prevented or compromised due to shortening, if the patient is symptomatic with low back discomfort due to LLD or he or she wants a lift, there is an indication for shoe raise. Complete equalization, however, is undesirable especially in cases of muscular weakness because this may make the limb so long that ground clearance is difficult. Large discrepancies, those in excess of 5 cm, require cumbersome and unattractive shoe alterations and are not recommended.

Surgical Methods

These can be classified under five main categories:

1. Conversion of limb with a terminal deficiency to an amputation followed by fitting of prosthesis.
2. Shorten the longer side (epiphysiodesis, epiphyseal stapling, resection of bone).
3. Lengthen the shorter side.
4. Use a combination of lengthening and shortening.

5. Surgical epiphysiolysis to restore growth.

Shortening of the long side

This can be done in three ways.

1. Premature physeal growth arrest of the proximal tibia and /the distal femur → epiphysiodesis

2. Temporary growth arrest by epiphyseal stapling.

3. Bone shortening by resection.

Epiphysiodesis Indications for epiphysiodesis include moderate limb length discrepancy about 5 cm, when there is sufficient anticipated growth in the opposite short limb and, when the expected adult height is equal to or above the normal standard. Pre-requisites for epiphysiodesis are that the discrepancy should not be more than 5 cm and there should not be significant discrepancy between the chronological age and the skeletal age. Epiphysiodesis is better avoided when the expected adult height is less than normal.

Technique Phemister originally described the technique. In his method, fusion is achieved by excising a block of cortex on either side of the growth plate, which is then reinserted with the ends reversed.

Advantages

The advantages of this procedure are:

1. It is technically relatively simple and has a low morbidity.

2. The correction of the inequality is achieved by the normal growth of the short side.

3. Success rate nears 90%.

4. Significant complications are rare.

Disadvantages

The disadvantages include the following:

1. The normal side is operated.

2. The ultimate height is decreased.

3. The procedure is virtually irreversible.

Complications

Apart from the usual complications of any major surgery on bone, there are specific potential complications inherent in this procedure including failure of correction, failure to achieve epiphysiodesis

and occurrence of angular deformity due to asymmetric growth arrest.

Epiphyseal stapling

Stapling is used only in selective cases for treatment of limb length discrepancy. The chief use of stapling remains in the correction of angular deformities.

Indications of epiphyseal stapling are:

1. Children with limb length discrepancy whose skeletal and choronologic age differ by more than 18 months.

2. Static limb length discrepancy in children too young for a permanent growth arrest.

Complications are more often with stapling than with epiphysiodesis due to the inherent uncertainties of this procedure. These include premature growth arrest with excessive shortening, asymmetric growth arrest, failure of the staples including breakage, loosening and extrusion and rebound increases in the length of the limb after removal of staples before skeletal maturity.

Resection of bone

The application of this technique is rare for obvious reasons. This procedure is indicated only in those patients with LLD who are nearing skeletal maturity or those who are skeletally mature.

As a general rule, such a major procedure as this is not justified unless the discrepancy exceeds 3 cm. The maximum shortening that can be tolerated in the femur is 5-6 cm, while that in the tibia is 3 cm.

The ideal indication of correction by resection of bone is a skeletally mature patient of acceptable height, whose limb length discrepancy can be fully corrected by femoral rather than tibial resection.

Femoral Vs Tibial Resection

Femoral resection is much easier and safer than the tibial and fibular shortening

Femoral resection is easier, internal fixation is possible, there is no weakening of the musculature of hip and thigh and union occurs rapidly. Correction up to 6 cm can be safely accomplished by femoral resection.

In the leg, two bones have to be dealt with, fascial planes are complicated, neurovascular bundle is more susceptible to injury and the possibility of weakness of leg musculature is more. A cast is usually necessary for stabilization and the maximum correction achieved is about 3 cm.

Correction of lower limb length inequality by lengthening

Conceptually, lengthening the shorter limb is the most attractive treatment modality for the correction of LLD. However the procedure has its own share of complications and should be approached with caution. There are two different methods of lengthening a limb.

1. Lengthening by stimulation of growth.

2. Mechanical lengthening.

1. Lengthening by Stimulation of growth

These are unpredictable and risky procedures, which have largely been abandoned. A mention is made only out of historical interest.

These include:

(a) Stimulation by creating an arteriovenous fistula

(b) Sub epiphyseal implantation of dissimilar foreign materials.

(c) Periosteal stripping

(d) Multiple surgical insult

(e) Sympathectomy

2. Lengthening by Mechanical means

Mechanical lengthening is the most proven and reliable method for the correction of LLD. It utilizes the principle of distraction osteogenesis and most commonly consists of lengthening by osteotomy and gradual distraction. Codville was the first to introduce the concept of femoral lengthening. Anderson and Wagner modified these techniques (Fig. 9.1). Wagner devised his apparatus, which could be applied to both the femur and tibia. The introduction of Ilizarov methodology has revolutionized the field of limb lengthening. The method uses tensioned crossed k wires with ring fixator used for stabilization to achieve multi directional stability and minimizes the complications of pin tract infection and loosening without compromising on the stability and stiffness of the fixation.

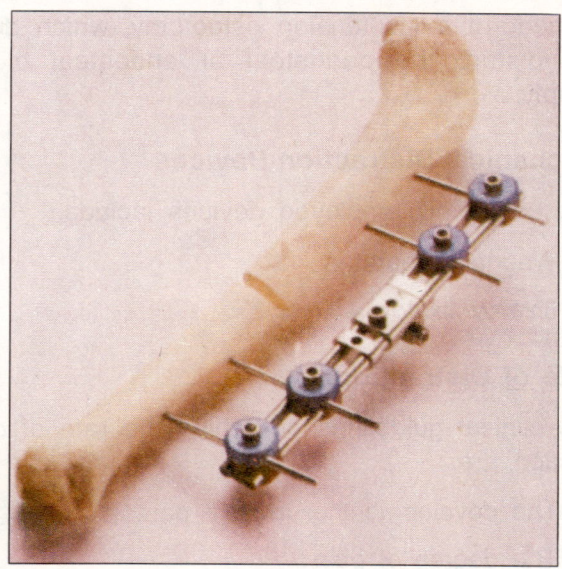

Fig. 9.1. Limb lengthening using Anderson apparatus

Ilizarov achieved lengthening up to 17 cm with his ingenious technique.

Lengthening by mechanical means can be done by the following methods:

(a) Lengthening by osteotomy and gradual distraction.

(b) Lengthening by osteotomy, sudden distraction, and implantation of bone or foreign materials, such as a "spacer".

(c) Trans iliac lengthening (modified Salter osteotomy).

The principles of osteotomy and gradual distraction include

(a) A semi open or open transverse, step cut or oblique osteotomy

(b) Application of a mechanical distraction device, and,

(c) Gradual distraction at the rate of 1–2 mm/day. It is preferable to distract in increments of 0.25 mm, 4 times daily. This is known as the rate and the rhythm of distraction respectively. A waiting period of 5–7 days is mandatory before starting the limb lengthening (distraction).

Corticotomy

Ilizarov introduced the concept of corticotomy or low-tension osteotomy.

This method employs 0.5-cm osteotome/ corticotome

to perform a low-tension osteotomy, which does not disturb the periosteal or endosteal blood supply.

Mechanical Distraction Devices

The commonly employed devices include

(a) Wagner apparatus

(b) Ilizarov fixator

Rate of Distraction

The clinical guidelines governing the rate of distraction are:

(a) The development of muscle paresis

(b) The degree of pain

(c) The development of sensory or motor neurologic deficit

(d) Any alterations in local circulation

(e) Any significant elevation of diastolic blood pressure (above 95 mm mercury)

These facts must be monitored at regular intervals throughout each day of lengthening, and, if adverse signs appear the distraction must cease or be reversed as necessary.

Complications of Limb Lengthening

Lengthening is an unphysiological operation and carries with it a variety of complications. The complications can be grouped into:

1. Systemic	Emotional lability, depression, Hypertension (more common with femoral lengthening), anorexia, weight loss	
2. Local	at the osteotomy site	– delayed union, nonunion, inadequate union
	pin tracts	– pin tract infection, loosening
3. Regional	adjacent bones and joints	(a) Knee flexion contracture
		(b) Equinus at the ankle
		(c) Valgus at subtalar joint
		(d) Valgus deformity of tibia
4. Neuromuscular	Sensory or motor neurologic deficit	
5. Vascular	Compartment syndromes	

Conclusion

LLD is a set of complex conditions where treatment options are many. The treatment protocol of any particular case should be devised to meet the individual requirements of that particular case. It is not possible to devise a "Cook book" equalization program based on x-ray films and physical examination alone. Thorough pre-operative planning and proper selection of procedure can go a long way towards the successful correction of a limb length discrepancy.

Amputations, Prosthetics and Orthotics

The word amputation is derived from the latin word "Amputare" which means "cutting around". Amputation is a procedure where part or whole of the limb is removed through one or more bones. The removal of limb through a joint is known as disarticulation. Amputations involve the lower limb in 60% of the cases. Males outnumber females in incidence of acquired limb loss by 3:2, a statistic probably attesting to the more hazardous work and recreational activities in which the males engage. It is important that both the patient and the surgeon have a realistic yet positive approach to amputation. The procedure should not be considered as a failure of treatment, it might be the treatment of choice to relieve pain, improve mobility and save life. Amputation is a reconstructive procedure aimed to help the patient resume his or her life by creating a new interface with the world.

Indications

The causes of amputations usually differ in different age groups. The various indications for amputations are listed in Table 10.1. The most common indication for amputation in the elderly patients is peripheral vascular disease including atherosclerosis, Raynaud's phenomenon and embolism. Diabetes mellitus is an important contributing factor. It contributes to ischemia and limb injury by two mechanisms:

1. Microangiopathy with vascular occlusion → ischemia

2. Neuropathy with impaired sensation → predisposition to trauma.

The causes in younger patients are related to trauma and its sequalae. These include road and rail traffic accidents, gunshot injuries and explosions, power tools and machinery.

Table 10.1. Indications for Amputation

1. Lack of Circulation	Injury • RTA • Gunshot injuries, explosions • Machines and power tools Peripheral vascular disease • Atherosclerosis • Burger's disease • Diabetes mellitus • Connective tissue disorders • Raynaud's phenomenon

2. Infections	• Acute fulminating infections
	  - gas gangrene
	• Chronic osteomyelitis
	  - infected non union of bone
	  - Madura mycosis

3. Malignant Tumours	• Osteosarcoma • Rhabdomyosarcoma • Malignant Melanoma • Synovial Sarcoma
4. Nerve Injuries	• Traumatic • Acquired • Leprosy (auto amputation)
5. Congenital Anomalies	
6. Electrical Burns, Extreme Heat and Cold Injuries (Frostbite)	

In children, limb deficiencies may be congenital or acquired. In developed countries congenital amputations account for as many as 60% of the amputations. Injury and malignancy account for a major share of the acquired amputations.

Types of Amputation

Amputations can be closed or open.

Open Amputations

Open amputations are usually done under emergency set up when there is risk of wound contamination or infection. In this procedure the amputation stump is left open (wound is not closed) after the first surgery. Open amputations can be of two types.

1. **Guillotine amputation** In this procedure all the tissues from skin to bone are cut at the same level and the wound is left open for further management. This is done as an emergency to save life in cases of gangrene, crushed limbs, etc. The problem with this procedure is of skin retraction. This can be prevented by

(a) applying stay sutures to the skin

(b) post operative use of skin traction

2. **Open amputation with flaps** In this procedure skin flaps are fashioned as done in a closed amputation but the wound is left open. The advantage of this procedure is that a longer length of stump can be retained, revision amputation at a higher level is not necessary and the closure becomes easier.

The open amputation stumps are closed after some time when the wound is healthy using one of the following techniques:

• Secondary closure :	Closure of the skin flaps after a few days.
• Plastic repair :	The soft tissues are repaired and skin flaps are closed without cutting the bone.
• Revision of stump :	The terminal granulation tissue, scar tissue and bone are removed, and skin flaps are fashioned to close the wound.
• Re-amputation :	The amputation is performed at a higher level.

Amputations can also be classified based on the timing of surgery

1. **Early amputations** are performed at the time of presentation as in severe crush injuries, trauma.

2. **Intermediate amputations** are done after a few days or weeks of presentation as in cases when efforts to salvage severely traumatized limb fail or attempts to salvage are long drawn and tedious with doubtful end result.

3. **Late amputations** are performed in cases such as infected non unions which have resisted all surgical efforts.

Levels of Amputation

In the past amputation through specific levels was essential for the proper fitting of prosthesis. The accepted ideal stump lengths are 25–30 cm below the greater trochanter in an above-knee amputation, 13–14 cm below the tibial articular surface in a below knee amputation, 20 cm stump length or 10 cm above elbow in an above elbow amputation and 17–20 cm from the olecranon in a below elbow amputation (Fig. 10.1). However, it is not always possible to achieve these standard stump lengths. The advent of

modern prosthetic designs allows prosthetic fitting to any well healed non-tender stumps.

Upper extremity

Fore quarter amputation

In this the upper limb along with part of the clavicle and scapula and the shoulder girdle muscles is removed.

Shoulder Disarticulation

Even in disarticulation of shoulder the humeral

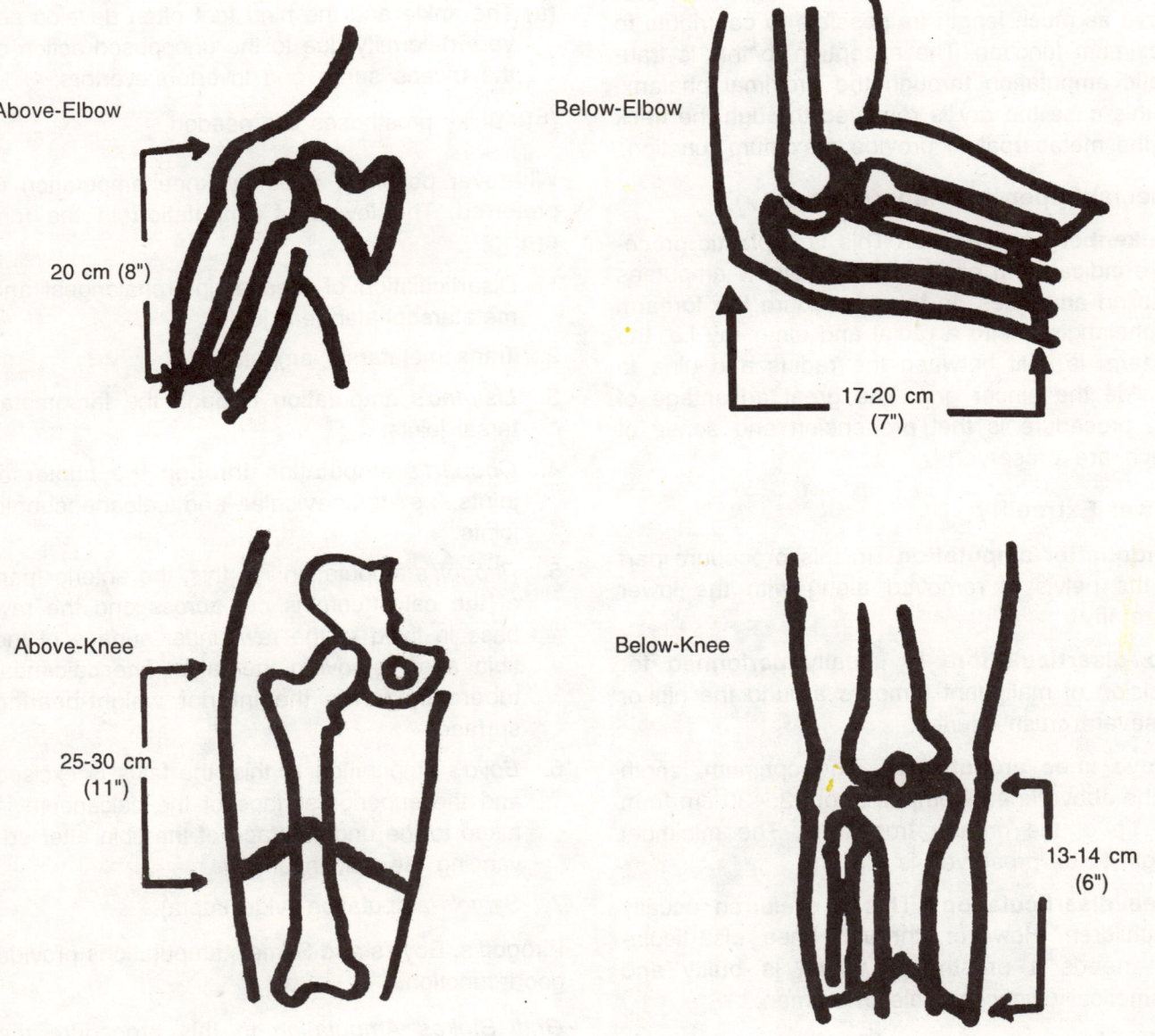

Above-Elbow

20 cm (8")

Below-Elbow

17-20 cm (7")

Above-Knee

25-30 cm (11")

Below-Knee

13-14 cm (6")

Fig. 10.1. Ideal amputation levels

head is preserved, wherever possible, to maintain the contour of the shoulder.

Above elbow amputation

A 20 cm stump from the tip of the acromion is ideal.

Below elbow amputation

The optimum length of a below elbow stump is 20 cm as measured from the tip of olecranon, with a minimum length of 7.5 cm.

Wrist disarticulation

Involves disarticulating the hand through the wrist joint.

Amputation through hand is designed to preserve as much length as possible to contribute to maximum function. The exception to this is traumatic amputation through the proximal phalanx. In this case the ray is removed through the neck of the metacarpal to provide maximum function.

Special upper limb amputations

Krukenberg amputation This is a plastic procedure indicated in bilateral below elbow amputees or blind amputees. In this procedure the forearm is phalangised into a radial and ulnar ray i.e. the forearm is split between the radius and ulna to provide the pincer grip. The great advantage of this procedure is that prehension and sense of touch are preserved.

Lower Extremity

Hindquarter amputation In this procedure part of the pelvis is removed along with the lower extremity.

Hip disarticulation is usually performed for excision of malignant tumours around the hip or in severe crush injuries.

Above knee amputation The optimum length of the above knee stump is about 25–30 cm from the tip of the greater trochanter. The minimum length to be preserved is 7.5 cm.

Knee disarticulation This is preferred usually in children. However, through knee disarticulation needs a prosthesis, which is bulky and cosmetically unacceptable in women.

Below knee amputation This is the most commonly performed amputation.

The amputation stump length is 14 cm below the tibial articular surface.

Special Lower Limb Amputations

Syme's amputation In this operation the tibia and fibula are divided first above the ankle joint. The heel flap is preserved and is sutured anteriorly to the end of the stump, after removing the talus and the calcaneum. This is a very good procedure especially in developing countries as it is suited for barefoot walking.

Amputations of Foot These procedures especially those proximal to tarso-metatarsal joints have almost become obsolete these days because:

(a) The ankle and the hind foot often develop severe deformity due to the unopposed action of the triceps surae and invertors/evertors;

(b) Bulky prostheses are needed.

Wherever possible, a below knee amputation is preferred. The levels of amputation in the foot are:

1. Disarticulation of toes at interphalangeal and metatarsophalangeal joints.

2. Trans metatarsal amputation.

3. *Lisfranc's* amputation through the tarsometatarsal joints.

4. *Chopart's* amputation through the midtarsal joints, i.e. talonavicular and calcaneocuboid joints.

5. *Pirogoff's* amputation In this, the anterior part of the calcaneum is cut across and the raw base in fixed to the raw under surface of the tibia after removing the talus. The calcaneal tuberosity forms the inferior weight-bearing surface.

6. *Boyd's* amputation In this, the talus is excised and the superior surface of the calcaneum is fused to the undersurface of the tibia after advancing the calcaneum.

7. *Syme's* amputation (vide supra).

Pirogoff's, Boyd's and Syme's amputations provide good function.

Gritti–Stokes Amputation In this procedure the bone is cut above the femoral condyles, the undersurface of patella is rawed and fixed to the raw surface of femur.

Basics of Surgical Technique

Amputation is the first step in the rehabilitation of an amputee and a meticulous attention to the following surgical principles is mandatory to ensure an optimal end result.

(a) **Tourniquet** The use of tourniquet is helpful in most cases to minimize the blood loss. It is recommended in all cases, the exception being an ischaemic limb. Exsanguination (with an Esmarch elastic bandage) of the limb prior to tourniquet inflation provides added advantage. This procedure is contraindicated in the presence of infection and malignancy for fear of spread of the disease proximally.

(b) **Level of Amputation** The cardinal dictum is to conserve all limb length possible, compatible with optimum function and consistent with appropriate treatment for the condition necessitating the amputation.

Ischemic limbs

In ischemic limbs, the ultimate decision about the level of amputation must be made according to the ability of the tissues to heal. In peripheral vascular disease healing is early with short stumps and rehabilitation is better with longer stumps. Clinical evaluation remains the mainstay for deciding the level of amputation in patients with ischemic limbs. The clinical guidelines of vascularity include peripheral pulse, color and temperature of the skin, free capillary bleeding from cut surfaces, and color, consistency and contractility of muscle. Other methods for evaluation of vascularity include doppler ultrasonography, A.B.P.I. (ankle brachial pressure index).

Myodesis should be avoided in ischaemic limbs. In below knee amputations in dysvascular amputees, since posterior skin is more vascular, long posterior skin flaps are fashioned. Immediate post surgical prosthesis fitting is generally avoided in these patients.

(c) **Skin flaps**

Good skin coverage is a very important aspect of amputation. The anterior and posterior flaps can be of equal lengths or the posterior flap can be longer. The scar should ideally not be located over weight bearing areas though the location of the scar is no more important with the advent of modern total contact prosthetic sockets. Atypical skin flaps are preferable to amputation at a more proximal level. The combined length of the flaps should be one-third of the circumference of the limb at the level of the bone section.

(d) **Muscles**

Muscles should be cut distal to the level of bone section.

The two techniques of muscle attachment are:

(i) Myoplasty

(ii) Myodesis

Myoplasty The muscles are trimmed and opposing groups of muscles are sutured to each other over the end of the bone.

Myodesis The muscles are anchored to the bone by means of drill holes.

This is contraindicated in ischaemic limbs.

The muscles should be cut at least 5cm distal to the level of the bone cut when these procedures are contemplated.

(e) **Nerves** The nerves are gently pulled down and cut with a sharp knife so that they can retract into the muscle mass. This minimizes the formation of painful neuromas. Large nerves such as sciatic nerve contain relatively large blood vessels and should be ligated before they are divided.

(f) **Blood vessels** Major blood vessels should be isolated and doubly ligated individually with non-absorbable sutures. Ligating the arteries and veins together may lead to the formation of an arterio venous fistula. The tourniquet should be released before the skin closure and meticulous hemostasis should be ensured.

(g) **Bone** During the bone section, muscles should be protected and excessive periosteal stripping should be carefully avoided to prevent the formation of a ring sequestrum.

The sharp bone edges are rasped and the subcutaneous bones beveled. Suturing of the periosteal flap over the medullary canal is supposed to maintain normal medullary pressure gradient. In below knee amputations the fibula is cut 2 cm proximal to the tibia to produce a conical stump.

(h) **A corrugated rubber drain** is used for 48 hours to prevent hematoma formation. In a guillotine amputation, a useful rule of thumb is to perform muscle section at the level of skin retraction and bone section at the level of muscle retraction.

Post Operative Treatment

The postoperative treatment is of two types:

1. Rigid dressing and Immediate Postoperative Prosthetic Fitting.

2. Soft dressing and delayed prosthetic fitting

1. Immediate Postoperative Prosthetic Fitting

This is indicated in young amputees with good vascular stumps. This method consists of the application of rigid plaster of paris dressing to the amputation stump on day 1 (followed by fitting of a temporary (endoskeletal)) prosthesis called as pilon prosthesis). The emphasis here is on early mobilization of the patient. The chief advantages of this method are:

(a) Less wound edema, better healing and early stump maturation due to the rigid dressing.

(b) Early bipedal ambulation helps in promoting better gait.

(c) Proprioception is retained due to early walking.

(d) Psychologically better for the patient as early walking restores confidence and self esteem to the patient.

2. Soft dressing and delayed prosthetic fitting

Immediate postoperative prosthetic fitting is contraindicated in elderly dysvascular amputees with underlying vascular disease either as a result of diabetes mellitus or atherosclerosis etc. In such patients soft dressing and late prosthetic rehabilitation are preferred for obvious reasons.

Complications Following Amputation

The common complications noted after amputation surgery are:

1. **Hematoma** occurs most commonly due to slipping of ligature or failure to secure adequate hemostasis. Hematoma delays wound healing and serves as a rich culture medium for microorganisms. Hematoma can be prevented by paying attention to meticulous hemostasis before stump closure. Use of penrose or suction drains minimize the risk of postoperative hematoma. Any hematoma must be aspirated and compression dressing should be given over the affected site.

2. **Failure of wound healing** is most often seen in amputees with diabetes and peripheral vascular disease. The failure is due to impaired vascularity, infection and/or poor surgical technique. Gaps of less than one cm are usually treated by dressing, while those greater than one cm may require revision amputation at a higher level. Wound healing failure with reamputation may occur in as many as 5–10% of patients.

3. **Infection** is more commonly seen in amputees with diabetes and peripheral vascular disease. Other factors are amputation at the infected level, near the zone of traumatic injury and presence of hematoma. The treatment is thorough debridement and antibiotic therapy. The stump may be left open and reassessed at a later date. Another method employed is that of partial closure where the middle one third of the stump is closed and the lateral and medial corners are packed open. This would allow closure of bone, and, at the same time, ensure adequate drainage.

4. **Phantom sensation/pain** Phantom sensation is the feeling that all or part of the amputated limb is still present. Phantom pain is a troublesome, painful or burning sensation in the part of the limb that is missing. The episodes of phantom pain are experienced by 70–90% of patients; fortunately these are brief. Trans cutaneous electrical nerve stimulation (TENS) is useful for treating this problem. Other modalities used include cold packs, acupuncture and regional sympathectomy. Pharmacologic treat-

ment with amitryptiline, carbamazapine, gabapentin, phenytoin and mexiletene has met with some success. Psychologic counselling may be helpful. Phantom pain in fact could be a variant of reflex sympathetic dystrophy which, when present, should be aggressively treated. It has been shown that the use of pre and post operative epidural analgesia reduces the incidence of phantom pain.

5. **Stump edema syndrome** refers to a condition caused by proximal stump constriction leading to stump edema, pain, ecchymosis and increased pigmentation. This can be treated by removal of prosthesis, elevation of limb and compression.

6. **Joint contractures** usually develop between the amputation and prosthetic fitting. These include flexion, abduction contracture of an above knee stump, flexion contracture at the knee (>15 degrees prevents prosthetic fitting) in below knee amputees and flexion contracture in above and below elbow amputations. These deformities are best prevented by aggressive physiotherapy soon after surgery.

7. **Skin problems** include contact dermatitis, superficial infections, reactive hyperemia, epidermoid cysts and verrucous hyperplasia. These can be prevented by good personal hygiene (includes keeping the residual limb and prosthetic socket clean and dry).

Amputations in Children

Congenital limb deficiencies, trauma and tumour constitute the main indications of amputation in children. Amputations in children present unique problems not seen in adults.

1. **Level of Amputation** It is important to keep in mind that there is a proportional change in the residual limb length with growth in a child amputee. A diaphyseal amputation removes one of the growth centers, thereby preventing the proportionate growth of the remaining limb. Disarticulation, which preserves the growth centers, is preferred to trans-diaphyseal amputation.

2. **Terminal Overgrowth** occurs in 8–12% of pediatric amputees. This is not due to overgrowth (longitudinal) from the proximal epiphyseal growth, but is due to appositional growth of bone at the transected end. This exceeds the soft tissue growth and leads to terminal overgrowth. When untreated the appositional bone can penetrate the skin. Terminal overgrowth occurs most commonly in the humerus, fibula, tibia and femur in that order. The best approaches for this problem include:

(a) stump revision with adequate bone resection

(b) stump-capping procedure (*Marquardt*)

In the stump capping procedure the bone end is split longitudinally into two and covered by autologous osteo-chondral graft (obtained from part of the amputated limb or posterior iliac crest)

3. **Spur Formation** occurs at the end of the stump but is not as troublesome as stump overgrowth.

The growth abnormalities in child amputees are given in Table 10.2.

Table 10.2. Growth abnormalities in amputation stump in children

General	Terminal over-growth, spur formation, growth arrest of the limb
Below knee	Anterior bowing of tibia, Varus angulation Fibular over-growth
Above knee	Coxa valga Hemiatrophy of pelvis
Below elbow	Radial over growth with pincer like contour
Above elbow	Humerus varus

However, because of growth factors, increased body metabolism and generally good vascularity, children often tolerate procedures on the amputation stump not tolerated by adults. These include closure of the stump under tension, use of skin grafts to cover the stump end and use of more forceful skin traction.

Complications after surgery are less severe in children. Painful phantom sensations are absent and neuromas are rarely troublesome. Psychologic problems are rare in children.

Children use prostheses very well and gait training is rarely required.

Prosthetics and Orthotics

Prosthetics is a branch of rehabilitation medicine dealing with the manufacture and fitting of artificial device to replace the function of a missing extremity. The artificial limb thus used is known as prosthesis.

In general prostheses can be grouped as lower limb prostheses and upper limb prostheses. The results following the use of lower limb prostheses are far superior to those following the use of upper limb prostheses. This is because sensation and dexterity are far more essential for the functioning of upper extremity than for the lower extremity.

Prosthesis can be internal as in total joint replacements or external as an artificial limb.

The rehabilitation of an amputee starts with the surgery itself and the postoperative care is of utmost importance. Rigid postoperative dressing constitutes the first step in the fitting of prosthesis. It is essential to retain as much residual limb length and as many functioning joints as possible to obtain best results with prosthetic fitting. This is especially true of upper limb amputation where artificial limbs can rarely substitute for the sensate functioning limb. Another important factor is to start the prosthetic fitting within 30 days of amputation wherever feasible. It has been shown that the outcomes are favorable in 70 to 85% when prosthetic fitting occurs within 30 days of amputation, as compared with 30% when started late.

Prosthetic fitting should be approached with caution in bilateral amputees with short stumps, elderly patients with dysvascular stumps, stumps with poor wound healing, presence of flexion contracture of greater than 45 degrees in an above knee amputee and in amputees with poor muscle power.

Classification

Prostheses may be classified based on the sources of power for the function. They are grouped into 2 categories.

1. **Body-powered devices** In these the power to move the prosthesis is provided by the remaining muscle groups of the same extremity or the opposite extremity.

2. **External-powered devices** In these the power source is external from a battery, which is rechargeable. Myoelectric prosthesis is a type of externally powered prosthesis where existing muscle action potentials are recorded by surface electrodes, which are then amplified and used to run a battery which provides the power for moving these prostheses.

Muscle Action Potential

↓

Amplification

↓

6 v Battery

↓

Movement of the Artificial Limb

Myoelectric prostheses are most suited for patients with transradial (below-elbow) amputations to provide a hand with ability to grasp. These prostheses have acceptable cosmesis and function but are expensive.

Aims of Prosthetic Fitting

The aim of prosthetic fitting is to substitute the function of a lost part. In the lower extremity the prosthesis must allow for ambulation with minimum energy expenditure.

The type of prosthetic fitting depends on

– age and general physique of the patient

– length of the stump

– status of circulation

– strength of remaining musculature, and

– requirements of job and activities of daily living of the patient.

Parts of a Prosthesis

The prosthesis consists of a socket, which is in contact with the amputation stump, a suspension to hold the socket, a prosthetic extension and a terminal device.

1. **Socket** Sockets are prosthetic components, which provide functional control and even pressure distribution over the amputation stumps.

Based on the contact between the socket and the stump the sockets can be classified into:

(a) End bearing (end of the stump bears the weight)

(b) Total contact (weight is distributed evenly throughout the surface)

(c) Total surface bearing (weight is distributed throughout the surface but different areas bear different loads) e.g. (i) Quadrilateral socket (ii) Patellar tendon bearing socket.

Prosthesis for lower limb amputations

Above knee amputation

1. **Socket** Two types of sockets are available: Quadrilateral (total contact) socket, and "CAT-CAM" socket.

   (a) **Quadrilateral socket** In this,

   (i) Ischial tuberosity bears majority of the weight.

   (ii) the proximal socket is contoured to maintain prosthesis under ischial seat.

   (iii) The disadvantage is that it does not prevent the tendency of the stump to go into abduction.

   (b) **"CAT-CAM" socket**

   (i) This is the contoured adducted trochanteric controlled alignment method.

   (ii) The advantage with this is the presence of wide anteroposterior and narrow mediolateral socket design which enables the stump to be placed in adduction for a more stable stance.

   (iii) The ischial tuberosity does not bear any weight.

2. **Suspension** The suspension attaches the prosthetic socket to the body

   (a) **Belt suspension** It is used prior to stump maturation or in very short stumps. e.g. Silesian belt
   Pelvic band - (double swivel pelvic band)
   - (rigid pelvic band)

   (b) **Suction suspension**

   Negative pressure through the swing phase is maintained by means of skin contact and a removable one-way valve, thus drawing the stump into the socket. This is ideal where a total contact prosthesis is used. The use with end bearing sockets may lead to terminal congestion. Suction suspension is contraindicated in flabby, short, ischemic stumps with severe scarring and with upper extremity involvement.

3. **Knee mechanism**

   Prosthetic knee mechanics can be:

   (a) Mechanical

   (b) Hydraulic

   (c) External hinge

   (a) **Mechanical**

   i) *Single axis, constant friction knee*

   It is a simple, durable and commonly prescribed design where a friction clamp is used to damp swing of the knee. The primary limitation of this design is a constant gait speed.

   ii) *Poly centric knee*

   The knee axis simulates the movements of a natural knee. The main indications of its use are knee disarticulation and amputees with weak hip extensors. The prosthesis provides better stance phase stability.

   iii) *Safety knee*

   This locks automatically if weight is borne on a semi flexed knee. It is useful in blind patients, those with weak hip extensors and in bilateral amputees.

   (b) **Hydraulic**

   Variable cadence knee

   This allows for varying walking speeds but has greater maintenance requirements. This leads to increased cost.

   (c) **External hinge** This is applied in patients with short stumps, persistent flexion contracture of the knee and in patients with ligamentous laxity of the knee.

4. **Prosthetic foot mechanics**

   (a) **SACH foot (Solid Ankle Cushion Heel)**

foot This is the most commonly used prosthetic foot design. It consists of a cushioned heel made of foam, which provides for shock absorption at heel strike. The stability is provided by solid wooden keel (Fig. 10.2). This design has great durability and low cost and is especially suited for walking in female and child amputees with low energy requirements.

The other foot designs include:

(b) Single axis It provides for dorsiflexion and plantar flexion only.

(c) Multiple axis This substitutes the motion of both ankle and subtalar joints. It is indicated for use on rough and uneven terrain.

(d) Seattle foot This is an advancement over SACH foot and has a *Delrin* keel instead of wood. It is useful for athletic patients.

(e) Stationary attachments, flexible endoskeleton (**SAFE**) foot.

(f) Flex foot This is made of graphite or fiberglass. It is lightweight, and durable but expensive. It is useful for athletic amputees.

(g) Jaipur foot was devised in SMS medical college, Jaipur. This prosthetic foot design was devised with the Indian patient in mind. The foot assembly is essentially a SACH foot but is made more cosmetic. It is fabri-

cated using locally available materials. The various materials used include tread rubber compound, rubber cushion compound, vulcanized rubber and microcellular rubber to construct the various parts of the prosthetic foot. Strength is provided by the wooden malleolar block (made of rosewood) while flexibility is provided by the metatarsal and heel sponge rubber blocks. The advantages with this design are that it is suited for bare foot walking, is less expensive, and provides better cosmesis and function including dorsiflexion, transverse rotation of the foot and inversion and eversion. This allows the patient to squat, sit crosslegged and walk on uneven ground.

(h) Elephant boot is a specially designed prosthesis for patients with Syme's amputation. It is spacious to accommodate the bulky stump and allows weight bearing on its sole.

(i) Kneeling boots are used by bilateral below knee amputees to kneel and work on the floor.

(j) Miscellaneous Peg legs are useful for bilateral above knee amputees for easy walking at home.

Other foot designs include Polyurethane, Dynamic foot, Dynamic Plus (with S shaped spring) and Griesinger foot (Ottobock).

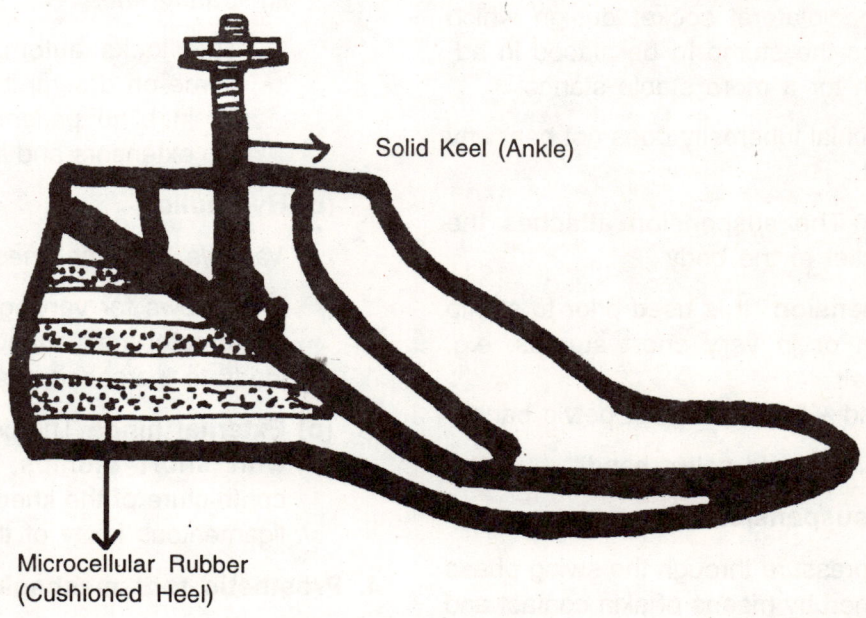

Solid Keel (Ankle)

Microcellular Rubber
(Cushioned Heel)

Fig. 10.2. SACH Foot

5. Prosthetic Shanks

There are two basic types of prosthetic shanks that are used:

(a) Modular assembly prosthesis or Endoskeletal prosthesis.

(b) Conventional or Exoskeletal prosthesis.

Endoskeletal prosthesis This consists of a metal tube with soft cosmetic covering. The inner metal tube supports the weight bearing. This provides good cosmesis, but is less durable than exoskeletal prosthesis. Endoskeletal prostheses are commonly made of titanium or aluminium but newer designs made of carbon are also available, which have the advantage of light weight.

Exoskeletal prosthesis This consists of a strong outer shell, which supports the body weight of the patient. This is less cosmetic, less expensive and more durable. Exoprostheses are usually made of willow wood or thermoplastic laminated material. These prostheses have pedilin insert and kemblo rubber mould lining inside.

Below knee amputation

Socket design for a below knee amputation prosthesis may be end bearing which is poorly tolerated (hence rarely employed) or patellar tendon bearing (PTB) which is a total contact prosthesis. The PTB prosthesis is now the accepted standard which functions through weight bearing over medial tibial tubercle and surrounding tissues.

Suspension The suspension mechanisms are fourfold:

1. Supracondylar strap
2. Thigh corset
3. Supracondylar socket
4. Suspension sleeve

The knee, foot and prosthetic shank designs are similar to the above knee prosthesis.

Other lower limb prostheses

Hemipelvectomy/Hip disarticulation

Socket Totally embracing socket is given which encloses both the iliac crests. In a patient with hemipelvectomy the weight bearing area is over the ischial tuberosity and buttock of the contralateral side, while in a hip disarticulation the weight bearing is on the ipsilateral ischium and buttock.

Suspension is through total contact with or without additional shoulder suspension.

The hip mechanism could be a standard hip joint, which locks automatically in extension or a Canadian tilting mechanism which is fitted anteriorly on the socket. It locks automatically when the patient stands. At the same time, it provides 20 degrees of hip flexion during the swing phase of gait.

The knee, foot mechanisms have been described previously.

Upper Limb Prosthetics

1. Body Powered Devices
2. Externally Powered Devices

   (a) Nickel, cadmium batteries.

   (b) Micro switch control

   (c) Myoelectric control

Upper limb prostheses are available for rehabilitation of wrist disarticulation, below-elbow, above-elbow amputees and those with shoulder disarticulation.

The terminal devices which are commonly used are :

1. **Hooks** These are more durable and easily maintained.

   They are of 2 types:

   (a) Voluntary opening

   (b) Voluntary closing

2. **Hands** These are superior to hook in cosmesis and for grasping large, cylindrical objects.

   They may be:

   (a) Passive

   (b) Voluntary opening

   (c) Voluntary closing

   It is essential to remember that the aim of

prosthetic devices in upper, limb is one of prehension and differs from the weight bearing function of lower, limb prosthetics.

Biceps Cineplasty refers to the surgical construction of a transverse canal through the biceps muscle. A pedicle flap is outlined and raised on the anterior aspect of the arm, which is then sewed in the form of a tube and inserted transversely through the biceps muscle. A split thickness skin graft covers the raw area. Into this canal is inserted a rod attached to a cable, which connects with the mechanism of the artificial hand. Contraction of the biceps is effective in producing flexion of the fingers of the artificial hand.

Orthotics

Definition

British Orthopedic Association Committee has defined orthosis as a "device or external appliance which promotes limb function, excluding prosthesis".

Orthotics is a branch of rehabilitation medicine, which deals with the assessment, prescription, manufacture, and fitting of an orthosis to the body. The terms splint, orthopedic brace or surgical appliance is presently covered by the term orthosis.

Orthosis functions by control of body motion and altera
tion of body shape.

Materials used

The Orthoses are made using two basic types of materials:

1. Conventional metal and leather
2. Molded plastics (Thermoplastics)

Plastic orthoses are more convenient because they are lighter and cosmetically more acceptable.

Classification

Orthoses can be classified broadly into 3 categories:

1. Upper limb orthoses
2. Lower limb orthoses
3. Spinal orthoses

Depending on the functions performed, orthotic devices may be classified into:

1. Devices which rest the joint / fracture in an acceptable position
   e.g. Thomas splint used for splinting fractures of the femur

2. Devices releasing weight
   e.g. Spinal braces, weight relieving calipers

3. Devices stabilizing unstable joints

Upper limb Orthotics

The common indication for use of orthotics in upper limb include:

1. Paralytic conditions

   (a) *Nerve palsies* Median, Ulnar and Radial nerve, brachial plexus injuries, stroke

   (b) *Poliomyelitis*

   (c) *Cerebral palsy*

2. Following fractures and dislocations

3. Soft tissue contractures (Post burn contractures, Volkmann's ischemic contracture)

4. Congenital anomalies e.g. Radial club hand

5. Following tendon repair / tendon transfers

6. Following reconstructive surgery, acute/sub acute phases of rheumatoid arthritis

7. Following total joint replacement

8. Conservative management of deQuervain's tenosynovitis, carpal tunnel syndrome

The upper limb orthoses may be classified as:

1. Static
2. Dynamic
3. Functional devices.

1. Static Devices

(a) Immobilize joint or body part.

(b) Position and maintain correct joint alignment.

(c) Protect recently injured or newly repaired tissues during healing.

(d) Prevent contracture of joints owing to muscle imbalance.

(e) Immobilize joints to improve function in the others joints.

2. **Dynamic devices**

   (a) Allows controlled motion of selected joints

   (b) Neutralize deforming process

   (c) Substitute for weakened or paralyzed muscle

3. **Functional devices**

   (a) Substitute for irreversible loss of function

   (b) Maximize hand function by maintaining useful joint position

   (c) Activate paralyzed or weakened joint function.

The Orthoses may be:

Temporary devices	e.g. in Fractures/dislocation, Peripheral neuropraxia
Semipermanent devices	e.g. in Tendon transfers, Reconstructive surgery in Rheumatoid arthritis
Permanent device	e.g. in Brachial plexus injury

The commonly prescribed orthotic devices in upper limb are

1. Cockup splint (WHO–Wrist Hand Orthosis)–can be of two types:

   (a) Dynamic (b) Static

2. Knuckle bender splint – functions to flex the MCP joints

3. Reverse knuckle bender splint – functions to extend the MCP joints

4. Mallet finger splint

5. Elbow control orthosis

6. Shoulder Abduction stabilizer orthosis (Aeroplane splint)

Lower Limb Orthotics

Several disorders interfere with walking, such as:

1. Neurologic dysfunction including poliomyelitis, cerebral palsy, myelomeningocele and stroke

2. Congenital anomalies

3. CTEV

4. Congenital metatarsus adductus

5. Congenital dislocation of hip.

6. Trauma

7. Degenerative arthritis

8. Muscular dystrophy

These conditions interfere with normal walking by creating deformities at the joints. The function of orthotics in lower limbs is to maximize gait efficiency by overcoming or minimizing the existing dysfunction.

The lower limb orthotics can be grouped into

1. Foot orthotics

2. Shoe Modifications

3. AFO (Ankle Foot Orthosis)

4. KAFO (Knee Ankle Foot Orthosis)

5. HKAFO (Hip Knee Ankle Foot Orthosis)

The nomenclature of the orthosis is based on the use of a system of standard terminology. This system uses the first letter of the name of each joint which the orthosis crosses in the correct sequence, with the letter 'O' for orthosis as mentioned above.

Foot Orthotics

These consist of removable appliances placed within the shoe and extend from the posterior border of the shoe to metatarsal heads. The main uses include arch support, mid and hind foot support and relief of pressure from metatarsal heads as and when indicated.

Indications

The common indications for use of various foot orthotics include:

1. Joint degeneration

   (a) Post traumatic

   (c) Osteoarthritis

   (c) Rheumatoid arthritis

The function of orthotics in joint degeneration due to trauma, osteoarthritis and inflammatory arthritis is three fold:

(a) Limit or prevent motion

(b) Correction/Prevention of progression of deformities

(c) To cushion impact loading

2. Arthrodesis

3. Instability

4. Pes planus/Plano valgus–useful for arch support and prevention of deformity.

5. Plantar calcaneal bursitis, spurs, fascitis.

The commonly used foot orthotics include

→ Whitman arch support

→ UCBL (University of California Biomechanics Laboratory) orthosis

→ Metatarsal bar

→ Heel cups (silicon heel)

→ Sesamoid platforms

Shoe Modifications

The main function of shoe modifications is to correct flexible deformities, accommodate residual deformities, transfer weight bearing from pressure sensitive to pressure tolerant areas and to help immobilize unstable and painful joints. e.g.

1. Medial/Lateral shoe wedges

2. Steel toe

3. Heal cushion

Ankle Foot Orthosis (AFO)

The primary function of AFO is to control alignment and motion of foot and ankle.

Conventional orthosis consists of metal upright attached proximally to calf strap, and distally to shoe via metal stirrup or shoe insert.

The use of stops is to prevent movement in unwanted direction, e.g. Plantar flexion stop is used in **equinus** deformity to prevent plantar flexion. The use of spring assists allows for compensation of motion deficit in specific direction e.g. Dorsiflexion Spring Assist is used in patients with weakness of dorsiflexors of ankle.

T-straps control valgus and varus instability.

AFO is used in

1. Spastic/Flaccid paresis/paralysis of plantar flexion and dorsiflexion.

2. Medial and Lateral instability.

AFO made of thermoplastic material can be used in place of metal. However, these materials should not be used in the presence of rapidly changing deformity, unreliable patients and in severe weakness of plantar flexors.

Floor Reaction Orthosis   This is a special orthosis used in patients with quadriceps paralysis.

Principle of FRO An imaginary line joining the centre of gravity to the point of contact of the foot at the floor is the weight line and its relationship to the axis of the knee joint determines the stability of the knee. At the time of heel strike the weight line passes behind the knee joint, which causes the knee to buckle or give-way in the absence of a normally functioning quadriceps muscle. One of the options to achieve alignment stability in these cases is to arrange the initial ground contact at the forefoot. This would result in the weight line passing anterior to the knee joint automatically stabilizing the knee. Many patients have a stable knee in spite of zero quadriceps because of an equinus deformity. This is the principle of a FRO.

FRO is a "one-piece laminated knee locking short leg brace". It consists of a knee crosspiece located in front of the patella, which is connected via lateral uprights to the ankle and foot assembly. The ankle is in 10 to 15° of equinus. The body weight acts through the lateral uprights to apply a posteriorly directed force in front of the knee, forcing it into extension. Thus the *floor reaction* is utilized to stabilize the knee (Fig. 10.3).

Knee-Ankle Foot Orthosis (KAFO)

The construction of KAFO is similar to the AFO with the addition of above knee extension with adjustable hinge.

Indications

1. Below knee weakness along with knee instability

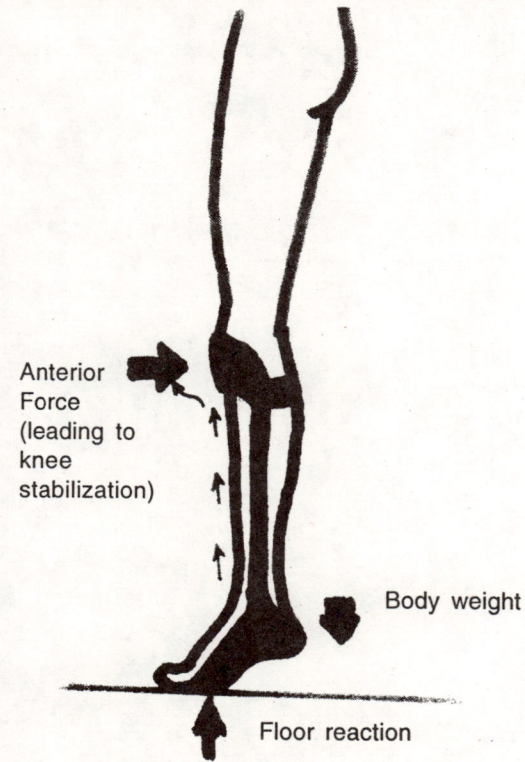

Anterior
Force
(leading to
knee
stabilization)

Body weight

Floor reaction

Fig. 10.3. Principle of Floor Reaction Orthosis

2. Weak/absent knee flexors/extensors (flaccid/spastic)

3. Long term non surgical management of limb deformities

4. Prevention of pathologic femur fracture

Contraindications

1. Absent active hip motion

2. Obesity

3. Poor cosmesis

4. Heavy weight of the orthosis

Moulded polypropylene can be used to construct KAFO where light weight and cosmesis is required.

Hip-Knee-Ankle-Foot Orthosis (HKAFO)

The HKAFO is constructed using a pelvic strap with single axis joint attached to conventional KAFO.

Indications

1. *Unilateral* HKAFO is indicated in

- Flail lower limb (weakness of hip musculature)

- Recurrent prosthetic hip dislocation

2. *Bilateral* HKAFO is indicated in

- Pediatric paraplegia (spastic/flaccid)

Spinal Orthoses

The spinal orthoses can be classified into:

1. Cervical Orthoses

   a) Flexion-extension control orthosis

   - Soft cervical collar

   - Philadelphia collar

   b) Flexion-extension Rotary control

   - SOMI brace(Sterno-Occipito-Mandibular-immobilizer)

   - Four Post Collar

2. Flexible Spinal Orthoses

   - Sacroiliac corset

   - Lumbosacral corset

3. Rigid Spinal orthoses for Thoracic, Lumbar, Sacral Spine

Nomenclature

CO → Cervical orthosis (commonly known as cervical collar)

CTLSO → Cervical Thoracic Lumbo Sacral Orthosis e.g. Milwaukee brace

TLSO → Thoracic Lumbo Sacral Orthosis e.g. Wilmington plastic jacket,

Charleston bending brace.

ASHE → Anterior spinal hyperextension brace.

The commonly used spinal braces in the current day orthopedics include the cervical orthosis in the treatment of cervical spondylosis and trauma. Spinal braces utilize the principle of three-point fixation and are useful in deformity correction e.g. in scoliosis and Scheurmann's disease. In addition, the various braces, such as ASHE brace, may be used in post surgical patients for immobilization, weight relieving and supporting purposes.

SECTION II
Regional Orthopedics

Cervical Spine

Relevant Anatomy

The cervical spine consists of eight functional units (each functional unit consists of any two adjacent vertebrae and their articulations with one another). Five of these units are alike and three, namely the first, second and the last (between the seventh cervical and the first thoracic vertebrae) are unique.

The typical features of the cervical vertebrae include foramen in each transverse process. The spinous processes are bifid and the vertebral foramina are triangular. The first cervical (C_1), also known as atlas, has no vertebral body and no spinous process. It contains two lateral masses. The second cervical vertebra (C_2), also known as axis, has a vertical projection called the dens, or the odontoid process. Dens articulates with the atlas and is believed to represent the vertebral body of the atlas. Dens has two primary ossification centres which fuse by 8 years. The seventh cervical vertebra is unique as it has a prominent nonbifid posterior spinous process and no anterior tubercle.

The first functional unit is Atlanto-occipital joint and its movement allows for about one third of full flexion and extension and for about 50% of lateral bending of head and neck.

The second functional unit is atlanto-axial joint and its movement allows for 50% of the rotations

of the head and neck. The weight across these two functional units is borne on the facet joints. The next five functional units (articulations between second through the seventh cervical vertebrae) contribute to 50% of rotation and 50% of lateral flexion. These five units bear weight on three surfaces-two facets and vertebral bodies. The posterolateral margins of the bodies project slightly beyond the disc to form bony pseudarthrosis (the uncovertebral joints of Luschka) across each of these functional units. Degenerative osteophytes forming at the uncovertebral joints or the facet joints compress cervical nerve roots, which exit through the foramen formed by the uncovertebral joint anteriorly and the facet joints posteriorly. The last functioning unit is the articulation between C_7 and T_1 which is similar to a thoracic unit in that the larger vertebral bodies of C_7 and T_1 bear the bulk of the weight across the unit, and the facet articulations are nearly at right angles to the intervertebral disc (thus allowing limited movements in flexion, extension and rotations).

Evaluation of a patient with neck symptoms

History

A meticulous history is imperative to define the specific lesion. The pathologic process may be local (trauma, tumor, infection) or referred from scalp, temporomandibular joint, teeth, upper extremities or thorax. The clinical characteristics include pain, abnormal posture or range of motion and neurologic or vascular dysfunction. Description of muscle weakness, gait abnormality or sphincteric disturbances is especially important. The physical examination must be complete to evaluate both the spine and the neurologic function of the extremities. Torticollis, facial asymmetry, other head and neck deformities and limitation of range of motion may be present. Palpation should be carried out to detect areas of tenderness, swelling, induration, asymmetry or malalignment in the bony and soft tissues of the neck. Anterior bony landmarks include the hyoid bone at C_3 level, thyroid cartilage at the C_4–C_5 level and first cricoid ring at C_6 level. The anterior neck is best palpated with the patient sitting and the examiner standing behind the patient. The posterior neck is best palpated with the patient in the prone position.

Motor Reflexes and DTR

- Roots C_3–C_5 via the phrenic nerve innervate the diaphragm

- C_5 innervate the deltoid and biceps muscle and is responsible for biceps reflex.

- C_6 supplies wrist extensors and abductors and extensors of thumb and is responsible for brachioradialis reflex.

- C_7 innervates the triceps, wrist flexors and finger extensors and controls the triceps reflex.

- C_8 innervates the finger flexors and has no definable reflex.

- T_1 innervates intrinsic muscles of the hand (including dorsal interossei) and has no definable reflex.

Radiologic Examination

Plain Radiographs

1. Flexion-extension (lateral) views to assess stability

2. Anteroposterior view to assess alignment of vertebrae, any destruction of vertebrae or cervical ribs.

3. Mouth open view (Fig. 11.1a) to assess odontoid and atlantoaxial rotatory instability.

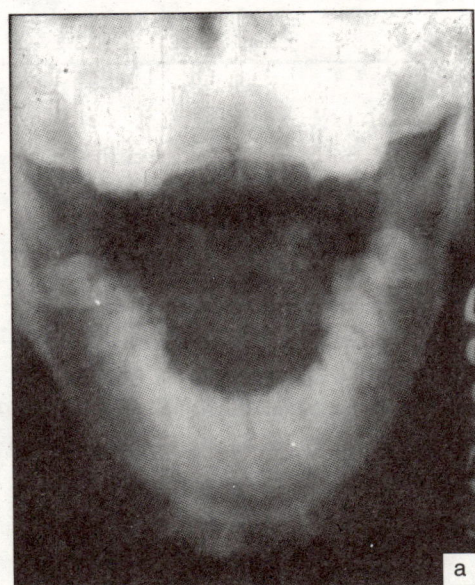

Fig. 11.1a. Mouth open AP view for upper cervical spine

4. Critical measurements on flexed lateral view

   (a) *Atlanto-axial interval (AAI)* up to 4.5 mm in children and up to 3.0mm in adults.

   (b) *Space available for spinal cord (SAC)* [not less than 13mm].

   (c) *Steel's rule of thirds* at the level of C_1, the one third space is occupied by the dens, one third by the spinal cord and one third is vacant.

Tomograms, Computerised Tomography (CT) or Magnetic Resonance imaging (MRI) when indicated are useful for making accurate diagnosis.

Congenital and Developmental Abnormalities

Basilar impression (basilar invagination, cranial settling) implies deformity of the bones at the base of the skull at the margin of the foramen magnum associated with upward migration of the odontoid. The odontoid can compress the brain stem, vertebral artery or obstruct the cerebrospinal fluid.

Types **Primary** basilar invagination is congenital and is associated with atlanto-occipital fusion, hypoplasia of atlas, bifid posterior arch of atlas, odontoid abnormalities, Klippel-Feil syndrome or Morquio's syndrome.

Secondary basilar invagination occurs with softening

of the base of the skull (or erosion and bone loss between the occiput and C_1/C_2) associated with osteomalacia, rickets, Paget's disease, osteogenesis imperfecta, renal osteodystrophy, rheumatoid arthritis, ankylosing spondylitis, achondroplasia and neurofibromatosis.

Diagnosis

1. **X-Rays** Many measurements have been proposed to diagnose basilar invagination on x-rays (Fig. 11.1b). The most commonly used ones are:

(a) Lateral Craniometry

(i) Chamberlain's line Line from posterior lip of foramen magnum to the dorsal margin of the hard palate. A vertical distance from the Chamberlain's line to the inferior edge of C_2 is abnormal if it is less than 33mm (Redlund-Johnell method). Chamber-lain's line is seldom used since posterior lip of foramen magnum is difficult to define on a standard X-ray.

(ii) McGregor's line Line from the upper surface of the posterior edge of the hard palate to the most caudad point of the skull. Tip of the odontoid more than 4.5 mm cephalad to this line is abnormal. McGregor's line is frequently used to screen basilar invagination.

(iii) McRae's line defines odontoid protrusion into the foramen magnum. Its significance lies in the fact that if the tip of the odontoid is caudal to the opening of the foramen magnum, the patient is not likely to have any complications of basilar invagination.

(iv) Ranawat Method measures C_1–C_2 index or the distance from the arch of C_1 to the center of C_2 pedicle. A distance less than 13 mm is abnormal.

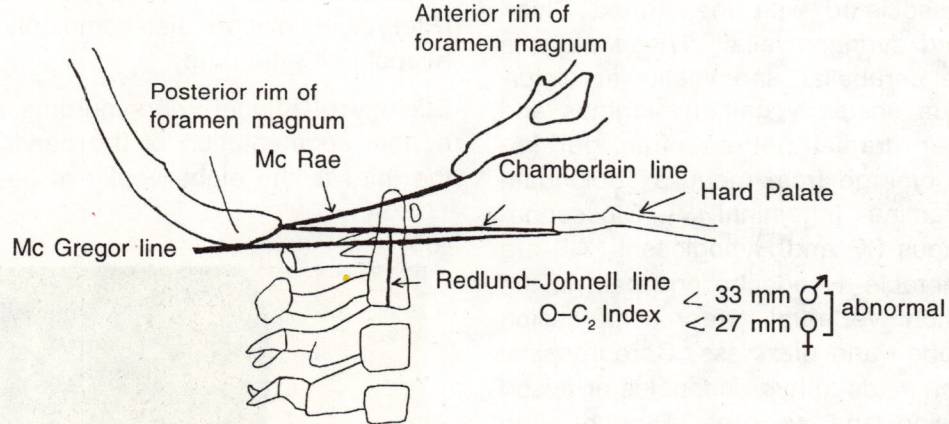

A. Lateral craniometry for diagnosis of basilar invagination

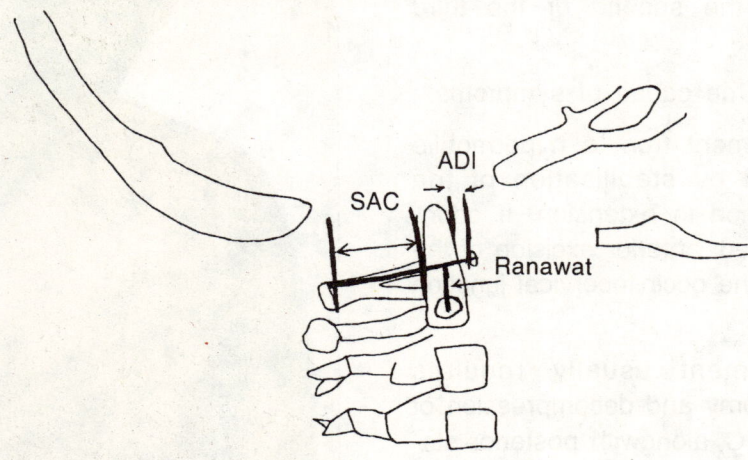

B. Ranawat method for diagnosis of basilar invagination

Fig. 11.1b. Common measurements in occipito-cervical disorders

(b) Anterior Craniometry

An objection to the lateral lines (McGregor's and Chamberlain's) is that hard palate may be distorted by abnormal facial configuration independent of the craniovertebral abnormality. Hence, Fischgold and Metzger defined a more accurate method.

(i) Fischgold and Metzger method

A line is drawn between the two digastric grooves on anteroposterior view of the skull (anteroposterior transoral tomogram). Normally this line passes 10.7 mm above the odontoid tip and 11.6 mm above the atlanto-occipital joint. This is the most accurate method but is impractical and expensive for routine use.

Clinically, the patients with basilar invagination frequently have a short neck, asymmetry of the face or skull, or torticollis. Weakness and paraesthesiae are common. Basilar invagination is frequently associated with the Arnold Chiari malformation and syringomyelia. These patients commonly have cerebellar and vestibular disturbances such as unsteady gait, nystagmus and dizziness. Lower cranial nerves often get impinged as they emerge from medulla oblongata and cranial foramina. Trigeminal (V), Glossopharyngeal (IX), Vagus (X) and Hypoglossal (XII) are particularly vulnerable. Headache and pain in the neck are common. Vertebral artery compression leads to syncope and dizziness. Cerebrospinal fluid compression leads to hydrocephalus or raised intracranial tension and seizures. Though often congenital, the patients with this condition do not develop symptoms till the second or the third decade.

Treatment depends on the cause of symptoms.

* An anterior impingement from a hypermobile odontoid is treated by stabilisation of the occipitocervical junction in extension. If odontoid cannot be reduced, anterior excision of the odontoid can follow the occipitocervical junction stabilization.

* Posterior impingement usually requires suboccipital craniectomy and decompression of the posterior ring of C_1 alongwith posterior stabilization.

Platybasia is a synonym of basilar invagination.

It is merely an anthropologic term used to indicate the flattening of the angle formed by the intersection of the plane of the anterior fossa with the plane of the clivus.

Platybasia has **no clinical significance.**

Klippel-Feil syndrome (Brevicollis, Congenital synostosis of the cervical vertebrae)

Klippel-Feil Syndrome is the condition of congenital fusion of two or more cervical vertebrae. In addition these patients have short neck (Fig. 11.2), low posterior hairline, restriction of neck motion and frequently associated abnormalities. These abnormalities include scoliosis (60%), genitourinary abnormalities, sprengel shoulder, deafness, ocular abnormalities, congenital heart disease and upper limb abnormalities (such as upper extremity hypoplasia, hypoplastic thumb, syndactyly, and super numerary digits).

Torticollis, facial asymmetry and webbing of neck (Pterygium colli) are also commonly associated with Klippel-Feil syndrome.

Etiology of Klippel-Feil syndrome is failure of the normal segmentation of the cervical spine during the third to the eight weeks of gestation.

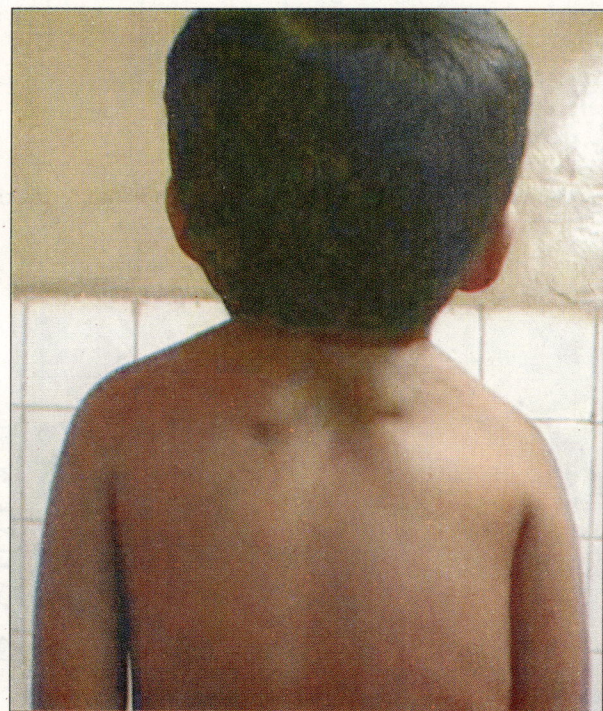

Fig. 11.2.   Klippel-Feil Syndrome. Note the short neck and low hair line

Radiographic features

Plain X-rays show vertebral synostosis with absent or hypoplastic disc spaces. Occipitalization of the atlas may be seen. Flexion-extension views and tomograms in flexion and extension are often required when fixed bone deformities (which prevent positioning) and overlapping shadows from mandible, occiput or foramen magnum (which obscure vertebrae) make the visualisation difficult on the routine X-rays.

Complications

Unfused segments often become hypermobile and lead to frank instability or degenerative osteoarthritis.

Note Unfused segments seldom give rise to pain.

Treatment

Majority of these patients are asymptomatic. Patients are advised to avoid activities which subject cervical spine to stress (to avoid trauma).When degenerative changes occur, conservative treatment is adequate for most patients. However, spinal fusion may have to be undertaken in selected unstable spines with spinal cord impingement. Treatment of cosmetic aspects of this deformity has met with limited success.

Congenital abnormalities of the Odontoid

Congenital abnormalities of the Odontoid include aplasia, hypoplasia and Os odontoideum. Os odontoideum results from the failure of fusion of the apex of odontoid (derived from pro-atlas) to the main body of the atlas and is the most common abnormality.This should not be mistaken for an odontoid fracture. *Odontoid hypoplasia is seen in Morquio syndrome.* Both the conditions can be acquired secondary to trauma or rarely, infection.

Clinically the patients may have various presentations from asymptomatic to atlantoaxial instability (AAI) leading to pain, torticollis, vertebral artery compression and neurologic symptoms. These symptoms arise usually around the third decade.

Radiographic findings

Recommended X-rays are open mouth anteroposterior and lateral. Tomograms are valuable because plain films may not always show abnormality. Lateral flexion - extension films with flexion-extension movements performed voluntarily by the patient are useful to demonstrate instability.

ADI (atlanto-dens interval)   measured from a line projected superiorly from the anterior border of the body of the axis to the posterior border of the anterior arch of the atlas should be less than 4mm.

Space available for the cord (SAC)   is the distance between the posterior aspect of C_2 to the nearest posterior structure, the foramen magnum, or posterior ring of C_1. SAC should be evaluated in all patients with craniovertebral abnormalities.

Treatment is conservative if the CV junction is stable. Surgery is recommended when ADI is more than 7–10 mm (even without symptoms), SAC is less than 13 mm or if neurological signs and symptoms are present. Surgical stabilisation consists of C_1–C_2 fusion, with preoperative traction and reduction if necessary. Occiput-C_2 fusion is done if C_1 ring is deficient. Postoperatively halopelvic stabilisation is provided till sound fusion occurs.

Atlanto-occipital fusion (Occipito-cervical Synostosis, Assimilation of Atlas, Occipito-cervical Fusion, Occipitalization of Atlas) is the most commonly recognized abnormality of the craniovertebral junction. It implies congenital union between the atlas and the base of the occiput, and is a failure of segmentation. It is frequently associated with basilar impression (50% cases; occurs due to diminished height of atlas ring), Klippel-Feil syndrome, occipital vertebrae and condylar hypoplasia. These patients are prone to C_1–C_2 instability if associated with C_2–C_3 fusion or abnormalities of the odontoid.

Other associated abnormalities include dwarfism, genitourinary abnormalities, funnel-chest, pes cavus and syndactyly.

Clinically the patients have short neck, torticollis and limitation of the neck movements. Neurological signs and symptoms due to basilar invagination occur usually around the 5th or 6th decade.

Radiologically the tomograms and CT scans reveal assimilation of the anterior arch of atlas into the occiput. Plain x-rays–lateral views in flexion and extension–are useful to determine ADI and SAC. MRI reveals posterior encroachment by the foramen magnum on the upper cervical cord or medulla oblongata.

Treatment may be hazardous and non-operative method such as cervical collar, brace, plaster and traction should be attempted initially in some patients. With neurological symptoms due to unstable atlanto-axial complex, a C_1–C_2 fusion with preliminary traction to attempt reduction is advised. Posterior signs and symptoms and MRI evidence of bony or dural compression may be indications for posterior decompression.

Torticollis (Congenital Muscular Torticollis, Congential Wryneck)

This is a common condition which manifests in the first 6–8 weeks of life. The deformity is caused by the ischemia and contracture of the sternomastoid muscle. The cause of ischemia has been proposed to be birth trauma (which is often associated with this condition). Head is tilted to the involved side and the chin is rotated to the opposite side (Fig. 11.3). If the infant is examined within the first four weeks of life, a "tumor" or mass (sternomastoid tumor) is usually palpable in the neck. This mass disappears by 4–6 months. Congenital dislocation of the hip may be associated in 20% cases. There is a preponderance of the right side involvement (in almost 85% cases).

Clinically the contracture of muscle is associated with typical deformity and reduced range of neck motion. Contracted sternomastoid is prominent. Facial asymmetry (Plagiocephaly) and mild dorsal compensatory scoliosis may be present.

Differential diagnosis includes congenital cervical spine abnormalities such as basilar impression, atlanto-occipital fusion, odontoid abnormalities etc. Tuberculosis of cervical spine, fractures of the cervical spine, inflamed cervical lymph nodes, cervical disc prolapse, extraocular muscle imbalance and hysteria are the causes of acquired torticollis and must be differentiated from the congenital variety.

X-rays are imperative to rule out bony causes of torticollis when suspected.

Treatment consists of stretching exercises, positioning and bracing and almost 85–90% patients respond within one year. Surgery should be undertaken after 1 year if head tilt, facial asymmetry and restricted neck motion persist.

Surgery consists of release of clavicular head and Z-plasty of sternal head (for better cosmesis, to preserve 'V' of neck especially in female patients). Mastoid head may be released in older patients while bipolar release or Z-plasty may be indicated in longstanding deformity. Posterior auricular and spinal accessory nerves should be carefully protected during surgery at mastoid attachment.

Facial asymmetry and limitation of motion of more than 30° usually precludes good result. However, cosmesis can be expected to improve if surgery is done even as late as upto 12 years of age.

Degenerative Conditions

1. Cervical Disc Disease (Acute Cervical Disc Herniation)

Acute disc herniation in the cervical spine is less common than in the lumbar region. It is more commonly seen in males between 30–50 years of age. The syndrome may be triggered by an acute injury to the disc with or without antecedent trauma

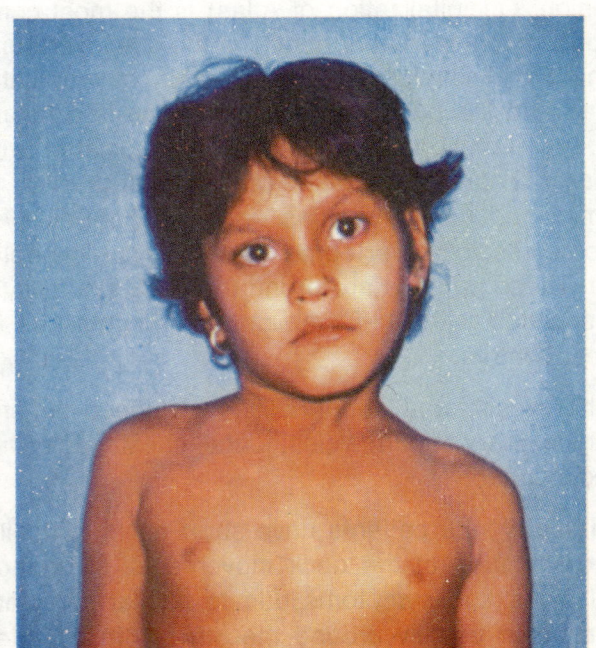

Fig. 11.3.   Right congenital torticollis. Note that head is tilted to right and chin is deviated to the left.

and when so, it is associated with degenerative changes in the disc.

Pathogenesis

Water content of the disc diminishes with age. Mechanical effects (particularly occupational, lifting etc) may be pathogenic. Soft disc herniation follows rupture of annulus and is usually posterolateral between the posterior edge of the uncinate process and the lateral edge of the posterior longitudinal ligament, resulting in acute radiculopathy (by impingement of the root below). Large central herniation, fortunately uncommon, may cause cord impingement. Anterior herniation may cause dysphagia.

Clinically the patient with cervical radiculopathy presents with pain, the location and radiation depending on the level involved. Pain is aggravated by coughing, sneezing, straining, lifting and pushing. Extension of neck and lateral bending to the same side aggravate the pain while deviation to opposite side and shoulder abduction relieve the pain.

There is spasm of the neck muscles and tenderness to palpation of the spinous processes of the involved vertebrae.

Neurologic findings vary with level of the disc and are enumerated in Table 11.1.

Radiologically plain x-rays may be normal or may reveal disc space narrowing. CT scan or MRI may be conclusive. Electromyography and nerve conduction studies are useful in delineating a specific radiculopathy.

Differential Diagnosis includes traumatic conditions (cervical sprain, traumatic neuritis of brachial plexus, instability), tumors (superior sulcus tumor with C8 radiculopathy), inflammatory conditions (e.g. tuberculosis of cervical spine), thoracic outlet syndrome, angina pectoris, reflex sympathetic dystrophy and neurologic conditions.

Treatment for acute cervical disc herniation is conservative. The keystone is rest. Cervical traction, collar, moist heat and muscle relaxants are useful adjuncts. Once the pain remits, exercises and physical therapy should be started. Most patients return to work in 2 to 4 weeks. Failure of

Table 11.1. Neurologic findings in Cervical Disc Prolapse

Nerve Root	Disc level	Location and Radiation of pain	Motor weakness	Reflex change
C_3	C_2–C_3	Back of neck especially around mastoid and pinna of the ear	none (readily detectable)	none
C_4	C_3–C_4	Back of neck radiating along levator scapulae muscle and anterior chest	none	none
C_5	C_4–C_5	Neck, shoulder and lateral arm. Sensations diminished over lateral deltoid	Deltoid	none
C_6	C_5–C_6	Neck, Occiput, interscapular area with radiation to thumb, index finger and numbness over dorsum of hand over first dorsal interosseous and tip of the thumb	Biceps	Diminished biceps reflex
C_7	C_6–C_7	Neck, occiput, interscapular area with radiation to volar forearm, ulnar aspect of hand and 4th and 5th fingers.	Triceps	Diminished triceps reflex
C_8	C_7–T_1	Neck, occiput, interscapular region with radiation to medial aspect of upper arm and forearm; numbness over IV & V fingers	Intrinsic muscles	none

conservative treatment to relieve pain (of radiculopathy and not the neck pain) and/or progressive signs of root dysfunction are indications for surgery. Discectomy and interbody fusion through anterior approach is the treatment of choice.

2. Cervical Spondylosis (Osteoarthritis of Cervical Spine)

Cervical spondylosis is the constellation of symptoms caused by chronic disc degeneration with associated facet arthropathy. Resultant syndromes encompass mechanical neck pain (discogenic), radicular pain (root impingement), myelopathy (cord impingement) or combination.

Cervical spondylosis typically is seen more commonly in males, between 40–50 years age. The most common level involved is C_5–C_6 followed by C_6–C_7 level. Frequent lifting, excessive driving and cigarette smoking have been identified as risk factors.

Pathogenesis

The pathology involves the intervertebral disc, paired uncovertebral joints and paired facet joints. With neck extension the cord is pinched between degenerated disc and osteophytes anteriorly and hypertrophic facets and infolded ligamentum flavum posteriorly. Spondylotic changes in the foramina comprise of osteophytes from uncovertebral joints leading to nerve root compression and restriction of neck motion. Ossification of posterior longitudinal ligaments, common in Asians, may result in cervical stenosis and myelopathy.

Clinically the discogenic neck pain is typically mechanical and is exacerbated by excessive neck movements. Occipital headache is common. Trapezius may be in spasm. Trigger points may be present in scapular muscles. Radiculopathy of one or more roots presents with typical dermatomal involvement. The lower nerve root at a particular level is usually affected. Myelopathy is characterised by quadriparesis, with upper limbs more involved than lower, ataxia, sensory changes, spasticity, and rarely, sphincteric involvement. Hoffman sign and 'Finger escape sign', where little finger spontaneously abducts because of weak intrinsics suggest cervical myelopathy.

Diagnosis is based primarily on history and examination. Plain x-rays show disc space narrowing and osteophytes formation (Fig. 11.4). Oblique views should be taken to assess foraminal compromise due to changes in joints of Luschka. The changes on plain x-rays, however, do not correlate with the symptoms; CT myelography or MRI are useful to delineate compressive pathology well.

Treatment

Conservative therapy is the mainstay of treatment. NSAIDs, exercises, cervical traction, cervical collar and physiotherapy are useful in most cases of discogenic and radicular pain. Changes in posture and specific measure to avoid neck strain should be encouraged.

Surgery is rarely needed for cervical spondylosis. Indications include myelopathy with motor or gait impairment or radiculopathy with persistent disabling weakness and pain. Anterior discectomy and fusion is performed to decompress the neural structures. In the presence of multi-level spondylosis and myelopathy, anterior approach to excise osteophytes and perform multiple vertebrectomies with strut graft fusion is undertaken. Posterior approaches include (trap door) laminoplasty to relieve cord compression without the instability associated with multilevel laminectomies.

Rheumatoid Spondylitis

Cervical spine involvement occurs commonly in

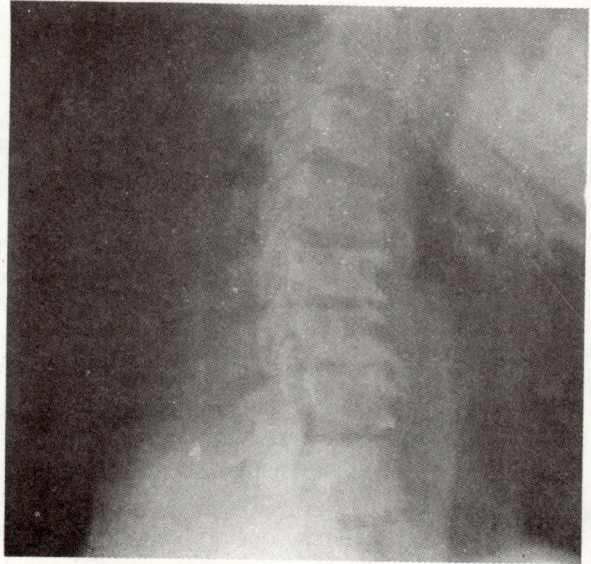

Fig. 11.4. Lateral X-rays of cervical spine showing reversal of cervical lordosis, reduced disc space between C_6–C_7 and C_5–C_6 with osteophytes formation

Rheumatoid Arthritis (RA) especially in severe cases and in longstanding disease. The most common complaints are neck pain, crepitus and decreased range of neck motion. The involvement of cervical spine in RA can be divided into atlantoaxial subluxation, atlantoaxial impaction and subaxial involvement of the cervical spine.

Atlantoaxial subluxation is the commonest involvement and occurs in 50–80% cases. Pannus formation at the synovial joints between the ring of C_1 and odontoid process destroys transverse ligament, odontoid process or both, resulting in atlantoaxial instability (AAI).

Patients present with neck pain, headache, restriction of neck movements and occasionally myelopathy. Increased atlantodens interval (ADI), more than 3.5 mm, and instability on flexion - extension views is seen. Most subluxations are anterior but posterior and lateral subluxations may also be seen.

An ADI of > 9–10 mm and SAC less than 13 mm is associated with marked risk of neurologic injury and is indication for surgical treatment. Posterior atlantoaxial fusion preceeded by preoperative halo traction for irreducible deformities is treatment of choice. Post operatively, halo immobilisation is continued for 3–4 months. The results of surgical treatment are poor once serious neurologic deficit sets in.

Atlantoaxial impaction (cranial settling, basilar impression) results from synovitis and cartilage destruction of occipitoatlantal and atlantoaxial joints. Patients present with occipital headache, myelopathy, or brainstem signs.

Diagnostic criteria

⇒ McGregor's line, > 4.5 mm odontoid projection above foramen magnum.

⇒ Ranawat's C_1–C_2 index < 13 mm is abnormal

⇒ Redlund-Johnell O–C_2 index < 33 mm men
      < 27 mm women is abnormal

Treatment

Progressive cranial migration (> 5 mm) or neurologic compromise is indication for Occiput-C_1–C_2 fusion. Preoperative halo traction may be necessary for irreducible deformities.

Anterior transoral excision of odontoid may be necessary in irreducible cases with anterior compression.

Subaxial Spine involvement occurs in 20% cases (Fig. 11.5a,b). Subluxations may occur at multiple levels due to the involvement of joints of Luschka and facet joints. Other subaxial problems include anterior spondylodiscitis with cord compression, compression from epidural rheumatoid granulation and subaxial hyperlordosis.

Treatment consists of posterior fusion and wiring

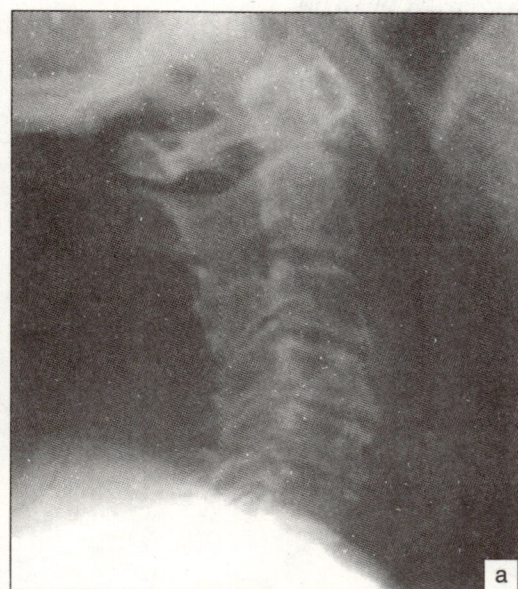

Fig. 11.5a. Lateral view of cervical spine with rheumatoid arthritis

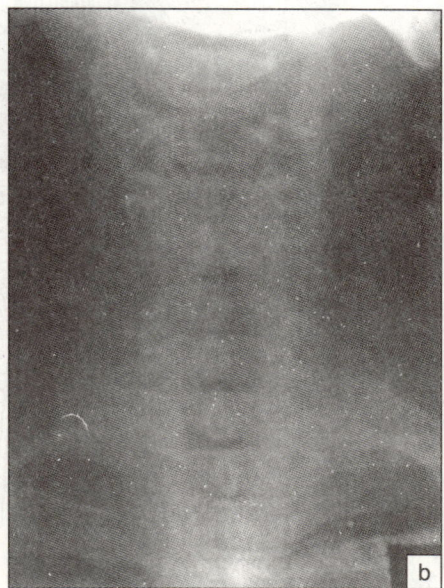

Fig. 11.5b. Anteroposterior view of cervical spine with rheumatoid arthritis

when subluxations more than 4 mm are present with intractable pain and myelopathy.

Thoracic Outlet Syndrome

Thoracic outlet syndrome (TOS) manifests as neck and shoulder pain radiating to the upper extremities with variable neurovascular signs and symptoms. Compression of the brachial plexus and the subclavian vessels is the cause of symptoms (Fig. 11.6). These structures are compressed at one of the three sites (Table 11.2).

Clinically the symptom complex remains similar regardless of the site of compression. Either vascular or neurologic features predominate the clinical picture. The condition is classified as given in the Table 11.3. Vascular compromise presents as non radicular referred pain associated with edema, dis-

Table 11.2. Sites and causes of neurovascular compression in TOS

Site	Etiology of compression
Supraclavicular	A cervical rib, degenerative arthritis of first costovertebral joint, Anterior and /or middle scalene muscles, Poor posture, Kyphosis, obesity.
Costo clavicular (between clavicle superiorly and first rib inferiorly)	Abnormal configuration of first rib or clavicle due to trauma, tumor or inflammation, Elevation of first rib, weight lifting.
Subcoracoid (between pectoralis minor and rib cage)	Shoulder hyperabduction and extension.

coloration, temperature changes and painful throbbing of fingers.

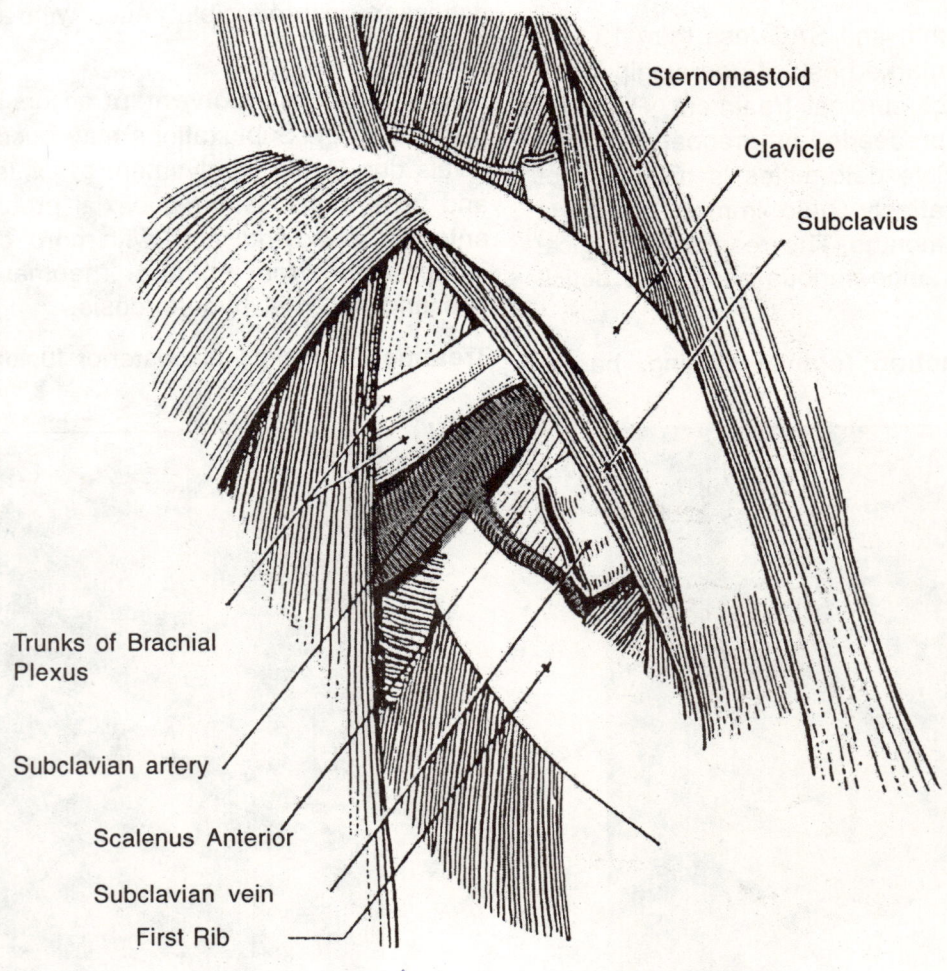

Fig. 11.6. Anatomy of Thoracic outlet showing possible sites of compression

Table 11.3. Wilbourne's Classification of TOS

1. Vascular	a)	Venous (Paget-Schroetter syndrome)
	b)	Arterial
2. Neurogenic	a)	Disputed neurogenic (most common)
	b)	Classical Neurogenic

Neurologic compromise presents as more defined radicular referred pain with associated specific motor, sensory and deep tendon reflex dysfunction.

More commonly however, patients present with vague symptoms which cannot be classified as either vascular or neurogenic. These patients are classified as disputed neurogenic, which is the most common presentation.

A positive Adson's test is often useful to confirm the diagnosis.

X-rays of neck, chest and shoulder should be obtained. A subclavian arteriogram may be indicated to rule out subclavian steal syndrome. The clinical tests used for evaluating TOS are given in the Table 11.4.

Table 11.4. Clinical tests for TOS

Site of compression	Clinical test
Supraclavicular	Adson's test: On extension of neck, deep inspiration and looking to the affected side, the radial pulse becomes feeble
Costoclavicular	Halstead (costo clavicular) manoeuvre: Symptoms appear when the shoulder is pulled downwards and backwards and the chest is protruded forwards
Subcoracoid	Wright's hyperabduction test: Symptoms appear / aggravate on hyperabducting the shoulder
Other tests	Roos test: arms are abducted and externally rotated, elbows are flexed and the fist is opened and closed for three minutes-Rapid fatigue/ reproduction of symptoms; Cervical flexion, lateral rotation test

Differential Diagnosis includes, in addition to subclavian steal syndrome, cervical disc syndrome, cervical spondylosis, Pancoast tumor, carpal tunnel syndrome, entrapment of ulnar nerve at elbow or wrist or reflex sympathetic dystrophy.

Treatment

Conservative treatment is the first choice. Programs to increase the space of the thoracic outlet and reduce pressure on neurovascular structures include correction of the faulty posture and body mechanics and manual stretching to increase the mobility of the neck, shoulder girdle and the first and second ribs. Strengthening exercises for the neck and shoulder girdle are helpful and correction of faulty posture is important.

Failure of conservative treatment with disabling symptoms is indication for surgical intervention. This may involve resection of cervical rib and its fibrous attachments, the first rib or a portion of the scalenus anterior and medius muscles. Trans axillary resection of first rib is the preferred surgical procedure.

Tuberculosis of Cervical Spine

Tuberculosis of the cervical spine may involve the atlanto axial joint or the subaxial spine. It is less common than the tuberculosis of the dorsal and lumbar spine. This fact, along with the frequently present spondylotic changes in adults over 40 years of age often leads to delayed diagnosis.

Pathogenesis

Tuberculosis of the cervical spine, like tuberculous spondylitis elsewhere, is secondary to a disease focus elsewhere in the body. The infection begins in paradiscal area of two contiguous vertebral bodies with rapid destruction and pus formation. Pus may track to the retropharyngeal area deep to the prevertebral fascia, to posterior triangle of the neck or to the suboccipital area. Spinal cord may be compressed by the pus and /or granulation tissue. Thrombosis of spinal artery may aggravate the neurological deficit.

Tuberculosis of the atlantoaxial joint may lead to atlantoaxial instability (AAI) due to destruction of transverse ligament and/or odontoid process and may culminate in serious neurologic compromise.

Clinically disease is more common in children and adolescents. Pain, fever and restriction of neck motion are common presenting symptoms.

Child often presents supporting his head with his hands to avoid movements which can be extremely painful. A large retropharyngeal abscess may produce dysphagia. Normal cervical lordosis is obliterated and spinous processes of affected vertebrae are tender to palpation. Quadriplegia may develop with spinal cord compression.

Radiologically plain x-rays show loss of disc space with destruction of the contiguous vertebral bodies and increased prevertebral soft tissue shadow. Increased atlantodens interval may be seen in disease involving C_1–C_2 area (Fig. 11.7a).

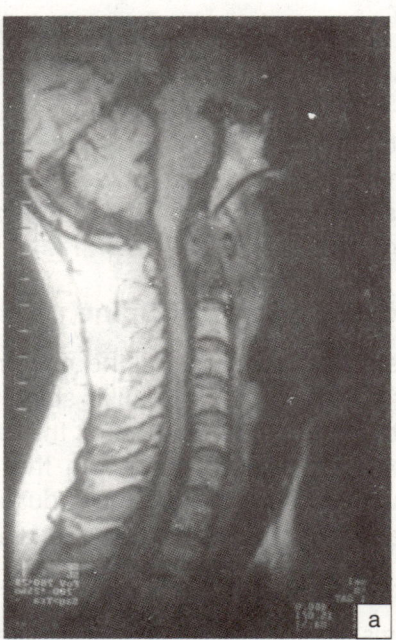

Fig. 11.7a. MRI picture of C_1–C_2 tuberculosis. Note the bony destruction and soft tissue swelling

MRI may be helpful in cases with neurological deficit to delineate site and severity of compression and the status of the spinal cord (Fig. 11.7b).

Treatment consists of antitubercular drugs. Usually four drugs are started in therapeutic doses. Rest is provided to the neck using a cervical collar or a four-post collar. The disease of C_1–C_2 area is best immobilised in skull traction using Crutchfield tongs or halo apparatus.

Large abscesses, which are threatening to rupture should be drained. A retropharyngeal abscess is best drained through the transoral approach.

Neurological improvement usually occurs with the rest and chemotherapy. However, the neurological deficit which does not improve after 4–6 weeks of treatment or worsens while on

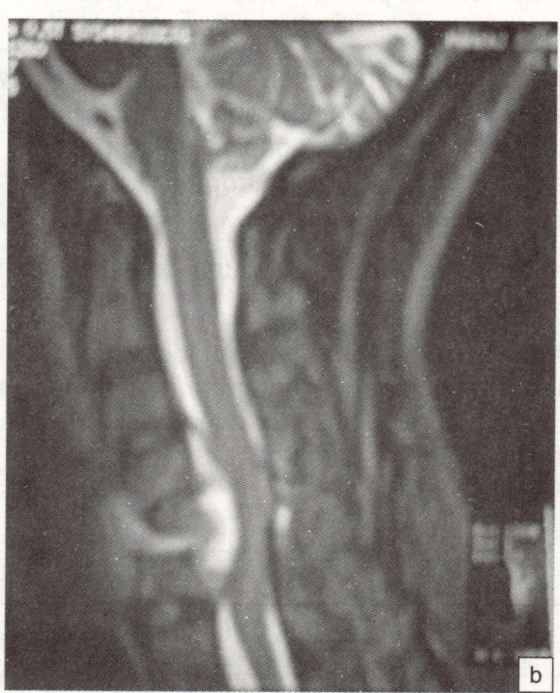

Fig. 11.7b. Tuberculosis of C_5–C_6 with Spinal Cord compression by the abscess (MRI–T_2 Weighted image)

treatment warrants surgical intervention. The disease at C_1–C_2 is approached through the transoral route while subaxial involvement is approached anteriorly. The debridement, drainage of pus and decompression of spinal cord is carried out. Corticocancellous grafts are used to bridge the defect created in the bone and to expedite fusion. Postoperative immobilisation is continued till the radiological evidence of bony fusion.

Any demonstrable AAI after healing of the disease at C_1–C_2 level is treated by occiput-C_2 fusion.

Shoulder

Relevant Anatomy

The shoulder joint is the attachment of upper humerus to the shoulder girdle (composed of scapula and clavicle).

Osteology

Clavicle is the first bone in the body to ossify and the last to fuse. It has two primary (appear in 5th to 6th fetal week) and one secondary ossification centre.

Scapula overlies second to seventh ribs, has two surfaces, three borders, three angles (inferior, superior and lateral) and three processes (spine, acromion and coracoid). It has one primary (appears in 8th fetal week) and six secondary ossification centres.

Humerus Proximal humerus is comprised of head, anatomic neck, surgical neck, greater and lesser tuberosities and bicipital groove. Humerus has eight centres of ossification, the first one of which appears in the 8th fetal week.

Arthrology

The shoulder complex has one major (gleno-humeral) and three minor articulations (sterno-clavicular, acromioclavicular, scapulothoracic).

Glenohumeral joint is a spheroidal, or ball and socket joint. It has minimal bony restraint as only one fourth of the articular surface of the proximal humerus is in contact with the shallow glenoid at any given time. It is the most mobile articulation in the body and also the one most prone to instability. The joint space is defined by the synovial membrane and the fibrous capsule. These are attached to the bony glenoid via the fibrocartilaginous glenoid labrum. Ligamentous restraint is minimal posteriorly; however, strong superior, middle and inferior glenohumeral ligaments stabilise the glenohumeral joint anteriorly.

Scapulothoracic joint is not a true joint. It allows scapular movements against the posterior rib cage. It is fixed mainly by the scapular muscles attachments.

Sternoclavicular joint is a double gliding joint with fibrocartilaginous articular disc. Its capsule is reinforced by the anterior and posterior sterno-clavicular ligaments and a very strong costoclavicular ligament. The sternoclavicular joint rotates 30 degrees with shoulder motion.

Acromioclavicular joint is a gliding joint that also possesses a fibrocartilaginous disc. Its ligaments include acromioclavicular ligaments and coraco-clavicular ligaments (with trapezoid—the anterolateral and conoid-the posteromedial and stronger).

Muscles

The deltoid muscle and the rotator cuff are the most important and the second most important dynamic structures in the shoulder complex respectively. The rotator cuff is the confluence of the tendons of four muscles namely, subscapularis, the supraspinatus, infraspinatus and teres minor. The rotator cuff functions as a "shock absorber" between the proximal humerus and the under-surface of acromion, stabilises the glenohumeral joint and firmly seats the humeral head within the glenoid cavity so that the deltoid can optimally move the arm.

Long head of the biceps originates from the superior margin of the glenoid to pass through the bicipital groove between the tuberosities before joining with the short head (arising from the coracoid process) to form belly of the biceps.

Evaluation of the Patient with Shoulder Symptoms

The evaluation of the disorders involving the shoulder region should begin with a good history. The pain in the shoulder disorders radiates up to the attachment of deltoid on the humerus. A more distal radiation along a particular dermatome suggests a cervical spine disorder. Pain in periarthritis persists even when patient is not using the shoulder and at night whereas pain due to post-traumatic conditions occurs only when the shoulder is moved.

Early restriction of shoulder movements may be realised by the patient as inability to hold overhead bar in public transport or inability to put the hand in the pocket of trousers. Patients with instability often complain of giving way or weakness of the shoulder while throwing.

Physical examination should include inspection of shoulder and the upper arm from all aspects. One should look for asymmetry, muscle atrophy, discoloration and deformities. The region is then palpated for tenderness, defects, deformities and masses. The active and passive range of shoulder movements is tested while one hand is kept on the shoulder to feel for associated crepitus. Loss of active motion when passive motion is normal suggests neuromuscular pathology or full thickness rotator cuff tear. A basic neurovascular evaluation should be done. Apprehension and stress testing should be performed for suspected instability. A brief examination of the cervical spine, ipsilateral elbow, forearm, wrist and hand should also be performed to rule out other causes of the symptoms.

Radiologic evaluation includes the basic shoulder series i.e. the true anteroposterior (AP) with arm in neutral rotation and the axillary views of the glenohumeral joint. Supplementary x-rays include the tangential or lateral scapular view, the transthoracic lateral view, and the AP projections of the shoulder with the arm in internal and external rotation. An anteroposterior view of the shoulders with the weights hung from the patient's wrists can be obtained when acromioclavicular joint injuries are suspected and integrity of acromioclavicular ligaments is doubtful.

Sophisticated diagnostic studies such as ultrasonography (for rotator cuff tears) or Magnetic Resonance Imaging (for rotator cuff tears or to assess musculoligamentous structures and labrum in shoulder instability) are available if warranted clinically. Arthroscopy of the shoulder is now routinely practiced as a diagnostic and therapeutic modality. Arthroscopy allows ready evaluation of joint and articular cartilage along with rotator cuff, subacromial bursa, biceps tendon, subscapularis muscle and glenohumeral ligaments. It has the added advantage that the pathology diagnosed can often be tackled at the same time.

Congenital and Developmental Conditions

Sprengel Shoulder (Congenital elevation of scapula) is the most common congenital abnormality of the shoulder in children. The condition is characterised by undescended scapula with elevation and medial rotation of its inferior pole. The affected scapula is small, relatively wide and its supraspinous portion is abnormally bent forward (Fig. 12.1a,b). The deformity is usually unilateral but may be bilateral. Almost 30% patients have omovertebral connections (i.e. bony, cartilaginous or fibrous connections to the cervical or upper dorsal spine). Sprengel shoulder has an increased association

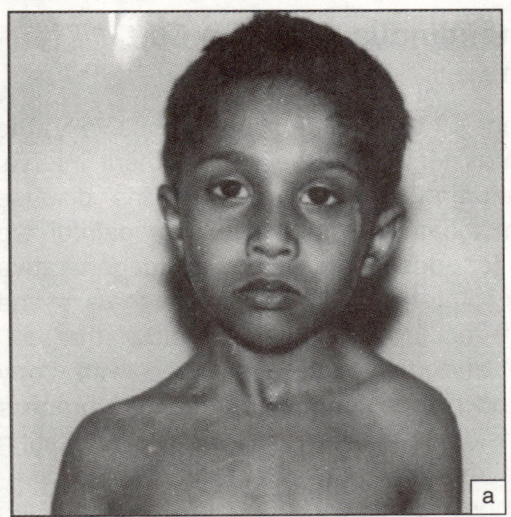

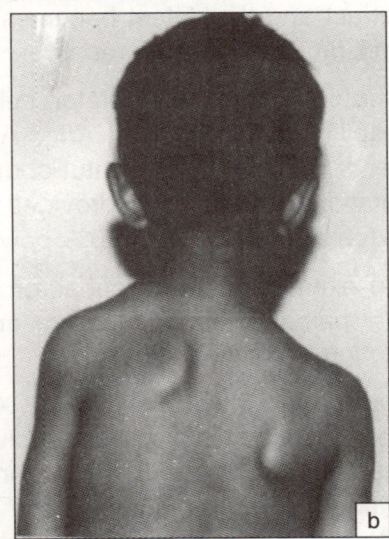

Fig. 12.1a,b. Sprengel shoulder left (a) Front view (b) Back view

with Klippel–Feil syndrome, kidney disease, scoliosis and diastematomyelia.

Pathogenesis Sprengel shoulder results from the interruption of the normal caudal migration of the scapula occurring between the 9th and the 12th week of gestation. There is also defective development of scapular muscles.

Diagnosis

Patients present with elevated scapula with or without associated torticollis. Severe cases have webbing of the neck (pterygium colli). Abduction at the shoulder is restricted in proportion to the severity of the deformity.

X-rays are necessary to assess the degree of the development of scapula, the degree of angular defor-mity of scapula, presence of omovertebral bone and diagnosis of associated abnormalities of the spine.

Treatment

Surgical treatment is needed for the cosmetic and the functional improvement as conservative treat-ment is ineffective. The two procedures, which have had the best results, are the Green and Woodward procedure. Traction type of brachial plexus injury may occur following the Green pro-cedure. This can be prevented by morcellization of the clavicle. The Green procedure consists of extraperiosteal detachment of muscles from scapula, resection of supraspinous portion of scapula and mobilisation of scapula inferiorly. Woodward pro-cedure involves release of (trapezius and rhom-boid) muscles from their origin along the spinous processes and resection of superomedial border, followed by lowering and derotation of the scapula.

The ideal surgical candidate is a child 3–8 years old with moderate to severe deformity and func-tional impairment (shoulder abduction less than 120 degrees).

Congenital Pseudarthrosis of the Clavicle

Congenital pseudarthrosis of the clavicle results from the failure of the union of the medial and lateral ossification centres of the clavicle. It is seen commonly on the right side. The condition presents itself as an enlarging, painless, non-tender mass. Rounded, sclerotic bone is seen at the pseudarthrosis site on x-ray.

Unacceptable cosmetic deformities or significant functional impairment (resulting from mobility of fragments or winging of scapula) are treated by open reduction and internal fixation with bone grafting. Successful union can be achieved fol-lowing surgery.

Degenerative Conditions

Impingement syndrome (Painful arc syndrome, Supraspinatus syndrome) is an extremely com-mon shoulder disorder resulting from narrowing of the space between the under-surface of the ante-rior acromion and the superior aspect of the proxi-mal humerus ("the impingement interval"). This space is normally at its narrowest in 60 degrees–

120 degrees abduction. The soft tissues in this space namely, the subacromial bursa, the long head of the biceps tendon, and the rotator cuff get impinged against coracoacromial ligament, undersurface of acromion and undersurface of acromio-clavicular joint (AC Joint). The conditions which can cause the narrowing of this space are subacromial bursitis, inflammation of supra-spinatus tendon, calcific deposits in degenerated supra-spinatus tendon, fracture of the greater tuberosity of humerus or the degenerative joint disease (of AC joint) resulting in osteophytes and subacromial impingement.

Clinically the patient complains of pain over the anterior aspect of shoulder. Palpation of the impingement interval elicits tenderness. The maximal pain is experienced on abduction of internally rotated shoulder between 60–120 degrees of elevation (hence the name "painful arc syndrome"). Pain is also experienced on forward hyper-flexion of the humerus. Injection of impingement interval with local anaesthetic relieves the patient's symptoms temporarily (impingement test).

If biceps tendinitis is present, the palpation over the bicipital groove elicits tenderness and biceps resistance test (Yergason's test) is positive. If associated with rotator cuff tear, typical clinical features as described in the later part of the chapter will be seen.

Radiologically the x-rays of the shoulder may show cysts, sclerosis or irregularity over the greater tuberosity, bony spurs along the undersurface of acromion or clavicle or the calcific deposits within the subacromial space.

Treatment

Conservative treatment is preferred initially. Hot fomentation, sling and NSAIDs are instituted. Avoidance of aggravating positions and activities are advised. Gentle shoulder exercises are advised to prevent stiffness. Occasionally, a subacromial injection of steroids is required if other modalities are not successful.

Surgery is reserved for recalcitrant cases and consists of open or arthroscopic decompression of the subacromial space (including anteroinferior acromioplasty and resection of the coracoacromial ligament).

Musculotendinous (Rotator) Cuff Syndrome

Impingement of the rotator cuff, especially the supraspinatus tendon in the impingement interval leads to attrition. The spectrum of the disease varies from inflammatory tendinitis or painful arc syndrome (as described above) to degenerative tear of the rotator cuff. Degenerative tears of the rotator cuff occur in individuals older than 40 years age and are often associated with bony changes and biceps tendon rupture. The process may be insidious or may follow a precipitating traumatic event of variable severity. Once a complete thickness tear occurs, the involved tendons retract and the defect becomes increasingly larger and more difficult to repair.

Clinically an *acute* rotator cuff tear presents as inability to abduct the arm. A *chronic* tear presents as weak and painful abduction and external rotation (Rotator cuff provides 80–90% power of external rotation and 50% power of abduction).

On examination, fine subacromial crepitus is usually palpable during passive and active range of motion of the shoulder.

Radiologically the plain AP X-ray of the shoulder reveals the superior subluxation of the humeral head. A shoulder arthrogram shows the leakage of dye injected in the glenohumeral joint into the subacromial bursa. Arthrogram, however, is not so useful in partial tears. Ultrasonography is reliable in detecting full thickness tears but is less reliable for partial thickness tears smaller than 1 cm. Magnetic resonance imaging is accurate at determining the extent of the tear. Arthroscopy allows direct visualisation of the pathology and repair of the tear.

Treatment of the acute tear of rotator cuff is surgical repair within 3 months for massive tear in young (less than 50 years) patients. Small and medium tears are repaired tendon to tendon or tendon to bone. Large and massive tears need mobilisation and transposition of existing cuff tissue, allograft cuff, fascia lata, or carbon fibre. (Impingement should always be tackled by acromioplasty).

Chronic tears are treated with NSAIDs, rehabilitation and subacromial steroids. If patients still remain disabled with pain, surgery should be considered. The results of surgery in longstanding tears are poor and the purpose is pain relief and not the functional improvement.

Cuff Tear Arthropathy

Cuff tear arthropathy implies degenerative osteoarthritis of shoulder following massive rotator cuff tear. The disease is characterised by rotator cuff tear, articular cartilage degeneration, and bone loss of humeral head, glenoid and acromion. X-rays show superior subluxation of humeral head, narrowing of joint space and altered bony contour of humeral head, glenoid and acromion.

Treatment is total shoulder arthroplasty with rotator cuff reconstruction. If rotator cuff is not reconstructible, the arthroplasty will fail; hence, only hemiarthroplasty should be considered in such cases. The aim of surgery is pain relief and the functional improvement is secondary.

Rupture of the long head of biceps tendon

Biceps tendon may undergo attrition as it passes through the shoulder impingement interval. In younger individuals (less than 40 year) it leads to bicipital tendinitis while in older individuals a complete rupture of the tendon may occur.

Clinically the patient is usually over 40 years of age and has history of episodes of impingement in the past. Tear presents with a sudden and painful popping sensation over the anterior aspect of shoulder during lifting. A concavity appears over anterior aspect of proximal arm while the retracted belly of biceps bulges over the anterior aspect of the distal arm (Fig. 12.2). Flexion of the elbow against resistance makes the swelling more prominent.

Treatment If diagnosed within the first week the treatment consists of surgical repair of tendon along with subacromial decompression. Repair is not possible after the first week due to marked retraction of the ruptured tendon. Though cosmetically objectionable, the function in these patients is good even without repair.

Frozen Shoulder (Adhesive Capsulitis, Periarthritis of shoulder) is a common affection of unknown aetiology resulting in symptomatic stiffness. Inflammatory process of the rotator cuff or immune mediated response are implicated. The disease is often initiated by coexistent cardiovascular or cerebrovascular disease, diabetes mellitus, thyroid disease, trivial trauma or any other painful shoulder condition.

Pathogenesis Disease starts with contracture of subscapularis and coracohumeral ligaments along with the thickening and loss of normal resilience of the joint capsule. The normal axillary recess gets obliterated and the joint volume is diminished (7–12 cc vis-a-vis normal of 25 cc).

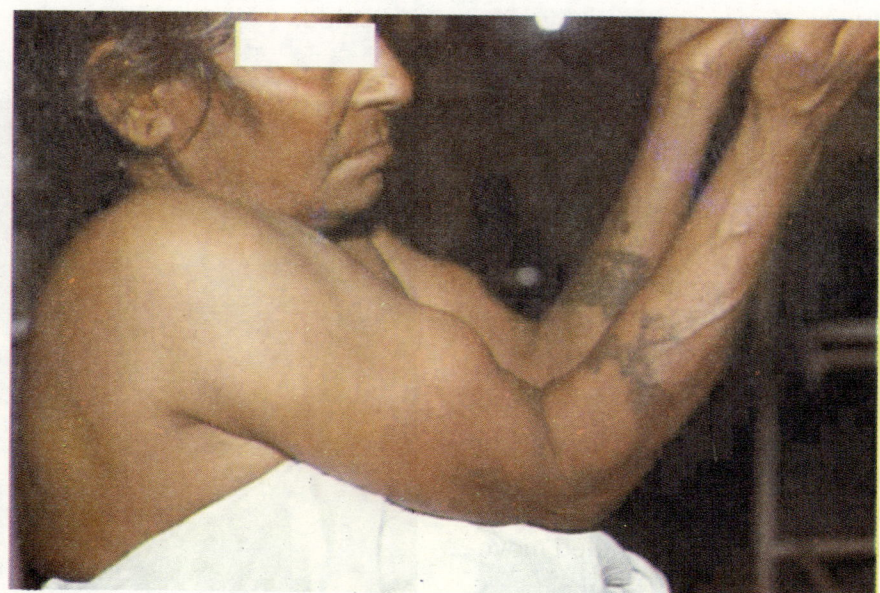

Fig. 12.2. Clinical photograph of a patient with rupture of the long head of the right biceps. Note the bunched up appearance of muscle belly and concavity over the proximal arm anteriorly

Clinically the patients are more commonly females between 45–60 years of age who present with gradual onset of pain and stiffness. Pain occurs at night also and patient is unable to lie on the affected side. Restriction of external rotation and abduction is typical though internal rotation also gets limited later.

Most patients have complete restoration of movements and relief of pain within 18 months.

Radiologically only finding may be sclerosis or cyst formation over the greater tuberosity. Arthrogram reveals decreased volume of the joint and loss of the axillary recess.

Treatment is by NSAIDs, local heat and gentle, regular exercises to regain movements. Rest in a sling is advisable if the pain is very severe. Local injection of hydrocortisone with xylocaine in the joint can be used to control pain. Hydraulic distension of the joint is described to break adhesions and loosen up the joint. Manipulation under anaesthesia is undertaken in recalcitrant cases but special care should be taken to avoid fracture of the humerus during manipulation. Surgery is indicated in cases where non-operative treatment has failed. Open or arthroscopic release of the contracted structures is done to gain movements.

Inflammatory Disorders

Infective

Tubercular Arthritis

Tuberculosis of the shoulder joint is less common than the tubercular infection of spine, hip and knee. Like elsewhere, the disease is secondary to a distant focus of infection. The disease can be synovial or osteoarticular. Pathologically the disease can lead either to copious pus formation and drainage through the sinuses or to the dry variety without any pus formation. The latter is called "caries sicca" and is peculiar to shoulder joint.

Clinically the patients are usually adults who present with pain, swelling and restriction of the shoulder movements. Marked wasting of periarticular muscles is present. Discharging sinuses may be present in the advanced disease. Attempted movements are painful.

Radiologically plain x-rays show marked osteoporosis, diminished joint space with destruction of joint surfaces and lytic areas in the humeral head and glenoid.

Treatment consists of anti-tubercular drugs and rest to the arm in a sling. Function remains poor if disease is advanced. Residual pain following anti-tubercular treatment is indication for shoulder arthrodesis.

Non Infective

Rheumatoid Arthritis (RA)

Shoulder joint and subdeltoid bursa are often involved in the polyarticular RA. Patients present with pain, swelling and restriction of movements.

Clinically it may be difficult to differentiate from tubercular arthritis unless polyarticular involvement or other stigmata of RA are present.

Radiologically plain x-rays show juxta articular osteoporosis, erosions of the joint margins and sometimes, superior subluxation of the humeral head (Fig. 12.3).

Treatment comprises of treating the systemic disease. Physiotherapy should be instituted to preserve and regain the range of movements. Local (intra-articular) injection of steroids may be required sometimes to control severe pain. When associated with functional disability due to the involvement of other joints in the ipsilateral extremity, total shoulder replacement arthroplasty is indicated.

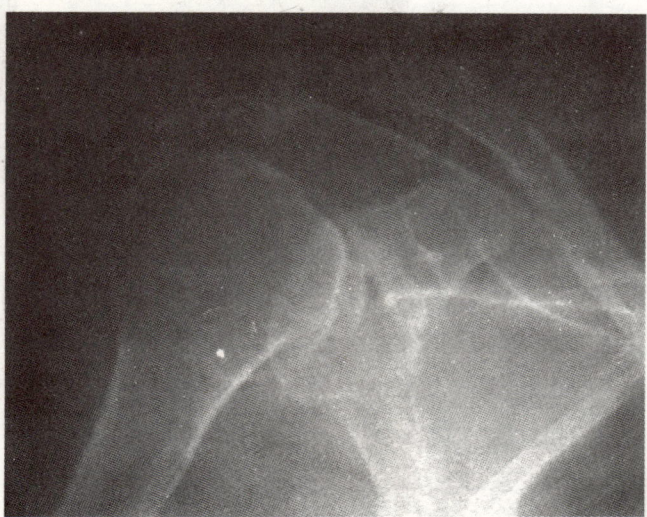

Fig. 12.3.   X-rays showing involvement of shoulder with rheumatoid arthritis

Chronic instability of the Glenohumeral joint can be of three types:

1. Chronic (Recurrent) Dislocation

Chronic (recurrent) dislocation is the chronic instability when apex of humeral head circumference moves beyond the rim of the glenoid. *It is anterior in most cases.* It usually follows an episode of acute, traumatic anterior dislocation in young adults (recurrence rate is 3–5 times more in those under 30 years than those over 30 years). Length of immobilisation has no effect on the recurrence rate. Usually if the first episode of dislocation occurs following severe trauma, the chances of recurrences are lesser. Other factors postulated to be contributing to chronic anterior instability are a detached labrum ("*Bankart lesion*"), depression in the posterolateral part of the humeral head ("*Hill Sach lesion*") and the laxity of capsuloligamentous structures and subscapularis muscle.

Clinically the patient complains of recurrent attacks of dislocation following increasingly trivial trauma (or even spontaneously) after an initial episode of posttraumatic dislocation. Patient avoids taking the arm to extension-abduction-externally rotated position.

Apprehension and stress testing in the anterior direction are positive.

Radiologically plain x-rays taken in 60° internal rotation show an impression defect (Hill Sach's lesion) on postero-lateral aspect of the humeral head (Fig. 12.4). CT or CT arthrogram when

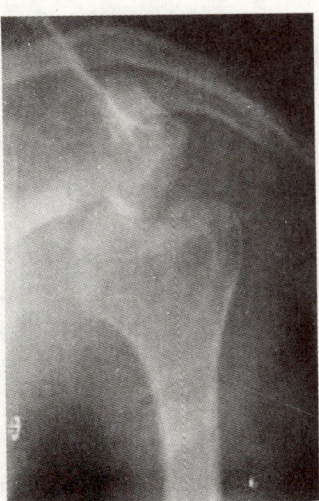

Fig. 12.4.   Dislocated shoulder with Hill Sach's lesion

indicated can be used to depict bony as well as soft tissue changes.

Treatment is essentially surgical. A large number of operations are described but three most commonly employed procedures are:

(a) Putti Platt Operation Consists of reefing and shortening the subscapularis muscle and anterior capsule to limit the external rotation.

(b) Bankart Operation aims to reattach the detached glenoid labrum to the roughened anterior rim of the glenoid (can be undertaken arthroscopically by the experts).

(c) Bristow Operation involves transfer of osteotomised coracoid process with its conjoint tendon attachment to anterior rim of the glenoid and fixation using a screw.

Chronic recurrent posterior dislocations are rare and when present, voluntary dislocations or psychiatric disorders should be ruled out. Patient typically is apprehensive and avoids forward flexion-adduction-internally rotated position of the extremity. X-ray/CT may show large anteromedial humeral head defect.

Treatment is surgical and consists of Putti Platt procedure (reefing of the infraspinatus tendon), reverse Bankart procedure or glenoid osteotomy.

2. Chronic (Recurrent) Subluxation

Chronic (recurrent) subluxation is milder form of instability and much more difficult to diagnose. The symptoms are milder and the patient may describe the shoulder as giving way, catching or slipping but it never actually dislocates. Apprehension and stress tests are often equivocal.

Treatment is conservative in most patients. Activities and exercises to strengthen the muscles around shoulder are encouraged. For those who do not respond to conservative treatment surgical repair of the damaged retaining structures may be indicated.

3. Functional Disability

Functional disability is the third type of chronic shoulder disability. It refers to situations where a fragment of tissues such as a displaced labral fragment, a loose osseous or cartilaginous body etc. may get interposed between the glenohumeral articulation, causing the shoulder to catch, slip or lock, not unlike the symptoms of a torn meniscus in the knee.

The patient may or may not be able to relate the symptoms to a particular shoulder position. Apprehension and stress tests are negative. CT, MRI and/or arthroscopy are often necessary to reveal intra-articular lesion responsible for the patient's symptoms. Definite treatment entails arthroscopic removal of intra-articular pathology giving rise to symptoms.

Arthrodesis and Arthroplasty of Shoulder

Arthrodesis of the Shoulder

Diseases for which arthrodesis was commonly performed in the past have become uncommon.

Indications

- Paralysis of deltoid and rotator cuff
- Severe destruction of the joint due to inflammatory disorders-Rheumatoid, treated tuberculosis
- Severe rotator cuff deficiencies
- Failed prosthetic reconstructions

Contraindications

- Absence of adequate power in scapulothoracic muscles viz. trapezius, serratus anterior.
- The presence of a prosthetic elbow is an absolute contraindication.

Position of Arthrodesis The most commonly recommended position is 30° flexion, 30° abduction and 30° internal rotation. Fixation is achieved with large cancellous screws or compression plates (Fig. 12.5).

Technique Intra-articular fusion with large cancellous screws or compression plating is treatment of choice.

Total Shoulder Replacement Arthroplasty

- Pain relief is the primary indication.

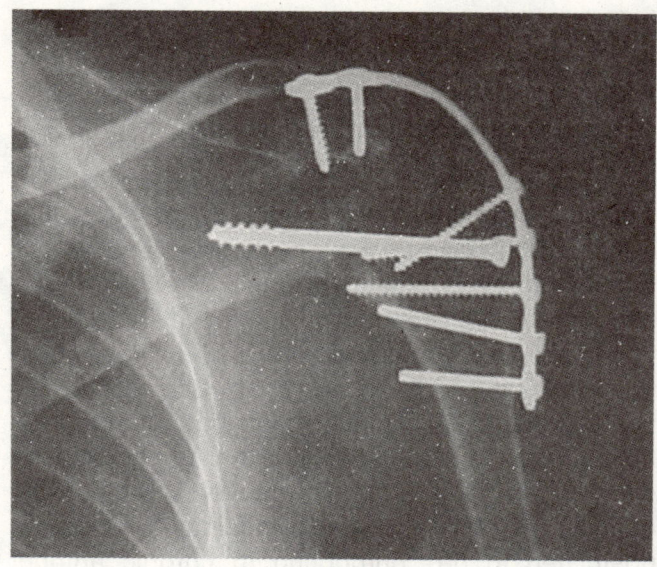

Fig. 12.5.   Arthrodesis of shoulder

- The improvement in function is less predictable, so limitation of function is secondary indication.

Indications

1. RA
2. Osteoarthritis
3. Fractures
   - acute, severe 3 and 4 part fractures
   - impression fractures of humeral head involving > 50% articular surface
4. Avascular necrosis
5. Malunion or non union of fractures (with painful joint)

Contraindications

1. Extreme Osteoporosis
2. Fulminant acute or recent infection
3. Paralysis of deltoid and rotator cuff
4. Neuropathic joint

Designs can be constrained, semiconstrained, and unconstrained. Most present day designs are unconstrained, surface replacements.

Relevant anatomy

The distal end of the humerus forms a complex articulation with the proximal radius and ulna to form the elbow joint. Humero-ulnar joint is a hinge joint between the trochlea and the proximal ulna. Humero-radial articulation is a pivot joint between the capitellum and the radial head. The radial head, in addition, also articulates with the proximal ulna to form the proximal radioulnar joint, which allows the rotation of the radius around the ulna.

Ligaments

The **Medial Collateral Ligament (MCL)** is the key stabiliser of the elbow joint. It consists of three parts: the anterior bundle, the posterior bundle and transverse ligament. The anterior bundle makes up the major portion of the MCL; it takes its origin just inferior to the medial apophysis and inserts into the medial aspect of the coronoid process. Since MCL originates slightly posterior and distal to the axis of rotation at the medial condyle, it shows increased tension with increased flexion.

The **Lateral Ligament Complex** is made up of the lateral (radial) collateral ligament and the lateral ulnar collateral ligament. Lateral collateral ligament is less well defined than the medial complex. It originates from the lateral epicondyle and inserts on the radial side of the proximal ulna and on the annular ligament.

The **annular ligament** originates on the proximal ulna, encircles the radial neck and then inserts on the proximal ulna.

Musculotendinous support is provided by the triceps, biceps, brachialis and the flexor and extensor muscle groups.

Carrying angle implies the normal valgus alignment of the long axis of the ulna with respect to the long axis of the humerus. It varies with respect to age and sex. The normal carrying angle is approximately 10°–15° in females and 5° in males.

Nerves coursing across elbow include Radial between the brachialis and brachioradialis; Median lies on the ulnar side of the brachial artery lateral to the biceps and Ulnar runs behind the medial epicondyle. Elbow range of motion is normally

0°–150° though, for function 30°–130° flexion and 50° each of pronation and supination are sufficient.

Evaluation of a Patient with Elbow Problems

The evaluation of a patient with elbow problem should begin with a careful and detailed history. Onset of symptoms may be important for elbow pathology as it can be acute with distal biceps avulsion or MCL injury while it would be chronic in lateral epicondylitis or arthritis. The aggravating symptoms should be enquired, as should be occupational activities. Baseball pitchers get MCL injury while factory workers are more prone to compression neuropathy. Tennis players and those lifting heavy weights get lateral epicondylitis while golfers are prone to medial epicondylitis. Age is important, as *little league pitchers* are prone to medial epicondyle stress fracture and osteochondritis dissecans while *major league pitchers* get MCL injury and ulnohumeral arthritis. Range of movement is important as progressive stiffness with swelling and constitutional symptoms may suggest inflammatory arthritis. History of cough, expectoration, weight loss, anorexia and contact with tubercular patient will suggest tubercular arthritis in these cases while involvement of multiple other joints especially those of hand and wrist, rheumatoid nodules and history of morning stiffness will suggest rheumatoid arthritis. History pertaining to cervical spine is important as pain from the cervical spine is often referred to the elbow joint. Similarly, pain of lateral epicondylitis often may be referred to dorsal forearm and wrist and confuse the examiner until the tenderness at the lateral epicondyle is elicited.

The physical examination of the elbow begins by inspection for the carrying angle, any swellings at or around the joint and deformities. Palpation of bony prominences of the distal humerus (medial epicondyle, lateral epicondyle, olecranon fossa), olecranon and radial head should be done. The three bony point relationship should be ascertained and compared with the normal side.

The range of flexion (normal, 0°–135°), extension (normal, 0°–5°), supination (normal, 90°) and pronation (normal, 90°) should be examined. A careful distal neurovascular examination should be done. Instability at the elbow joint should be tested by the varus / valgus stress test. Elbow is stressed in both full extension and 30 degrees of flexion to test the MCL and LCL.

Imaging

An antero-posterior (forearm supinated) and a lateral (with forearm neutral and elbow flexed 90 degrees) x-rays are routinely employed to assess the elbow joint. Special oblique views to assess specific regions, radial head view (45 degrees caudal-tilt lateral view) and stress radiographs to assess instability are performed when indicated.

Computerized tomography is indicated to evaluate complex fractures and intra-articular loose bodies. Magnetic resonance imaging is useful to evaluate collateral ligament injuries and tendon ruptures.

Arthroscopy of the elbow joint is now routinely employed at many centres to visualise articular cartilage, remove loose bodies, perform synovectomy and even perform arthrolysis for the stiff elbow.

Congenital Conditions Affecting Elbow

1. Congenital Radio-Ulnar Synostosis is characterised by bony fusion/ fibrous union between the proximal radius and ulna, placing forearm in pronated position. It is of two types: In the more common variety the synostosis is limited to the proximal third of the radius and ulna (Fig. 13.1a,b), while the other variety has extensive radio-ulnar synostosis.

It is often bilateral. The condition may be associated with the developmental dysplasia of the hip, clubfoot, chromosomal abnormalities or syndactyly and camptodactyly. Clinically the child presents with lack of the forearm rotations. Proximal dislocation of the radial head (anterior or posterior) may also be present.

Treatment is difficult. Recurrences are common after surgery. Surgery should be considered if motion, function and potential growth of fused segments are interfered with. Osteotomies are performed for disabling pronation deformities. If bilateral, the dominant arm should be left pronated and the non-dominant arm is osteotomized distal to the fusion to achieve 20–30 degrees of supination.

2. Congenital Dislocation of the Radial Head is characterised by congenital dislocation of an

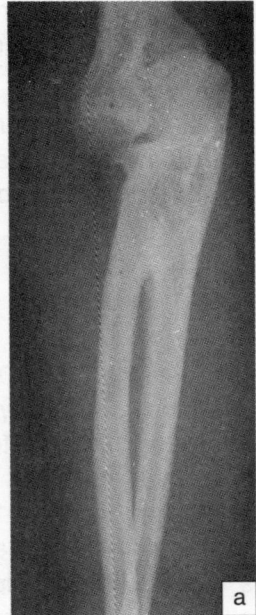
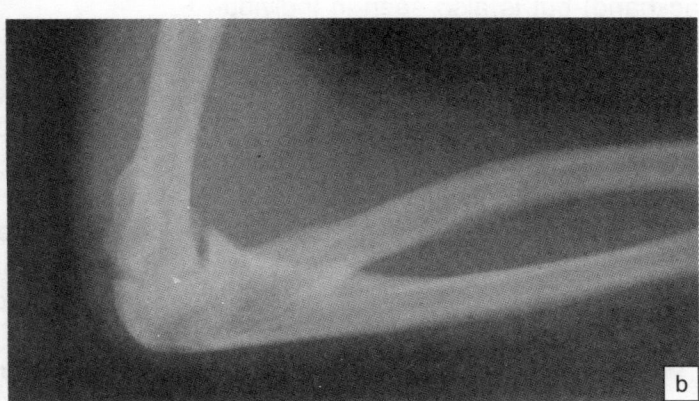

Fig.13.1a,b. Congenital radio-ulnar synostosis

supination.

2. Congenital Dislocation of the Radial Head

is characterised by congenital dislocation of an abnormally formed radial head (Fig. 13.2a,b). Ulna is short and bowed. The shape of capitellum is abnormal (as compared to the normal shape of capitellum in traumatic dislocation). The condition is sometimes bilateral.

Treatment consists of the resection of the radial head once the growth is complete.

3. Congenital webbing of the elbow (Pterygium Cubitale)

is characterised by a broad skin web spanning the front of elbow along with flexion deformity of the elbow. The forearm is pronated. Other webbing disorders may sometimes be associated. Underlying muscles (especially biceps and brachioradialis) may be abnormal.

Treatment is difficult and risky. The shortened

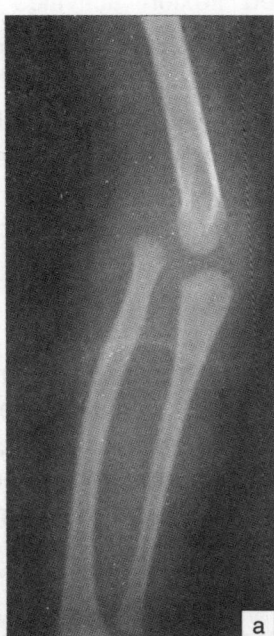
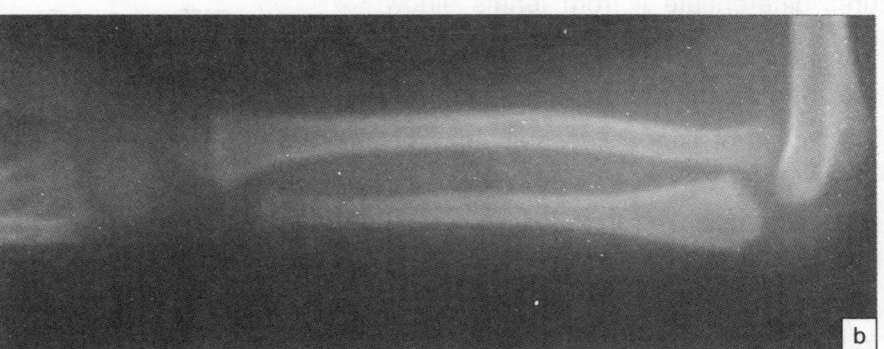

Fig. 13.2a,b. Congenital dislocation of radial head

Common Elbow Conditions in the adults

Inflammatory and overuse disorders around elbow

Lateral epicondylitis (*Tennis elbow*) is classically related to poor technique in racket sports (especially backhand) but is also seen in individuals whose occupations require repeated extension of the wrist or rotation of the forearm such as carpenters, electricians etc.

The disorder is caused by chronic degeneration of the extensor carpi radialis brevis (ECRB) at the common extensor origin.

Clinically the patient presents with pain at the lateral epicondyle but, in chronic cases, the pain may be referred to the extensor aspect of the forearm. The pain is exacerbated by resisted wrist extension and by palpation over the lateral epicondyle. Pain is also exacerbated by passively flexing the fingers and wrist with the elbow fully extended. The range of elbow movements is full.

Radiological examination X-rays are usually normal but calcific deposits may be noted adjacent to the lateral epicondyle in chronic cases.

Differential Diagnosis Conditions such as cervical spondylosis with cervical root compression, compartment syndrome of the anconeus and intra-articular abnormalities of the elbow may show presentations similar to the tennis elbow and must be ruled out. A particularly important condition to differentiate from tennis elbow is the *posterior interosseous entrapment syndrome* or the *Radial Tunnel Syndrome*. Radial tunnel syndrome is most frequently caused by compression neuropathy of the posterior interosseous nerve at the arcade of Frohse as it enters the proximal border of the supinator muscle. The following features differentiate it from tennis elbow:

1. Dysesthesia or reduced sensations over dorso-radial aspect of wrist or hand may be present.

2. Weakness of finger extensors may be present in severe cases.

3. Resisted supination from fully pronated position reproduces pain of radial tunnel syndrome.

4. Maximal tenderness is 4 cm **distal** to the lateral epicondyle between the heads of the extensor digitorum communis and ECRB. Palpation at this point may also elicit paraesthesiae in addition to pain thus duplicating the patient's symptoms.

5. Injection of 0.25% sensorcaine into the area of posterior interosseous nerve and arcade of Frohse relieves the symptoms for a few hours.

Treatment

Acute onset condition with mild to moderate pain is treated conservatively with rest, avoidance of aggravating conditions and NSAIDs. A counter-force brace (tennis-elbow strap) worn about the proximal forearm may reduce the force absorbed at the lateral epicondyle. Physical therapy in the form of stretching, heat modalities, activity modifications and strengthening exercises of involved muscle group is helpful. If physical therapy is ineffective a local hydrocortisone injection (along with 1 ml of 1% xylocaine) in the area just anterior to the lateral epicondyle below the origin of ECRB muscle is able to provide relief. No more than three injections are advisable.

Surgery is indicated when conservative treatment fails or the patient experiences recurrent episodes of disabling pain. The debridement of degenerated ECRB muscle is performed.

Medial Epicondylitis (Flexor origin syndrome, *Golfer's elbow*) is an overuse syndrome of the flexor-pronator group, especially pronator teres resulting from repeated flexion activities of the wrist and fingers (seen in many athletes and labourers).

Clinically the patients present with pain and tenderness at the medial epicondyle exacerbated by flexor-pronator stress (resisted flexion of fingers). Swelling and erythema at medial epicondyle may be seen.

Differential Diagnosis

1. **Cubital Tunnel Syndrome** or entrapment of the ulnar nerve at the elbow may present with medial elbow and forearm pain. However, Tinel's sign over ulnar nerve, paraesthesiae elicited by prolonged hyperflexion and electromyography (EMG) help in differentiating it from golfer's elbow.

2. **Median nerve entrapment** may be confused with golfer's elbow but patients often complain

of night pain and tenderness over the median nerve. EMG can help confirm or exclude the diagnosis.

3. Stress fracture of the epiphysis of the medial condyle in adolescents.

Treatment is similar to that for lateral epicondylitis, starting with rest and anti-inflammatory drugs, and heat therapy; steroids can be injected locally with care to avoid adjacent ulnar nerve. Recalcitrant cases can be taken up for surgical treatment, which involves debridement of degenerated tissues and repair of pronator teres muscle.

(Distal) Biceps tendon rupture

Distal rupture of biceps tendon is rare. It is caused by sudden force overload with the elbow in midflexed position. Middle aged males are most commonly affected.

Clinically the patients present with acute onset of pain, swelling and ecchymosis in the antecubital fossa. The patients have weakness of elbow flexion and forearm supination.

Treatment is operative reattachment to restore supination and flexion strength. Early repair within 7–10 days after injury provides nearly full recovery. Radial nerve should be carefully protected during the repair.

Distal triceps avulsion is a rare entity. It is caused by decelerating counterforce during active elbow extension.

Clinically the patient presents with sudden loss of active elbow extension. A defect is palpable in the triceps tendon.

Treatment consists of operative reattachment to enable the patient to perform overhead activities.

Olecanon Bursitis (*Student's elbow,* miner's elbow)

Olecranon bursitis is the most common superficial bursitis about the elbow. The cause of bursitis can be septic or aseptic (more common).

The onset of painful swelling of the olecranon bursa is usually the result of repetitive mechanical stresses. An underlying olecranon spur may predispose to bursitis.

Clinically the full range of motion at the elbow is usually present though a tensely swollen bursa may sometimes limit flexion due to pain (Fig. 13.3). During evaluation, careful attempt should be made to rule out septic process, gout, hydroxyapatite crystal deposition, chondrocalcinosis, rheumatoid arthritis and tubercular bursitis all of which can present with olecranon bursitis. An aspiration of bursa from the lateral approach under strict aseptic condition can provide invaluable specimen for analysis to rule out septic, rheumatoid, tubercular or crystal deposition disorder.

Treatment of aseptic bursitis consists of rest, splints, NSAIDs and avoidance of irritating factors. Elbow pads may be worn in cases of traumatic bursitis. Aspiration followed by compressive dressing may be done for tense bursae. Occasionally steroid injections following aspiration may help. Recalcitrant/chronic cases sometimes require operative excision. The treatment of olecranon bursitis associated with a systemic inflammatory disease is directed at the control of the underlying disease.

In cases of septic bursitis, treatment starts with aspiration and antibiotics. Appropriate modifications in the antibiotic regimen are made once the culture report is available. Aspiration and irrigation are repeated if the fluid reaccumulates. If aspiration, irrigation and antibiotics fail to control the disease, incision and drainage along with excision of the bursa should be performed.

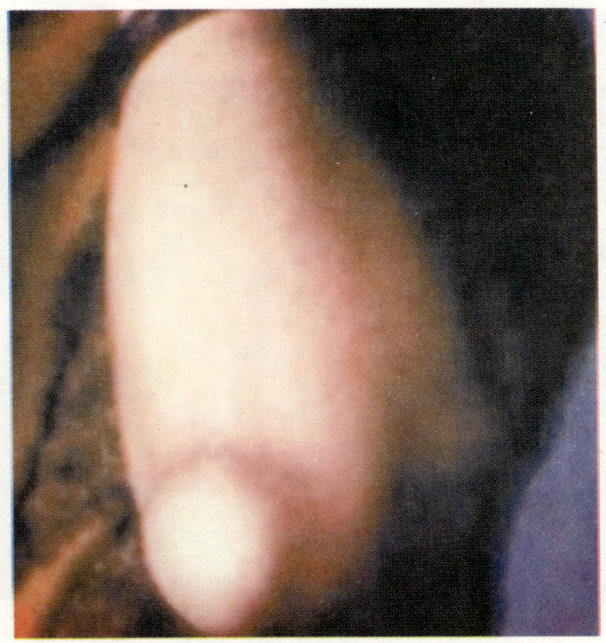

Fig. 13.3. Olecranon bursitis

Ulnar Nerve Neuritis occurs due to repeated mechanical stretching and friction. Progressive cubitus valgus, direct trauma, recurrent subluxation and osteophytes are some of the causes, which lead to ulnar nerve neuritis. Clinically the patient presents with an elbow deformity (congenital or posttraumatic) which is longstanding (at least for 10–15 years: hence the term *Tardy ulnar nerve palsy)* and signs of ulnar nerve dysfunction. EMG and NCV can be used to confirm the diagnosis.

Treatment is anterior transposition of the ulnar nerve.

Inflammatory Arthritides

Rheumatoid elbow

Elbow joint is frequently involved in polyarticular rheumatoid arthritis. Pain on movements and swelling are often the initial symptoms. Olecranon bursitis is common. Subcutaneous nodules are frequently seen on the extensor aspect of ulna.

Radiocapitellar arthritis is often the predominant feature of elbow involvement (Fig. 13.4a-c). Decrease in motion results. Marked pain occurs, especially during the forearm rotations. Ulnohumeral joint is also involved leading to swelling, pain, loss of motion and crepitus. Severe wasting around the joint is often seen. Radiologically, plain X-rays show osteoporosis, reduction of joint space and erosions.

Treatment The goal of treatment of rheumatoid elbow is to maintain painless arc of motion since the elbow is the most important joint for positioning

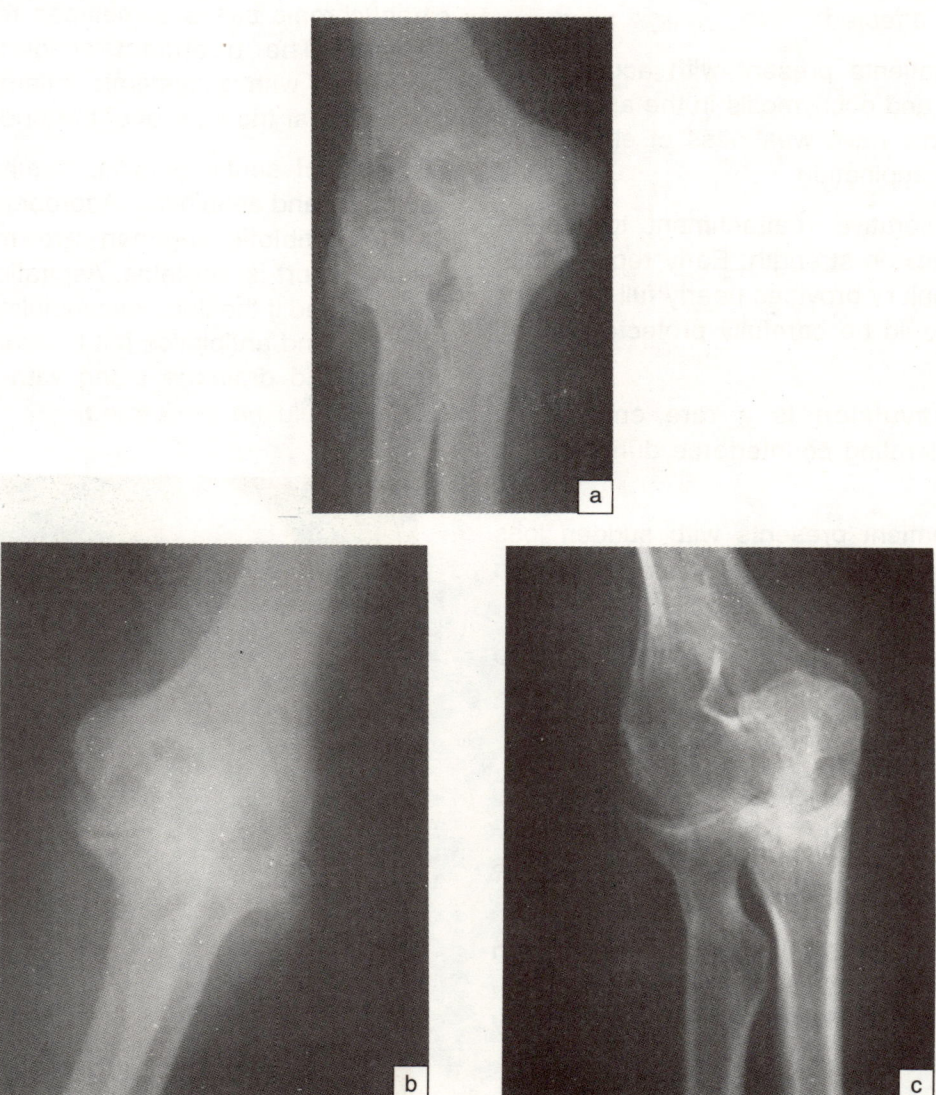

Fig. 13.4a-c. Elbow arthropathy caused by rheumatoid arthritis. Note the loss of joint space, osteoporosis and erosions

show osteoporosis, reduction of joint space and erosions.

Treatment The goal of treatment of rheumatoid elbow is to maintain painless arc of motion since the elbow is the most important joint for positioning of hand. A stiff elbow leads to great functional loss unlike the shoulder or the wrist joints.

Conservative treatment consists of symptomatic treatment, non-steroidal anti-inflammatory drugs (NSAIDs), intermittent splintage and active exercises. Steroid injections are often given in the joint or in the olecranon bursa.

Surgical treatment may be directed towards excising recalcitrant olecranon bursa or painful rheumatoid nodule or may be directed at arthritis where three primary methods of treatment are available.

1. **Synovectomy with radial head excision** is effective in relieving pain and improving arc of motion especially if done early in the disease process.

2. **Excisional arthroplasty** with interposition of various substances (Fascia, cutis or part of triceps muscle) is useful when ulnohumeral joint shows severe destruction but ligament stability is preserved. Interposition arthroplasty provides good motion but particularly in rheumatoid patients leads to a very unstable elbow.

3. **Total elbow arthroplasty** is indicated for stiff and painful joints with advanced disease particularly with involvement of other joints in the limb. An unconstrained elbow design is preferable, as it is less likely to loosen. Shoulder should be carefully evaluated before elbow arthroplasty. A patient with limited shoulder motion will exert greater forces on elbow and the prosthetic joint is more likely to become loose.

Tuberculosis of elbow

Involvement of elbow joint in tuberculosis is not common. The disease, like osteoarticular tuberculosis elsewhere, occurs by secondary spread from a focus elsewhere. Elbow involvement leads to progressively increasing pain, swelling and loss of motion. Muscles around the elbow undergo wasting. Sinus may form commonly as the joint is superficial.

Radiologically, plain x-rays show rarefaction of

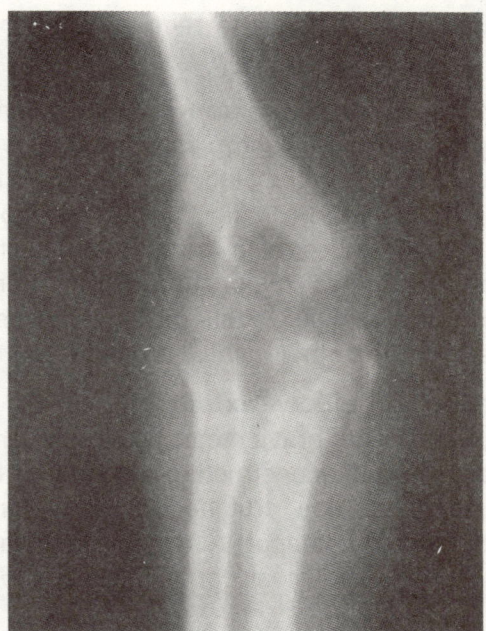

Fig. 13.5. Tubercular arthritis of elbow

bones and areas of lysis. Reduction or obliteration of joint space eventually occurs (Fig. 13.5).

Treatment consists of anti-tubercular drugs and splintage of the elbow. Movements are encouraged when the disease is controlled and pain subsides. If, after healing, the joint remains painful and/or stiff, excision arthroplasty can be used to regain useful motion. However, such an elbow remains weak and unstable and is not suitable for manual work.

Haemophilic elbow Elbow is commonly involved in hemophiliacs, especially those who use crutches for ambulation due to the involvement of the lower limbs. Acute hemarthrosis presents with sudden onset of pain, swelling and inability to move the elbow. Recurrent episodes of hemarthrosis lead to chronic hemophilic arthropathy.

The elbow is wasted and stiff.

X-rays show generalised reduction of bone density, erosion, reduced joint space and subchondral cysts. Osteophyte formation may occur in longstanding cases.

Treatment of acute hemarthrosis is splintage and factor VIII infusions. As the pain and swelling reduce, gentle intermittent active exercises are encouraged. Synovectomy is a useful procedure in hemophiliacs with refractory hemarthrosis. Elbow replacement is indicated in severely de-

It is important that hand be reconstructed before elbow.

Restoration of elbow flexion is most commonly done by Steindler's flexoroplasty, which involves proximal and lateral advancement of the flexor mass on humerus. Pronation contracture of the forearm is an undesirable consequence of this operation. Pectoralis major and minor transfer, after elongation with fascia lata graft and Latissimus dorsi transfer are other useful procedures.

Restoration of elbow extension is not commonly required as gravity can extend even the paralysed elbow. Reconstruction is required if the patient needs to use crutches or for overhead activities. Use of posterior third of deltoid transfer to the triceps is the most commonly done procedure.

Elbow Disorders in Children

Little leaguer's elbow is seen in adolescents involved in throwing activities, particularly Little League pitching in North America.

Little Leaguer's elbow results from the compressive forces at the radiocapitellar joint and distraction forces in the medial aspect of the elbow. Articular damage to the capitellum, ligamentous laxity of medial elbow ligamentous complex and ulnar nerve neuritis leading to tardy ulnar nerve palsy may result.

Clinically the patient may present with medial and/or lateral elbow pain. Locking of elbow may occur in severe cases by the loose bodies formed by fragmentation of the capitellum. X-rays may show resorption and fragmentation of capitellum.

Treatment consists of change in throwing activities. Elbow should be splinted for rest and comfort. Arthrotomy or arthroscopy to excise the incarcerated loose fragment may be required.

Osteochondritis dissecans of the capitellum denotes osteochondral defect resulting from repetitive microtrauma or a vascular insult. In the elbow it most commonly involves capitellum (*Panner's disease*). Clinically the patient presents with pain and swelling over the lateral aspect of the elbow.

Radiologically the plain x-rays show osteochondral fracture of the capitellum, intra-articular loose bodies and capitellar deformity. Treatment consists of rest and avoidance of throwing activities if fragment is intact and not separated.

Arthroscopic removal is indicated for intra-articular loose bodies. Drilling and bone grafting may help in selected cases.

Arthrodesis and Arthroplasty of Elbow

Arthrodesis of elbow is an uncommon procedure as motion at the elbow is absolutely necessary for the proper functioning of the upper extremity. Fusion causes severe functional limitation and is reserved for patients with painful arthrosis with high activity demands such as manual labourer. Infections such as tubercular arthritis are also indications for fusion.

Good bone stock is an important pre-requisite for achieving elbow fusion.

Position of Arthrodesis is 90° of flexion and in mid-prone position. Radial head excision may be necessary to allow rotations.

Resection/Excision Arthroplasty (with or without fascial interposition)

Indications

- elbow ankylosis after infection or trauma
- failed elbow arthroplasty

Resection arthroplasty is not preferred in rheumatoid arthritis as it leads to great instability and in patients who often are dependent on upper extremity to ambulate with walking aids. Complications of excision arthroplasty are instability and re-ankylosis.

Total Elbow Arthroplasty

Indications

- Pain unresponsive to medical treatment (following trauma and RA)
- Instability

Stiffness per se is not an indication for the total elbow arthroplasty. Gross deformity or significant cartilage erosion should be evident before deciding on surgery.

Contraindications

- Acute sepsis
- Neuropathic joint

- Heavy activity requirement
- Elbow arthrodesis
- Poor bone stock

Design Constrained designs offer intrinsic stability but are more prone to loosening.

Semiconstrained implants with a linked hinge which provides less constraint ("*Sloppy Hinge*") and permit varus, valgus and rotatory forces are the preferred implants.

Other Important Considerations

- Re-balancing of soft tissues is absolutely mandatory
- Lower extremity joint surgery should be completed first (if indicated) to avoid stress on elbow implant while crutch walking.

Complications

- Transient ulnar nerve paraesthesiae
- wound dehiscence and hematoma (10–15%)
- Infection
- Triceps weakness
- Epicondylar fracture
- Loosening
- Instability/dislocation

Results Elbow replacement can be relied upon to provide durable relief of pain, functional status and range of motion in carefully selected cases.

Wrist

Relevant Anatomy

Wrist or the radiocarpal joint consists of radius, scaphoid and lunate and is closely related structurally and functionally to the ulnocarpal joint.

Osteology

Distal radius consists of styloid process, lunate fossa and scaphoid fossa. The sigmoid notch on the ulnar side articulates with the ulnar head. The distal articular surface of radius faces volarwards (11°) and ulnarwards (21°) and is approximately 11mm distal to the distal articular surface of ulna in majority of people (ulnar minus variant).

Distal ulna consists of styloid process and the head (or the articular surface). Ulnocarpal joint includes the triangular fibrocartilage complex (TFCC). TFCC is also an important stabiliser of distal radio ulnar joint.

The proximal row of carpal bones consists of scaphoid, lunate, triquetrum and pisiform while the distal row consists of trapezium, trapezoid, capitate and hamate. Transverse articulation between the proximal and the distal carpal rows constitute the midcarpal joints.

Ligaments

Ligaments of the wrist provide interosseous stability to an inherently unstable bony arrangement. The ligaments are divided into dorsal and palmar—the palmar ligaments stabilising proximal carpal row to the distal radius being thus far the most important for stability. The major palmar ligaments are radiocapitate, radiolunotriquetral and radio scaphoid. Distally the most important palmar ligament is capitotriquetral which is primarily involved with stabilising the distal to the proximal carpal row. Radial collateral ligament and ulnar collateral ligaments are specialised condensations of the wrist capsule and are not true wrist ligaments. Dorsal ligaments are less strong and less distinct structures and include radioscaphoid, radiolunate and radiotriquetral. The remaining dorsal ligament is the scapholunate interosseous ligament, which is commonly injured in dorsiflexion wrist injuries. Main ligaments are palmar ligaments stabilising proximal carpal row to distal radius. The scaphoid tends to tether the lunate in flexion through the scapholunate (SL) ligament, while the triquetrum tends to extend the lunate through lunotriquetral ligament. When the SL ligament is disrupted, the scaphoid flexes excessively and lunate is dorsiflexed by the unopposed effect of the triquetrum leading to DISI (Dorsal Intercalated Segmental Instability) pattern. When LT ligament is disrupted, lunate is flexed by the scaphoid resulting in VISI (Volar Intercalated Segmental Instability) pattern of instability. There are fewer ligaments stabilising the distal to proximal row i.e. midcarpal joints. The symptomatic wrist instability, therefore, is common at midcarpal joints.

Kinematics

Motions at the wrist include flexion (normal 0°–65°), extension (normal 0°–55°), radial deviation (0°–15°) and ulnar deviation (normal 0°–35°). Flexion and extension are mainly at radiocarpal joint (two-third) but also at intercarpal joint (one-third). The instant centre for wrist motion is at the head of the capitate but is variable (Fig. 14.1a,b).

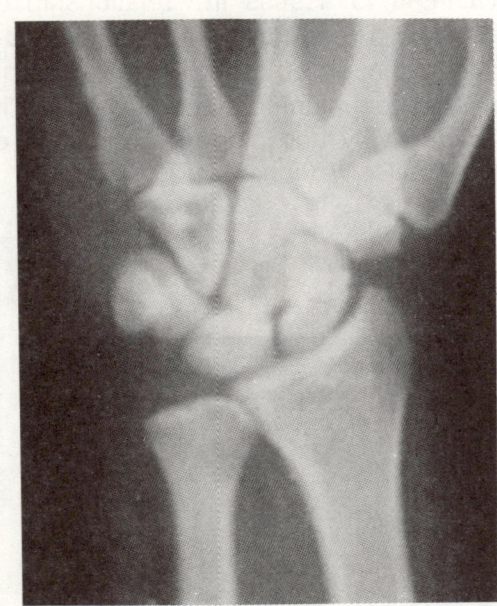

Fig. 14.1a. X-ray of normal wrist (centre of motion is the centre of capitate)

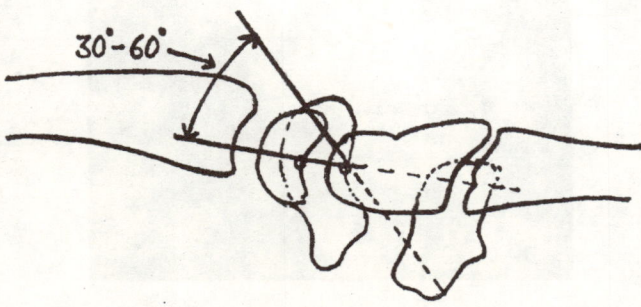

Fig. 14.1b. Balanced carpus

Muscles Extensor tendons at the wrist are divided into six compartments (Table 14.1). Flexor tendons of the fingers pass through the carpal tunnel at the wrist. Flexor retinaculum (Transverse carpal ligament), extending from the hook of the hamate and pisiform ulnarly to the trapezius and scaphoid laterally) makes up the roof of the carpal tunnel which contains median nerve and 9 tendons (8 finger flexors + flexor pollicis longus). Flexor carpi radialis, Flexor carpi ulnaris, palmaris longus, ulnar nerve and ulnar and radial arteries lie outside the carpal tunnel.

Table 14.1. Dorsal extensor compartments of the wrist and common extensor tendon afflictions

Compartment	Tendons	Common Associated Pathologic Conditions
1.	EPB, APL	deQuervain's tenosynovitis
2.	ECRL, ECRB	
3.	EPL	Rupture (in Colles' #, RA*)
4.	EDC, EIP	Extensor tenosynovitis
5.	Ext. Digiti minimi	Rupture (in RA*
6.	ECU	Snapping (at ulnar styloid)

*Rheumatoid arthritis

Nerves

Median nerve enters the wrist through the carpal tunnel and supplies the radial two **L**umbricals, **O**pponens pollicis, **A**bductor Pollicis Brevis (APB) and the superficial head of the **F**lexor pollicis brevis (**LOAF** muscles). Median nerve provides sensation to the radial three and half digits in hand and its autogenous sensory zone is index finger pulp.

Ulnar nerve enters the wrist through the Guyon's canal. The roof of Guyon's canal is volar carpal ligament and the floor is transverse carpal ligament. Ulnar nerve supplies lumbricals to the ring and little fingers, all interosseous muscles, hypothenar muscles, adductor pollicis and deep part of the Flexor Pollicis Brevis. Ulnar nerve supplies sensation to the ulnar one and half digits and the autonomous zone is small finger pulp.

Vessels Radial artery lies between the brachioradialis and flexor carpi radialis (FCR) at the wrist. It then enters the anatomic "snuff box" between the extensor pollicis longus (EPL) and extensor pollicis brevis (EPB). Ulnar artery lies between the flexor carpi ulnaris (FCU) and the flexor digitorum superficialis (FDS) at the wrist and enters the wrist through Guyon's canal.

Evaluation of Patient with Wrist Problem

Evaluation of suspected wrist pathology should begin with a detailed history. The age, dominant hand (handedness) and occupation should be always asked. The history of injury, if any, is important and attempts should be made to ascertain the mechanism of injury including the direction of forces involved. Onset of symptoms is usually acute following injuries while the onset is chronic in cases of arthritis, tendinitis and carpal instability. The location of pain can provide a clue to the possible aetiology. Pain localised to the radial side of the wrist occurs following scaphoid fracture or avascular necrosis, lunotriquetral strain, deQuervain's tenosynovitis, intersection syndrome (vide infra), FCR tendinitis, scapho-lunate advanced collapse (SLAC) and dorsal intercalated segmental instability (DISI) type of carpal instability pattern. Pain on the ulnar side of the wrist can be due to extensor carpi ulnaris (ECU) or flexor carpi ulnaris (FCU) tendinitis, extensor digiti minimi tendinitis, ulnar-carpal abutment, TFCC tear and volar intercalated segmental instability (VISI) type of carpal instability pattern. Pain over the dorsum of the wrist is commonly seen in association with dorsal ganglion, Kienbock's disease or rarely, avascular necrosis of capitate, while pain on the volar aspect occurs in carpal tunnel syndrome, volar ganglion and ulnar tunnel syndrome. History of a painful click suggests carpal instability or TFCC injury.

Examination of the wrist should begin with careful inspection of the attitude, contour and overlying skin. Bony palpation, including palpation of the radial styloid and bones of the carpus, yields specific information regarding disorders of the wrist. The normal movements permitted at the wrist viz. Flexion (normal, 0°–80°), extension (normal 0°–70°), ulnar deviation (normal, 0°–30°) and radial deviation (normal, 0°–20°) should be tested. Distal neurovascular examination should always be performed. Tinel's sign and test of strength of individual muscles should be performed in suspected nerve injuries / entrapments.

Radiologic examination Routine radiographic examination of the wrist includes a posteroanterior (PA), lateral and oblique (45° pronation posteroanterior) radiographs. Scaphoid is better visualised when PA view is taken with the wrist in ulnar deviation. Carpal tunnel view, taken with wrist extended at right angle with the palm resting on x-ray cassette and the beam directed at 45° to the wrist in a proximal to distal direction, visualises the carpal tunnel encroachment and the fractures of the hook of the hamate. In cases with suspected wrist instabilities and normal radiographs, stress radiographs taken as PA views of clenched fist in maximal radial and ulnar deviation can help visualise subtle instabilities (when standard antero posterior x-ray is normal but anteroposterior x-ray with the fingers squeezing tightly to form a fist reveals an abnormal gap, the condition is called *dynamic scapholunate dissociation*). Normal carpal arcs of Gilula (Gilula's Lines) should be carefully evaluated to assess the relationship of the carpal bones. These are three concentric arcs drawn along the proximal and distal cortical outlines of scaphoid, lunate and triquetrum (lines I and II respectively and along the proximal edges of distal carpal row (line III) (Fig. 14.2).

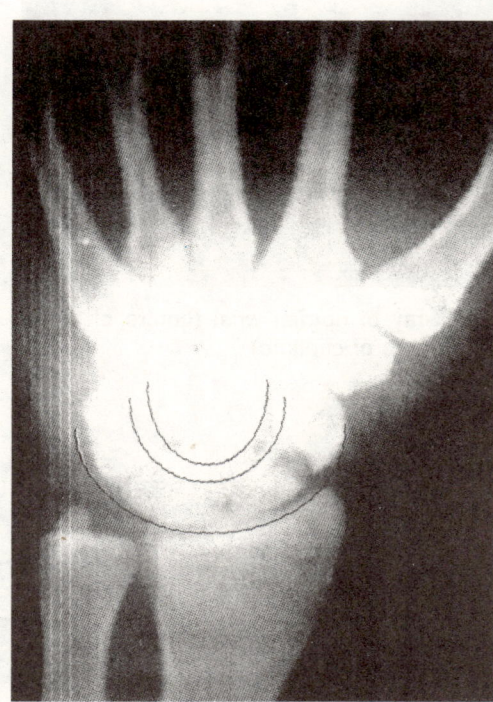

Fig. 14.2.   Anteroposterior x-ray of wrist showing Gilula's lines

Wrist instabilities can also be evaluated using fluoroscopy.

Arthrography is useful, especially in cases with chronic wrist pain, to evaluate ligamentous tears, TFCC injury and cartilaginous injuries. Bone scan can be useful for wrist injuries especially carpal bone fractures and for the diagnosis of Reflex Sympathetic Dystrophy (RSD). Computed tomography (CT) is best for the fracture visualisation; CT is also useful to evaluate distal radioulnar joint. Magnetic Resonance Imaging is extremely useful for early diagnosis of scaphoid fracture and evaluation of TFCC and ligamentous injuries.

Arthroscopy is fast proving to be an extremely useful tool in the diagnosis and management of wrist disorders. It is more sensitive than MRI in the diagnosis of ligamentous injuries and is very useful in the diagnosis and treatment of the pathologies of TFCC.

Congenital Abnormalities of the Wrist

1. Madelung's Deformity is an autosomal dominant disorder seen more frequently in females. It is characterised by abnormal growth of the anteromedial portion of distal radial epiphysis with premature fusion of the ulnar half of the distal radius and results in progressive ulnar and volar tilt. Ulnar growth is not affected. Radial head subluxation and/or bowing of radius may be associated. Ulnar head subluxates and becomes prominent. The deformity can be unilateral or bilateral. Early treatment consists of observation especially in mild, asymptomatic patients. Operative treatment includes ulnar shortening with or without the dorsal radial close wedge osteotomy for severe cases. In adults, Darrach procedure (excision of the distal 2.5 cm of ulna) can improve functional ability. Epiphysiolysis of the ulnar/palmar aspect of the radius may also be successful.

2. Congenital Absence of the Radius (C.A.R.) (Radial Club Hand) is the most common long bone deficiency in the upper extremity. Disorders of the radial development lead to radial deviation of the hand, absent scaphoid and sometimes a hypoplastic thumb. Right hand of males is most commonly involved and the deformity is bilateral in 50% cases. Partial or complete absence of the radius, with or without adjacent hand deficiencies can be seen as an isolated finding or in association with several syndromes. Fanconi's syndrome and VATER syndrome should be considered when the radial dysplasia is bilateral. Fanconi's syndrome is an autosomal recessive disorder with pancytopenia, brown skin pigmentation, hip dislocation and aplastic thumb. The prognosis in these cases is poor.

VATER syndrome comprises of vertebral anomalies, imperforate anus, tracheo-oesophageal aplasia and renal abnormalities. Other syndromes associated with C.A.R. are thrombocytopenia (alongwith knee dysplasia), heart abnormalities (Holt-Oram-Lewis syndrome) and chromosomal abnormalities (trisomy 17). The terminal variety of C.A.R. has absent radial ray and abnormalities of radial artery and median nerve; while the intercalary variety includes an absent radius with normal carpus and first ray.

The wrist in these patients is in radial deviation and flexion and the thumb may sometimes be rudimentary or absent (Fig. 14.3a-d).

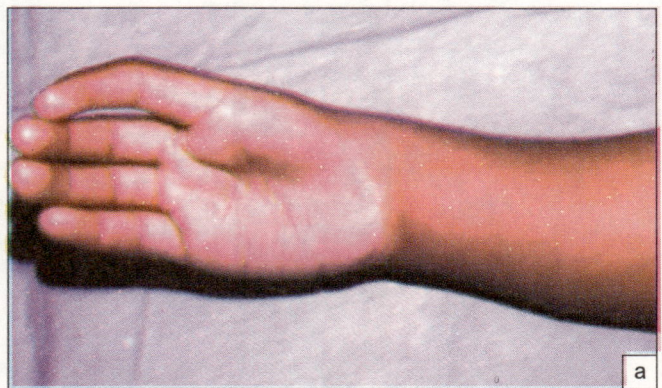

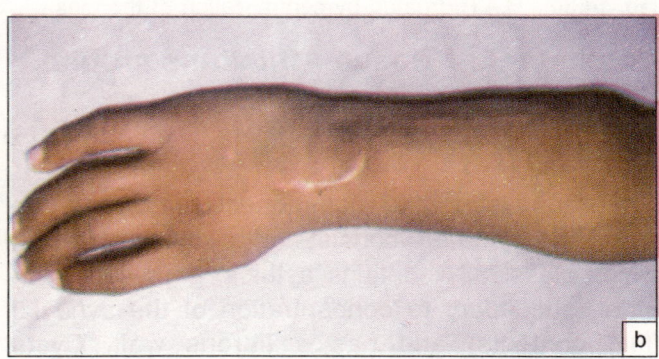

Fig. 14.3a,b. Congenital absence of radius and the thumb (a) Volar view (b) Dorsal view

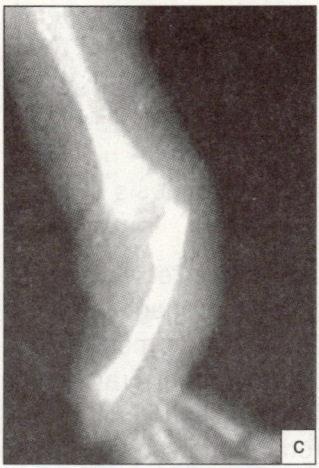 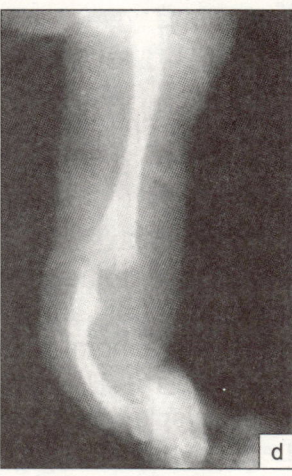

Fig. 14.3c,d. X-rays of patient with C.A.R. (c) Lateral and (d) AP

Treatment consists of early splinting and passive stretching. Later, centralization of the distal wrist and hand over the ulna is performed (Fig. 14.3e). Pollicization is needed for the patient without a functional thumb. A stiff, nonfunctional elbow and associated medical problems are contraindications to the surgery.

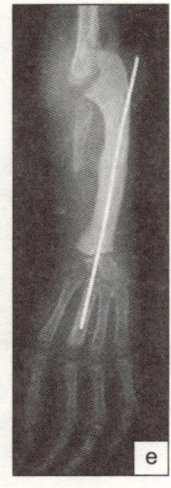

Fig. 14.3e. C.A.R. treated by centralization of the ulna

Common Soft Tissue Afflictions around the Wrist

1. Ganglion

Ganglion cyst is the commonest mass seen in wrist and hand. It consists of a cystic swelling which classically contains a thick, gelatinous material (secondary to concentration of the synovial fluid contents) and has a fibrous wall. Cysts usually have a long stalk which originates from one of the carpal joints. The ganglion at the wrist

most typically occurs on the dorsal aspect of the wrist, emerging from the scapholunate joint capsule. It can also present on the radial volar aspect of wrist, from either the tenosynovium of the radial wrist flexors or the joint capsule of the wrist.

Clinically, ganglion usually presents as visible swelling and is often painless and causes no functional limitation. However, if the cyst becomes large it can be painful. Though the ganglion is cystic, it often presents as hard nodule. The size of the cyst can often wax and wane. A ganglion on the dorsum of the wrist becomes more prominent on flexion of the wrist and nearly disappears on the extension.

Treatment of a small cyst comprises of the aspiration with a large bore needle followed by injection of a soluble steroid to facilitate cyst wall sclerosis. Injection of hyaluronidase is sometimes used instead of steroid to achieve the same effect. Recurrences are extremely common. If recurrences are frequent, there is pain, cyst is large or the diagnosis is doubtful, surgical excision should be considered. Meticulous dissection is needed for complete excision of the entire cyst along with its stalk down to the wrist joint.

2. deQuervain's tenosynovitis

deQuervain's syndrome is stenosing tenosynovitis of the first dorsal compartment over the radial styloid. The tendons involved are APL and EPB. It is commonly seen in patients who use their hands and thumbs in a repetitive fashion e.g. golfers, players of racket sports and clerical workers.

Clinically, the patients present with localised pain and swelling in the vicinity of radial styloid. If the inflammation is severe, the patients may also complain of pain and paraesthesiae radiating distally into the thumb and over the dorsum of the hand and index finger due to irritation of dorsal sensory branch of radial nerve which passes directly over the inflamed tendons. Patients have a positive *Finkelstein test*. This test is performed by the ulnar deviation of the wrist with the thumb in the palm; severe pain in the region of thumb and radial aspect of the wrist implies a positive test.

Radiological examination of the wrist (PA view) should be performed to rule out the fracture of the radial styloid or bony protuberances as the cause of mechanical irritation of the first dorsal compartment.

Treatment is conservative initially. Thumb spica splinting, NSAIDs and local steroid injection in the first dorsal compartment are the treatment modalities. If the patient still remains symptomatic, surgical decompression is done by dividing (and excising a part of) thickened tendon sheath of the first dorsal compartment. Special care should be taken to avoid injury to the superficial branch of the radial nerve.

3. Flexor carpi ulnaris/Flexor carpi radialis tendinitis

Flexor carpi ulnaris/Flexor carpi radialis tendinitis present with pain especially when lifting weights and flexing the wrist against resistance. Local tenderness over the affected tendons is common. FCU can sometimes undergo calcific tendinitis. Treatment consists of rest, NSAIDs and splinting. Recalcitrant cases can be treated by tenolysis.

4. Intersection Syndrome

Intersection syndrome is caused by the inflammation at the junction of the tendons of the first (EPB, APL) and second dorsal compartments (ECRL, ECRB) of the wrist proximal to the extensor retinaculum. The patients present with localised pain and crepitus (*squeakers*) on wrist flexion and extension. Treatment is conservative initially in the form of splinting, NSAIDs and local injection. Decompression is required rarely and is reserved for the recalcitrant cases.

5. Extensor Pollicis Longus Tenosynovitis

EPL tenosynovitis presents with pain in the region of Lister's tubercle on the dorsum of the wrist. Thumb movements aggravate pain. Tenderness is elicited on palpation of EPL tendon at Lister's tubercle. Treatment is rest, NSAIDs and splinting.

6. ECU Subluxation

Extensor carpi ulnaris tendon can subluxate from its groove in the sixth dorsal compartment. It is associated with snapping and discomfort. Treatment consists of immobilisation of the wrist and forearm in pronation. If the nonoperative treatment is unsuccessful, operative reconstruction of the fibroosseous tunnel should be done.

7. Wartenberg's Syndrome (*Cheiralgia Paraesthetica*)

Wartenberg's syndrome (*Cheiralgia Paraesthetica*) is isolated neuritis of the superficial radial nerve from the compression. The compression can be extrinsic (by bangles) or intrinsic (anomalous muscles, fascial bands). Treatment is expectant with rest and splintage and removal of extrinsic compression. Resistant cases need operative decompression of the nerve.

Inflammatory Conditions

1. Tubercular Arthritis of Wrist

Tuberculosis of the wrist is not common and as in the case of osteoarticular tuberculosis at the other sites, is usually secondary to a focus elsewhere in the body. Tuberculosis of the wrist presents with swelling, increasing pain and stiffness of the wrist. There is marked wasting of the forearm muscles and the grip is weak. All the movements are painfully restricted. Advanced cases may present with sinuses or ulcers over the dorsum of the wrist. The joint gets disorganised and carpus may subluxate from the radius.

Radiological examination reveals the generalised osteoporosis of the wrist and carpal bones, with or without the areas of destruction in the wrist

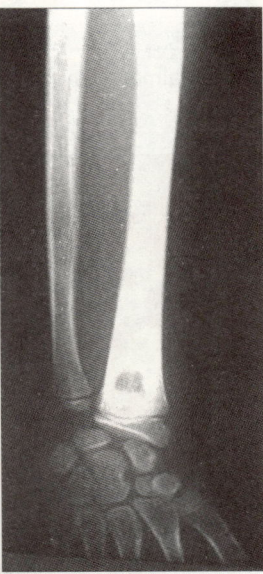

Fig. 14.4.   Tuberculosis of wrist joint. Note the lytic lesion in metaphysis with osteoporosis of carpal bones

bones (Fig. 14.4). Intercarpal joints are invariably involved and diminished intercarpal joint spaces with crowding of carpals is seen. Carpal bones appear indistinct and hazy.

Treatment consists of antitubercular drugs alongwith immobilization of the wrist in 20 degrees dorsiflexion in a POP slab. Mobilization of the wrist is started once the pain and swelling subside and sinuses heal. Some restriction of wrist movements persists invariably. Painful stiff wrist after the drug treatment of advanced tubercular arthritis is best treated by wrist arthrodesis.

2. Compound Palmar Ganglion

Compound Palmar Ganglion is the tubercular bursitis of the ulnar bursa (also known as great palmar sheath). It presents as a fluctuant swelling on the volar aspect of the wrist under the flexor

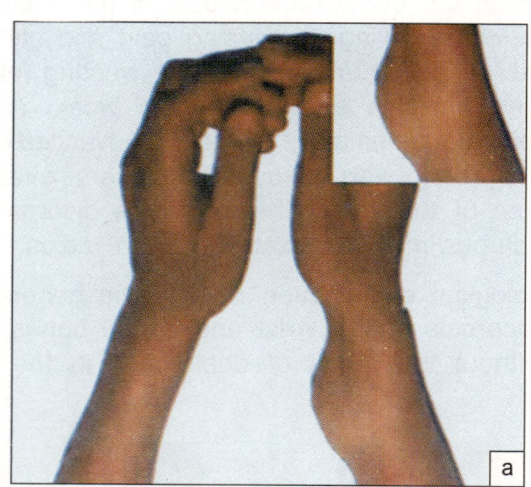

Fig. 14.5a. Compound palmar ganglion (*Inset:* Close up view)

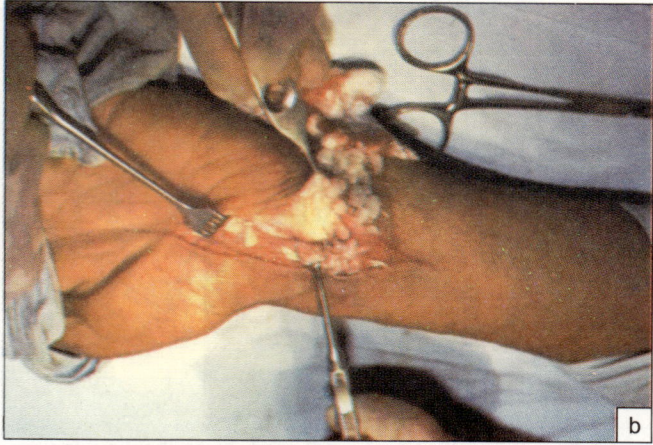

Fig. 14.5b. Compound palmar ganglion–intraoperative picture

retinaculum extending proximal and distal to flexor retinaculum (Fig. 14.5a,b). Cross fluctuation is positive. The condition is initially painless and does not interfere with finer movements. Later on as the flexor tendons get adherent, fingers become stiff. Treatment is administration of antitubercular drugs. Resistant cases are treated with surgical excision of the infected tissue in addition to administration of anti tubercular drugs.

3. Rheumatoid Arthritis (RA)

Wrist is one of the commonest and the earliest joints to get involved in Rheumatoid Arthritis (Fig. 14.6). The involvement is bilateral and symmetrical. The wrist involvement in RA occurs in a predictable fashion. On the radial side the radio-scaphocapitate and radio lunatotriquetral ligaments are attenuated leading to rotatory displacement of scaphoid. Scapholunate dissociation leads on to radio carpal collapse. Carpus supinates and subluxes around the stronger radial dorsal ligaments. On the ulnar side attenuation of the ulnar carpal ligaments leads to radial drift of the carpus. Distal radioulnar joint is involved and dorsal subluxation of the ulnar head occurs producing *caput-ulnae syndrome*. The ECU tendon displaces volarward leading to unopposed action of extensor carpi radialis longus and brevis, ulnar translocation of carpus and radial ward displacement of the metacarpal. Ulnar and volar aspects of radius are eroded resulting in further ulnar and volar

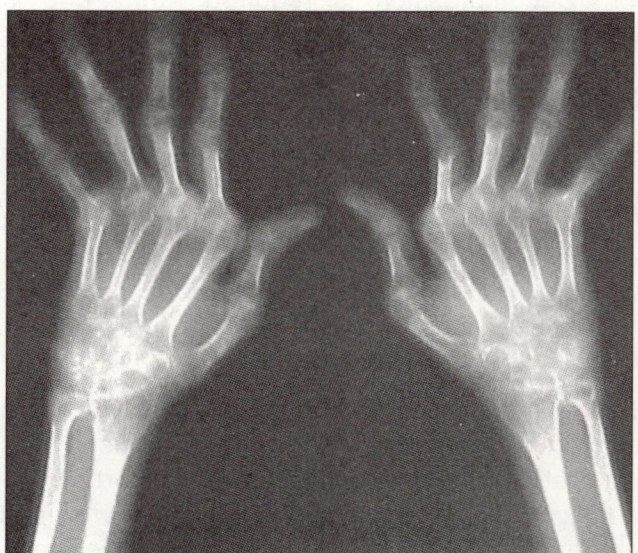

Fig. 14.6. Rheumatoid arthritis with severe involvement of both wrists

extensor tendons to little and ring fingers from a sharp prominence of distal ulna (Vaughn-Jackson syndrome). Extensor carpi radialis brevis ruptures when the wrist is dislocated volarwards.

Treatment consists of extensor tenosynovectomy and wrist synovectomy. ECU tendon can be relocated to a dorsal position. When pain is present over the distal ulna, the Darrach's resection of distal ulna may be performed. Painful, unstable wrist is best tackled by wrist arthrodesis, which provides stability and improves function.

The ideal position of wrist fusion is in 10°–20° dorsiflexion; but if bilateral wrists are to be fused, the other wrist should be fused in 10° palmar flexion.

Avascular Necrosis of Carpal Bones

1. Kienböck's Disease

Kienböck's disease is osteonecrosis of the lunate. Though its exact aetiology is unknown, it is believed to be caused by repetitive compressive forces on the wrist. These patients usually have negative ulnar variance (i.e. distal ulna is proximal to distal radius; distal ulna is relatively short compared to the distal radius). Lunate undergoes avascular changes and gets softened, fragmented and deformed. Necrosis of overlying cartilage occurs. Devascularization takes place slowly over a period of two years but the bone does not regain its normal shape and cartilage.

Clinically patients are young adults, usually manual labourers or heavy workers who complain of dorsal wrist pain in the dominant hand. Stiffness of the wrist is often associated with greater restriction of dorsiflexion. Localised tenderness over lunate may be elicitable. Radiographs reveal increased sclerosis, fragmentation and collapse of lunate depending on the stage of advancement (Fig. 14.7). Note is made of negative ulnar variance on X-rays in most patients. MRI is an extremely useful investigation for early diagnosis.

Treatment in early cases consists of splinting the wrist. Cases with advanced disease are treated with ulnar lengthening or radial shortening to reduce the stresses on the lunate. Triscaphe fusion (Scaphoid - Trapezium - Trapeziod: STT) is also recommended to achieve the same goal. Excision of lunate and its replacement with silastic

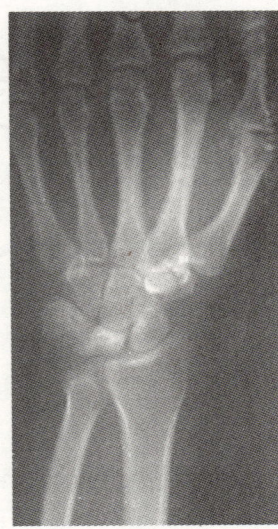

Fig. 14.7. Kienböck's disease

implant and wrist arthrodesis are rarely indicated in the treatment of Kienbock's disease.

2. Presier's Disease

Presier's disease is avascular necrosis of the scaphoid often seen in the proximal fragment after scaphoid fracture since the blood supply enters the scaphoid distally. Bone scan, CT scan and MRI are extremely useful in the diagnosis of avascular necrosis. Resultant non union following avascular necrosis can give rise to SLAC (vide infera). Treatment consists of Matti Russe bone grafting. Presence or absence of punctate bleeding when the proximal fragment is curetted at the time of bone grafting is the most important prognostic factor.

Carpal Instability

Carpal instability implies the disruption of the normal relationship of the carpal bones caused by intercarpal ligament injury. Functional range of motion at the wrist is 5 degrees of palmar flexion, 30° of dorsiflexion, 10 degrees of radial deviation and 15° of ulnar deviation. Most wrist instabilities are based on scapholunate angle (normal 30°–60°). Clinically, carpal instability leads to pain and abnormal motion. The carpal ligament injuries leading to carpal instability can occur either alone or in combination with fractures of the scaphoid, triquetrum, radial styloid and distal radius. Injuries leading to carpal instability can be acute or may not be recognised initially and present as chronic carpal instability. The various patterns of carpal instabilities are:

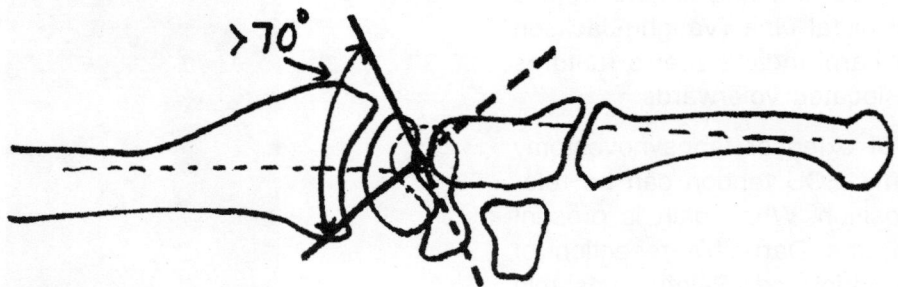

Fig. 14.8. Dorsal Intercalated Segmental Instability (DISI)

1. DISI pattern (Fig. 14.8)

Dorsal Intercalated Segmental Instability pattern results from radial-sided inter carpal ligamentous injury, scapholunate ligament being the most important ligament injured. Scaphoid fracture or scapholunate dissociation is the most common precipitating injury. The injury results from a fall on the out stretched hand leading to dorsal tilt of carpal bones. On the clenched fist AP view, Scapholunate gap is increased (normal up to 2 mm) and lunate is tilted dorsally. The scaphoid is palmar flexed and the scapholunate angle measured on the lateral X-ray of the wrist is increased (normal, 40°–60°). Also, the radiolunate angle (normal, 0–11°) and lunato-capitate angle are increased. On examination, Watson's test is positive i.e. there is a palpable clunk with passive radial deviation of the wrist with the scaphoid stabilised volarly. A positive test suggests scapholunate instability. Treatment of the injuries in acute stage (within 3–6 weeks) is immobilisation or, if ligaments are completely torn, repair through a dorsal approach and stabilisation with K wires. Arthroscopic repair of the ligaments is now possible.

Late reconstruction (after 6 weeks) usually consists of a salvage procedure such as STT fusion, Scaphocapitate fusion, proximal row carpectomy, or wrist arthrodesis.

2. VISI pattern (Fig. 14.9)

Volar Intercalated Segmental Instability results from ulnar sided ligamentous injury, the most important ligament injured being lunotriquetral. Examination includes the ballotment test. The lunate is stabilised with the examiner's thumb and index finger of one hand and the triquetrum and pisiform are passively pistoned anteroposteriorly with the other hand. Pain, crepitus and laxity indicate a positive test and imply triquetrolunate dissociation.

Radiographs show increased volar tilt of the lunate on the x-ray. Scapholunate angle is decreased (<30 degrees). MRI can show ligamentous injury but is not very sensitive. Arthroscopy is the best modality for diagnosing these injuries.

Treatment of the acute injury is closed reduction and plaster immobilization with or without K-wires. Chronic instability is treated by ligament reconstruction or limited intercarpal fusion.

3. Midcarpal instability– TriquetroHamate (TQH) Instability (Clunk and pain on ulnar deviation of wrist)

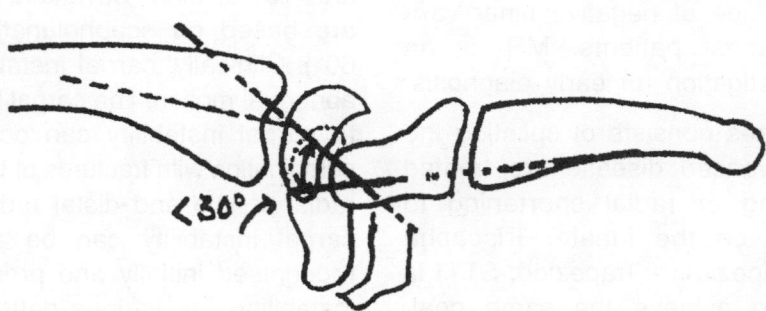

Fig. 14.9. Volar Intercalated Segmental Instability (VISI)

Midcarpal instability is the instability at mid carpal joints and can be intrinsic (i.e. due to laxity at triquetro - hamate articulation) or extrinsic (secondary to the fracture of the distal radius). Often there is no history of specific injury.

Normally, the proximal row of carpals is in volar flexion in radial deviation. This position of carpals changes to dorsiflexion by a smooth transition when the wrist is ulnar deviated.

In mid carpal instability the proximal row reduces suddenly into a dorsiflexed position resulting in a catch-up "clunk". The wrist in these cases at rest shows a VISI pattern on neutral lateral x-ray.

Pain and the wrist clunk can be corrected by dorsally directed pressure on pisiform which corrects proximal row palmar flexion deformity. The contralateral side may often have same asymptomatic deformity.

Treatment of the acute injury is immobilisation in a long arm cast in supination and ulnar deviation.

The chronic injury is treated conservatively by a splint, putting pressure on pisiform. If conservative treatment fails, Triquetrohamate or a four corner fusion (capitate, lunate, hamate and triquetrum) is undertaken.

Degenerative Conditions

1. **Osteoarthritis** of the wrist is extremely uncommon.

2. *SLAC* (Scapho Lunate Advanced Collapse) is a pattern of degenerative arthritis, often seen after non union of scaphoid fracture or scapholunate dissociation. Typical SLAC wrist shows loss of radial columnar height with arthritis progressing from radio scaphoid joint leading on to destruction at capitolunate because of the shear forces (Fig. 14.10). The joint between the lunate and hamate is the next one to be involved.

However, the pathology never involves radiolunate articulation.

The patient typically presents with pain and stiffness of the wrist. The radiographs show reduced joint space between radius and scaphoid, and capitate, and lunate and hamate.

Treatment of SLAC without the involvement of

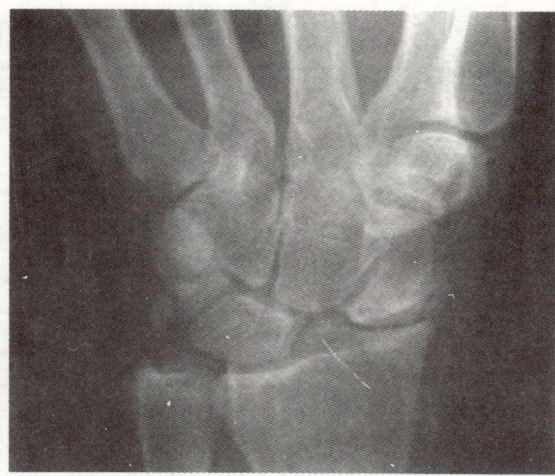

Fig. 14.10.   Anteroposterior x-rays showing SLAC wrist

lunato-capitate cartilage is proximal row carpectomy. The capitate head in these cases shifts proximally to articulate with lunate fossa and allows preservation of wrist movements. Lunato-capitate cartilage involvement is treated by 4 corner fusion between capitate, lunate, hamate and triquetrum (CALTH). Complete wrist arthrodesis provides pain relief but permanently sacrifices wrist motion.

3. **Triscaphe Degeneration** (Scaphoid-Trapezium-Trapezoid) is the next most common degenerative pattern of the wrist. Triscaphe fusion (STT Fusion) is the treatment of choice when indicated.

Ulnar abutment (ulnar impaction) is defined as impaction of ulnar head against the triangular fibrocartilage complex and ulnar carpus leading to painful degeneration of TFCC. Malreduction of distal radius fracture, premature closure of radial physis and Madelung deformity can be the underlying causes. The patients complain of ulnar side wrist pain. Diagnosis of ulnar impaction syndrome is made by testing the forearm pronation -supination with the wrist in ulnar deviation as well as by compression of the ulnar side of the wrist against the distal ulna with forearm in pronation. Radiological examination reveals lytic lunate along with chondromalacia of triquetrum and ulnar plus variant. Wrist arthroscopy is a useful diagnostic tool.

Treatment is arthroscopic debridement of TFCC with or without ulnar shortening. "Matched" distal ulna resection described by Bower (Bower's hemiresection arthroplasty) preserves the ulnar styloid and TFCC and is an extremely useful procedure.

Hand

Relevant Anatomy

Thorough knowledge of the anatomy of the hand is a must for accurate diagnosis and treatment of disorders of hand.

Osteology

The *metacarpals* articulate with the carpus at the carpometacarpal joints. These are gliding joints, which have relatively little motion and usually are not commonly involved in any clinical pathology. However, carpometacarpal joint (CMC) of the thumb is a mobile saddle joint. It frequently develops degenerative arthritis due to its high joint reaction forces and wide arc of motion. The metacarpophalangeal joints (MCP) are ellipsoid joints. A thick fibrocartilagenous portion of the volar capsule (volar plate) connects the metacarpal neck to the base of the proximal phalanx. Volar plates of the four (IInd-Vth) metacarpals are connected by deep transverse metacarpal ligament. Collateral ligaments of MCP joints are under tension with the joint in flexion and lax with the joint in extension due to the eccentric shape of the metacarpal head ("cam effect"). MCP joints should, therefore, always be immobilised in flexion to prevent shortening of collaterals and resulting stiffness. Interphalangeal (IP) joints are hinge joints with volar plate and all collateral ligaments. Unlike MCP, IP joints are bicondylar and hence, more stable. IP joints have no "cam effect".

Flexor Tendon System

The flexor pollicis longus (FPL) is the deepest and most radial tendon in the carpal tunnel and inserts onto the base of the distal phalanx of the thumb. The tendons of the flexor digitorum superficialis (FDS) are the most superficial tendons in the carpal tunnel and palm. FDS tendon of each digit splits into two slips at the level of the proximal phalanx. These slips insert along the palmar aspect of the middle phalanx.

The flexor digitorum profundus (FDP) lies deep to FDS and emerges between the two slips of FDS, inserting at the base of the distal phalanx. The flexor tendons are tethered to the volar aspect of the phalanges by a series of fibro-cartilaginous pulleys, which have dual function. They provide mechanical stability by preventing bowstringing and provide nutrition to the tendon by synovial diffusion. There are four annular pulleys and three cruciate pulleys. Annular pulleys are more important particularly the second (A2) and fourth (A4). The odd numbered annular pulleys overlie joints (A1, the first annular pulley is most proximal and overlies MCP joint while A3 overlies PIP joint) while the even numbers annular pulleys and all cruciate pulleys overlie the phalanges (A2 is proximal to C1, both of which overlie proximal phalanx while C2, A4 and C3 overlie middle phalanx in that order from proximal to distal) (Fig. 15.1).

Extensor Apparatus

Extensor apparatus has a complex anatomy. This

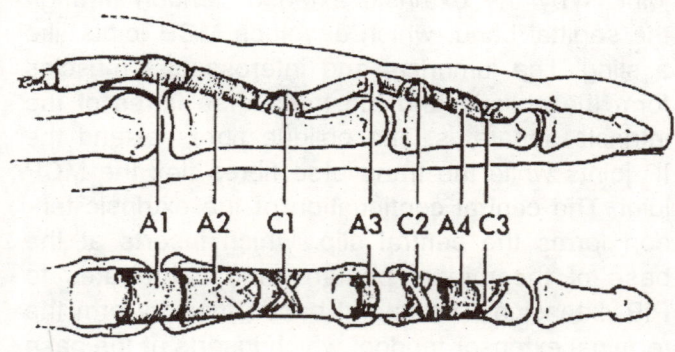

Fig. 15.1. Anatomy of flexor tendon sheath. This diagram is helpful in understanding gliding of tendon

is required because the extrinsic tendons of the fingers (Ext. digitorum communis) terminate proximal to the PIP joint and also because only one extrinsic tendon exists for each finger as compared to two extrinsic flexor tendons (FDP & FDS). Dorsal extensor apparatus is formed by contributions from extrinsic extensors (Extensor dig. communis, extensor indicis proprius and extensor digiti minimi) as well as intrinsic extensors (lumbricals and interossei) (Fig. 15.2). The extension at the MCP

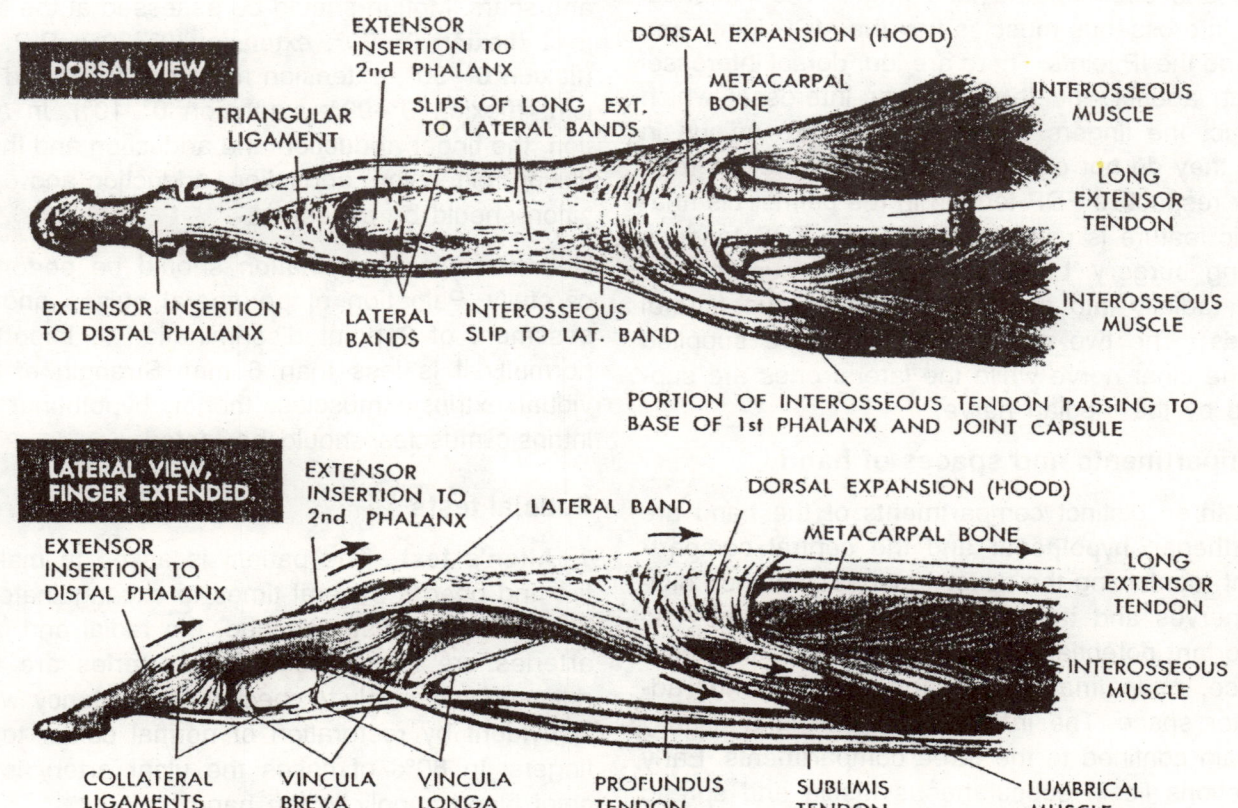

Fig. 15.2. Dorsal digital expansion

joint is by the extrinsic extensor tendon through the sagittal band, which envelops MCP joints like a sling. The lumbrical and interosseous muscles form the oblique and the transverse fibres of the intrinsic apparatus. The oblique fibres extend the IP joints while the transverse fibres flex the MCP joint. The central continuation of the extrinsic tendon forms the central slip, which inserts at the base of the middle phalanx and contributes to PIP extension. The lateral bands fuse to form the terminal extensor tendon, which inserts at the base of the distal phalanx and extends the DIP joint.

Intrinsic muscles of hand

Intrinsic muscles originate and insert within the hand and include thenar, hypothenar, interosseous and lumbrical muscles. Thenar muscles cover thumb metacarpal and include abductor pollicis brevis (APB), opponens pollicis (OP), flexor pollicis brevis and adductor pollicis muscles. The first three muscles oppose the thumb and are innervated by the median nerve while adductor pollicis is supplied by the ulnar nerve. The hypothenar muscles comprise of abductor digiti minimi, flexor digiti minimi and opponens digiti minimi. These muscles abduct and supinate the little finger. The lumbrical and interosseous muscles flex the MCP joints and extend the IP joints. There are four dorsal interossei which abduct and three palmar interossei which adduct the fingers. The lumbricals are unique in that they do not originate from any bone but from their respective FDP tendon in the palm. This anatomic feature is used to identify the FDP tendons during surgery. Lumbricals (four in number) insert radially into the extensor apparatus (lateral bands). The two medial lumbricals are supplied by the ulnar nerve while the lateral ones are supplied by the median nerve.

Compartments and spaces of hand

The three distinct compartments of the hand are the thenar, hypothenar and the central compartment (containing the flexor tendons, common digital nerves and the superficial palmar arch). The important potential spaces of the hand are thenar space, midpalmar space and the posterior adductor space. The infections in the hand usually remain confined to the three compartments. Early infections lie in subcutaneous fascia and spread into synovial and deep fascial spaces only when neglected or inadequately treated.

Neurovascular structures

Digital nerves are located volar to digital arteries and arise from median and ulnar nerves. The superficial palmar (arterial) arch is distal and volar and is supplied by ulnar artery. The radial artery supplies deep palmar arch. Digital arteries arise from the superficial palmar arch. Unlike the fingers, in the palm, the digital arteries are volar to the digital nerves.

Approach to a patient with hand problem

History of a patient with complaints pertaining to hand should take into consideration the age, occupation, handedness, activities and chronicity of symptoms. It is important to know the exacerbating activities and the functional impairment due to the problem.

Physical examination begins by inspection of the attitude of the hand. Skin should be inspected for thickness, irregularities and scars. Asking the patient to make a fist inspects knuckles. Muscle wasting should be looked for. Web spaces and nails should be inspected. Palpation includes feeling the skin for thickness, assessment of temperature, dryness and scars. Motion should be assessed at the MCP joint (flexion 0°–90°; extension 0°–30°); PIP joint (flexion 0°–90°; extension none normally) and DIP joint (flexion 0°–90°; extension 0°–10°). In addition, the finger abduction and adduction and thumb flexion, extension, abduction, adduction and opposition should be assessed.

Neurovascular examination should be performed carefully. Palpation of peripheral pulses and assessment of 2 point discrimination is important; normally it is less than 6 mm. Strength of individual extrinsic muscles, thenar, hypothenar and intrinsic muscles should be tested.

Special tests

1. Allen's test The patient is asked to make a fist and open it several times to exsanguinate the hand. With the fist clenched, the radial and ulnar arteries are compressed. The arteries are then released selectively to check for the patency, which is evident by restoration of normal colour to the fingers. In 80% of cases the ulnar artery is the chief blood supply to the hand.

Allen's test should be performed in every case

suspected of having T.O.C.S (See chapter 11). It is also useful in evaluating the patency of arterial supply to hand in cases of ulnar artery aneurysm, thrombosis, also when microvascular surgery or tumour excision is contemplated. Allen's test for fingers is performed by occluding the two digital arteries at the base of the finger and releasing them one after the other to look for the vascularity of the finger.

2. Extrinsic Muscle tightness (Volkmann's sign)

Contracture of flexor muscles is evident by possible passive extension of IP joints with the wrist in flexion while the same is not possible when the wrist is extended.

Contracture or adhesions of EDC to bone or retinaculum at wrist is evident by possible passive flexion of PIP joint when MCP is extended but inability to do so when the MCP is held in flexion.

3. Intrinsic muscle tightness (Bunnell's test)

With the MCP flexed, it is possible to passively flex PIP joint but with MCP extended, it is not possible. Sometimes intrinsic tightness is manifested only after surgical treatment of co-existing extrinsic tightness.

Radiological examination

Posteroanterior, lateral and oblique radiographs are routinely taken. Individual digits should be x-rayed for suspected pathology in any one of them.

Congenital disorders of hand

The cause of congenital hand disorders can be genetic (30%) or environmental (10%). However, almost in two third cases the cause is unknown. The congenital hand disorders can threaten the extremity (as in case of constriction bands), can cause tethering and disorders of growth (as in club hand), or can compromise appearance and function.

1. Syndactyly

Syndactyly is one of the commonest congenital hand deformities. It involves ring and middle fingers most commonly. Syndactyly can be simple, involving only the skin, or, complex involving the bones. The fingers may be joined over the entire length of digits (complete) (Fig. 15.3) or over partial length (incomplete). Syndactyly can be asso-

ciated with several syndromes such as *Apert Syndrome* (syndactyly of all digits, mental retardation, skull and facial abnormalities), *Poland syndrome* and *Streeter's dysplasia*. Apert's syndrome is classically associated with acrosyndactyly (tips of the fingers are fused). Treatment is release done between 18 months to 5 years of age. Skin grafting in usually required to cover areas of skin defect after release.

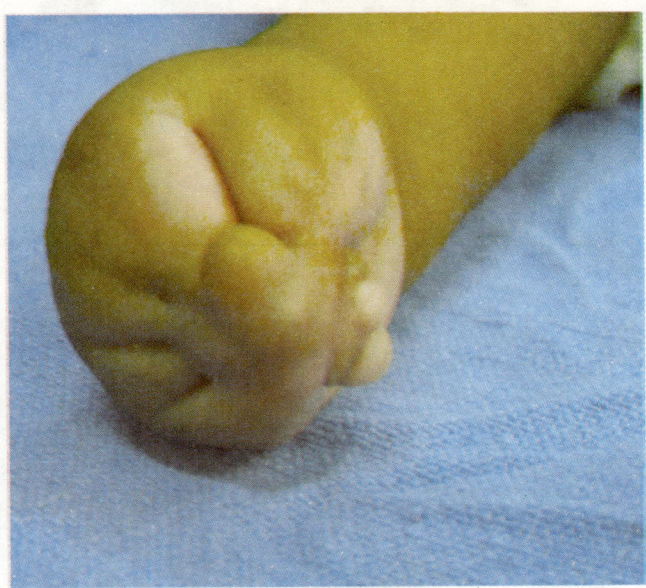

Fig. 15.3.   Complete syndactyly of the hand

2. Polydactyly

Polydactyly usually involves ulnar digits. It can be one of the three types :

a) presence of only extra soft tissues; b) extra digit with its own bone, tendon and cartilage (Fig. 15.4a-d), and c) complete with its own metacarpal. Polydactyly of thumb is usually associated with a generalised syndrome. The presence of a flail extra digit is treated by excision whereas the treatment of a separate digit is for cosmetic reasons. The least developed digit is amputated; care must be taken to ligate neurovascular. bundle and protect the ulnar collateral ligament.

3. Deformity of digits

a) **Clinodactyly**   involves lateral deviation of the small finger at the DIP joint caused by trapezoid shaped middle phalanx. It can also occur in the triphalangeal thumb. Patients are often mentally retarded. Treatment is for cosmetic reasons and

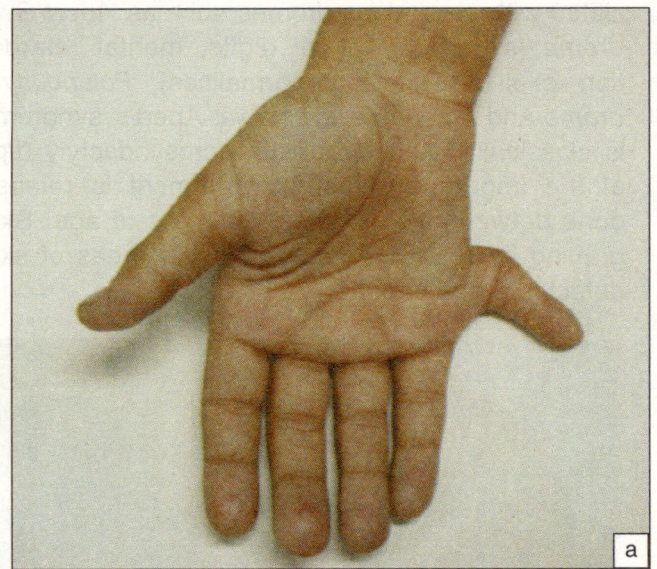

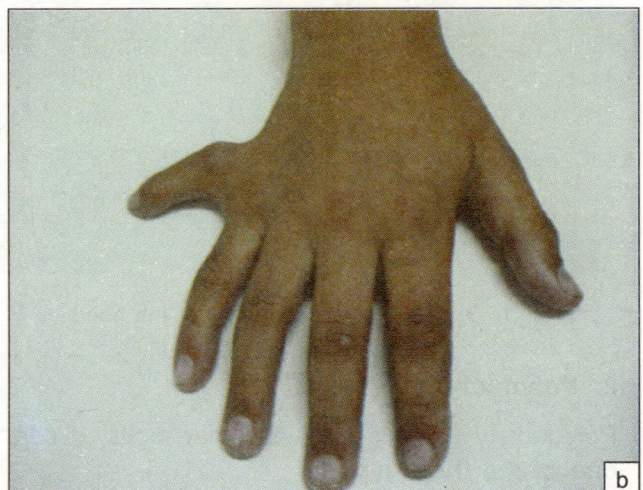

Fig. 15.4a,b. Clinical photograph of polydactyly.
Note the involvement on the ulnar side

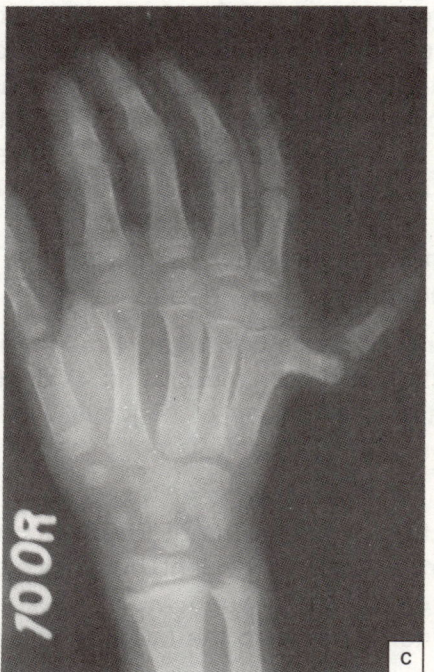

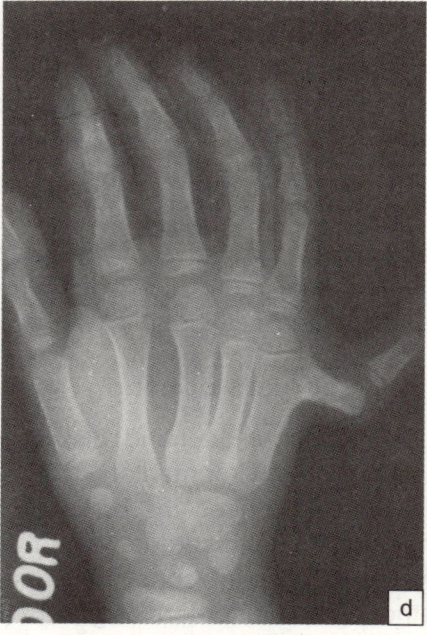

Fig. 15.4c,d. X-ray picture of the same patient.
Note the extra digit with its own bone.

involves closing wedge osteotomy of the middle phalanx.

b) Delta phalanx is a variety of clinodactyly and results from an abnormal epiphysis which is 'J' shaped or 'C' shaped with longitudinally bracketed diaphysis either in the middle phalanx of little finger or the proximal phalanx of the thumb. When the deformity is severe, it should be treated by realignment procedures.

c) Kirner's deformity is characterised by in curling of small finger DIP joint usually in peripubertal girls. Osteotomy can be performed if patients are seen late and want correction.

d) Camptodactyly (Non traumatic flexion deformity of PIP) is familial abnormality with flexion contracture of PIP joint usually involving the little finger. It is often bilateral though not necessarily to equal degree. The common underlying causes can be abnormal FDS, abnormal extensor apparatus or aberrant lumbrical insertion. It can be distinguished from other finger contractures by the facts that it is present from birth and only PIP joint of the little finger is involved.

Treatment is passive stretching and splinting in early stages. If the deformity is passively correctable, FDS transfer to the extensor hood can be undertaken.

e) Symphalangism is hereditary stiffness of PIP along with varying degree of shortness of middle phalanx secondary to congenital ankylosis of the joints. It is often associated with syndactyly, Apert syndrome and Poland syndrome. Treatment in children is observation. In adolescents, angulation osteotomy after epiphysis has fused can be tried.

f) Cleft hand A cleft hand is a V shaped congenital defect of hand (Fig. 15.5) which can vary in severity from a) a simple cleft between middle and ring finger; b) absent ray, usually middle ray,

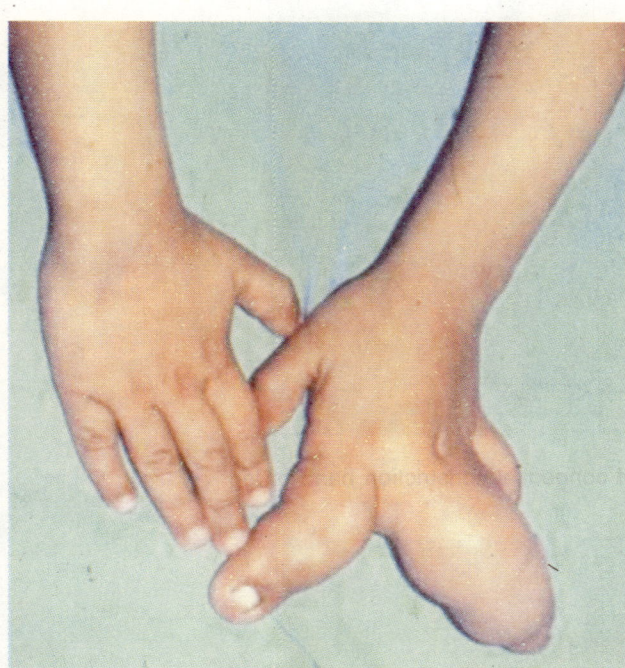

Fig. 15.5. Child with cleft hand (left). Note the presence of concomitant macrodactyly and absent middle ray.

sometimes index; c) hypoplasia of radial digits; to, d) syndactyly of remaining digits.

'Lobster claw' hand is the most severe variety where only border digits (only one radial and one ulnar rays) are present. Treatment is required only if grasp and pinch are not possible; when there is hypoplasia of thumb or impaired movements of

the digits. Syndactyly release, thumb reconstruction, cleft closure, first space widening and tendon transfers to restore function are commonly employed procedures.

g) Congenital trigger thumb Congenital trigger thumb is caused by the stenosing tenosynovitis at A1 pulley. It presents with fixed flexion contracture of the thumb at birth and is often bilateral. It should be differentiated from the clasped thumb in which the flexion contracture is at IP as well as MCP joint of thumb and is caused by deficient extensors of the thumb. The condition should be differentiated from the congenital contracture of flexor pollicis longus muscle. Trigger thumb can be left for one year when nearly 30% will resolve spontaneously. Splinting and passive stretching should be tried. Recalcitrant cases should be treated by surgical release of A1 pulley at the MCP joint.

h) Macrodactyly is non hereditary congenital enlargement of one or more digits corresponding to the distribution of one or more peripheral nerves; thus it is also called nerve oriented macrodactyly. It occurs most commonly in the territory of the median nerve (Fig. 15.6). The enlargement affects distal part more than proximal and phalanges are affected more frequently than metacarpals. Joint stiffness is often present as is deviation of digits due to uneven overgrowth of the borders of the digits. Condition should be differentiated from cavernous hemangioma clinically (consistency and vascular examination) and radiologically. Treatment is difficult and consists of

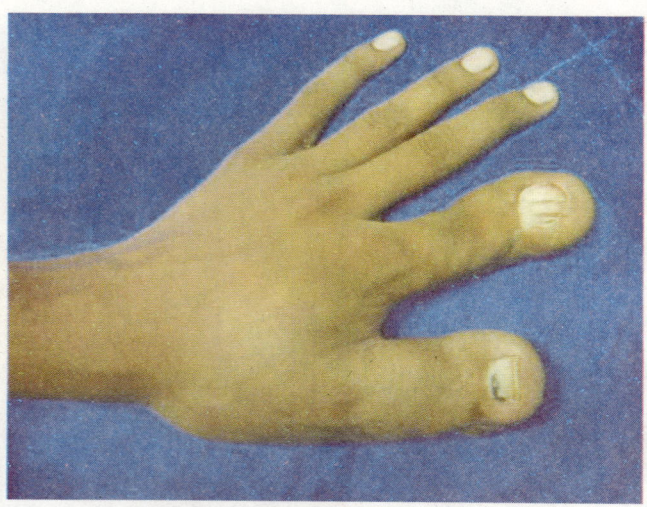

Fig. 15.6. Clinical photograph of macrodactyly

reduction of the size of digit (osteotomies, defatting, epiphyseodesis) or amputation of the affected digit.

4. Constriction Ring Syndrome (*Streeter's dysplasia*)

Constriction ring syndrome consists of congenital constriction ring / band affecting digits or more proximal part of limb (Fig. 15.7a). When severe these cause severe lymphoedema or even amputation. Constriction rings are associated with club feet, syndactyly or acrosyndactyly (distal fusion of digits with cleft or separation proximally) and neurological abnormalities. Treatment consists of early release of constriction rings with multiple, circum-ferential Z-plasties if the oedema is gross (Fig. 15.7b).

5. Congenital Amputations

Congenital amputations can result either from failure of development or Streeter's syndrome. Amputations often involve only one or two fingers when associated with congenital constriction rings and good function is usually achieved with remaining digits. Amputation of the thumb, however, requires reconstruction with metacarpal lengthening, toe transfer or index finger pollicization. Complete absence of the hand in blind children is classically treated by a Krukenberg procedure, which involves creation of a radio-ulnar claw.

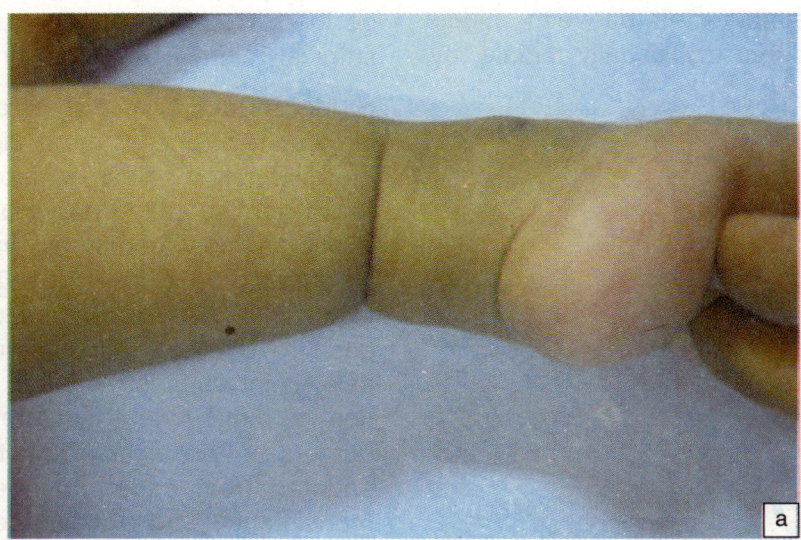

Fig. 15.7a. Pre operative clinical picture of congenital constriction band of leg

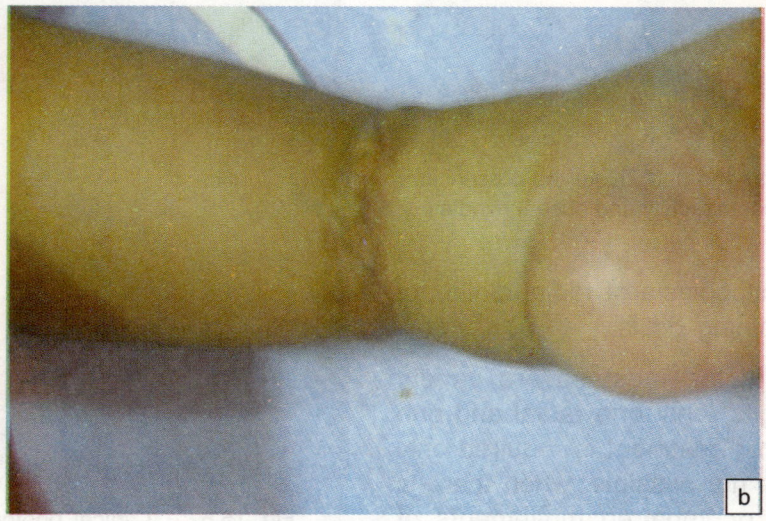

Fig. 15.7b. Post operative clinical picture following constriction band release in the same patient

Common soft tissue disorders of the hand

1. Ganglion

Ganglion cyst is the most common mass in hand. It can present on the dorsal aspect of hand in relation to the sheath of extensor tendons of the hand or on the palmar aspect of the fingers at A1 pulley (volar retinacular ganglion). Ganglia are usually soft, non tender and transilluminant but when present in relation to flexor tendon sheath (seed ganglion) they can be tender and hard. The size of ganglion may wax or wane. Treatment includes aspiration, rupture or surgical excision.

2. Mucous Cysts

Mucous cysts are ganglia arising from the dorsal aspect of DIP in association with osteoarthritic dorsal spurring of the DIP joint. They are frequently associated with Heberden's nodes. Cysts are painful and protrude between the proximal nail fold and the attachment of the terminal extensor tendon of the DIP joint. Pressure on the germinal matrix may lead to abnormal nail production. Overlying skin often becomes attenuated and shiny and occasionally gives way spontaneously leading to discharge of mucinous contents. Treatment consists of meticulous surgical excision of the cyst along with the overlying skin and debridement of the associated marginal osteophytes.

3. Epidermoid (inclusion) Cyst

Epidermoid (inclusion) cyst results from penetrating injuries leading to implantation of epithelioid tissue into deeper areas. These cysts present as painful, usually palmar subcutaneous nodules which are not transilluminant. The lesion may sometimes involve the distal phalanx and show cystic lesion on x-ray. Treatment is excision along with overlying adherent skin.

4. Trigger finger/Trigger Thumb

Trigger finger is caused by the irritation or inflammation of the fibro-osseous tunnel and tendon system, which results in a nodule on the FDS tendon. Ring and middle fingers are most commonly involved. The swelling snaps to and fro through the opening of the sheath (at the site of A1 pulley) resulting in triggering, i.e. locking of the finger in flexion. Triggering can also occur in the thumb at the level of A-1 pulley and involves the FPL tendon. The disorder may be an early manifestation of the rheumatoid disease but is most commonly seen as an isolated condition caused by degenerative changes or chronic irritation. Treatment in early cases consists of NSAIDs, splinting and injection of soluble steroid with local anaesthetic in the fibro-osseous sheath at the level of A1 pulley (and not in the tendon !). Recalcitrant cases are treated by division of the A1 pulley.

5. Dupuytren's contracture

Dupuytren's contracture is proliferative fibrodysplasia of subcutaneous palmar fascia, which leads to contractures due to progressive development of nodules and cords. The etiology is uncertain but the disorder occurs more commonly in alcoholics, diabetics, smokers, epileptics and in those with liver disease.

The disorder usually affects men (ten times more commonly than women) between the ages of 40 and 60 years. Ring and the little fingers are most frequently involved. The disorder is usually bilateral but more advanced in one hand. The patient presents with painless palmar nodules and flexion contractures (Fig. 15.8), which limit the hand function. Other areas which show involvement include the dorsum of PIP joint (where thickening of subcutaneous tissues leads to formation of knuckle pads or *Garrod's pads*), plantar fascia (fibrous nodular

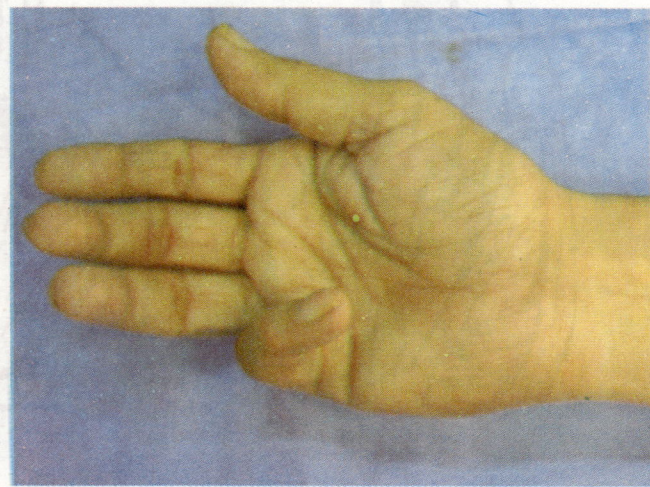

Fig. 15.8. Clinical picture of a patient with Dupuytren's contracture. Note the flexion at MCP and PIP joints of the little finger

thickening-*Ledderhose's disease*) and penis (*Peyronie's disease*).

Pathologically, the disease begins in the distal palm as a nodule of dense fascia often adherent to the overlying skin. This can result in puckering of the skin at the distal palm. The pretendinous bands of the palmar aponeurosis cause MCP joint contracture. As the degenerative process continues, the distal slips of palmar fascia pull PIP joint into flexion.

Luck described three stages in the pathogenesis of Dupuytren's contracture (Fig. 15.9).

Treatment of Dupuytren's contracture in early cases limited to simple palmar nodularity is observation. MCP joint contracture beyond 30° and any PIP joint contractures are indications for surgery. The surgical options available include percutaneous fasciotomy, subtotal fasciectomy and total fasciectomy. Subtotal palmar fasciectomy of the involved fascia is treatment of choice. Prognosis is better when MCP joint alone is involved. PIP joint flexion has a poor prognosis. Results of attempts to correct PIP joint flexion deformity are not satisfactory and often lead to loss of flexion at PIP joint.

Mcgash procedure involves excision of contracted skin also along with the fascia and leaving the wound open.

Salvage procedures for the severe PIP contractures are skeletal shortening, arthrodesis and amputation.

Infections of the hand

Infections of the hand are uncommon but are very important since they can lead to complications and functional impairment. Diabetes, pin pricks and bites during fights are important predisposing factors. Though staphylococcus aureus is responsible for most hand infections, polymicrobial infections (including anaerobic species in almost one third cases) are also common. The patients present with acute pain and constitutional symptoms. Examination reveals tenderness over the affected area and over enlarged proximal lymph nodes (axillary and epitrochlear lymph nodes). The general principles of the treatment of hand infections include rest, elevation, splinting, broad spectrum systemic antibiotics (adequate alone only in cases with cellulitis) and drainage of pus.

Common hand infections

1. Paronychia / Eponychia

Paronychia is the most common infection of the hand and involves the soft tissue fold around the fingernail. An eponychia involves the eponychial fold at the base of the nail and the lateral fold.

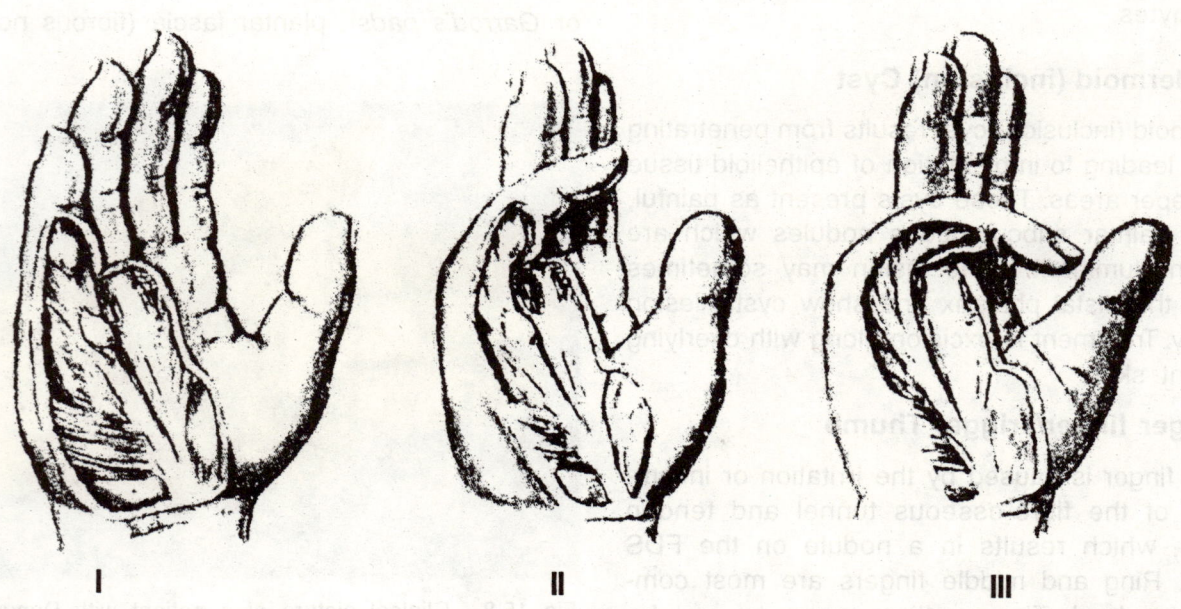

I   II   III

Fig. 15.9.   Stages in Dupuytren's contracture
I - Contracture of palmar aponeurosis; II - MCP flexion; III - PIP flexion

Infection is usually by staph. aureus and is often introduced in the paronychial tissue by hang nail, tooth or manicure instrument.

The condition presents with exquisite tenderness. In early stages elevation, splinting, warm saline soaks and oral antibiotics may suffice. In extensive lesions, incision and drainage (including complete unroofing of paronychia along with removal of a portion of nail, loose packing and soaks) is performed.

2. Felon

A felon is a subcutaneous abscess involving the distal pulp of the digit. Felon may follow a penetrating injury or spread from paronychia. Pulp normally has dense collection of fibrous septae which divide the pulp into many small unyielding compartments. The pus collection in the pulp, therefore, results in: i) excruciating pain; ii) necrosis of terminal phalanx due to excessive pressure in pulp interrupting vascular supply; and, iii) a residual focus of infection frequently unless drainage is meticulous and complete.

Clinically, a felon presents with swelling, tenderness and cellulitis on palmar aspect of the fingertip involving the entire pulp. The infection progresses rapidly and can lead to osteomyelitis of distal phalanx or can penetrate the skin. Involvement of neurovascular bundles can lead to sloughing of distal portion of finger. The infection can spread to flexor tendon sheath or DIP joint.

Treatment of felon is an emergency and is always surgical. Following principles should be observed:

- Flexor sheath should not be opened.

- Injury to digital nerve and vessels should be avoided.

- Incision should be lateral/dorsal. Lateral incisions should be ulnar except in thumb and little finger where they should be radial.

- All the vertical septae must be divided.

After I & D the wound should be loosely packed (pack is removed at 36 hours) and wound allowed to heal by secondary intention. Intravenous antibiotics must be given for at least 48 hours followed by oral antibiotics for two weeks.

3. Herpetic Whitlow

Herpetic Whitlow is a viral infection caused by herpes simplex virus. It is seen especially in medical/dental personnel and small children. It usually involves thumb or index finger and may be preceded by viral illness. Patients present with pain and clear, fluid filled vesicles or bullae of the distal finger. The tenderness however, is not as much as with pyogenic infections. Over a period of time crust formation over the lesion occurs and superficial epidermis desquamates. The condition is self-limiting and resolves over 3-4 weeks. Treatment consists of splintage, elevation and acyclovir. **I&D is contraindicated** as it may lead to systemic dissemination (leading to secondary viral encephalitis) and secondary bacterial infection. The disease is known to recur.

4. Suppurative Flexor Tenosynovitis

Suppurative flexor tenosynovitis is the suppurative infection of the flexor tendon sheath. It is a surgical emergency because if untreated it can lead to adhesions (leading to stiffness of finger) and necrosis of the flexor tendon.

The four classical *Kanavel's signs* described to make the diagnosis are a) tenderness along the tendon sheath; b) finger held in flexed position; c) pain on passive extension of the finger; and, d) symmetric swelling of the digit (sausage shaped digits).

The infection can spread to the deep spaces; index finger and thumb flexor tendon infections spread to thenar space; those of middle, ring and small fingers spread to midpalmar space while that from the small finger can also spread to the ulnar bursa.

The treatment of suppurative tenosynovitis is surgical drainage through a midlateral incision or closed sheath irrigation.

5. Radial and Ulnar Bursa Infections

FPL and FDS (little finger) sheath infections with proximal extension lead to radial and ulnar bursa infections respectively. These proximal extensions make it mandatory to give additional proximal incisions to drain the pus.

6. Deep Fascial Space Infections

Deep fascial space infections occur in the palm

and may be limited to web space (*collar button abscess*), or may extend to midpalmar space. The latter presents with swelling and loss of contour of palm, and painful movements of middle, ring and little fingers. Thenar space infection leads to swelling and pain on movements of thumb and index finger. Hypothenar space infections are rare.

Treatment of deep space infections includes I & D and intravenous antibiotics.

Arthritis of hand

Osteoarthritis (Degenerative joint disease-DJD) of hand

Osteoarthritis is characterised clinically by pain, weakness, deformity and limitation of movements and radiologically by focal erosions, loss of articular cartilage space, subchondral sclerosis, osteophytes and cyst formation. The females are more commonly affected than males. The most frequently affected hand joints are the distal interphalangeal joints and the carpometacarpal joint of the thumb. The distal interphalangeal joint involvement results in tenderness and bony enlargements called *Heberden's nodes* (Fig. 15.10a,b) and mucus cyst. Thumb CMC involvement results in pain and decreased pinch strength. Adduction of the thumb is particularly painful. Grind test, performed by axial compression with rotation of the thumb causes pain at the CMC joint. With advanced disease, adduction deformity of thumb may result from radial subluxation of the metac-

arpal on the trapezium. The proximal interphalangeal joints are rarely involved by DJD and when affected, have tenderness and bony enlargement at PIP joint called *Bouchard's nodes*.

Treatment is conservative in most cases and consists of NSAIDs, splint, physiotherapy and intraarticular steroid injections. Surgical options include excision of osteophytes, mucus cysts, arthroplasty and arthrodesis. The primary indication for surgery is pain unresponsive to conservative treatment. Severe involvement of DIP joint is treated by fusion in 10–15 degrees of flexion. Arthrodesis of DIP relieves pain, corrects deformity and stabilises the joint.

CMC joint osteoarthritis is treated by resection arthroplasty (excision of distal half or entire trapezium) with or without interposition of tendon (FCR or portion of APL). Arthrodesis of CMC joint should be performed only if it is the only joint involved and MCP joint is normal. DJD of radial sesamoid of the thumb can sometimes cause pain at CMC joint with narrowing of the space between the radial sesamoid and radial condyle of metacarpal. Excision of the sesamoid ameliorates the symptoms.

Proximal interphalangeal joint involvement of the ring and little fingers is best addressed by implant arthroplasty. Implant arthroplasty is not advised for the index and the middle fingers as it does not allow a good lateral or key pinch due to residual instability. Arthrodesis of PIP joint is useful for

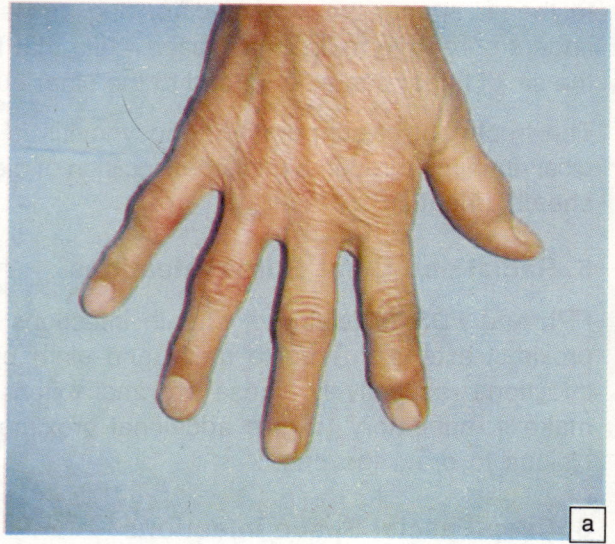 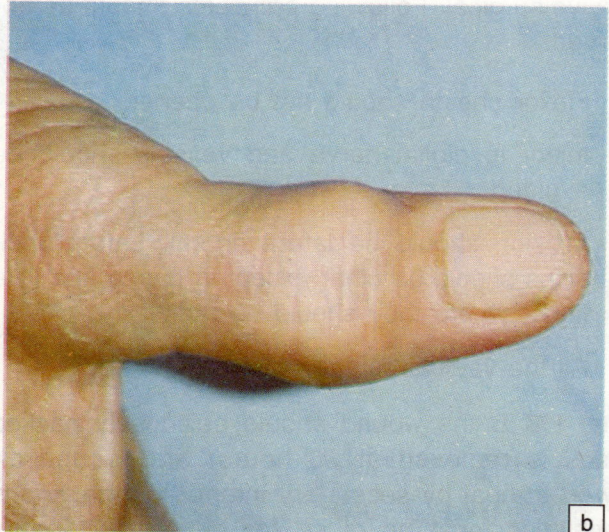

Fig. 15.10a,b. Heberden's Nodes. Note the swelling of DIP joints

pain relief and providing stable pinch. The position of PIP joint fusion varies as follows: Index 30° flexion; middle 35° flexion; ring 40° flexion, and little finger 45° flexion.

Inflammatory arthritis of hand

Rheumatoid Arthritis (RA)

RA of the hand occurs early in the course of the disease. Progressive joint destruction and deformity occurs frequently due to the combined effect of tenosynovitis and synovitis. Hypertrophic synovitis destroys cartilage and erodes bone, compresses nerves, leads to entrapment or rupture of tendons and destroys supporting periarticular structures leading to instability of the joints. Compensatory deformities occur frequently. Clinically the patients present with pain, weakness and mechanical dysfunction. Tenosynovitis (esp. deQuervain's), trigger finger / thumb, and carpal tunnel syndrome are common. Tenosynovitis is characterised by passive flexion more than active flexion at the finger joints. The tendon ruptures may occur following tenosynovitis. Flexor pollicis longus is the most commonly ruptured flexor tendon as it rubs at an osteophyte over anterior aspect of scaphotrapezial joint (Mannerfelt lesion). EDC tendons to ring and little fingers are commonly ruptured extensor tendons as they rub on distal ulna (*Vaughn-Jackson Syndrome*). EPL can rupture over Lister's tubercle.

Classical deformities of the rheumatoid hand are ulnar drift deformity (Fig. 15.11c-e), intrinsic plus deformity, boutonniere deformity (Fig. 15.11a), swan neck deformity and Z-thumb (Fig. 15.11b). The common deformities of the hand joints in rheumatoid hand are shown in Table 15.1. The pathogenesis of these deformities is discussed below along with their treatment modalities.

Table 15.1. Deformities in the hand in Rheumatoid Arthritis

PIP Joint	Boutonniere (commonest) , swan neck, unstable PIP
MCP Joint	Volar subluxation, ulnar drift, dislocation of MCP joints
Thumb	Boutonniere (commonest), Flail IP joint, Duck-bill thumb or Z thumb (dislocated CMC joint, hyperextended MCP and flexed IP joint)

Treatment of RA in early stages is splinting and physiotherapy in addition to the medical treatment.

The surgical treatment aims to relieve pain, improve function, prevent further damage and, improve cosmesis. The treatment depends on the structures and/or joints involved. Surgical indications include pain, chronic synovitis (synovectomy if there is no destruction or loss of cartilage and the disease is unresponsive to medical treatment for 6 months), nerve entrapment, tendon rupture and deformities limiting the function.

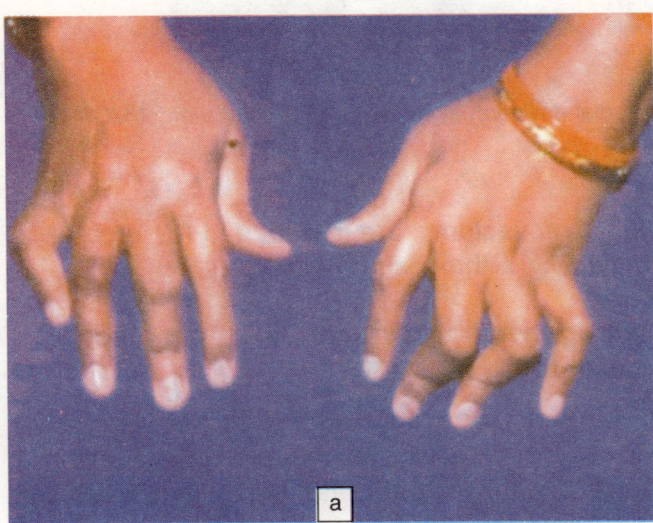

Fig. 15.11a. Boutonniere deformity. Note the flexion at PIP joints

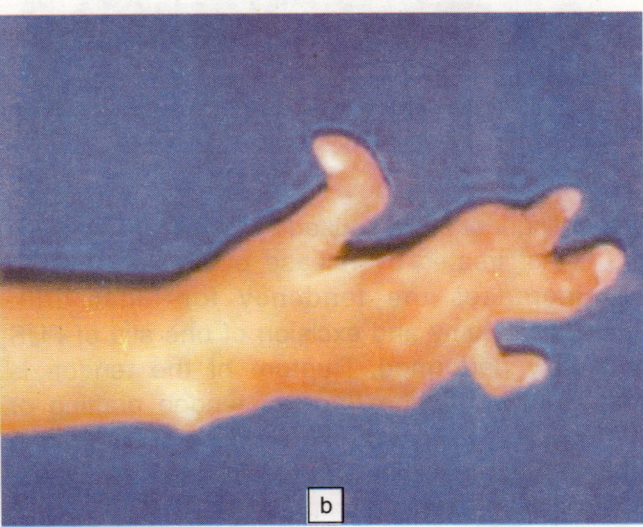

Fig. 15.11b. Swan neck deformity. Note the hyperextension of PIP joint and flexion of DIP

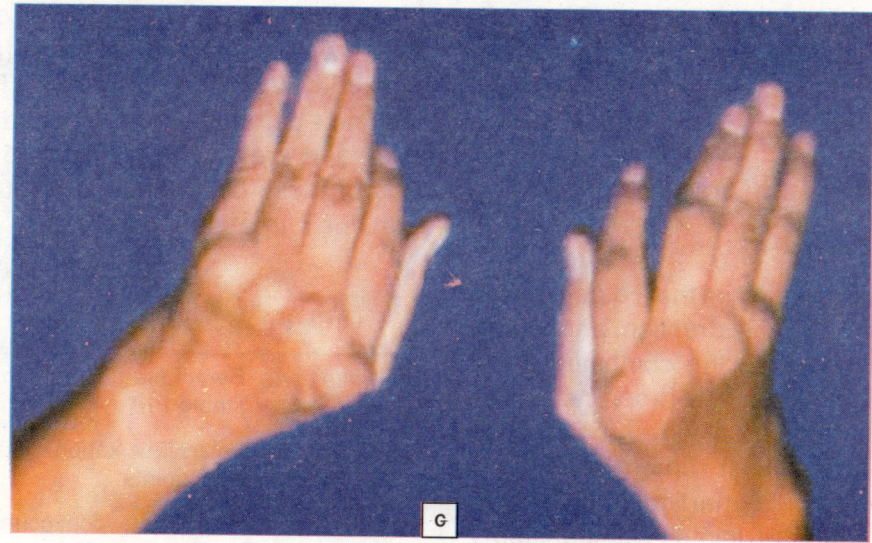

Fig. 15.11c. Ulnar drift at the MCP joints

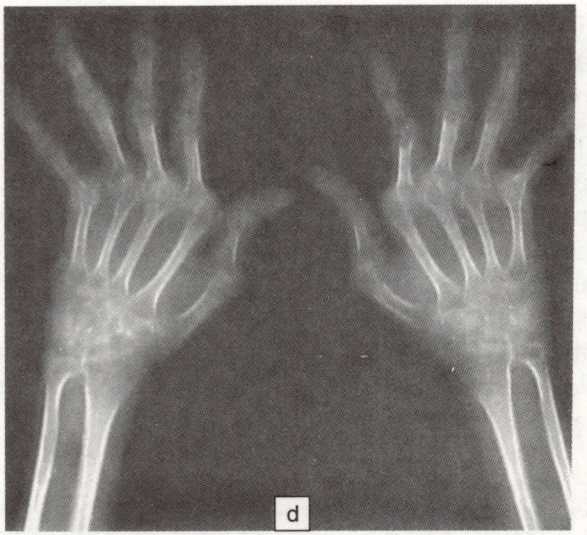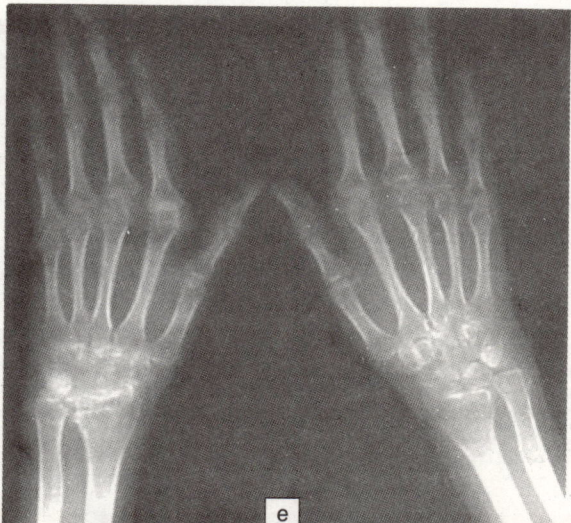

Fig. 15.11d-e. Radiographs of a patient with Rheumatoid arthritis.
Note the symmetrical juxta articular osteoporosis, radial deviation at wrist and ulnar deviation of MCP joints and carpal coalition

Trigger finger of RA is caused by flexor tenosynovitis and is not treated by release of A1 pulley since that increases the tendency for ulnar drift. Tenosynovectomy and excision of one slip of FDS is usually performed. Rupture of the tendon is addressed by tendon transfer, tendon grafting or arthrodesis. Tenosynovectomy can prevent tendon rupture and may also be required at late stage along with tendon grafting.

EDC (to IV & V) rupture is treated by repair during early period (4–6 weeks). Later, tendon grafting with synovectomy are required. FPL rupture is treated by arthrodesis of PIP joint.

Pathogenesis and treatment of specific deformities

1. Intrinsic plus deformity presents with flexed MCPs and extension at interphalangeal joints. It leads to weakness of grasp and stiffness. Flexion of MCP joints improves flexion of IP joints. Treatment is physiotherapy in early stages and intrinsic muscles release/transfer in late stages.

2. Boutonniere deformity (Flexion at PIP and hyperextension at DIP) is the most common deformity at PIP. Synovitis of PIP joint leads to elongation or rupture of the central slip of extensor tendon. PIP joint flexes as a result and lateral bands sublux volarwards. The latter in their new position become active flexors of PIP (rather than extensors) and hyperextend the DIP (by relative shortening of extensor mechanism). Lack of passive flexion at DIP with PIP in extension is the earliest sign of boutonniere deformity.

Treatment of mild deformities, which are passively correctable, is by synovectomy and splinting. Tenotomy of terminal slip of extensor tendon relaxes extensor mechanism and prevents hyperextension of DIP joint.

Late reconstructions for significant deformities require the central band reconstruction as well as lateral band transfer. Severe fixed deformities need arthroplasty or fusion.

3. Swan Neck Deformity indicates PIP hyperextension and DIP flexion caused by dorsal subluxation of the lateral bands following laceration, rupture or tenosynovitis of FDS, laxity of ligaments/capsule of PIP or intrinsic tightness. Early cases are treated by splintage, PIP synovectomy, mobilisation of lateral bands with or without intrinsic release, tenotomy or lengthening of central slip or tenodesis of FDS proximal to the PIP joint. Recurrences are common after the correction of swan neck deformity in RA.

4. Ulnar drift occurs at the MCP joints due to several factors. Synovitis of the MCP joints weakens the dorsal and radial structures and leads to lengthening of collateral ligaments (radial more than ulnar as the former are longer and more oblique). Mechanical factors then result in the ulnar drift. Ulnar subluxation of extensor tendons occurs during the power grip of the hand due to the ulnar sloping of the metacarpal heads. Extensor carpi ulnaris and extensor digiti minimi subluxate early due to the involvement of distal radioulnar and wrist joints. The transverse linkage of the extensor tendons then pulls all the extensor tendons ulnarwards. Pull of the long flexor tendons is fixed to the proximal phalanx due to the firm attachment of the volar plate and displaces the proximal phalanx in ulnar and volar direction. Radial deviation deformity at the wrist aggravates the ulnar drift of the fingers and vice versa. Severe cases with ulnar drift deformity may result in MCP joints dislocation.

Early cases can be treated by rest, splintage and synovectomy. Surgery comprises of intrinsic balancing (crossed intrinsic transfer shifts the attachment of ulnar intrinsics to the radial collateral ligament of the adjacent ulnar finger) and realignment of extensor tendons. Severe cases may need silastic arthroplasty of MCP joints.

5. Thumb deformities in RA can be boutonniere (due to MCP synovitis), swan neck (Fig. 15.12), combination of boutonniere and swan neck, Gamekeeper's thumb (due to ulnocarpal ligament laxity) or arthritis mutilans due to severe destruction at MCP and IP joints. Swan neck deformity is treated by CMC joint arthroplasty while the fusion of MCP joint is the most useful procedure for other deformities.

Tendon injuries

Tendon injuries are commonly associated with open, closed or penetrating injuries. The injuries must be recognised and diagnosed early because it is necessary to repair them primarily within the first few days. Digital nerves and vessels are frequently injured along with the tendons and careful examination must be performed to rule out neurovascular injuries.

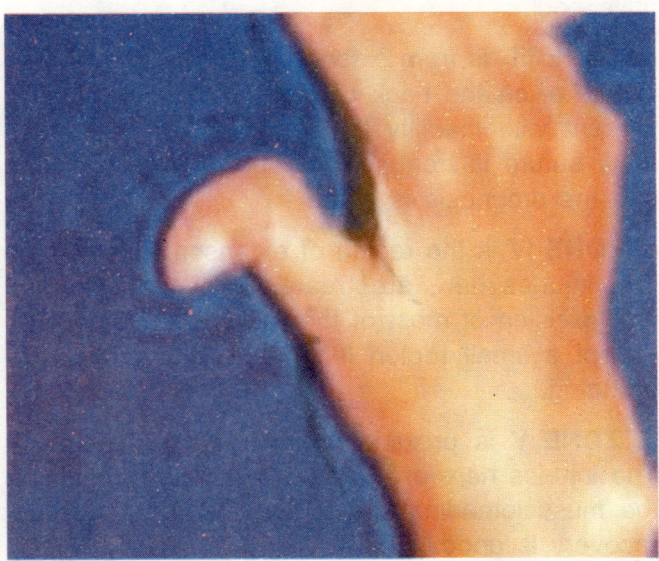

Fig. 15.12. Swan neck deformity of thumb

Extensor tendon injuries

Extensor tendon injuries are divided into various types according to the location of the laceration.

1. Zone I injuries are distal to the insertion of the central slip of the extensor tendon. Avulsion of the extensor tendon from the distal phalanx with or without a bony fragment leads to the mallet finger. On examination, finger is held in an attitude of slight flexion at DIP and there is loss of extension at DIP joint. Splinting the DIP in hyperextension for 6-8 weeks can usually treat mallet finger injuries. If a piece of bone is avulsed and the joint is subluxated, open reduction and internal fixation is recommended. If the lateral bands are injured they should be repaired primarily. Chronic mallet fingers often end up with a swan neck deformity (Fig. 15.13a,b).

2. ZONE II extends from MCP joints to the insertion of central slip. Avulsion of the central slip from the base of middle phalanx leads to boutonniere deformity. The lateral bands displace anteriorly and hyperextend DIP by tenodesis effect. Diagnosis can be made early by Elson's test wherein the patient is unable to extend the PIP joint over the edge of the table. Early cases are treated by splinting the PIP in extension for 6–8 weeks. Late cases need repair of central slip with or without reconstruction of lateral bands.

Extensor injuries over the MCP joint are treated by primary repair using roll stitch which is later pulled out.

3. ZONE III is from extensor retinaculum to MCP joints i.e. on the back of hand. The injuries here present with inability to extend MCP joints. Primary suture is treatment of choice in this region and the prognosis is good.

4. ZONE IV is the region of extensor retinaculum. The injuries here are treated by primary repair and excision of most of the overlying retinaculum except a small region left intact to prevent bow stringing.

5. ZONE V is proximal to extensor retinaculum. The injuries here are treated by primary repair of the musculotendinous unit and the prognosis for recovery is good.

6. Injuries to EPL EPL can be lacerated following injury or may rupture spontaneously following

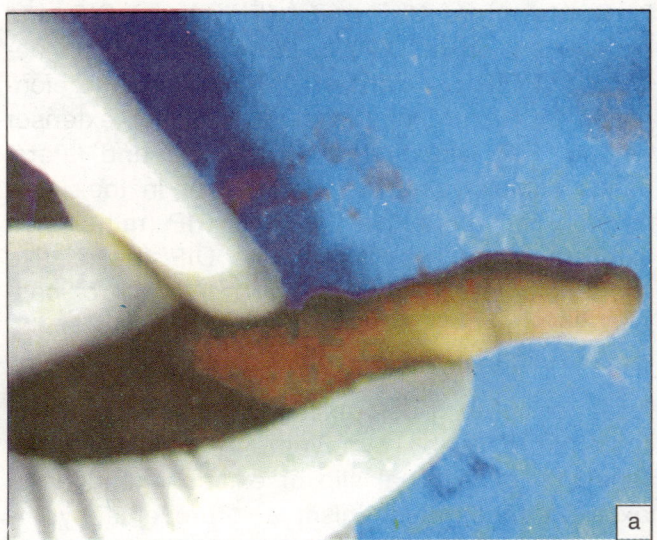
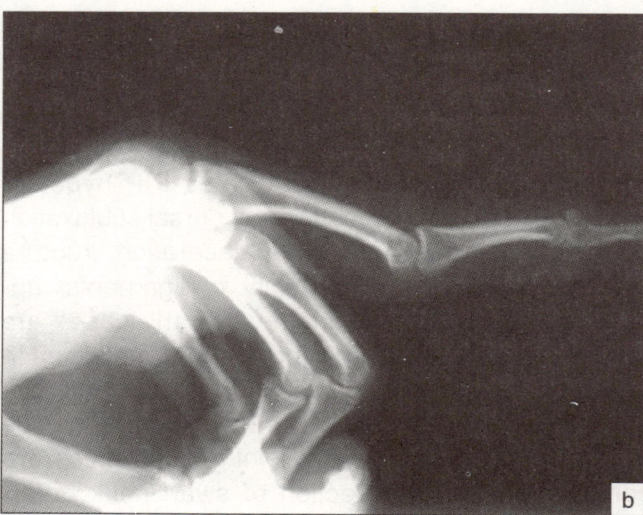

Fig. 15.13a,b. Clinical and radiographic picture of a patient with chronic mallet finger causing swan neck deformity

Colles' fracture. While the primary repair is ideal for acute laceration, spontaneous ruptures or old lacerations are best treated by extensor indicis proprius (EIP) transfer to the distal stump of EPL.

Flexor tendon injuries

Flexor tendon injuries are also divided into various types depending on the location of the injury. A2 and A4 flexor pulleys should always be preserved or reconstructed if injured.

1. ZONE I is distal to the insertion of FDS tendon. Avulsion of FDP insertion on distal phalanx is commonly seen with sports injuries (*Jersey finger*). The finger during sports is caught in opponent's jersey and forcibly extended. Ring finger is most commonly affected. The injury is diagnosed by asking the patient to flex DIP with PIP stabilised in extension to eliminate the effect of FDS. Treatment is direct repair whenever possible. A4 pulley should be preserved. If recognised late in young patients, the operative reconstruction using graft may be done. If the longstanding injury is present in older patients, DIP fusion / tenodesis can be performed in 30 degrees flexion.

2. Zone II (*No Man's Land*) extends from the metacarpal neck to FDS insertion and is the region of fibro-osseous tunnel. It is called no man's land because the flexor tendon repairs in this region are associated with marked adhesions and successful repairs are difficult. Both FDS and FDP should be repaired and A2 and A4 pulleys should be preserved. Late tenolysis is often required. Neglected injuries are treated with two stage reconstruction. The first stage involves excision of fibrous flexor sheath (except A2 and A4 pulleys) and placement of silastic rod for 6 weeks. After 6 weeks the silastic rod is replaced by a tendon graft to substitute for FDP.

3. ZONE III extends from transverse carpal ligament to the metacarpal neck. Cut tendons in this area, especially FDP do not retract proximally too far due to lumbrical attachment. Direct repair is method of choice to treat lacerations in this area.

4. ZONE IV underlies the transverse carpal ligament. Primary repair of the tendons is the method of choice. Transverse carpal ligament may need complete or incomplete incision for repair of tendons with subsequent repair to prevent bowstringing.

5. ZONE V extends from the transverse carpal ligament proximally to the musculotendinous units. End to end repair is recommended in this zone after carefully identifying the respective proximal and distal stumps.

6. Injuries to FPL are treated using the same principles. Primary repair should be done as there is little risk of adhesion formation. Cruciate pulleys are more important in thumb than fingers and should be preserved.

Replantation

Replantation implies reattachment of a part of the body partly or totally severed from the body. The success of replantation has increased dramatically in recent years with advancement in microsurgical techniques.

Indications for replantation include all thumb amputations, multiple digits amputation, single digit amputations distal to FDS insertion, all amputations proximal to digits and amputations in children. Single digit amputations in no man's land (from distal palmar crease to PIP joint) are contraindications for replantation. Other contraindications are mangled or crushed digits, prolonged warm ischemia time, severe de-gloving injuries and patients with arteriosclerotic vessels.

Preservation and transport of amputated part

Amputated part is transported cold to reduce its metabolic demands and slow cell necrosis. The maximum warm ischemia time is 6 hours while the maximum cold ischemia time is 12–18 hours. The amputated part is preserved and transported with dry cooling. The part is placed in a polyethylene or cellophane bag and this bag is then placed in a container filled with ice and transported. This procedure ensures cooling without freezing which leads to crystallisation of cells and fluids and precludes replantation.

Procedure of replantation involves isolation of neurovascular bundle followed by debridement of wound, fixation of bone, repair of extensor and flexor tendons and anastomosis of veins in that order. Postoperative care includes rest, monitoring and anticoagulants. Thrombosis of vascular repair is the most common cause of failure. Results following replantation are much better in children than adults.

Reflex Sympathetic Dystrophy

Reflex sympathetic dystrophy (RSD) is a syndrome characterised by intense burning pain, vasomotor disturbance and trophic changes in the extremity. RSD follows trauma especially to nerves, surgery or disease. The predisposing causes are a painful lesion in a person with diathesis or particular personality. Excessive efferent activity from sympathetic fibres is the pathological mechanism.

Clinically the patient presents with pain, swelling, discoloration and stiffness. Relief with sympathetic blockade is diagnostic as well as therapeautic. Triple phase bone scan helps in early diagnosis and shows increased uptake in all the phases.

X-rays show ground glass appearance along with patchy osteoporosis in late stages.

Treatment comprises of physical therapy and analgesics. Sympatholytic medicines are quite useful. Stellate ganglion block can be curative.

Raynaud's Disease

Raynaud's disease is occurrence of Raynaud's phenomenon (hyperemia, pallor and cyanosis of the digits on exposure to the cold) without any underlying disease. It typically occurs in young females. It can lead to distal trophic changes or even gangrene. Treatment involves avoiding exposure to extreme cold, digital protection, calcium channel blockers, beta blockers and sympathetic blockade.

CHAPTER 16

Thoracolumbar Spine

Relevant Anatomy

The thoracolumbar spine consists of 12 dorsal and 5 lumbar vertebrae joined together by discs anteriorly and facet joints posterolaterally. It protects and surrounds the thoracolumbar spinal cord, which gives off segmental nerve roots. These roots leave the spinal canal through the intervertebral foramina to innervate the chest wall, abdominal cavity, lower extremities and perineum.

The thoracic spine has a sagittal curve convex posteriorly called kyphosis. Lumbar spine has a normal curve convex anteriorly called lordosis. Any curvature in the coronal planes is abnormal and is termed scoliosis.

Osteology The vertebrae become progressively larger from upper dorsal to lower lumbar spine. The vertebral bodies are convex anteriorly, and concave posteriorly. The outer shell of vertebral body is thin cortical bone called end plate. The end plates are in contact with intervertebral discs superiorly and inferiorly and supply nutrition to the disc via diffusion. The inner part of vertebral body is filled with trabecular bone along with hematopoietic marrow.

Thoracic vertebrae (in contrast to lumbar vertebrae) have costal facets present on all the twelve vertebral bodies and transverse processes of T_1-T_9 to provide attachment to ribs. The lumbar vertebrae are the largest. They are more mobile because of lack of support from the rib cage.

Sacrum consists of fusion of five vertebrae. There are usually four pairs of pelvic sacral foramina on anterior as well as posterior aspect that transmit the respective branches of the upper four sacral nerves. Sacrum acts as the keystone in the pelvis and transfers the weight from spine laterally through the sacroiliac joints into the pelvis.

Coccyx is the vestigial tail bone, consisting of fused four lowest spinal elements. The joint between coccyx and sacrum is a true diarthrodial joint. Coccyx provides attachment to gluteus maximus, external anal sphincter and the coccygeal muscles.

Joints Each vertebra articulates with the next adjacent vertebra by two paired facet joints and one intervertebral disc. Facet (apophyseal) joints are oriented 60 degrees in the sagittal plane and 20 degrees posterior in thecoronal plane in dorsal spine. The orientation changes to 90° in the sagittal plane and 45° anterior in the coronal plane in the lumbar spine.

The superior articular facet (SAP) is anterior and lateral to the inferior articular facet of the vertebra above in dorso-lumbar spine, unlike the cervical spine where it (SAP) is anterior and inferior.

Intervertebral disc is a fibrocartilaginous structure like a jelly filled donut. Disc has outer, obliquely oriented annulus fibrosus made up of type I collagen and a softer inner nucleus pulposus made of type II collagen, embedded in a matrix of proteoglycan and water. The combination of collagen for strength and water and proteoglycan for cushioning gives the disc its unique mechanical properties viz. load bearing, motion and limited compressibility. Discs are avascular in adults.

Ligaments

All the vertebrae are connected by strong anterior longitudinal ligament (ALL) – the primary stabiliser of the throaco-lumbar spine and the weaker posterior longitudinal ligament (PLL). Interspinous ligaments extend between the spinous processes and facet capsules. ALL resists excessive extension while PLL limits flexion.

The ligamentum flavum is a strong, yellow, elastic ligament connecting the laminae. It protects spinal contents posteriorly and its overgrowth results in spinal stenosis. The supraspinous ligaments lie dorsal to the spinous processes and the interspinous ligaments. Iliolumbar ligament is a stout ligament, which connects the transverse process of L_5 with the ilium. Vertical shear type of unstable fractures of the pelvis may avulse the transverse process of L_5 through tension on this ligament.

Spine Musculature

The thoracolumbar spine is blanketed superiorly by trapezius and inferiorly by latissimus dorsi. Deep to these superficial muscles are the rhomboids and levator scapulae. The intrinsic muscles of the spine are deep to this layer and comprise of the erector spinae, interspinalis and transversalis muscles. They act to extend, rotate and laterally flex the spine. The deep muscles of the back are innervated by dorsal primary rami of spinal nerves.

Nerves

The spinal cord ends at the lower border of L_1 in 90% of people. The individual nerve roots continue as the cauda equina below that. As the nerve root enters the foramen to leave the spinal canal, it is bordered superiorly by the pedicle of the same named vertebra (i.e. L_5 root exits below the pedicle of L_5), posteriorly by the superior articular facet of the next vertebra below and anteriorly by the vertebral body. The nerve root occupies the superior portion of the foramen and reaches the level of the next disc far laterally, outside the foramen. Thus, the L_4 nerve root is not compressed by the L_4/L_5 disc herniation. In fact, a particular disc herniation affects the next lower nerve root before it exits the spinal canal through the foramen. For example, in L_5/S_1 disc prolapse, S_1 nerve root is involved while in L_4/L_5 disc prolapse, L_5 nerve root is involved.

Vascular Supply

The arterial supply to the spine comes as direct branches from the aorta and iliac arteries. The segmental arteries cross anteriorly at the level of midpoint of each vertebral body. There are approximately eight anterior medullary feeder arteries arising from segmental arteries, which enter the spinal canal to supply the vertebrae and spinal cord. The largest of these anterior medullary feeder vessels is the artery of Adamkiewicz, which enters between T_4 and T_{10}, usually on the right side. However, it is often neither large nor consistent in location. Thus there is significant risk of ischemic insult to the cord during surgery on dorsal spine.

The venous drainage of the spine is profuse and occurs through a large network of veins in the epidural space called Batson's plexus. The latter drains the vertebral bodies, dural space, muscles, facet joints and segmental nerve roots. It also receives tributaries from the pelvis and abdomen in the lumbar spine and thoracic cavity in the thoracic spine. These venous channels lack valves and allow metastatic cancer cells/infections from genitourinary, gastrointestinal and respiratory tracts to get deposited in the spine.

Evaluation of patient with spinal problem

A complete history is essential to evaluate the complaints pertaining to the back. The age is an important factor. Children may be affected by congenital or developmental disorders, infections or primary tumors. Young adults are more commonly affected by instability due to degenerative disc disease, spondylolisthesis or traumatic fractures. Elderly people are most commonly affected by degenerative disorders (such as lumbar spondylosis and/or lumbar canal stenosis), metastases or osteoporotic fractures.

The onset of symptoms (whether acute or chronic), their progression, the aggravating and relieving factors and the concomitant presence of constitutional symptoms are useful facts to elicit in history. Presence of radicular symptoms should be ascertained. Girdle pains are often the earliest presentation of the dorsal spine tuberculosis. Sphincteric incontinence and saddle anaesthesia may point towards the cauda equina syndrome. Careful assessment should be made of any history suggestive of visceral or vascular origin of symptoms or the disease related to other skeletal areas masquerading as spinal disease (Referred pain). Careful psychological evaluation is important in some patients with chronic low back disorders who may be deriving secondary gains out of the illness.

Physical examination should start with inspection of the overall alignment in sagittal and coronal planes, posture of the patient and the presence of any tilt or list to one side. Back should be inspected for scars, hairy patches or skin dimples, any area of redness, unusual swellings, deformity (scoliosis, increased or decreased lordosis or exaggerated dorsal kyphosis), shoulder alignment, balance and pelvic obliquity.

Normal thoracic kyphosis is 20°–45° (mean 34°) while the normal lumbar lordosis is 30°–50°. Normal lumbo-sacral junction (L_5–S_1) angle measures 12°–14°. Spasm of paraspinal muscles should be noted. Gait should be observed carefully; a wide based gait is seen in myelopathy while patients with stenosis lean forward while walking. The spasticity is often made out on seeing the patient walking. An antalgic gait may suggest a hip pathology, which may be responsible for the symptoms.

Palpation of the spinous processes, coccyx and sacroiliac joint should be done for tenderness. A 'step-off' of midline spinous processes may be seen in spondylolisthesis. Acute gibbus deformity or posttraumatic swelling should be palpated for tenderness. Regional lymph nodes and paraspinal muscles should also be palpated. A rectal exami-

nation should be done in all cases. Pain on pressure over the renal angle may suggest urinary system as the cause of pain in the back. Other problems causing referred pain such as abnormalities of the gallbladder, pancreas and menstrual cycle disturbances should be ruled out.

Range of motion should be tested in all directions for any limitation. Flexion (normal: able to touch the toes), Extension (normal: 30°–40°), Lateral bending (normal: 30 degrees to each side) and rotations (normally symmetric) should be tested. Range of motion of hips should also be evaluated. Chest expansion should be noted.

Neurological examination involves examination of sensations, strength testing of muscles and reflexes. The sensations are tested based on the fact that segmental nerves form predictable patterns of innervation. The sensory dermatomal pattern comprises of T_4 innervation at nipple level, T_{10} at the umbilicus level and L_1 at groin. The dermatomes in leg wrap laterally to medially so that L_3 innervates inner thigh, L_4 the medial aspect of the knee and anteromedial leg, L_5 the anterior calf and dorsal aspect of foot and S_1 the posterior calf and sole of the foot. Motor function is assessed by the fact that thoracic nerve roots innervate the intercostal muscles. In the lower limbs, L_3 and L_4 supply the hip flexors, L_4 and L_5 supply knee extensors, L_5 foot dorsiflexors and S_1 root supplies plantar flexors of the foot. Sacral nerve roots S_2 to S_4 control the sphincter tone and transmit perineal and perirectal sensations.

Deep tendon reflexes are innervated by L_4 (knee jerk), and S_1 (ankle jerk). Bulbocavernosus reflex is innervated by sacral roots S_2–S_4.

Special Tests

1. **Straight leg raising (SLR)** is a test for the tension on the nerve root. Passive lifting of the leg leads to the pain radiating down the posterior or lateral aspect of the leg distal to the knee and often into the foot. Bringing the leg down to a less elevated position relieves the pain. *Lasegue manoeuvre* consists of dorsiflexion of foot to further tension the root and it aggravates the symptoms and brings about the pain in a less elevated position.

2. **Contralateral (or cross) straight leg raising** Raising the contralateral leg can cause the pain

in the affected leg. It indicates a large central disc herniation.

3. **Bowstring test** After the straight leg raising, knee is flexed to reduce the tension on nerve root and the pain and pressure is applied in the popliteal fossa by hand. Return of pain suggests tension on the nerve root.

4. **Femoral nerve stretch test** The patient lies prone and the knee on the affected side is flexed. The development of the radicular pain suggests disc herniation in upper lumbar spine.

5. **Burn's test** is done for malingering. The patient is asked to touch the floor while kneeling on a chair. An inability to do so suggests malingering.

Investigations Plain x-rays (AP and lateral) are most commonly performed investigations in spinal disorders. The lateral films should be taken erect when evaluating spondylolisthesis and in flexion and extension when suspecting instability. The AP views should be taken both erect and supine (in right and left bending positions) when evaluating the scoliotic deformities. The right and left obliques for evaluation of pars interarticularis should be taken when spondylolysis is suspected. A concomitant AP x-ray of the pelvis can help in diagnosing hip and sacroiliac pathologies, ankylosing spondylitis, metabolic bone disease and the metastatic bone disease. Myelography outlines the spinal cord and nerve roots but is seldom indicated these days due to the availability of better and non-invasive investigations.

Computed Tomography (CT) should be done when evaluating the fresh or old fractures of the spine to delineate osseous pathology. CT myelography can help in evaluation of compressive myelopathies or intraspinal space occupying lesion (SOL) but MRI has replaced it this present day for all such indications.

Magnetic Resonance Imaging (MRI)

MRI is invaluable in the assessment of disc disease (especially after failed disc surgery), ligamentous injuries, intraspinal SOL, compressive myelopathies, spinal cord pathologies, spinal tumors and for identifying infections around the spine such as tuberculosis and discitis.

Bone Scan

Technetium pyrophosphate radiolabelled bone scan is useful to diagnose spinal disorders associated with activation of osteoblasts, which pick up radiotracer preferentially. Examples are osteoblastic tumors (primary as well as metastatic), fractures (including stress fractures), bone or disc infections and Paget's disease.

Nerve Conduction Studies and EMG are indicated for evaluation of radiculopathies as in cases of degenerative disc disease. They can be used to confirm clinical impression but are non-specific.

Psychological Evaluation such as Minnesota Multiphasic Personality Inventory (MMPI) should be employed when a functional cause for back pain is suspected and patient is likely to be unsuitable for surgery.

Congenital and Developmental Disorders of Thoracolumbar Spine.

1. Spina Bifida

Spina Bifida implies failure of the fusion of the posterior elements. It is most commonly seen at the lumbosacral junction and is seldom responsible for the low back pain attributed to it. It may be associated with a tell tale lesion in the skin over the lower back. It may sometimes be associated with spinal dysraphism and has been discussed in detail elsewhere.

2. Transitional Vertebra

There is sometimes an additional lumbar (lumbarisation of first sacral vertebra) or sacral (sacralisation of the fifth lumbar vertebra with presence of only 4 lumbar vertebrae) vertebra.

The sacralisation or lumbarisation can be partial (fusion of the transverse process to that of vertebra above or below only on one side) (Fig. 16.1) or complete (on both sides of the midline). The transitional vertebrae (especially unilateral or partial ones) have been claimed to alter biomechanics of the spine and have been believed to cause backache. Most workers present day, however, consider them only as incidental findings.

3. Block Vertebra

Block vertebra is most commonly an incidental

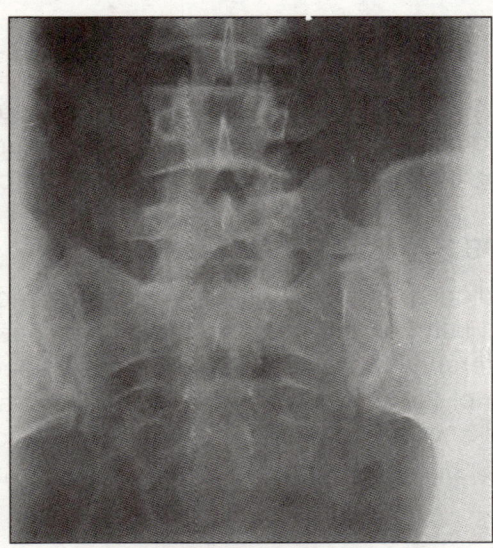

Fig. 16.1. Transitional vertebra (partial–left sided) at lumbo-sacral junction

finding on radiographs but should be differentiated from bony ankylosis following the healed tubercular disease. The block vertebra implies fusion of the two adjacent vertebrae with an absent or rudimentary disc without any loss of the height of the vertebral body. Condition needs no treatment.

Scoliosis

Scoliosis is an abnormal lateral curvature of the spine. The scoliosis can be classified into two main categories:

1. Non structural Non structural scoliosis is caused by a number of conditions, which produce an apparent scoliosis without rotation of the vertebrae, and in the absence of a true, intrinsic spinal deformity. These conditions include poor posture, hysteria, limb length discrepancy, hip deformity, muscular spasm (sciatic scoliosis) and inflammatory conditions. Non structural scoliosis is often mobile and disappears on the treatment of the underlying disorder.

2. Structural Structural scoliosis is associated with rotation of the vertebrae, is fixed and is a true, intrinsic spinal deformity. Structural scoliosis can be further divided into various types depending on the etiology:

(a) **Idiopathic** (when no primary cause is found) accounts for 85% of all cases. A genetic influence is strongly suggested in these cases. There is a female preponderance for curves

(5:1) and a familial tendency. It is believed to be a sex-linked trait or autosomal dominant pattern with variable expression and incomplete penetrance.

Idiopathic scolisis is divided into three types depending on the age of the patient at the time of onset of scoliosis:

i) Infantile (before 3 years of age)

ii) Juvenile (3–10 years of age)

iii) Adolescent (from 10 years to skeletal maturity)

(b) **Congenital** scoliosis is caused by congenital bone malformations (Fig. 16.2) and the causes include diastematomyelia, hemivertebra, wedge vertebra, unilateral unsegmented bar etc.

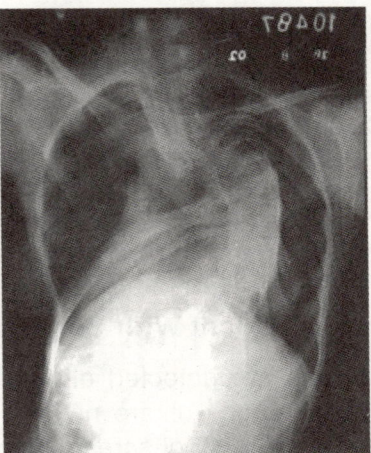

Fig. 16.2. Congenital dorsal scoliosis. Note the congenital rib abnormalities

(c) **Neuromuscular** or paralytic scoliosis is caused by neuropathic causes (such as cerebral palsy, poliomyelitis, syringomyelia, spinal muscular atrophy, Fredrich's ataxia) or myopathic causes (such as arthrogryposis, muscular dystrophy).

(d) **Neurofibromatosis**

(e) **Mesenchymal disorders** such as Marfan's Syndrome and Ehlers-Danlos Syndrome.

(f) **Trauma**

(g) **Metabolic disorders**

(h) **Rare causes** such as bone dysplasias, extraspinal contractures, thoracic surgery, infections, tumors etc.

Pathoanatomy

Scoliosis is characterised by the lateral curvature

of the spine. There is an associated vertebral rotation with the spinous processes of the vertebrae within the curve rotated towards the concavity. The ribs within the curve are also rotated and become prominent on the convex side giving rise to an unsightly hump. The curve showing the rotation of the vertebrae is called the primary curve and it never disappears completely on forward bending or longitudinal traction. Often, to keep the trunk balanced, extra curves develop above and below the primary curve. These are called secondary curves. The secondary curves do not show rotation of the vertebrae and disappear on forward bending/ longitudinal traction. The vertebrae at the either end of the curve whose end plates are first to become horizontal are called the end vertebrae.

There may be an associated alteration of the sagittal plane curvatures, the most common being thoracic hypokyphosis or lordosis. When kyphotic deformity is associated with scoliosis, it is termed kyphoscoliosis. Scoliotic curve at cervico-dorsal and lumbosacral junction are particularly bad as they lead to unsightly cosmetic deformity and pelvic obliquity respectively.

Evaluation of a Patient With Scoliosis

These deformities are detected either incidentally on x-ray in early stages or are noticed by patient or the parents. The school-screening programme for scoliosis practised abroad has considerably improved the early detection of these cases. The important facts to elicit in the history are age, sex, menarche, history of pain, progression and family history of scoliosis.

These patients as asymptomatic and only rarely present with pain. In fact, presence of back pain warrants thorough investigation to rule out other aetiologies (such as infection, osteoid osteoma).

On physical examination, the patient presents with asymmetry in the level of the shoulders and waist crease. Scapula may be prominent on one side and inequality of breasts is present. The iliac crest is higher and more prominent on one side.

A posterior rib hump is present and becomes exaggerated on forward bending. The flexibility of the curve should be assessed by longitudinal traction and asking the patient to bend forwards.

Any paraspinal spasm or mass should be noted and tenderness over the spinous processes should be elicited. Leg length measurements should be taken for any discrepancy. A complete neurological examination should be performed in all cases.

Imaging

The radiographs of the spine (AP views-erect and supine, latter in right and left bending positions and lateral views) establish the extent, severity, rotation of vertebrae, presence of any bony abnormalities and flexibility or correctability of the curve. (Fig. 16.3). Radiographs of the spine also permit

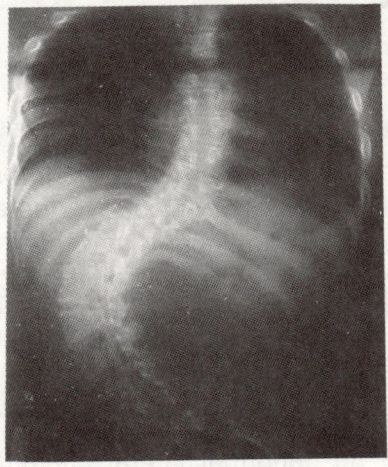

Fig. 16.3.   Right sided idiopathic dorsolumbar scoliosis

measurement of the angle of the curve (Cobb angle is the most often used method) for recording (Fig. 16.4).

Ferguson angle is the other angle measured. Mini Mehta's rib-vertebra angle difference is used to predict the progression of infantile idiopathic

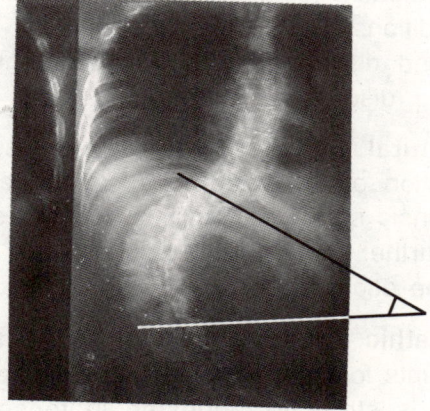

Fig. 16.4.   Measurement of Cobb's angle

scoliosis (a difference of > 20° between the convex and concave sides is significant). Additional x-rays can be taken to establish the skeletal maturity or the skeletal growth remaining. Various methods used for the purpose are pelvis x-ray (Risser sign), ring apophysis of the vertebra and x-ray of the wrist for bone age.

MRI may be indicated when spinal dysraphism, diastematomyelia (Fig. 16.5), infection or tumor is suspected to be the cause of scoliosis.

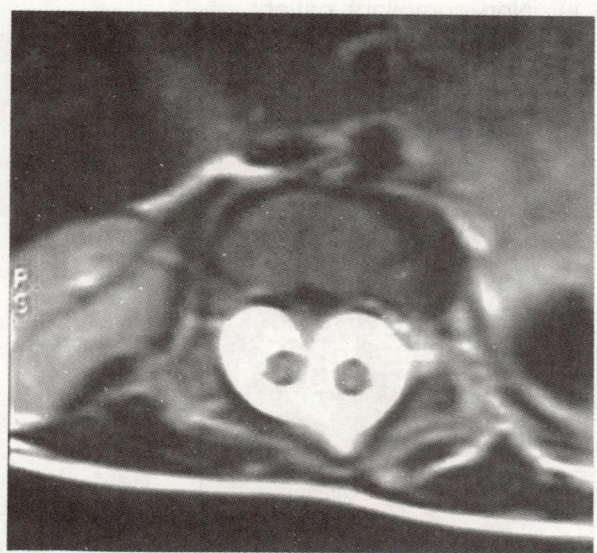

Fig. 16.5.   MRI of a patient with Diastematomyelia showing split cord

Pulmonary Function Test should be performed in all cases with curve measuring more than 60° to document decreased vital capacity seen in these cases.

Prognosis

Scoliosis is a progressive disorder in skeletally immature patients.

1. Younger the age more is the risk of progression.

2. Severity of curve: More severe the angulation and rotation, more is the tendency for progression.

3. Shorter curves progress more than longer curves. Harrington Factor has been calculated to predict the risk of progression depending on degree of curve and number of vertebrae in the curve.

4. Female sex and onset before menarche are associated with more progression.

5. Positive family history has worse prognosis.

6. Higher the curve in the spinal column, greater is the deformity and progression e.g. thoracic curves progress more than lumbar curves.

7. Rigid curves and curves associated with neurofibromatosis and poliomyelitis are associated with worse prognosis.

Treatment

The treatment of scoliosis aims to reduce the progression of curve, correct the curve and maintain the correction. Cosmesis is often the primary concern of the patient. Respiratory function usually does not improve after the surgery but the correction of the severe curve may check the deterioration of the respiratory function. Pain and neurologic problems are unusual and should be thoroughly investigated to rule out any intraspinal pathology. The following treatment modalities are commonly employed for the treatment of scoliosis:

1. Observation   A curve less than 20° in skeletally immature patients and less than 50° in mature patients is observed. Patients are asked to follow up for clinical examination and radiographs every 4–6 months. If a curve in skeletally immature patient shows progression of more than 5°, these children are braced.

2. Exercises are advised as an adjunct for the patients who are under observation or mature patients with less than 30° curve where the surgical treatment is not contemplated. Exercises are particularly useful for patients with obesity, back pain and exaggerated lumbar lordosis. Postural exercises, lateral bending and pelvic muscles exercises are commonly prescribed.

3. Orthosis A curve more than 30° (but less than 45°) at the initial visit or more than 25° with documented progression in an immature patient is an indication for the brace treatment. The goal of brace treatment is to prevent progression of the curve. The spinal orthosis or brace is contoured to provide a corrective force to the spine while the child grows. Hence, the curve should be flexible and more than one year of skeletal growth should be remaining before the brace treatment can be instituted. Braces are not very effective for cervicothoracic curves. The following types of braces are commonly used:

a) *Milwaukee brace* or Cervico-Thoraco-Lumbo-Sacral Orthosis (CTLSO) is used for dorsal curves. It has adjustable supports made of steel and is distracted periodically (Fig. 16.6a-d). It has a chin support which can cause deformation of teeth and malocclusion. Hence careful supervision and orthodontic care is required. CTLSO is used in curves above D_9 vertebra.

b) *Boston brace* or Thoraco-Lumbo-Sacral Orthosis (TLSO) is used for thoraco-lumbar or lumbar curves. This type of brace has polypropylene shell, which is contoured to provide corrective force to the spine. It does not have the chin support. TLSO is used in curves below D_9 vertebra.

The braces are worn 23 hours a day till skeletal maturity and then are weaned off.

Contraindications to brace treatment are:

i) Curve more than 40°

ii) Non compliant patient

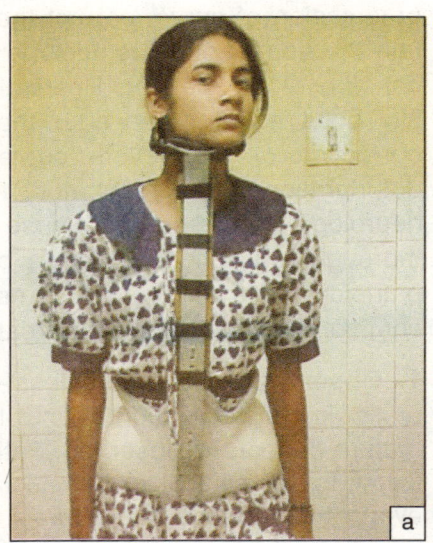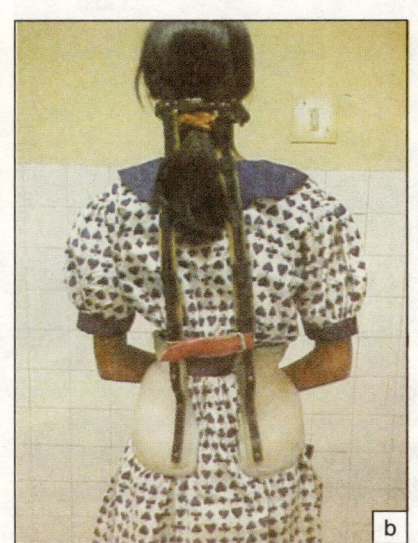

Fig. 16.6a,b.   Scoliosis patient treated with a Milwaukee brace

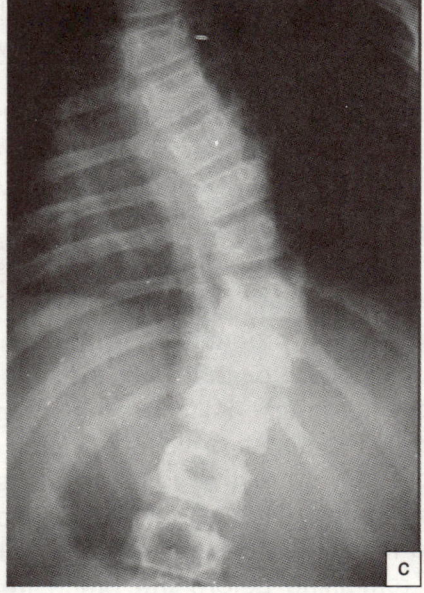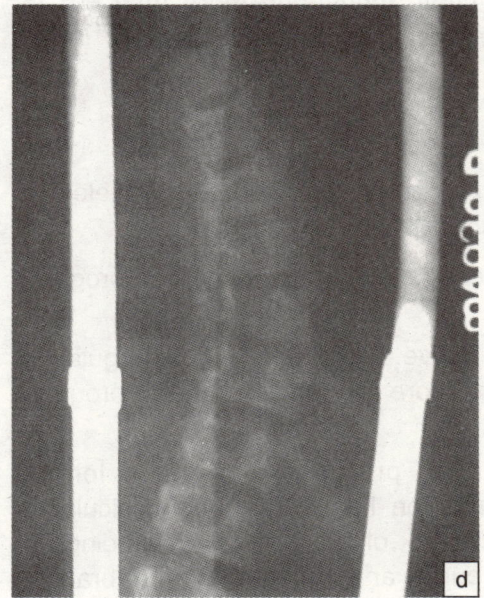

Fig. 16.6c,d.   Pre and post treatment X-rays following use of Milwaukee brace

iii) Thoracic lordosis; and,

iv) Less than one year of growth remaining.

Considerable guidance, direction and emotional support is required to the patient and family to ensure compliance with brace treatment.

4. Plaster

Localiser casts are applied on special tables where head and pelvic traction reduce the curve. POP jacket is applied to maintain the correction.

Alternatively, hinged casts are applied with turn-buckle, which allows gradual correction of the deformity.

5. Electrical treatment

Electrical stimulation of paraspinal muscles has been described to correct the scoliotic curve but has been shown to be less effective than brace treatment.

6. Halo-Pelvic traction

Halo-Pelvic traction is effected through adjustable steel rods fixed to the pelvis through a hoop with pins passing through the ilium and to skull using halo ring. Gradual distraction of these steel rods gradually corrects the curve (Fig. 16.7).

7. Operative treatment

Operative treatment is indicated for thoracic curves more than 40°, progressive curves and curves which fail the brace treatment. Curves, which are not cosmetically deforming especially when congenital, can be fused in situ when they show progression. Usually a posterior spinal fusion is done but when the posterior elements are deficient, anterior fusion using a rib graft can be done. The extent of fusion is decided by extent of the curve and must include neutral or non-rotated vertebrae on either end of the curve. Surgical stabilisation often has to be supplemented with corrective instrumentation.

Various anterior (Zielke, Dwyer) and posterior (Harrington, Luque, CD, Hartshill, Moss Miami) instrumentation systems are available to correct the scoliotic curves (Fig. 16.8a,b). The newer instrumentation systems provide segmental fixation, which is more secure and derotate the curve to provide improved cosmetic results.

Kyphosis

Kyphosis is a deformity in sagittal plane, which is convex posteriorly.

Types of Kyphosis Thoracic spine has a normal kyphosis but a curve measuring more than 50° is pathological. *Any* kyphosis in thoracolumbar junction or lumbar spine is abnormal. A sharp *angular* kyphosis is caused by the involvement of one or

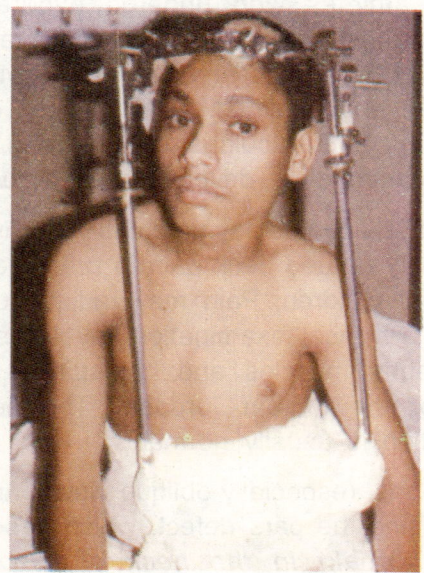

Fig. 16.7. Halo-Pelvic traction for the correction of spinal deformities

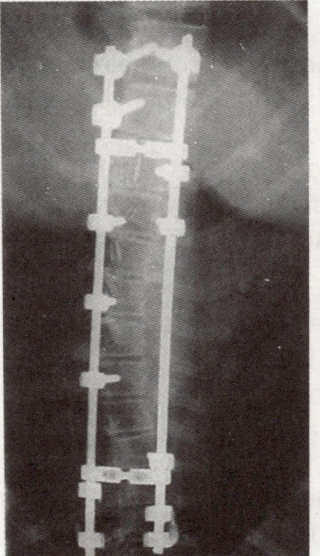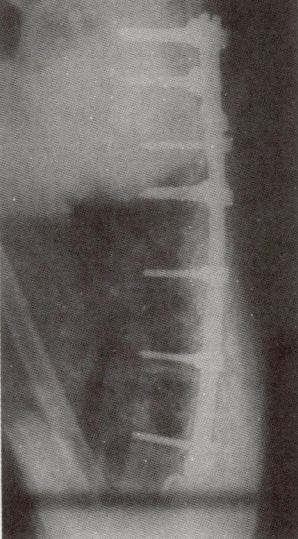

Fig. 16.8a,b. Moss Miami instrumentation for Scoliosis correction

two vertebrae and is often the result of trauma (compression fracture), tuberculosis, congenital malformation, post surgical and Calve's disease. Tuberculosis and neurofibromatosis can sometimes give rise to somewhat rounded *gibbus* deformity. A more generalised kyphosis (*roundback*) involving long segment of spine is generally due to faulty posture, ankylosing spondylitis, Scheurmann's disease, metabolic disorders (e.g. senile osteoporosis–*Dowager's hump*) and Paget's disease.

Most curves are treated by observation and extension exercises. Braces can be used in skeletally immature patients. However, severe curves or curves with refractory pain are treated with posterior spinal fusion with or without anterior decompression.

Adolescent Kyphosis (Scheurmann's Disease)

Adolescent kyphosis, also called Scheurmann's disease, is thought to be secondary to repetitive trauma and stress fracture of the anterior aspect of vertebral bodies in the growing adolescents. Genetic factors are also implicated, as sometimes the disease tends to be familial. Collagen weakness, stunted ossification of the vertebral end plates, osteopenia, nutrition and endocrine factors are also implicated. Adolescent kyphosis can occur in thoracic spine (most common) or thoracolumbar or lumbar spine.

Clinically, the patient presents in early adolescence (between 12–14 years of age) with thoracic or lumbar back pain. The pain is usually aggravated by prolonged standing or activity and is relieved by rest. Examination reveals an increased thoracic kyphosis or abnormal flattening of the normal lumbar lordosis (when the disease affects lumbar spine). There may be local tenderness. The paraspinal muscles and hamstrings are in spasm and often contracted. The neurological examination is normal.

Plain radiographs (lateral radiographs with patient standing) reveal an increase in the kyphosis at least 5° in three or more consecutive vertebral bodies with associated anterior wedging of the vertebral bodies. X-rays taken in hyperextension help in assessing the rigidity of the curve. Other findings on x-rays are irregularity of end plates, narrowing of intervertebral disc space and herniation of disc material into the weakly ossified vertebral end plate called Schmorl's nodes.

Differential diagnosis of Scheurmann's disease includes postural kyphosis (flexible, no radiological changes), spondylitis (infective or inflammatory), trauma, congenital kyphosis and tumors.

Treatment of mild deformities with minimal symptoms is observation. Active physical therapy program is initiated in all cases. Brace treatment is recommended if the curve is more than 45° but less than 65°, vertebral wedging measures more than 5° and there is at least 1 year of growth remaining. Milwaukee brace (CTLSO) is given if the apex of the deformity is at or above D_9 while underarm brace (TLSO) is given for curves with a more caudad apex.

Surgery is indicated for severe curves (>70° with >10° wedging), painful curves, curves which are refractory to bracing for more than 6 months, and curves with neurologic signs or symptoms. A posterior spinal fusion with or without instrumentation is performed. Severe rigid curves often need combined anterior and posterior fusion and instrumentation.

Spondylolysis and Spondylolisthesis

Spondylolysis implies a break in the pars interarticularis resulting in the loss of bony continuity between the superior and inferior articular processes. Condition occurs most commonly at L_5 vertebra. Spondylolysis is believed to be the results of non-union of stress fracture. Spondylolysis is commonly seen in athletes who undergo hyperextension stress activities (gymnasts, football linemen). There is also high incidence among soldiers with heavy backpacks and Eskimos. Other causes of defect in the pars interarticularis are infection, trauma, tumor, congenital or developmental defects.

Spondylolysis can be asymptomatic or may present with activity related back pain in preadolescent or adolescent children. Pain may radiate to buttock or thigh. Physical examination reveals spasm in paravertebral muscles and hamstrings and flattening of the lumbar lordosis. The neurologic examination is usually normal.

Radiographs, (especially oblique views) are helpful in visualising the pars defect, which is seen as a *"Collar" (break) in the neck of "Scotty dog"* (Fig. 16.9). Bone scan is extremely useful investigation for screening in a child with back pain before the plain radiographs show the bone

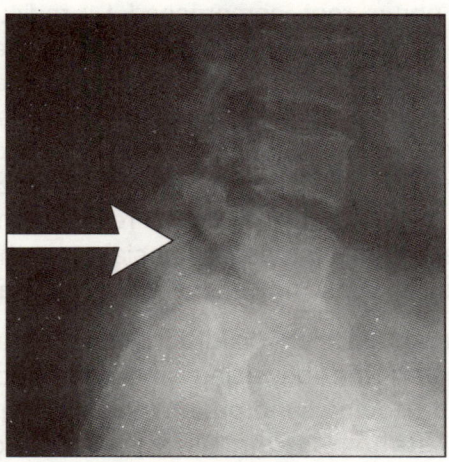

Fig. 16.9. Spondylolysis L_5–S_1 showing break in pars interarticularis (Arrow)

defect. CT Scan can help in identifying the pars defect.

Treatment of spondylolysis is restriction of activities (especially hyperextension), stretching, abdominal strengthening and spinal flexion exercises and bracing for severely symptomatic patients. Severe unrelenting pain may need L_5–S_1 fusion rarely.

Spondylolisthesis implies an anterior displacement of the vertebral column on a lower vertebra resulting from spondylolysis, articular process malformation or elongation of the pars interarticularis. The condition is seen most commonly as anterior slippage of L_5 vertebra over S_1. Spondylolisthesis is classified, depending on aetiology, into dysplastic, isthmic, degenerative, traumatic and pathologic. The severity of slip is graded according to the percentage of the superior anteroposterior extent of the vertebra below by which the vertebral column has slipped forward; Grade I is 0--25% slip, Grade II is 25–50% slip, Grade III is 50–75% slip, Grade IV is 75–100% slip while Grade V is >100% i.e. spondyloptosis when the vertebra above slips completely and comes to lie in front of the vertebral body below.

Spondylolisthesis occurs commonly around the adolescent spurt and progression occurs during 10–15 years of age (degenerative and pathologic varieties present late). Patients may be asymptomatic but low back pain or L_5 radiculopathy may develop. A prolapsed intervertebral disc is commonly seen one level above the listhesis. Examination reveals restricted forward flexion of hips and back, hamstring tightness, flat buttocks (due to vertical sa]crum)

and lumbosacral kyphosis with compensatory hyper-lordosis of lumbar spine. A pelvic waddle gait may be seen. Palpation of lumbosacral junction may reveal a step and an attempt to press spinous process from side to side elicits pain (due to loose lamina). Female patients may present with obstetric problems due to reduced anteroposterior dimensions of the pelvis.

Radiographs reveal the characteristic "*Beheaded Scottish Terrier* "sign.

Treatment The goals of treatment are pain relief, return to activity and prevention of deformity. Grade I & II slips are treated with observation especially if they are asymptomatic. Symptomatic Grade I & II slips are treated by restriction of activities, brace and physical therapy. Surgical treatment is required when patient is unresponsive to conservative treatment, shows progression of slip (especially in skeletally immature patient), when the patient has neurological deficit or when a severe degree of spondylolisthesis exists. Surgical treatment consists of in-situ posterolateral fusion (from tip of transverse process to alae of sacrum-Transalar fusion) from L_4 to S_1. Decompressive procedures, such as laminectomy (for radiculopathy or cauda equina), or Gill's procedure (removal of loose lamina) are required for neurological deficit. Gill's procedure (operculectomy) alone is contra-indicated in children as it can lead to rapid worsening of the slip. Decompression in adults is combined with posterolateral fusion or pedicular screws and segmental fixation (Fig. 16.10a,b). The availability

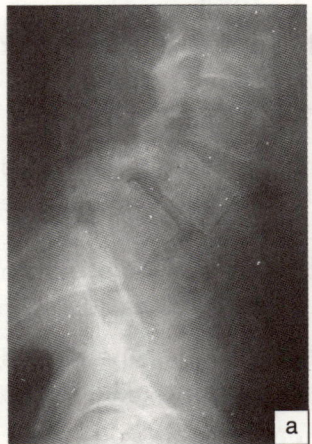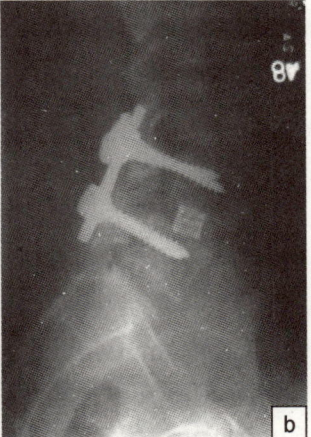

Fig.16.10a,b. Spondylolisthesis L_4–L_5 treated by decompression, segmental fixation and spinal fusion using cage (a) preoperative (b) postoperative x-rays

of modern instrumentation has made it possible even to reduce the slip and fix it in the reduced position. Surgical fusion should always be combined in these cases to control pain and progression.

Degenerative conditions

Lumbar Disc Disease

1. Herniated Nucleus Pulposus

Displacement of the nucleus pulposus resulting in impingement of a nerve root is most common at L_4–L_5 level followed closely by L_5–S_1 level.

Types of herniation are:

Protrusion   annulus tear but posterior longitudinal ligament (PLL) is intact.

Extrusion   Tear of PLL with herniation of disc through it but herniated portion remains attached to the parent disc.

Sequestration   Complete displacement with free disc fragment in the spinal canal.

Pathology The mean age of patients with prolapsed disc is 35 years and the disease is uncommon below 20 and after 60 years of age. It is seen more commonly in certain occupations involving lifting heavy objects and vibration, certain sports such as diving from a board and driving certain motor vehicles. Other causes, which predispose to herniated disc, are cigarette smoking, sedentary life style and anxiety and depression.

Disc herniations follow tear of annulus fibrosus and classically occur posterolaterally with impingement of nerve below (L_5 root in L_4–L_5 disc prolapse, S_1 in L_5–S_1 prolapse). Central herniations cause back pain without radiculopathy or cauda equina syndrome (12%).

Following disc herniation, facet joints get involved and synovitis, cartilage destruction, osteophyte formation, capsular laxity and subluxation occur. Spinal stenosis may occur following disc degeneration due to facet joint subluxation and hypertrophy.

Cysts or tumors such as synovial cyst, perineural cyst or neurofibroma may mimic a herniated disc.

Evaluation of a Patient with Intervertebral Disc Prolapse

Clinically the patient presents with low back pain radiating to leg (along a dermatome depending on the nerve root compressed–L_5 radiculopathy causes pain down the back of thigh to the lateral calf and anterior foot while S_1 radiculopathy results in pain over posterior calf and sole of the foot). The leg pain is more than the back pain. Pain is worse with sitting, coughing, sneezing and forward bending. Lying down relieves the pain. Numbness, tingling, paraesthesiae or other neurologic symptoms may accompany the pain.

Bowel and bladder disturbances are rare and should alert the physician about the possibility of a cauda equina syndrome. While eliciting history, mental status, drug history and industrial or medicolegal status must be accurately determined.

Examination reveals muscle spasm and a list or bend. Spinal movements, especially flexion are reduced. The straight leg raising (SLR) test is usually positive in lower lumbar disc herniations. Contralateral (or crossed) SLR (pain on the affected side while raising the opposite leg) is pathognomonic of prolapsed large central disc with root impingement. Flip test, i.e. positive SLR while lying down but negative SLR on sitting suggests malingering. Reverse SLR (Femoral stretch test), elicited in prone position, suggests L_3 or L_4 nerve root involvement.

Depending on nerve root involved, various combinations of weakness may be encountered such as inability to walk on heels in L_4–L_5 protrusion and inability to walk on toes in L_5–S_1 herniation. Specifically, tibialis anterior weakness occurs in L_4 root compression while extensor hallucis longus weakness occurs in L_5 nerve root compression. Sensory disturbances are common in the affected dermatome. Reflex loss may occur in L_4 radioculopathy (knee jerk) and S_1 radiculopathy (ankle jerk).

Pain drawing and MMPI (Minnesota Multiphasic Personality Inventory) should be done in patients with chronic low back pain.

Investigations for prolapsed intervertebral disc prolapse should be deferred until 6-8 weeks after initial conservative treatment. Plain x-rays are not useful as discs are not visualised on plain x-rays but serve to rule out spondylolisthesis, tumor, infection and spondylosis.

The MRI has become the gold standard for visualising the cord, dura, nerve roots and disc but has high false–positive rate. Any findings on MRI should be correlated with the history and examination.

CT scan is useful for herniated disc and stenosis and can be combined with myelogram for additional information. MRI, however, has replaced most imaging modalities like myelographs, CT, etc. for prolapsed disc (Fig. 16.11a.b).

Discography is rarely useful except to confirm the disc as the cause of symptoms in patients without radiculopathy.

Bone scan can help to rule out tumor, infection or spondylolysis.

Electrodiagnostic studies can be useful to rule out other neurologic disorders and if there is lack of clinical correlation.

Injection of facets, root sleeves or epidural space can help in diagnosis of cause of pain and temporary pain relief.

Differential Diagnosis

Pain due to prolapsed intervertebral disc should be differentiated from viscerogenic pain (due to kidney, uterus or prostate problems), vascular pain (aortic aneurysm), neurogenic (spinal cord tumors or cysts), psychogenic, or spondylogenic (tumors, osteoporotic compression fractures, tuberculosis, ankylosing spondylitis etc.).

Treatment

Most patients' symptoms resolve with time.

Conservative treatment consists of short duration of bed rest, NSAIDs, and physical therapy and is successful in 80–90% patients. Modalities such as local heat, ultrasound, massage, Transcutaneous electrical nerve stimulation (TENS) and electrical stimulation make the patient subjectively feel better though they are not scientifically proven.

Once the acute symptoms subside patient is subjected to gradual increase in mobilisation, advised correct posture and back stabilising (extension) exercises.

Invasive treatment such as epidural steroids are rarely useful (used for refractory leg pain) while chemonucleolysis in not popular because of the complications of anaphylaxis and neurological complications.

Surgery is indicated for failure of conservative treatment, radicular pain or neurologic deficit, positive nerve root tension signs and any positive imaging studies that correlate with symptoms. Frequent recurrences which interfere with patient's ability to work also indicate need for surgical treatment. Functional overlay must be ruled out before surgery.

Laminotomy and discectomy without fusion is the procedure of choice. Microdiscectomy, and Laser assisted surgery are minimally invasive and are associated with quick recovery. However, associated pathologies such as sequestered disc, facet impingement and foraminal stenosis are often missed.

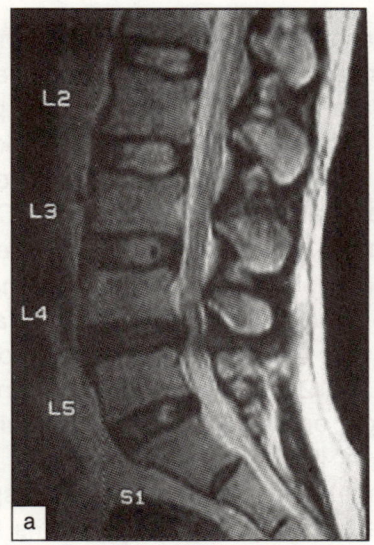 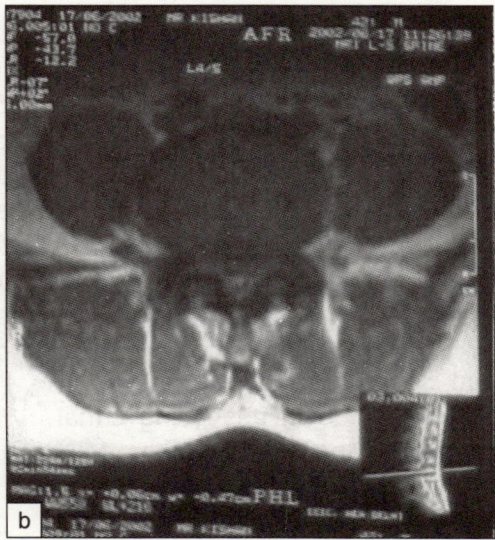

Fig. 16.11a,b. MRI showing prolapsed intervertebral disc between L_4 and L_5 (a) sagittal (b) axial cut

Recently endoscopic discectomy techniques have been developed for removal of prolapsed disc.

2. Spinal Stenosis

Spinal stenosis is defined as narrowing of the spinal canal (central stenosis) or lateral recess (lateral stenosis) with neural impingement that produces symptoms of radiculopathy. Central stenosis can be congenital (as in achondroplasia) or acquired (more common). The narrowing of the central canal is due to facet joint hypertrophy or hypertrophy of the supporting soft tissues. Acquired stenosis is usually due to degenerative changes as mentioned above, due to degenerative spondylolisthesis or due to combination of these two. Other causes of stenosis are iatrogenic (following spinal fusion, laminectomy or disc surgery), post traumatic, fluorosis and Paget's disease.

Spinal stenosis is an ageing process and therefore, is significant only if it is clinically symptomatic. It is more common after the fifth decade.

Clinically the symptoms of spinal stenosis are insidious pain, typically in lower back, buttock and the lower extremities and associated paraesthesiae. Pain is worse with standing, hyperextension and walking but is relieved by rest, sitting and forward flexion. Neurogenic claudication is seen in about 50% patients and should be differentiated from vascular claudication. Neurogenic claudication is not relieved just by standing and patient has to sit or lie down to get relief. Also, it takes longer time to abate as compared to vascular claudication. The peripheral pulses are palpable in neurogenic claudication.

Physical examination reveals paucity of objective findings; spinal movements are good; sciatic tension signs are absent and neurologic deficit may or may not be present. Sometimes it is a good idea to make the patient walk for a while and examine again when neurologic deficit may become apparent.

Investigations

Plain x-rays reveal spondylosis. CT scan is an extremely useful investigation in assessing canal dimensions, particularly of the lateral recess. MRI is becoming more useful but it does not delineate bony details as well as the CT Scan. Myelography shows hourglass constriction or complete block and root impingement but is rarely performed present day due to the availability of non-invasive investigations.

Treatment is non-operative in most cases and consists of rest, exercises, NSAIDs, lumbosacral corset and epidural steroids. Conservative treatment is not usually helpful in severe cases.

Operative indications are significant symptoms compromising the quality of life. Decompression with or without fusion is the treatment of choice. Lateral recess stenosis needs removal of overgrown superior facet by undercutting. If the nerve root is tight after laminectomy and facet undercutting, it may be compressed between superior facet and posterior vertebral body, between superior facet and pedicle, superior facet or pedicle against bulging lateral annulus, inferior facet and vertebral body (in degenerative spondylolisthesis) or between transverse process of L_5 and sacral ala (extraforaminal lateral root compression – *FAR-OUT SYNDROME*).

3. Facet Syndrome

Facet syndrome occurs due to inflammation or degeneration of the facet joints. Patients are usually elderly, over 50 years of age and present with lower back pain, which becomes worse with hyperextension. Patient sometimes may have referred pain to buttock and posterior thigh. There may be tenderness in paraspinal area. Facet joints injections confirm the diagnosis and are also therapeutic.

4. Lumbar Spondylosis (Osteoarthritis of spine)

Lumbar spondylosis implies degenerative changes in lumbar spine. These patients are usually over 50 years of age. They commonly present with low back pain referred to the buttocks and posterior thigh. Morning stiffness is common. Pain is usually aggravated by extension. On examination, the range of motion of spine is restricted. Neurologic examination is usually normal. Radiographs show severe degeneration of facet joints and discs and may suggest associated spinal stenosis (Fig. 16.12). MRI is indicated only if neurologic findings or symptoms are associated. Investigations in lumbar spondylosis are needed to rule out more serious spinal or extraspinal causes as the cause for patient's symptoms before ascribing them to osteoarthritis of spine.

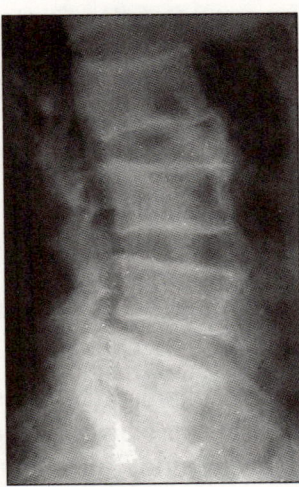

Fig. 16.12. Lateral lumbar spine X-rays showing extensive spondylotic changes with lumbar canal stenosis

Treatment includes local heat, NSAIDs and lumbar corset. Modification of daily activities to avoid aggravation should be emphasised. Exercises and hydrotherapy are quite helpful. Patient education can help the patient to understand and live with the disease.

Surgery is rarely indicated except in cases of concomitant stenosis or associated neurological deficit.

Inflammatry Disorders of Spine

Infective

1. Tubercular Spondylitis

Spine is the most commonly affected part of skeleton with tuberculosis and accounts for more than 50% cases of osteoarticular tuberculosis. Infection of spine is always secondary to a focus elsewhere and the spread is via blood. Infection of the lumbar spine most often occurs from a focus in genitourinary tract via Batson's venous plexus. The infection, travelling via the hematogenous route, involves the adjacent end plates of two vertebral bodies with disc between them. The anterior part of the vertebral bodies is affected first and the paradiscal disease soon compromises the nutrition of the disc (which derives its nutrition by diffusion from the adjacent end plates) and results in diminished intervertebral disc space. The posterior elements are rarely involved in tuberculosis.

The disease occurs most commonly in dorsolumbar spine. When it involves the dorsal spine, destruction of anterior part of vertebral bodies along with the normal kyphosis of dorsal spine gives rise to unsightly kyphotic deformity. Copious suppuration occurs following tuberculous infection and a cold abscess may be the only presenting symptom without any radiologically demonstrable lesion. Pus can be limited around the spinal column (paraspinal abscess) or can track along the spinal nerves or along the various fascial planes to chest, pelvis, inguinal region, thigh or buttock.

Tubercular infection can sometimes involve more than one area of spine with normal vertebrae in between. Such skip lesions are reported in 7% cases.

The pus, granulation tissue, sequestrae, sequestrated disc or thrombosis of arteries can result in neurological deficit (Pott's paraplegia) early in the course of the disease. This type of paraplegia (occurring within one year of onset) is called *Early onset paraplegia. Late onset paraplegia* occurs later (after more than one year) either due to reactivation of a previously healed disease or due to mechanical factors (internal gibbus, instability etc.). Causes of Pott's paraplegia are shown in Table 16.1.

Table 16.1. Causes of Pott's Paraplegia

Early Onset (less than one year)	Late Onset (more than one year)
1. Inflammatory Oedema	1. Reactivation of Disease
2. Cold Abscess	2. Internal Gibbus (stretching of cord)
3. Tubercular Granulation Tissue	3. Myelomalacia
4. Tubercular Debris	4. Constrictive Scarring Around Cord
5. Coke Sequestra	5. Anterior Transverse Bony Ridge
6. Pathological Subluxation/Dislocation	
7. Tubercular Meningitis/Arachnoiditis	
8. Infective Thrombosis/Endarteritis of spinal vessels	

Healing of tubercular spondylitis occurs by bony ankylosis between the affected vertebrae. (Note: Spine and short long bones of hands and feet are the only sites where healing of the tubercular lesions occurs by new bone formation).

The paraspinal abscess may resolve completely or may undergo fibrosis or calcification and may persist on radiographs without suggesting residual disease.

Residual kyphotic deformity after disease has healed may progress relentlessly in growing children and surgical intervention is needed to check the progression (Fig. 16.13a-d).

Evaluation of a Patient with Pott's Paraplegia

Clinically the patients present with insidious onset of pain and constitutional symptoms. Pain increases progressively and is aggravated by spinal movements. Anorexia, loss of weight and night sweats may be present. An abscess may sometimes be the presenting symptom.

Examination reveals marked restriction of spinal movements and painful muscle spasm. Angular kyphosis is often appreciable and is tender on palpation. One must palpate for cold abscess in groin, thigh, buttock and chest wall.

Detailed neurologic examination must be done is all cases. Earliest neurological deficit occurs in the form of spasticity and gait abnormality. Weakness of muscles subsequently may make walking difficult. Sphincteric control is lost with further progression of neurological deficit. Further progression of spinal compression leads to flaccid

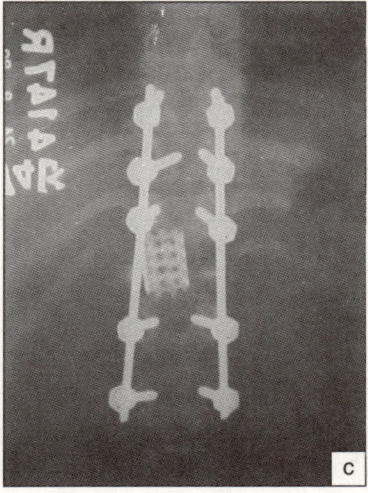

Fig. 16.13a.　Residual kyphotic deformity following healed Pott's spine

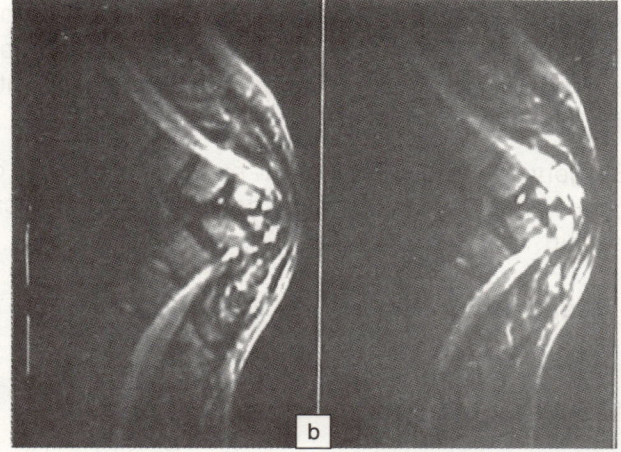

Fig. 16.13b.　MRI of the same patient showing stretching of the cord.

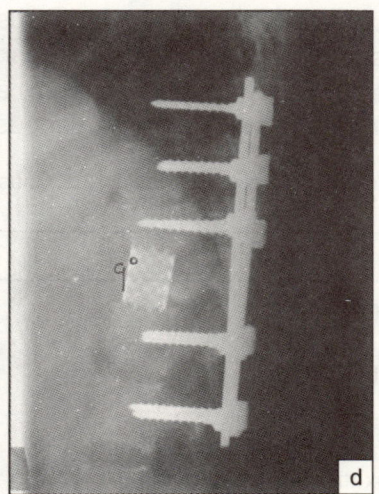

Fig. 16.13c,d. X-rays following surgical correction of the deformity, posterior instrumentation and cage fixation

paraplegia. Sensory deficit can occur though it occurs late.

Radiologically, plain radiographs reveal loss of intervertebral disc space, irregular destruction of adjacent vertebral bodies, generalised osteoporosis, destruction and collapse of vertebral bodies with resultant kyphosis and paravertebral soft tissue shadow (Fig. 16.13e,f).

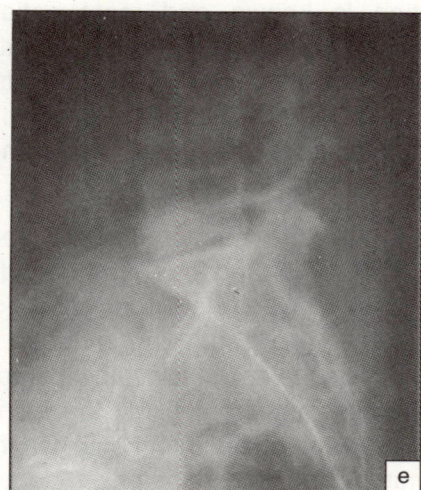

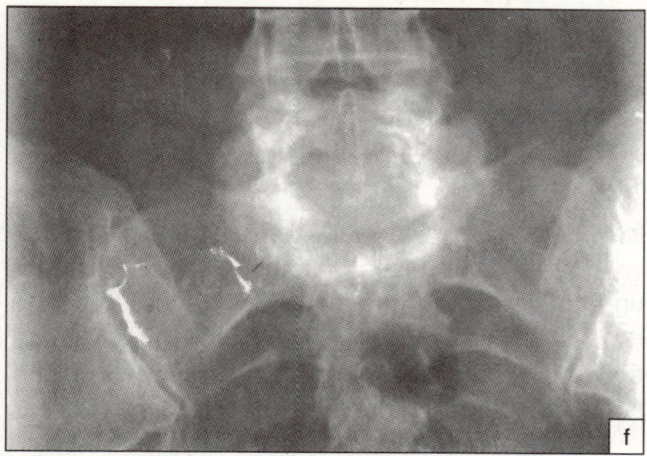

Fig. 16.13e,f. Tuberculosis L_5–S_1. Note the disc space narrowing

Erythrocyte Sedimentation Rate is elevated. It is rarely possible to isolate AFB from the pus aspirate. MRI is extremely useful to assess the status of spinal cord and to evaluate severity and the extent of spinal cord compression (Fig. 16.13g,h). It can also help to pick up skip lesions and rule out trauma or tumors as the cause of paraplegia. Infective nature of the pathology can be further confirmed by performing

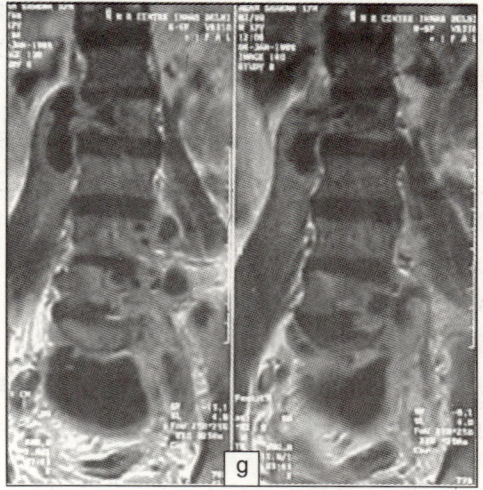

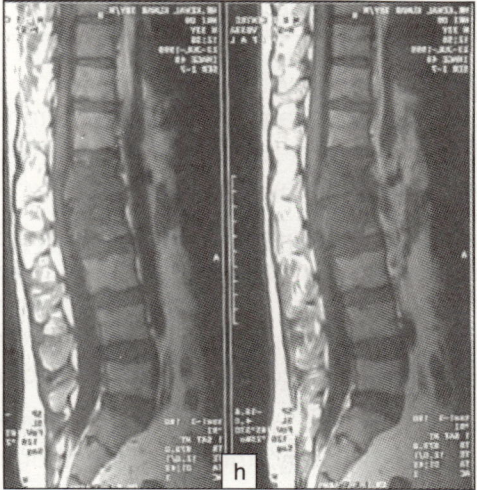

Fig. 16.13g,h. MRI picture of Pott's spine L_1–L_2 showing destruction of vertebral bodies and soft tissue shadow

contrast (gadolinium) enhanced MRI, which shows rim enhancement in tuberculosis and diffuse enhancement in pyogenic lesions.

Treatment of tubercular spine without neurological deficit consists of administration of antitubercular drugs and spinal support or rest if the pain is severe. The abscess is initially kept under observation as most abscesses resolve with 6 weeks of antitubercular treatment. However, pointing or rapidly enlarging abscess despite treatment needs to be drained surgically.

Treatment of Pott's spine with early onset paraplegia consists of antitubercular treatment along with close observation. If, however, patient does not improve with 4–6 weeks of conservative treatment, if paraplegia occurs or worsens while on treatment, if sphincters are involved, if paraplegia is painful or if paraplegia occurs in elderly, the surgical treatment is indicated (Table 16.2).

Table 16.2. Indications for surgical treatment in Pott's Spine

– Failure of conservative treatment for 6 weeks
– Worsening neurologic deficit on ATT
– Fresh neurologic deficit on ATT
– Painful paraplegia, paraplegia in elderly
– Late onset paraplegia due to instability of spine
– Respiratory difficulty due to progressive kyphotic deformity(>70°)
– Tubercular abscess causing dyspnea/dysphagia (retropharyngeal abscess)

Costo-transversectomy where head, neck and a part of posterior rib is removed along with transverse process of the affected vertebra is sufficient to drain the pus and relieve compression in children.

Anterolateral decompression is an extrapleural retroperitoneal approach to spine wherein anterolateral part of body, pedicle, transverse process and posterior part of rib (up to the angle) are excised and the cord is decompressed.

Anterior decompression involves anterior approach to the vertebral body through transthoracic or transabdominal route to curette out diseased bone and granulation tissue. Bone grafts are often used to fill up the bony defect.

Treatment of Pott's spine with late onset paraplegia needs comprehensive investigation including MRI. While the cases with gliosis or atrophy of cord are associated with poor prognosis, attempt can be made to relieve compression on the cord caused by the internal gibbus. Those cases where late onset paraplegia is due to recrudescence of the disease, antitubercular drugs can suffice to aid complete recovery.

2. Disc Space Infection (Pyogenic discitis)

Discitis occurs usually in young adults and invariably follows an invasive procedure (discectomy, lumbar puncture etc). Clinically, patient presents with severe back pain, tenderness and spasm and is prostrated.

Laboratory investigations reveal leucocytosis, raised ESR and positive technetium bone scan. MRI is diagnostic.

Treatment consists of rest, immobilisation and antibiotics. Healing is with bony ankylosis.

Non Infective Inflammatory Spondylitis

Ankylosing Spondylitis (Marie-Strumpell disease, Bechterew's disease) is a disease of unknown aetiology involving sacroiliac joints and spine. Genetic predisposition is known and most patients are HLA B-27 positive. It is an enthesopathy and inflammatory joint disease of synovial joints, which develop bony ankylosis. Hips are involved in 50% cases and 50% cases of hip involvement are bilateral.

Clinically the disease has predilection for males (M:F ratio is 9:1) in 2nd and 3rd decades. The disease presents with insidious onset of back pain along with marked morning stiffness. Though the disease affects the entire spine, the thoracolumbar spine is often the first region of the spine to be involved. Recurrent chest infections can be seen due to limited chest expansion. Iridocyclitis is seen in some cases.

Examination reveals marked stiffness of lumbar and, if involved, cervical spine movements. Chest expansion and forward flexion are reduced. Patient often has a kyphotic deformity affecting whole spine.

Schrober's test Normally on bending forwards, two fingers (one placed at the level of posterior superior iliac spine and the other 10 cm above the first) move apart at least 15 cm (so the distance between them becomes 25 cm). In ankylosing spondylitis this is markedly reduced.

Radiological examination reveals haziness of articular margins, erosions and sclerosis on either side of the sacroiliac joints. The spine looks like bamboo (*"bamboo spine"* due to ossification of ligaments with discs looking as nodes and vertebral bodies as internodes) (Fig. 16.14a,b). There is calcification of sacrotuberous and sacrospinous ligaments and also at the insertion of tendo-achilles and plantar fascia on the calcaneus. Hips may show reduced joint space or ankylosis on radiographs (Table 16.3).

Complications There is a higher incidence of

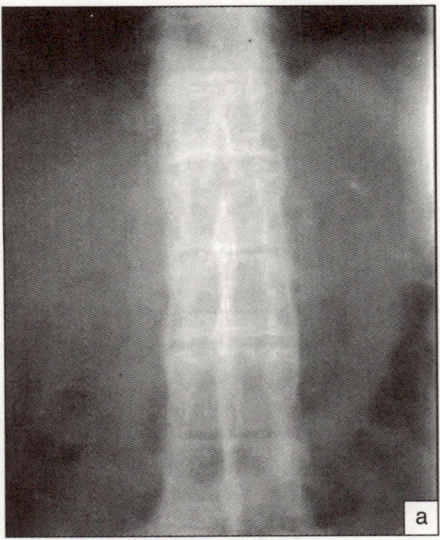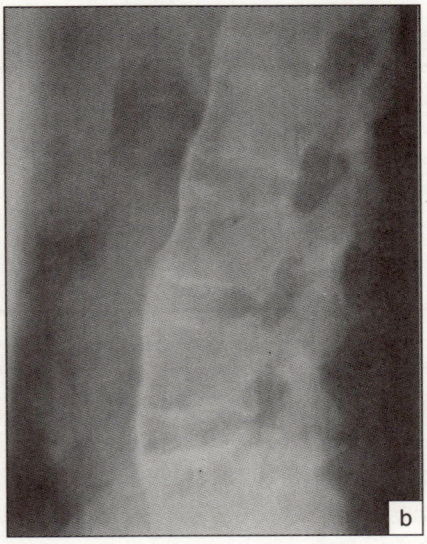

Fig. 16.14. (a) AP and (b) Lateral view x-rays of spine with Ankylosing spondylitis

tuberculosis, both pulmonary and extrapulmonary, in these cases. There is severe locomotor disability due to ankylosis of the hips as well as the spine.

Table 16.3. Radiologic features of Ankylosing Spondylitis

- Shiny corner sign
- Squaring of vertebra (due to calcification of ALL)
- Progressive kyphosis
- Ossification of ALL, interspinous, supraspinous ligaments–*Bamboo spine*
- Syndesmophyte formation (bone formed at right angle to the vertebral body)
- Anderson's lesion: Pseudarthrosis of spine (radiolucent lesion extending from vertebral body through the posterior elements)
- Bilateral sacroilitis : fusion of the sacroiliac joints eventually
- Concentric narrowing/obliteration of hip joint space
- Enthesopathy: bone formation at soft tissue attachments on bone (whiskering of ischial tuberosities, calcaneal spurs)

Sometimes stress fractures develop in completely ankylosed spine due to repetitive cyclic stresses (*"Pseudarthrosis"* or *Anderson lesion*). It is important to differentiate this lesion from tuberculosis. It is treated by orthotic support and if the problem persists, the spinal instrumentation and posterior fusion may have to be undertaken.

Treatment of ankylosing spondylitis is NSAIDs, physical therapy and hydrotherapy to relieve pain. Yoga can help a lot of patients to regain movements and control pain. Radiotherapy to relieve pain and control disease has been abandoned due to the risk of radiation injury to gonads and development of radiation induced leukaemia. Patients should be educated about the disease and its natural history. Regular exercises are recommended to preserve movements and prevent deformities. Patients with severe flexion deformity should have evaluation of hips. If the hips are involved, they should be replaced first. However, if the patient still has severe flexion deformity of spine, spinal osteotomy should be done below the L_2 level to correct the dorsal/dorsolumbar spine deformity.

Relevant Anatomy

Hip is a ball and socket joint, like shoulder, that attaches to the body axis through a bony girdle.

Osteology

Acetabulum is formed superiorly by ilium, posteroinferiorly by ischium and anteroinferiorly by pubis. The surface of acetabulum is composed of an incomplete ring of hyaline cartilage that surrounds the central acetabular fossa. The acetabular fossa merges with the acetabular notch inferiorly. A transverse acetabular ligament completes the acetabulum inferiorly. Acetabular labrum is a fibrocartilaginous inferior extension of the walls of acetabulum which deepens the acetabulum and provides increased coverage of femoral head. *Proximal femur* consists of femoral head, which articulates with the acetabulum, femoral neck and greater and lesser trochanters. The neck of femur forms an angle of nearly 135° with the femoral shaft in frontal plane and 15° in sagittal plane (angle of anteversion).

Joint Hip joint is a ball and socket joint and allows flexion, extension, abduction, adduction, external rotation and internal rotation. The hip joint capsule attaches to acetabular rim and inserts on intertrochanteric line anteriorly and on the distal aspect of the femoral neck one finger breadth above the intertrochanteric crest posteriorly. The capsule is composed of three distinct ligaments. Iliofemoral (or Y ligament of Bigelow) is the main capsular restraint to extension and internal rotation. It is the strongest ligament in the body. Other ligaments are pubofemoral and ischiofemoral. Ligamentum teres extends from acetabular notch and transverse ligament to fovea of femur. The synovial membrane lines the capsule completely. Entire femoral head and most of the neck are intrasynovial.

Muscles

The main function of muscles acting on hip is to permit efficient walking by maintaining the stability of the weight bearing leg in spite of continued change in the position of body and limb. Muscles acting on the hip can be divided into following functional groups:

1. Abductors Gluteus medius and minimus arise from outer ilium and insert on the greater trochanter. The superior gluteal nerve (L_4–S_1) supplies these muscles. Tensor fascia lata arises from anterior iliac crest and inserts on to iliotibial band and is also supplied by superior gluteal nerve.

2. Adductors Adductor longus arises from the front of pubis and inserts on to linea aspera. Adductor brevis extends from inferior pubic ramus to linea aspera / pectineal line of femur while adductor magnus extends from inferior ischiopubic ramus to adductor tubercle. Gracilis extends from lower symphysis to proximal medial tibia or pes anserinus. Pectineus extends from pubis to pectineal line.

The anterior division of obturator nerve (L_2–L_4) supplies the adductor longus and gracilis while most of the adductor magnus and adductor brevis are supplied by the posterior branch of the obturator nerve (L_2–L_4). Posterior part of adductor magnus is supplied by sciatic nerve while pectineus is supplied mainly by femoral nerve.

Note Adductor magnus has dual nerve supply (like Brachialis, which is supplied by radial and musculocutaneous nerves). Pectineus also has dual nerve supply (femoral as well as obturator).

3. Hip Flexors The primary flexors of the hip are iliopsoas (strongest), rectus femoris, and sartorius. Pectineus and tensor fascia lata also function as flexors of the hip. All these muscles except tensor fascia lata are supplied by the femoral nerve (L_2–L_4).

4. Hip extensors are gluteus maximus (which extends from ilium to gluteal tuberosity and is supplied by inferior gluteal nerve L_5–S_2) and hamstrings (semimembranosus, semitendinosus and biceps femoris–all supplied by sciatic nerve-L_4–S_3)

5. Internal Rotators of hip are gluteus medius and minimus and tensor fascia lata.

6. External Rotators of the hip are gluteus maximus (supplied by inferior gluteal nerve-L_5–S_2), obturator internus and superior gamellus (both supplied by nerve to obturator internus-L_5–S_2), inferior gamellus and quadratus femoris (both supplied by nerve to quadratus femoris-L_4–S_1), obturator externus supplied by obturator nerve and piriformis supplied by nerve to piriformis (S_1–S_2).

Blood supply to femoral head is from three sources (Fig. 27.4a,b). Medial femoral circumflex artery is a branch of profunda femoris and is most important. Lateral femoral circumflex artery is also a branch of profunda femoris and supplies the inferior part of the femoral head. Artery of the ligamentum teres is a posterior branch of obturator artery. It is an important vessel in children though it contributes only minor blood supply in adults.

Approach to a patient with hip disorder

Evaluation of a patient with symptoms pertaining to hip begins with history. Pain is one of the main complaints in hip joint disorders and can be felt over anterior or lateral aspect of the hip, in the groin or over the knee. Pain is usually aggravated with activity. Pain even at rest suggests inflammatory pathology. Pain progressively increases with time in conditions such as osteoarthritis. Sometimes pain in the hip may be secondary to spinal disorders. Stiffness, limping, limitation of the walking distance, inability to sit cross legged or squat are the other common complaints in a patient with hip disease. Age (younger patients are more likely to have hip dysplasia, Perthes', SCFE, avascular necrosis, or tuberculosis while the older patients are more likely to have osteoarthritis or hip fractures), onset of symptoms and duration of symptoms are important facts to elicit. History of excessive alcohol or steroid intake or previous history of trauma may suggest avascular necrosis.

Examination of a patient with hip disease should be done after the patient is adequately undressed. Observation should assess the gait, levels of anterior superior iliac spines, contours, resting posture of hip, wasting and leg length inequality. *Trendelenberg gait* is seen in patients with gluteus medius weakness and in this kind of gait the patient lurches towards the weak side during the stance phase of gait to place centre of gravity towards the weak hip. The *antalgic gait* results from reduced time in the stance phase on the painful side. The *short limb gait* is characterised by an obvious up and down movement of head and shoulders.

Palpation of greater trochanter, trochanteric bursa and ischial bursa is done for tenderness. Presence of pelvic obliquity is confirmed by palpation. Scarpa's triangle is palpated for tenderness. Tenderness over posterior superior iliac spine or sacroiliac joint suggests spinal or sacroiliac disease. Tenderness may be present in various muscles such as tensor fascia lata or gluteus maximus.

Movements at hip are tested for range and pain. Flexion (normal 0°–125°), extension (0°–30°), abduction (0°–45°), adduction (0°–30°), external rotation (0°–45°), and internal rotation (0°–30°) are tested.

Leg lengths are measured after palpation and testing range of motion. True leg length is measured by noting the distance from ASIS to medial malleolus when the pelvis is level. In the presence of deformity, the affected limb is placed in position of deformity and limb length measured. For measurement of unaffected limb, it should be placed in position identical to the affected limb and limb length measured. Apparent leg length discrepancy is measured from xiphisternum to the tip of medial malleolus when both the legs are parallel.

Neuromuscular examination should be done in all cases. Spine, ipsilateral knee and contralateral hip should be examined in all cases. Strength should be tested in all the muscle groups around hip. Telescoping should be performed to determine stability of the hip.

Special tests

1. Trendelenberg test The patient is asked to stand on one leg and lift the other leg with the hip and knee flexed. When standing on normal limb, the pelvis gets lifted on the opposite side (Negative Trendelenberg test). Patients with deficient abductors, fracture neck of femur or dislocated hip allow the pelvis to drop on contralateral side when standing on the affected leg (positive Trendelenberg test) (Fig. 17.1). Normally during stance phase of one limb, pelvis on the opposite side is lifted up by contraction of the abductors to maintain the position of centre of gravity. This requires normal fulcrum (centre of femoral head), lever arm (neck of femur) and motor power (abductors). Dysfunction of any/all the three leads to the Trendelenberg gait.

2. Thomas's test is done for flexion deformity of hip. The patient lies supine and the hip not being tested is passively flexed as far as possible. This is done to obliterate lumbar lordosis. The hip being tested remains flat on the examination table if there is no flexion deformity while if a flexion deformity is present, the patient's thigh on the affected side rises off the table. The angle between the thigh on the affected side and the table gives the angle of deformity.

3. Ober's test is done for iliotibial band contracture. The patient lies on the side with affected side up. The examiner flexes the normal side to obliterate lumbar lordosis. The affected side is then flexed, abducted, and extended at the hip (with knee flexed) and then allowed to fall. If the iliotibial band is normal, the thigh should drop to the adducted position. In the presence of iliotibial band contracture, the thigh remains abducted when the leg is released.

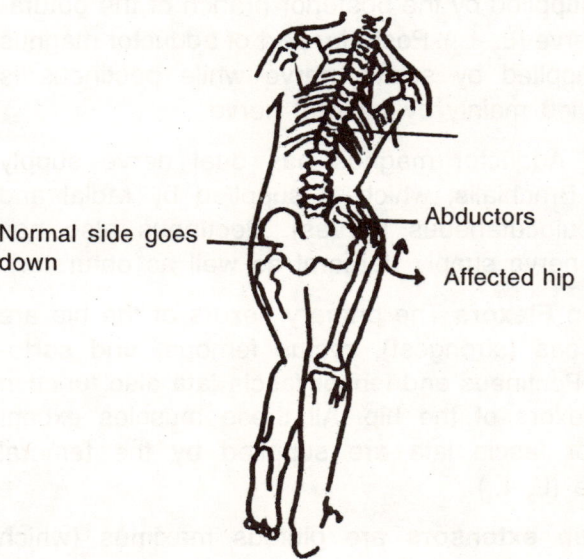

Fig. 17.1. Positive Trendelenberg test

Investigations for Hip Disease

Plain radiographs including AP and Lateral (translateral and frog leg) are obligatory to evaluation of any hip pathology.

Oblique (Iliac and obturator) views are essential for evaluating fractures/pathologies of walls/columns of the acetabulum.

Computerised Topography is helpful for evaluation of the complex fractures and dislocations and for evaluation of other (non traumatic) pathologies of femoral head and acetabulum.

Magnetic Resonance Imaging is extremely useful for earliest diagnosis of avascular necrosis, occult hip pain, pseudofractures, hip infections and synovial pathologies.

Bone Scan is useful for early detection of infections and for diagnosis of subtle fractures.

Arthroscopy of the hip is both diagnostic as well as therapeutic. It is extremely useful to diagnose labral lesions, articular cartilage lesions and synovitis and can be useful for synovial biopsies and removal of loose bodies.

Congenital and Developmental Disorders of the Hip

Developmental Dysplasia of Hip (DDH)

DDH is the most common disorder of the hip presenting during the first 3 years of life. The term DDH is used to include dysplasia without subluxation, subluxatable hip and the dislocated hip. This spectrum has been identified because of the fact that a hip dysplastic at birth may become normal in early months of life. Also, a dysplastic hip which is without subluxation or is subluxatable at birth may dislocate later. Congenital dislocation of hip may be teratologic (occurs at 12–18 weeks of intrauterine life) or typical (occurs in perinatal period).

Incidence of congenital dislocation is 4–10 per 1000 live births with considerable racial variation. DDH is more commonly associated with intrauterine crowding (other uterine packing problems such as metatarsus adductus, torticollis and calcaneovalgus are commonly associated), breech presentation, hyperextension at knees, oligohydramnios, twins and ligamentous laxity. Genetic predisposition is known and the disease often has a familial pattern. Postnatal factors are also involved in causation especially when infants are carried in a position of extension and adduction at the hips.

Almost 60% of cases of congenital dislocation of hip (CDH) are first born and it affects females more frequently than males (6:1). The left hip is more commonly affected (60%) while 20% cases are bilateral.

CDH is often associated with diseases like Ehlers-Danlos syndrome, Larsen's syndrome, myelomeningocele, arthrogryposis etc.

Pathological Changes in Congenital Dislocation

CHD is characterised by marked laxity of hip joint capsule and defective acetabular growth (acetabular roof is excessively sloping). The proximal femur has a small ossific nucleus, which appears late. There is excessive proximal femoral anteversion. Labrum is inverted in cases with dislocation and transverse acetabular ligament is shortened. The capsule may have an hourglass constriction often caused by a tight iliopsoas tendon traversing the front of the hip joint. The hip joint is filled with pulvinar, the hypertrophic fibrofatty tissue. Ligamentum teres is hypertrophied.

Clinical features

The clinical features of CDH depend on age at diagnosis and the severity of dysplasia. CDH is diagnosed most commonly in infants by positive *Barlow test* and *Ortolani's test*.

Barlow's test is a provocative test to detect a dislocatable or subluxatable hip. Adduction and axial loading (or depression) of the femur dislocates the hip.

Ortolani's test is a reduction manoeuvre for a dislocated hip in a newborn (Fig. 17.2). Elevation and abduction of the femur relocate the hip, often with an audible or palpable "clunk". In a child older than 2 months of age, the best test is demonstration of reduced abduction (especially with hips flexed) as the Barlow and Ortolani's tests may no longer be positive. In older children there may be asymmetry of the gluteal, inguinal and thigh skin folds. Bilateral dislocations usually are associated with widened perineum. The limb is shortened and externally rotated. The greater trochanter on the affected side is higher. With the knees and hips flexed and feet together, the knee on the affected side is lower (*Galeazzi sign*). Telescoping is strongly positive.

When the child presents after walking, limp is the main complaint. Trendelenberg test is positive. There is increased lumbar lordosis and scoliosis convex towards the affected side. The adaptive changes are generally more marked in teratologic dislocations and occur at an earlier age.

Radiographic examination

Ultrasonography of hip should be obtained in infants with suspected CDH, as it is the most sensitive investigation in the newborn.

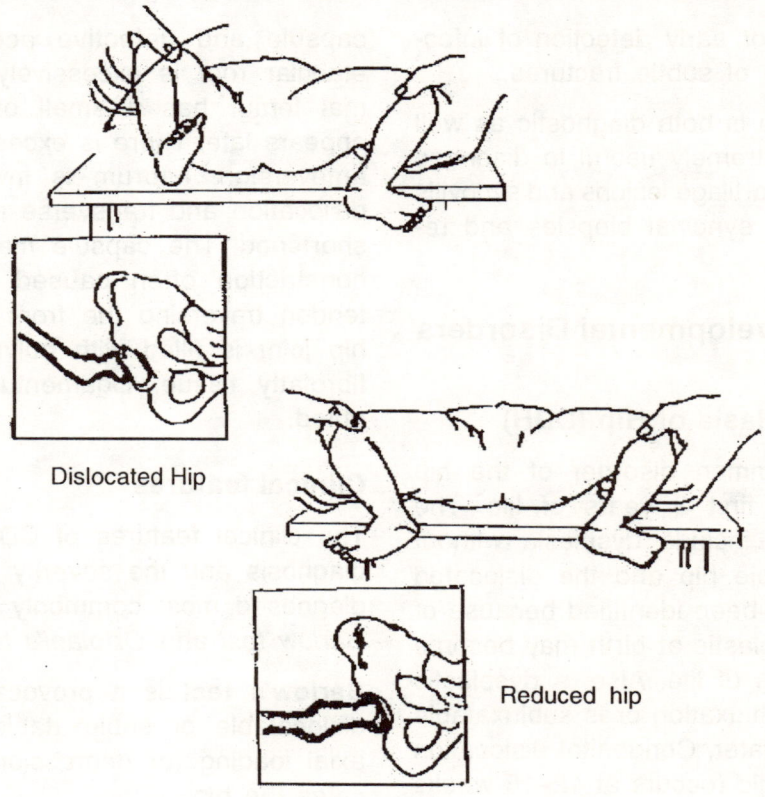

Dislocated Hip

Reduced hip

Fig. 17.2. Ortolani Test

Plain x-rays are useful in children over 3 months of age. The radiological features seen on plain radiographs are (Fig. 17.3a,b).

1. Delayed appearance of femoral ossific nucleus on the affected (left) side. (Normally appears by 6–12 months. Compare with opposite side).

2. Lateral and superior migration of proximal femur

3. Shenton's line is broken

4. Increased acetabular index (>30°).

5. Centre Edge (CE) angle of Wiberg is less than 20°–25°

6. Femoral neck-shaft angle is increased (coxa valga)

7. Delayed ossification of the triradiate cartilage.

8. Ossific nucleus of femoral head lies in upper and outer quadrant (cf: lower and outer quadrant in subluxation and, lower and inner quadrant in normal hip)

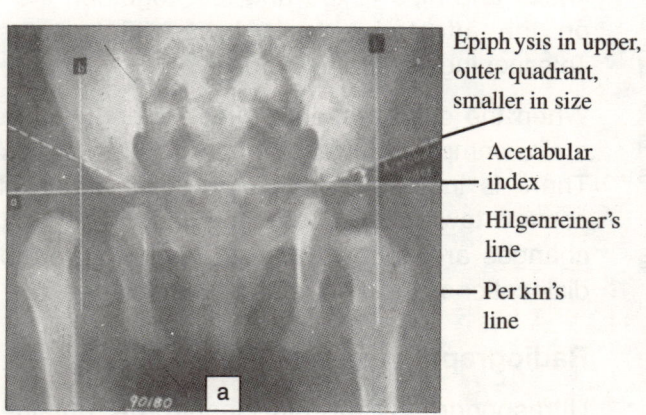

Epiphysis in upper, outer quadrant, smaller in size

Acetabular index

Hilgenreiner's line

Perkin's line

a

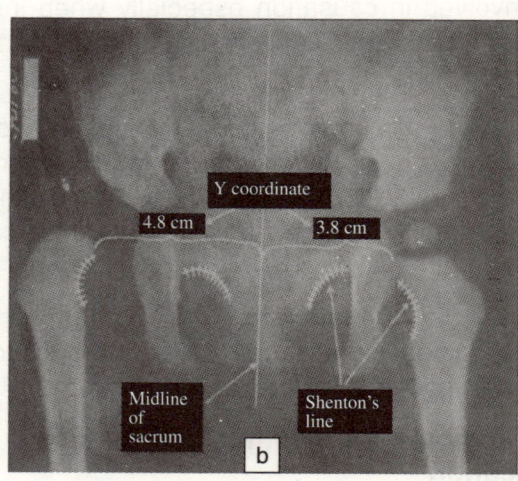

Y coordinate

4.8 cm   3.8 cm

Midline of sacrum

Shenton's line

b

Fig. 17.3a,b. Plain x-ray features of CDH

(*Note* **Hilgenreiner's line** is a horizontal line passing through the triradiate cartilage on both the sides. **Perkin's line** is a vertical line along the lateral acetabular margin and perpendicular to Hilgenreiner's line).

Arthrography is useful in diagnosing mechanical blocks to reduction and in confirming shape and congruence of femoral head and the acetabulum. It can also be used post operatively for evaluation of the adequacy of reduction.

CT Scan is useful after ossification of femoral ossific nucleus, in children older than 6 months of age. Its real usefulness, however, remains in documenting concentric reduction when the patient is in a plaster cast.

MRI is now becoming popular as the investigation of choice before 6 months age when the proximal femoral ossific nucleus is still cartilaginous. It is useful to diagnose CDH as well as to confirm concentricity of reduction during treatment.

Treatment

The principle of treatment of dysplastic hip is to obtain and/or maintain reduction to allow for normal development and it should be achieved as early as possible. Treatment of CDH is categorised according to the age of presentation (Fig. 17.4).

1. Birth to 3 months of age Children with CDH in this age group are treated by gentle manipulation and reduction. The reduction is maintained in a *von Rosen* or other suitable splint. *Pavlik harness* is used frequently in the west to achieve and maintain reduction. Splintage should be continued for duration of twice the age of infant with a minimum of 2 months. Pavlik harness should not be used in teratalogic dislocation of the hip(is ineffective in this type and may cause avascular necrosis).

2. Three months to 18 months of age Children with CDH in this age group need adductor tenotomy as the hip contracture is developed. Closed reduction under anaesthesia with adductor tenotomy if necessary and spica cast is the treatment of choice. Hip spica cast is applied in 110° flexion and *safe zone abduction* (30°–60°) and 10°–20° internal rotation. The spica cast is kept for 6 months. A single cut CT scan may be done to confirm reduction where plain radiographs look doubtful. Occasionally open reduction may be necessary in a child older than one year if closed reduction fails or when extreme positioning is required to maintain reduction, thus subjecting the femoral head to the risk of avascular necrosis.

3. Between 18 months to 3 years In children in this age group, traction and gentle attempt at reduction after adductor tenotomy may be made but usually does not succeed. Open reduction, usually by anterolateral approach is required. Femoral varus derotation osteotomy may sometimes have to be done in cases with excessive femoral anteversion. Postoperatively patient is kept in spica cast for 6–12 weeks followed by abduction splint for 6–12 weeks.

4. Between 3 years to 6 years of age Children in this age group need open reduction along with an acetabular osteotomy to improve shape of the acetabulum and/or coverage of the femoral head as the capacity for acetabular remodelling is diminished by this time. After 4 years of age, acetabular osteotomy is preferred to femoral osteotomy. Most commonly performed acetabular osteotomy is Salter's osteotomy which is useful for mild to moderate acetabular dysplasia. Salter's osteotomy improves anterior (20°–30°) and lateral (10°–15°) coverage. Other pelvic osteotomies performed for CDH are Pemberton osteotomy, Steele (triple innominate) osteotomy, Sutherland (double innominate) osteotomy, Wagner (dial) osteotomy and Ganz osteotomy.

In older children (above 5 years) with bilateral CDH, no surgical treatment should be attempted in view of poor results. Unilateral cases, however, can be salvaged with *Chiari osteotomy* or acetabular augmentation by shelf procedure (*Staheli*).

Congenital Coxa Vara

Congenital coxa vara is a disorder characterised by a decreased neck shaft angle at proximal femur caused by a defect in the ossification of the femoral neck. Unilateral cases are diagnosed by shortening and reduced abduction on the affected side. Bilateral cases are associated with widened perineum. Plain radiographs show reduced neck shaft angle (Fig. 17.5) and a triangular radiolucent area of defective ossification abutting inferior neck (*Fairbank's triangle*).

Treatment depends on severity. Mild cases may

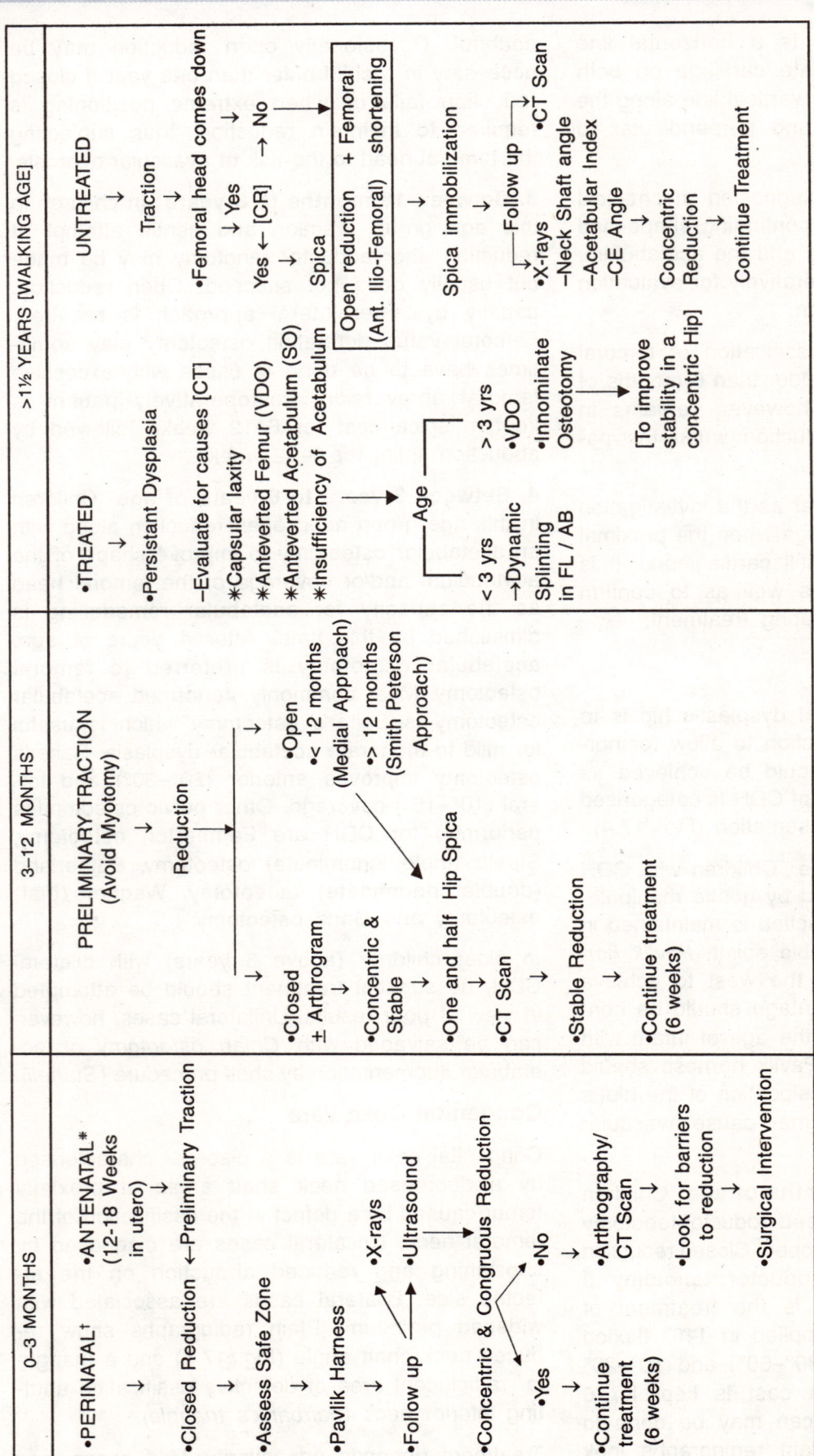

* Antenatal: or teratologic dislocation occurs between 12-18 weeks in utero and has soft tissue contractures at birth.
†Perinatal: dislocation occurs in the perinatal period.

CR : Closed Reduction   CT : Computerised Tomography
FL : Flexion   AB : Abduction
VDO: Varus Derotation Osteotomy   SO : Salter's Osteotomy

Note : Difficulty in Reduction ↑ with Age • Early diagnosis is the key to success

Fig. 17.4. Algorithm for treatment of CDH based on age of presentation

correct spontaneously. The severe cases, especially when neck shaft angle is less than 100 degrees, should be treated by valgus osteotomy.

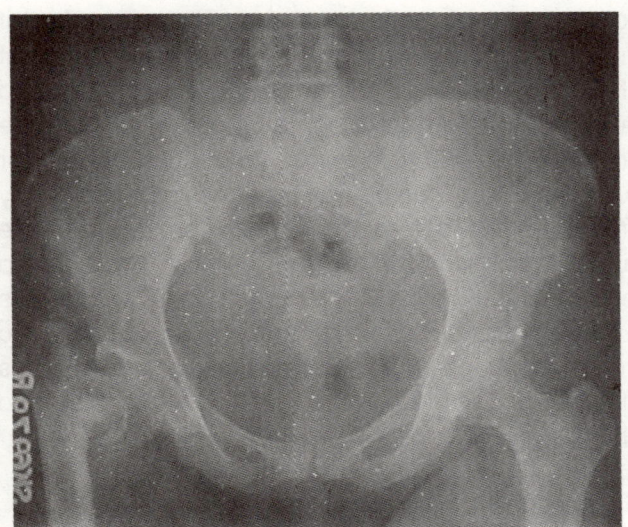

Fig. 17.5.   Congenial coxa vara affecting the right hip. Note the reduced neck shaft angle

Legg-Calve Perthes' Disease

Perthes' disease is a non-inflammatory condition leading to deformity of the weight-bearing surface of femoral head. It arises as a result of repeated vascular insults leading to avascular necrosis of the proximal femoral epiphysis.

The Perthes' disease occurs between 4 - 8 years of age and is much more common in males (M:F=4:1). Almost 10% cases are bilateral though usually not simultaneous. Perthes' disease has a higher incidence among children with older parents, children of maternal smokers during pregnancy, breech delivery, low birth weight and delayed skeletal maturation.

Pathogenesis

Idiopathic avascular necrosis of the femoral head occurs followed by subchondral fracture, revascularization (by creeping substitution), and healing ossification processes. The disease is divided into avascular necrotic stage, fragmentation stage and reparative stage. The process of necrosis and reconstitution takes about 2 years.

Clinical features

Clinically the disease varies in severity. Patient usually presents with limp, often without pain.

Limping increases with activity and may be intermittent. Pain when present is usually in the groin, anterior thigh and sometimes in the knee. Sometimes the disease presents with synovitis with associated muscle spasm. Decreased range of motion is found in almost all patients and abduction and internal rotation are mainly restricted.

Radiologically the plain x-rays show increased joint space (because of increased cartilaginous growth) and subchondral lucency. The femoral head shows increased density, fragmentation and is deformed (Fig. 17.6). Based on plain radiographs, the extent of involvement can be graded according to the Catterall classification:

1. Group I Anterior head involvement (less than 1/2 femoral head affected) without any sequestrum or subchondral fracture.

2. Group II Anterior and central half of head involved (more than 1/2 but less than 3/4th) with intact lateral margin. Sequestrum, subchondral fracture and anterolateral metaphyseal lesions are present.

3. Group III Almost 3/4th of femoral head is involved including the posterior half of epiphysis - only posteromedial segment is spared. Large sequestrum forms along with subchondral fracture and diffuse metaphyseal changes.

4. Group IV Entire head is involved.

The disadvantage of Catterall classification is that these changes take up to 8 months to appear.

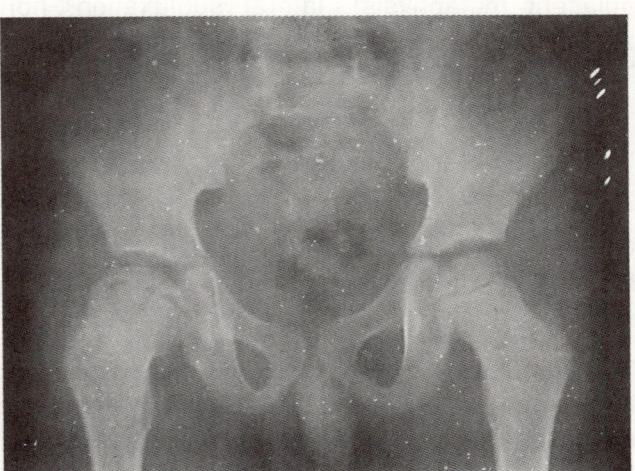

Fig. 17.6.   Perthes' disease of right hip. Note the increased sclerosis and flattening of the capital femoral epiphysis

Lateral pillar classification is more useful. Group A: Lateral pillar intact; Group B: less than 50% lateral pillar is collapsed; Group C: greater than 50% lateral pillar is collapsed.

Arthrogram can be used to assess containment of head and its deformity and subluxation.

Bone scan can be used to diagnose the condition early.

MRI is a non-invasive investigation, which is extremely useful for early diagnosis, and can differentiate between live and dead marrow.

Differential Diagnosis Perthes disease should be differentiated from transient synovitis, septic arthritis, blood dyscrasias (especially sickle cell disease), lymphoma, trauma, tumour and rheumatic fever. Bilateral cases must be differentiated from multiple epiphyseal dysplasia, spondyloepiphyseal dysplasia, pseudoachondroplasia, sickle cell disease and hypothyroidism.

Prognosis

Clinical and radiological prognostic factors have been recognised.

Clinical Age more than 6–8 years, obesity, decreased range of movements especially presence of adduction contracture, and female sex are associated with poor prognosis.

Radiological *"Head at risk"* signs are identified as calcification lateral to the epiphysis, *Gage's sign* (V-shaped lucent area in lateral epiphysis and adjacent metaphysis), lateral subluxation, horizontal physis and diffuse metaphyseal reaction. The presence of these signs indicates impending extensive osteonecrosis of femoral head.

Uncovering of the femoral head by >20% is a bad prognostic indicator.

Greater the Catterall group (more extensive the femoral head involvement), worse is the prognosis.

Treatment of Perthes' disease is aimed at maintaining the sphericity of the femoral head and is based on the principle that hip mobility and containment of the femoral head within the acetabulum will lead to the best healing and remodelling of the avascular femoral head. Young patients (4 to 6 years age) with involvement of less than 50%

of the head (Catterall I) are observed without active treatment. Catterall II group patients less than 6 years of age are observed if they have a good range of motion. Intermittent traction and active range of motion exercises are prescribed if there is limitation of movements. Aim of treatment of Catterall III and IV groups is to achieve good range of motion and containment. This can be achieved by orthotic devices (abduction braces) or surgery. Surgery can be Salter's innominate osteotomy or a femoral osteotomy. These procedures are suitable only for those cases where there is no femoral head deformity. In group III & IV patients where the head is deformed or collapsed, no treatment is possible. Catterall IV group patients older than 6 years are treated with traction and abduction bracing.

Slipped Capital Femoral Epiphysis
(Adolescent Coxa Vara)

Slipped capital femoral epiphysis (SCFE) is a condition wherein the femoral neck displaces through the growth plate in anterior and superior direction while the femoral head remains in the acetabulum. The condition is caused by weakness of the perichondrial ring and the zone of hypertrophy in the growth plate. The exact cause is unknown. Various aetiologies have been suggested including hormonal dysfunction.

The incidence of SCFE is 1–3 per 100,000. Males are affected more commonly than females (2.5:1). Almost 25% cases are bilateral. SCFE is common during 13 to 16 years age in males and 11 to 13 years in females. There is an increased incidence in overweight as well as slender tall patients, hypothyroidism, hypopituitarism, renal osteodystrophy, hypogonadism, Down's syndrome and in the presence of a positive family history.

Classification

*   An *acute* slip occurs suddenly
*   An *acute on chronic* slip presents with acute exacerbation of symptoms, which have been present for more than 3 weeks.
*   A *chronic* slip is the one where history of symptoms is of more than 3 weeks' duration

Pathogenesis

Slip occurs through the *zone of hypertrophy* and the

displacement occurs due to body weight and muscle action. Epiphysis displaces posteriorly and inferiorly while the neck displaces in anterior and superior direction. The leg rotates externally under the effect of these displacements. Progressive apparent coxa vara and shortening of the leg result.

Clinical features

Clinically the patient, usually between the age of 10 and 16 years, presents with a history of chronic or intermittent pain of insidious onset in groin, thigh or medial knee associated with a limp. Patient may also present with acute pain after an injury with a history of intermittent pain previously (acute on chronic). In the acute phase, there is significant muscle spasm and synovitis with restricted range of motion. Gait is antalgic with externally rotated foot progression angle. There is decreased internal rotation, abduction and flexion. Hip flexion produces external rotation with knee pointing towards the axilla during flexion (other causes of knee pointing towards the axilla during flexion include coxa magna and gluteus maximus contracture). Severe cases may be associated with shortening of femur.

Radiologically the earliest changes are seen only on lateral x-ray. On AP view, a line along the superior neck does not intersect any part of epiphysis (*Trethowen's sign*) (Fig. 17.7a,b). The medial and proximal part of femoral neck does not overlap the ischium (Capener's Sign).

Chronic changes are seen in longstanding cases and can be widening of physis, sclerosis, and ossification at the junction of medial femoral neck. Narrowed joint space and osteopenia of femoral head are seen in chondrolysis.

Treatment in mild to moderate cases is in situ pin fixation. A single pin or titanium screw is passed from close to base of neck anteriorly towards posteroinferiorly. Patient is mobilised partial weight bearing with crutches for 6 weeks. Aim of pinning in situ is to prevent further progression of slip and to achieve early closure of physis.

Attempts to reduce the physis in longstanding cases leads to avascular necrosis.

In cases of severe slip primary epiphysiodesis is described as a method of treatment.

Compensatory transcervical and basal neck osteotomies are described to correct the deformities. These procedures are technically demanding and associated with increased incidence of avascular necrosis. Contralateral hip should be closely observed till physeal closure. Prophylactic pinning is indicated only in cases with renal osteodystrophy, which are associated with increased incidence of bilateral slip.

Complications

Chondrolysis may be associated with forceful manipulation or after surgery when pin penetrates the head to enter the joint. Clinically, the patient presents with stiffness, severe pain and muscle

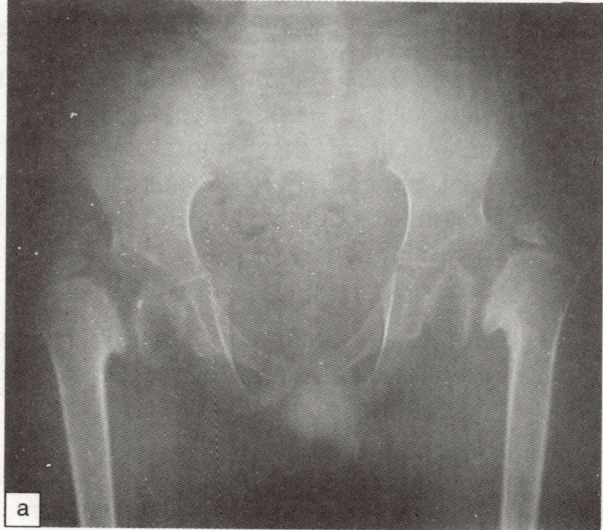
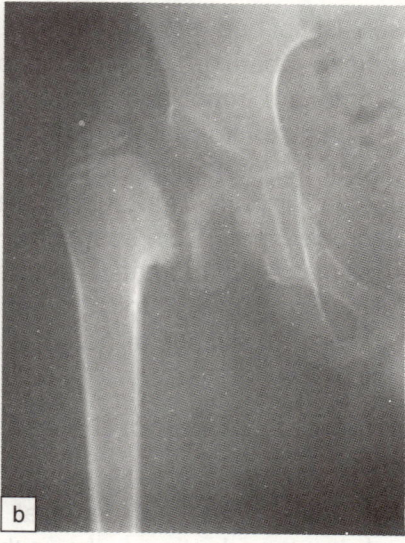

Fig. 17.7a,b. Radiographic appearance of slipped capital femoral epiphysis. Note the apparent coxa vara

spasm. Hemogram and other laboratory parameters are normal. Radiographs show joint space narrowing. Bone scan is positive with increased uptake in the region of acetabulum and femoral head. It may recover completely in 6-12 months but may cause degeneration or ankylosis of the joint. Treatment is traction, range of motion exercises, NSAIDs and salvage operations such as arthrodesis or arthroplasty. Other complications are avascular necrosis and secondary osteoarthritis.

Transient Synovitis of Hip (Observation Hip, Toxic Synovitis, Coxitis Fugax)

Transient synovitis is a self-limiting condition seen in children between 3 to 5 years of age. Synovitis of the hip joint occurs without any obvious etiology.

The child presents with complaints of limp and pain in groin, anteromedial thigh or knee. The duration of symptoms varies from a couple of days to a fortnight. The affected hip is in attitude of flexion and external rotation. All the attempted movements are painful near the extremes. There may be history of sore throat, tonsillitis or low-grade fever. Leukocytosis and slight increase in sedimentation rate may be present. Radiographs are normal but may show soft tissue swelling in the region of gluteus medius, obturator internus and psoas. Aspiration of hip under aseptic conditions should be performed if differentiation from infective hip arthritis cannot be done.

Toxic synovitis must be differentiated from septic arthritis, tubercular arthritis, avascular necrosis of femoral epiphysis and Perthes' disease.

Treatment consists of bed rest and traction. Patient's symptoms quickly abate on elimination of weight bearing. Patients are mobilised when they have regained full, painless range of motion and can ambulate without pain and limp. If pain persists or recurs, pyogenic arthritis, tubercular arthritis or avascular necrosis should be suspected. Even if the child becomes asymptomatic and returns to activity, a follow up visit at 8 to 12 weeks should be advised to rule out avascular necrosis clinically and radiologically.

Avascular Necrosis of Femoral Head (Osteonecrosis)

Avascular necrosis (AVN) of femoral head is characterised by the death of the subchondral bone of femoral head caused by vascular insult.

The exact pathogenesis is not known though the infarction theory (due to incompetent blood supply to femoral head) as well as progressive ischemia theory (reduction in blood flow subsequent to increase in bone marrow pressure) has been postulated. Recently interest has been generated in increased *free fatty acids* found in the circulation in these patients and fat embolism leading to thrombosis of the vessels supplying blood to the head is being advanced as a cause of AVN.

Risk Factors for AVN include trauma (femoral neck fracture, hip dislocation, fracture of acetabulum), steroid use, alcoholism, post-irradiation, sickle cell disease, Caisson disease (dysbarism), and Gaucher's disease. Several cases however, may be idiopathic.

Classification AVN has been classified into five stages (Ficat and Arlet) based on clinical, radiologic, pathologic and bone scan findings.

Stage 0 refers to the asymptomatic hip in a patient with established AVN of the other side.

Stage 1 The patient is normal clinically and radiologically and the bone scan may show a cold spot. Pathologic findings include infarction of the weight bearing part of the femoral head with abundant dead marrow cells and osteoblasts.

Stage 2 Patients are mildly symptomatic, x-rays show increased density in the femoral head. No flattening of the head is seen in stage 2A, while flattening (crescent sign) is seen in stage 2B. Bone scan shows increased uptake and biopsy shows deposition of new bone over the necrotic trabeculae signifying reparative process.

Stage 3 The changes in this stage are advanced with mild to moderate pain, collapse and loss of sphericity of the femoral head, with preserved joint space. There is subchondral fracture with collapse, compaction and fragmentation of the necrotic segment. Bone scan shows increased uptake.

Stage 4 In this apart from all the above changes there is involvement of the hip joint by secondary osteoarthritic process.

Clinical Features

The patients are often asymptomatic in early stages of the disease. Pain is the usual presenting complaint. Limited hip range of motion occurs late in the disease. The disease is often bilateral but may be asymptomatic on one side. Early diagnosis of AVN needs a high index of suspicion.

Radiological Features

Radiological changes usually lag behind the pathological changes. X-rays are often normal until late in the disease. Comparison with opposite side is often useful in early disease. Subchondral lucency and loss of sphericity heralds the beginning of collapse of the femoral head. A sclerotic sequestrum forms (Fig. 17.8a). Changes of secondary osteoarthritis are seen in late stages.

Magnetic Resonance imaging is the earliest test to become positive even before the onset of symptoms. It is also useful to rule out pre-clinical disease on the normal side.

Bone Scan is also useful but is not as sensitive as the MRI.

Treatment varies according to the presence or absence of the femoral head collapse. In cases where the contour of the femoral head is maintained, core decompression of the femoral head is done. An 8–10 mm diameter core of bone is removed from the anterolateral part of the femoral head. Core decompression aids revascularisation by providing a channel for vascular ingrowth. It also relieves pain by decompressing intraosseous compartment (intra osseous hypertension is believed to be one of the causes of pain in AVN).

Other techniques used for early disease are fibular (Fig. 17.8b) or tibial strut grafts, vascularised fibular bone grafts and osteotomy of the proximal femur to bring a relatively normal (less affected) portion of the femoral head against the weight bearing region of the acetabulum.

Treatment of the late disease with secondary osteoarthritis of the hip (Fig. 17.8c) is arthrodesis

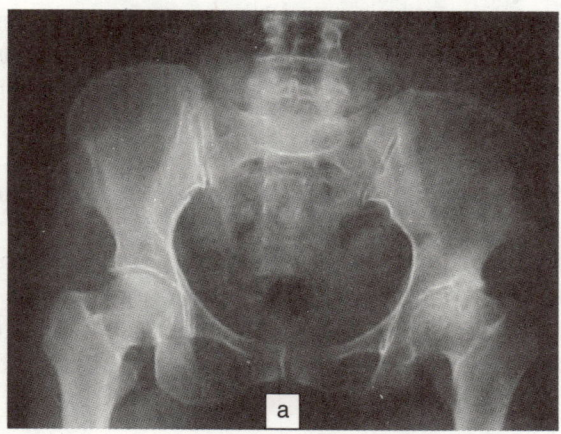

Fig. 17.8a. Avascular necrosis of left femoral head

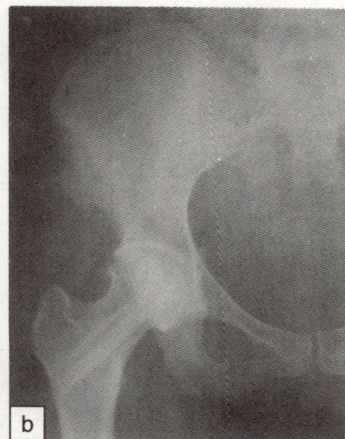

Fig. 17.8b. Early AVN treated by core decompression and fibular grafting. Note that the contour of the femoral head is maintained

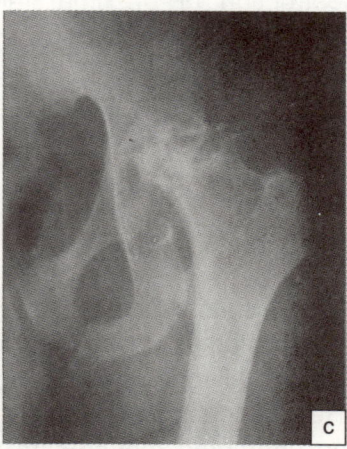

Fig. 17.8c. Advanced AVN in a patient with SLE. Replacement arthroplasty remains the only possible treatment in this case.

(for unilateral disease in young and active patient with normal ipsilateral knee and spine) or arthroplasty. Arthroplasty is the preferred option for advanced AVN because of its ability to relieve pain and provide mobility.

Infective Disorders

Pyogenic Arthritis of the Hip Joint

Pyogenic arthritis of the hip is common in infants and children. Adult patients rarely develop pyogenic arthritis of the hip. Those adults who develop septic arthritis of the hip are frequently immunocompromised intravenous drug abusers, diabetics, patients with renal failure or those taking corticosteroids or chemotherapeutic drugs.

Pathogenesis Staphylococcus aureus is the most common pathogen. Gram negative organisms may cause the infection in neonates. Septic arthritis of the hip joint in a neonate may develop following femoral venipuncture, umbilical vein sepsis or hematogenous spread from a distant infective focus. Pyogenic osteomyelitis of proximal femur may lead to septic arthritis due to intracapsular location of the proximal metaphysis (cf. Shoulders, knee, ankle). Suppuration in the hip joints leads to increased intrarticular pressure, distension of the joint, osteonecrosis of proximal femur and pathological dislocation. Femoral head in the new-borns and infants is mostly cartilaginous and undergoes rapid dissolution under the effect of enzymes released in the joint. This leads to classical sequelae of septic arthritis of infancy (*Tom Smith arthritis*) which is characterised by extensive destruction of proximal femur leading to hypermobility of hip and severe shortening of the limb.

The disease in the older children destroys the femoral head and acetabulum and leads to bony ankylosis.

Clinical features

Clinically, septic arthritis of the hip presents with constitutional symptoms. A high index of suspicion is required to diagnose the condition in the new-borns. Reluctance to move the affected limb and crying on attempted movements may be the only symptoms. Where the differentiation between the septic arthritis of the hip and osteomyelitis of proximal femur is difficult, presence of rotations of the hip rules out septic arthritis.

The onset in older children can be acute or subacute. Constitutional symptoms are more prominent than in the new-borns. Patients have pain in the hip and limping. Pain gets worse with activity. There is restriction of all the movements of the hip.

Psoas abscess is often confused with septic arthritis in young children. The presence of tenderness in the gluteal region, normal examination of the spine, and restriction of all movements of the hip especially rotations favour the diagnosis of septic arthritis. Though the extension of hip is painful in psoas abscess, rotations are typically painless and free.

Radiological Examination

Plain x-rays in early stages are normal. X-rays do not help much in the newborns where ultrasound may be a useful investigation to demonstrate the effusion in the joint. Plain x-ray in the newborn may show pathological dislocation of the hip. In young children with Tom Smith arthritis, differentiation from CDH can be made on plain x-rays by failure of proximal femoral epiphysis to appear and by the presence of a normal acetabulum (with normal shape, slope and capacity not unlike the opposite hip) (Fig. 17.9a). In older patient, x-rays in septic arthritis of the hip show rarefaction of the bone, loss of joint space, bony destruction

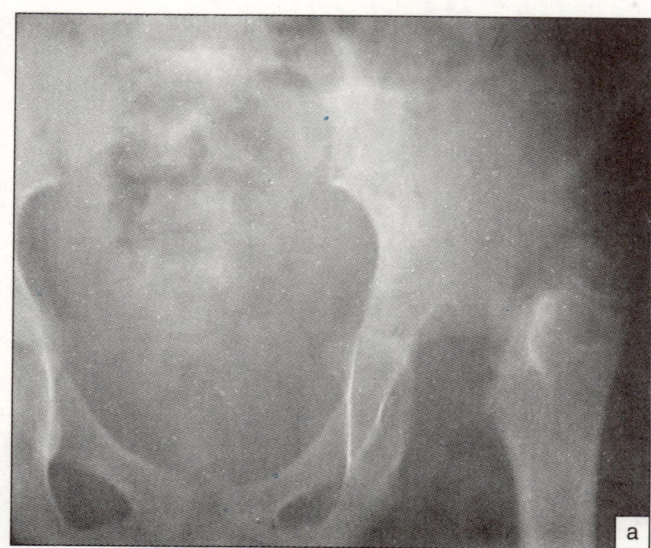

Fig. 17.9a. Tom Smith arthritis of left hip

along with sclerosis and in late stages, bony ankylosis (Fig. 17.9b).

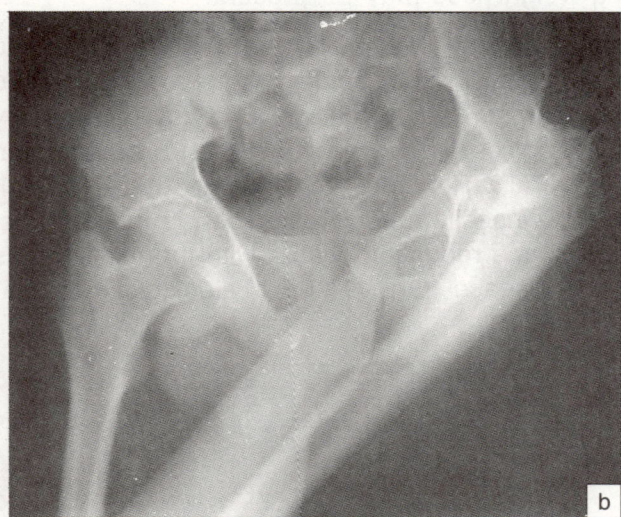

Fig. 17.9b. Sequelae of septic arthritis—bony ankylosis in severe degree of adduction

Diagnosis

In addition to clinical and radiological features a patient suspected of having septic arthritis of the hip must have aspiration of the joint and joint fluid sent for cell count and chemical analysis. Hemogram including total and differential leukocyte count, blood culture and WBC labelled scan can all help in diagnosis but clinical diagnosis remains the most important consideration.

Treatment of septic arthritis of the hip begins with institution of parenteral antibiotic therapy depending on the suspected or known sensitivity pattern of the pathogenic organism. Skin traction provides rest, relieves pain and spasm and prevents and corrects deformity. If the disease is early and responds to antibiotic therapy by resolution of local and constitutional symptoms, gradual mobilisation of the joint is started.

Most cases, however, present late and drainage of the hip joint should be undertaken as soon as possible to prevent further destruction of the hip joint. Posterior approach to the hip joint is used and the joint is washed out. Postoperatively, the patient is kept in skin traction till the symptoms settle down.

Joints with severe damage due to septic arthritis are immobilised in hip spica to achieve the bony ankylosis in functional position.

Treatment of sequelae

- Bony ankylosis in good position needs no treatment

- Bony ankylosis with deformity needs corrective subtrochanteric osteotomy to enable the child to stand and walk.

- Bony ankylosis with discharging sinus tract is treated with debridement and curettage of sinus tracts and cavities if any and removal of sequestrae.

The unstable hip in Tom Smith's arthritis is treated by either a valgus (pelvic support osteotomy) or varus (placing the greater trochanter in acetabulum after osteotomy) osteotomy of the proximal femur to treat instability. The latter procedure is useful in young children with complete destruction of femoral head and remaining growth in the trochanteric apophysis. Trochanteric arthroplasty is done, i.e. trochanteric apophysis is kept in the acetabulum and it acts like capital femoral epiphysis. Severe shortening may require limb lengthening.

Tuberculosis of the Hip Joint

After the spine, the hip joint is the most commonly affected part of the skeleton in tuberculosis. Tuberculous arthritis of the hip occurs following the hematogenous spread from a pulmonary, gastrointestinal or urogenital focus. Tuberculosis of the hip was earlier said to be the disease of children but the increased incidence of HIV has made tuberculosis a disease affecting all age groups of immunocompromised patients. The incidence of Multi Drug Resistant (MDR) tuberculosis is also on the rise.

Pathogenesis

The disease can be juxta-articular, synovial or osteoarticular. The lesion starts most commonly in the acetabulum (superolateral part), femoral head, femoral neck (Babcock's triangle) and the greater trochanter, in the orders of decreasing frequency. The extent of destruction of the cartilage and bone determine the fate of the joint.

The earliest stage of tuberculosis of the hip is the stage of synovitis wherein the limb lies in an attitude of flexion, abduction and external rotation; *the stage of apparent lengthening*. Further progression of the disease to arthritis leads to an attitude of flexion, adduction and internal rotation—*the stage of apparent shortening*. When extensive destruction of articular cartilage occurs, it results in the *stage of true shortening*.

The disease heals with fibrous ankylosis. In some cases, erosion of superior margin of acetabulum occurs with proximal migration of the femoral head on dorsum ilii resulting in wandering acetabulum.

Clinical Features

Pain in the affected limb and limp are the most common presenting features. Night cries also occur commonly – the child wakes up from sleep with severe pain as the muscle spasm which keeps the damaged joint surfaces apart during the day, relaxes at night allowing the damaged joint surfaces to come together and cause severe pain. Wasting is seen in the thigh and gluteal regions. All the movements at the hip joint are painfully restricted. The deformity at the hip is according to the stage of the disease as described above. Presence of flexion, abduction and external rotation may occur in the arthritic stage when the iliofemoral (*Bigelow's*) ligament is destroyed or when the patient is treated in a spica or by traction. A cold abscess may present in the buttocks or in proximal thigh. Discharging

sinuses may be present in advanced cases. Constitutional symptoms of anorexia, night sweats and weight loss may be present.

Radiologically the plain x-rays show increased joint space in the earliest stages. Generalised osteoporosis soon follows and is followed by localised bony destruction in the acetabulum (Fig. 17.10a) or proximal femur (Fig. 17.10b). There is usually no sclerosis seen in tuberculosis. Joint space reduction occurs with further progress of the disease (Fig. 17.10c). Pathological disloca-

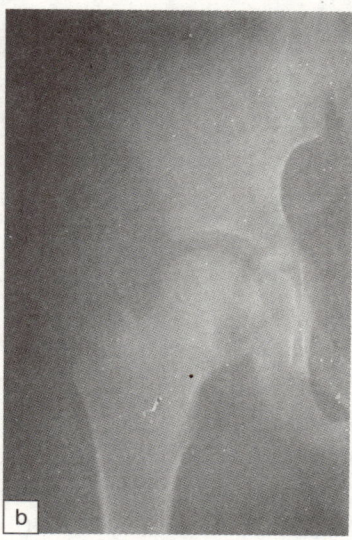

Fig. 17.10b. Tubercular involvement of femoral head

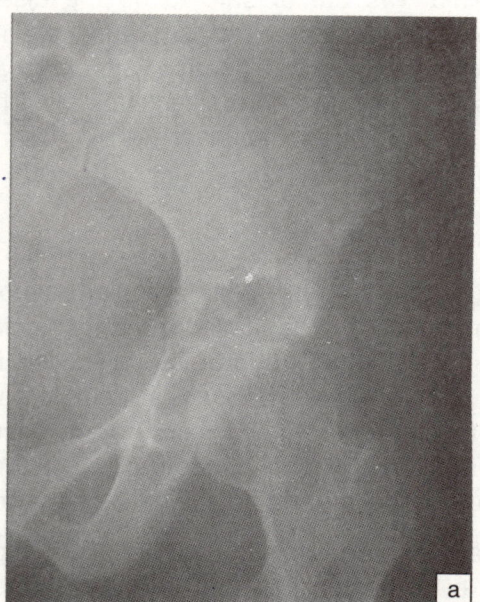

Fig. 17.10a. Tuberculosis left hip with superolateral acetabular involvement

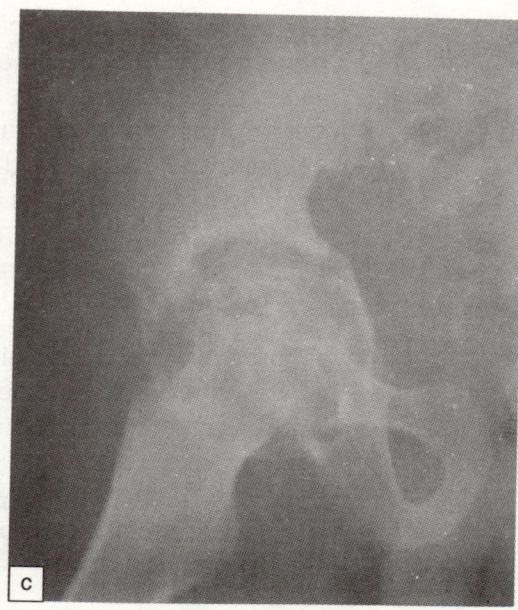

Fig. 17.10c. Arthritic stage of tuberculosis causing destruction of the right hip joint

tion .may be seen. Fibrous and not the bony ankylosis is the rule in tubercular arthritis. The presence of sclerosis and/or bony ankylosis suggests secondary pyogenic infection via the discharging sinuses.

Treatment of tuberculosis of hip joint begins with institution of antitubercular treatment. Early cases with synovitis are treated with traction with an aim to preserve the joint and its mobility. With abatement of symptoms, the joint is gradually mobilised.

Joint debridement is undertaken when the disease has not destroyed articular cartilage and control of disease with return of joint mobility can be expected after debriding the joint. Loss of articular cartilage manifested by loss of joint space on plain radiographs is a contraindication to joint debridement.

Girdlestone arthroplasty i.e. resection of the head and neck of femur is undertaken in tuberculosis of the hip joint with the following aims:

- To confirm the diagnosis by retrieving tissue for histopathological examination

- To reduce the disease burden

- To improve vascularity and improve penetration of antitubercular drugs

- To correct the deformity at the joint

- To improve mobility at the joint

However, shortening, instability and persistence of pain are major drawbacks of Girdlestone arthroplasty.

In joints where the joint is not salvageable, the aim is to achieve a stable painless hip in good position. Fibrous ankylosis in functional position is achieved by applying hip spica after correction of deformities is obtained by traction or under anaesthesia. One of the treatment related complication includes frame knee in children (stiffness of the knee associated with premature epiphyseal fusion in patients treated with hip spica).

Corrective Osteotomy to correct the deformity is a useful procedure in an otherwise painless hip, which is stiff in non-functional position.

Arthrodesis of the hip was classically performed extra-articularly in older days (Ischiofemoral or *Brittain's arthrodesis* done for adduction deformity and Iliofemoral arthrodesis done for abduc-

tion deformity) due to the fear of disseminating the disease by operating on a tubercular joint. With the availability of effective antitubercular drugs today, even intraarticular arthrodesis can be performed. The arthrodesis is performed to achieve a stable, painless hip in functional position.

Arthroplasty in treatment of hip should not be done till a disease free period of at least 10 years has elapsed, due to the fear of reactivation of disease.

Degenerative Arthritis of the Hip

Primary degenerative arthritis of the hip is extremely rare in our country. It is usually seen in western countries. Mselini, Kashin-Beck diseases and Handigodu are rare endemic osteoarthritic conditions, which are seen in Africa, China and India respectively. The disease in our set-up is often secondary to trauma, infection, avascular necrosis, rheumatoid arthritis, developmental dysplasia of the hip, spondyloarthropathies, crystal deposition disease, SCFE, storage diseases, collagen vascular diseases, Perthes' disease etc. A rare rapidly progressive osteoarthritis of hip has been reported with analgesic (indomethacin) abuse the so-called "*Analgesic hip.*"

Clinically, the patient with osteoarthritis presents with pain in groin, buttock and front of the thigh or knee. Pain is usually activity related but even comes at rest as the disease progresses. Patients often start limping and have an antalgic gait. Restriction of movements occurs and internal rotation is the earliest movement to be lost. The limb often has an adduction – external rotation deformity. Flexion deformity may also be present. This results from inflammatory products gravitating to the dependent inferior area of the joint and causing capsular contracture in this area first. The shortening (supra trochanteric) occurs with advanced disease.

Radiologically the plain x-rays show reduction of joint space, irregularity of subchondral bone, subchondral sclerosis, cyst and osteophyte formation and lateral or superolateral subluxation of the femoral head (Fig. 17.11). Based on the radiographic appearance osteoarthritis of hip has been classified into superolateral, inferomedial, and protrusio types.

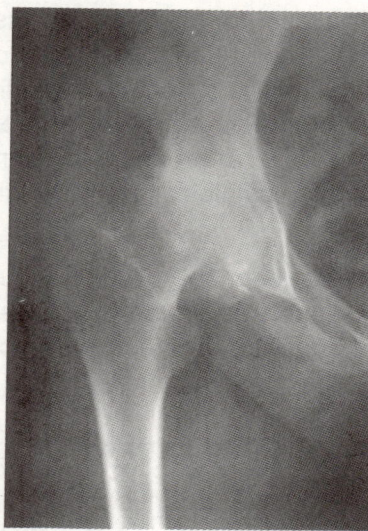

Fig. 17.11. Radiologic features of osteoarthritis of hip

Treatment of osteoarthritis is conservative initially. Exercises (occupational, aerobic), alteration of activities of daily living, use of cane or other walking aids and weight reduction are important non-pharmacological measures to control symptoms. The use of heat or cold may reduce symptoms. Paracetamol should be used initially and NSAIDs can be added in gradually increasing doses if needed. Intraarticular steroid injections can be beneficial but should be used cautiously and sparingly to avoid damage to cartilage, infection and occurrence of neuropathic joint.

Surgical treatment consists of arthrodesis in young patients with unilateral hip disease and normal ipsilateral knee, spine and contralateral hip. Osteotomy of femur or pelvis attempts to improve the weight bearing condition of hip by altering the weight bearing relationship of the femoral head and acetabulum. Total hip arthroplasty is the most common treatment for osteoarthritis. It mainly aims to relieve pain though it also corrects mechanical derangement and improves motion. Both cemented and cementless implants are available, the latter are used in young patients with good bone stock.

Common Operations Performed on the Hip Joint

Osteotomy

Aim Reduces joint reaction forces by increasing weight bearing surface and restoring joint congruity.

Indications

Varus (adduction) Osteotomy

- Spherical femoral head
- Little or no acetabular dysplasia
- Abduction deformity with painless, adequate abduction
- Antalgic gait
- Apparent lengthening of affected extremity
- Lateral overloading of the hip joint
- Residual subluxation or neck shaft angle > 140°

Valgus (abduction) Osteotomy (More commonly needed)

- Adduction deformity with adequate adduction.
- Trendelenberg gait
- Short limb gait

Pre-Requisites for Osteotomy

- At least 70° of flexion must be possible for a satisfactory result.
- Only for young patients preferably non-obese with non-deformed femoral heads and preserved joint space
- Unilateral involvement with underlying mechanical cause

Arthrodesis

Aim To achieve stable, painless hip in functional position.

Indications

Unilateral hip disease in a young patient (Fig. 17.12a) such as

1. Infection
   i) Pyogenic
   ii) Tubercular
2. Trauma
3. Sequelae of childhood hip disease.

Arthritis in young active patients–in bilateral cases,

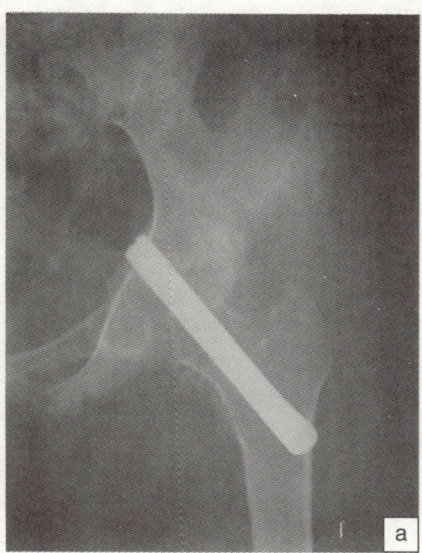

Fig. 17.12a. Unilateral hip arthrodesis using Smith Peterson nail

arthrodesis can be done on one side and THR on other (Fig. 17.12b).

Pre-requisites Freely mobile ipsilateral knee, spine and contralateral hip.

Position of Fusion 30° flexion, 0°–5° adduction (abduction causes more back and knee problems subsequently) and 0°–5° external rotation.

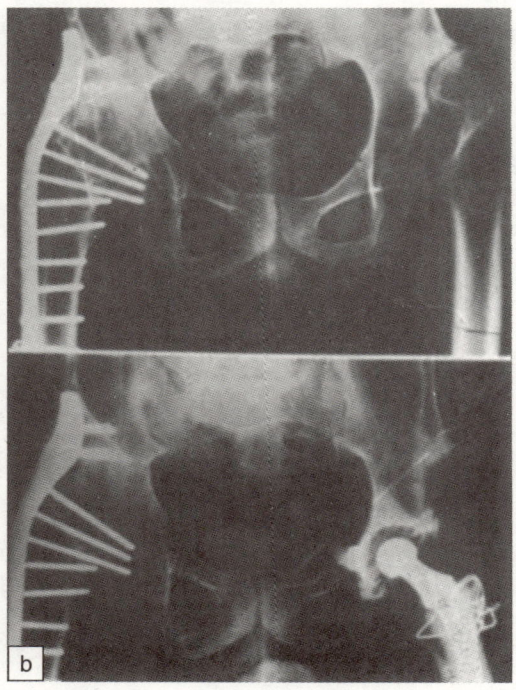

Fig. 17.12b. Hip arthrodesis using plates and screws on the right side and total hip replacement on the left side

Girdlestone Arthroplasty

is a salvage procedure (Fig. 17.13). It can be done in bilateral cases with severe arthritis/hip disease if the patient cannot afford THR.

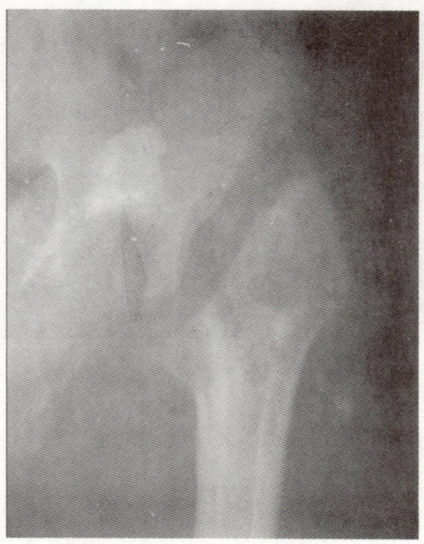

Fig.17.13. Girdlestone arthroplasty of left hip

Indications

- Tuberculosis of hip (vide supra).
- Bilateral severe arthritis of hip joint (Bilateral Girdlestone or Girdlestone on one side can be done).
- Can be used in patients with cerebral palsy or paraplegia to improve sitting.

Problems

- Shortening
- Pain
- Instability

Total Hip Arthroplasty

Aim To eliminate pain and restore function.

Indications

Painful hips due to primary or secondary osteoarthritis, rheumatoid arthritis and ankylosing spondylitis.

Types

a) **Cemented** (Fig. 17.14a,b)
- For older patient

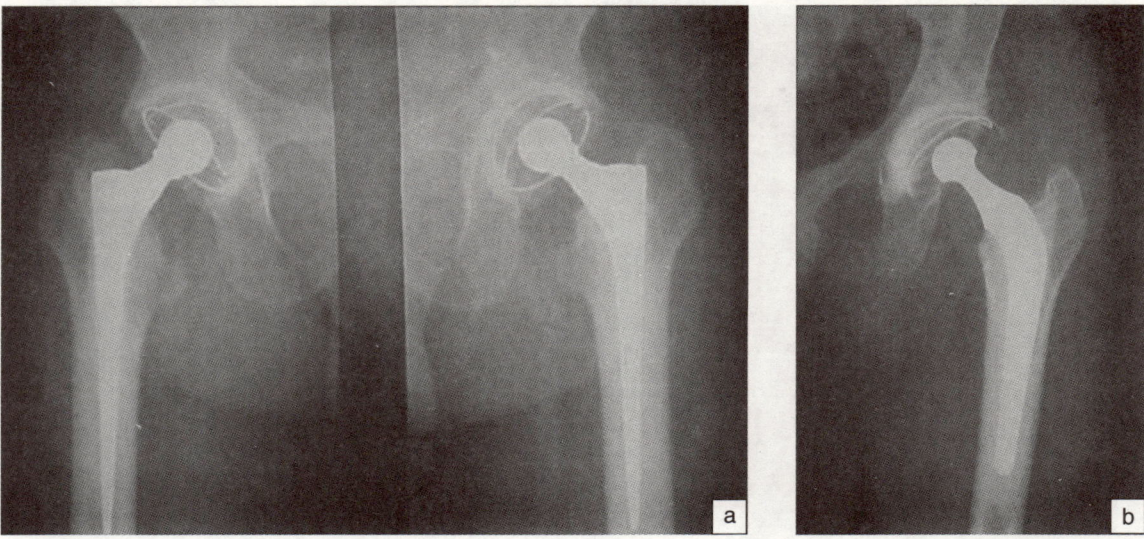

Fig. 17.14a,b. X-Rays appearance of cemented total hip replacement

- Poor bone stock
- Short life expectancy
- Obese patient

b) Uncemented

- Young patient
- Good bone stock

Bearing Most commonly used bearing is metal on polyethylene.

Polymethyl methacrylate (PMMA) is used to fix the cemented components in bone.

Hybrid hips are now popular which use cement less acetabular component and cemented femoral component.

Relevant Anatomy

The knee is a hinge joint, which provides support for the body.

Osteology

Distal femur contributes to the knee joint in the form of two rounded ends called condyles of the femur. The medial condyle is larger in surface area than the lateral condyle. Anteriorly, the condyles merge to form the articular surface for the patella. Distal femur provides attachment for anterior cruciate ligament (ACL), posterior cruciate ligament (PCL), tibial collateral ligament and fibular collateral ligament. The femoral condylar epiphysis is present at birth and ossification of distal femur is complete by 20 years age.

Proximal Tibia The condyles of tibia are widened platforms for articulation with the condyles of femur. The medial plateau is larger and concave while the lateral plateau is smaller, convex and higher. The two tibial condyles are separated by the intercondylar eminence. ACL attachment lies anteriorly on intercondylar eminence while PCL attachment site is more posteriorly. Tibial plateau has a posterior inclination of 10°. The proximal tibia has two tubercles: tibial tubercle, which is the site for patellar tendon insertion and Gerdy's tubercle which gives attachment to iliotibial band. The tibial condylar epiphysis is usually present at birth and completes ossification by the age of 20 years.

Patella is the largest sesamoid bone in the body. Its lateral facet is concave and larger while the medial facet is usually convex and smaller. Odd facet makes contact in extreme flexion. Patellofemoral contact is largest in 45° flexion. Patella acts as a fulcrum for quadriceps and protects the knee joint. Ossification centre for patella appears in the second year and closes at puberty.

Joint Tibiofemoral joint is a combination of a hinge, sliding and a gliding joint. It allows flexion, extension and slight rotation. The menisci are included within the synovial space of the tibiofemoral articulation whereas the cruciate ligaments are excluded. Within the synovium, there can be shelves or bands called *plicae* which are the remnants of membranes which separate the compartments of the knee during embryonic development. Three types of plicae can be present: the suprapatellar plica, the infrapatellar plica and the medial plica (medial plica often becomes symptomatic by getting caught between patella and medial femoral condyle).

Ligament The ligaments of the knee guide knee movements and provide stability. The medial collateral ligament (MCL) extends from the medial femoral condyle to the medial tibial condyle and has two parts. The superficial MCL is a broad, triangular ligament while the deep MCL blends intimately with capsule and also attaches to the medial meniscus. *Posterior oblique ligament* is the posterior portion of MCL located on the medial posterior corner. MCL resists the valgus angulation at the knee.

The lateral collateral ligament (LCL) is a cord like structure extending from the lateral femoral condyle to the fibula. The LCL resists the varus angulation. Other important lateral stabilising structures are popliteus tendon, arcuate ligament, iliotibial band and lateral head of gastrocnemius.

Anterior cruciate ligament (ACL) extends from the anterior intercondylar area of the tibia to the medial aspect of the intercondylar area of the lateral femoral condyle. It is 40mm × 10mm, extrasynovial and intra-articular. It has two bundles, the anteromedial which is tense in flexion and posterolateral which is tense in extension. ACL resists anterior displacement of tibia on the femur.

Posterior cruciate ligament (PCL) extends from the posterior intercondylar area of the tibia to the intercondylar surface of the medial femoral condyle. It measures 38 × 13mm on an average. PCL resists posterior displacement of the tibia on the femur.

Meniscofemoral ligaments are *ligament of Humphry* anterior to PCL and *ligament of Wrisberg* posterior to PCL. These ligaments extend from posterior aspect of the lateral meniscus to embrace PCL.

Meniscotibial ligaments or coronary ligaments attach menisci to tibia. The lateral and medial patellar retinacula are continuations of fascia lata and quadriceps tendon respectively. Retinaculae reinforce anterolateral and anteromedial aspects of knee capsule and merge with it.

Menisci

Menisci are crescent shaped fibrocartilages, which deepen the articular surfaces for load transmission, reduce stresses on the joint surfaces, provide stability and function to transmit load and absorb shock. Menisci are attached to borders of tibia by coronary ligaments. Each meniscus has an anterior, a middle and a posterior horn. Only outer one-fourth of the meniscus is vascularized (red zone) while the inner three-fourth is avascular (white zone). Menisci are pushed back in flexion and pushed forward in extension.

Medial meniscus is "C" shaped and is wider posteriorly and anteriorly. It inserts anterior to ACL anteriorly and anterior to PCL posteriorly. Medial meniscus is less mobile than lateral meniscus.

Lateral meniscus is more circular. It inserts posterior to ACL anteriorly and anterior to posterior horn of medial meniscus posteriorly. Lateral meniscus has weaker attachment to lateral capsule and has deficient attachment where popliteus tendon passes through the capsule. Since the lateral meniscus is less firmly attached to the capsule and freer to move about, it often escapes injury.

The order of arrangement of ligamentous structures and meniscus of the knee on the tibial plateau is, from before backwards:

- Anterior horn of medial meniscus
- ACL
- Anterior horn of lateral meniscus
- Posterior horn of lateral meniscus
- Posterior horn of medial meniscus
- PCL

(From anterior to posterior the mnemonic to remember the attachments is *Medical College Lahore, Lahore Medical College*).

Muscles

Extensors Quadriceps is the major extensor of knee and consists of four parts: rectus femoris, vastus lateralis, vastus medialis and vastus intermedius. Quadriceps is supplied by branches of femoral nerve (L_2–L_4). Tensor fascia lata also acts as extensor of the knee. It is supplied by the superior gluteal nerve.

Flexor Medial hamstrings flex and internally rotate the knee. These include gracilis, semitendinosus and semimembranosus. While branches of obturator nerve supply gracilis, the other two are supplied by the sciatic nerve.

Lateral hamstring, namely biceps femoris flexes and externally rotates the knee; the sciatic nerve supplies the biceps.

Posterior muscles, which flex the knee, are gastrocnemius, plantaris and popliteus.

Nerves Tibial nerve lies medially in the popliteal fossa and supplies branches to the two heads of gastrocnemius and branch to soleus. Common peroneal nerve lies laterally in the popliteal fossa, winds around the fibular neck and passes through peroneus longus. In the surgical correction of flexion deformity of the knee, the nerve must be released especially at origin of peroneus longus to prevent tethering of nerve during extension and subsequent palsy.

Vessels Popliteal artery gives medial (superior and inferior), lateral (superior and inferior), and middle genicular branches, anterior tibial branch and then continues as posterior tibial artery. Peroneal artery is a branch of posterior tibial artery or less commonly the popliteal artery.

Evaluation of a Patient with Knee Symptoms

History in a patient with knee symptoms should elicit the information about the age, chronicity and the type of symptoms. Pain and swelling are the two most common complaints in disorders of the knee. Other symptoms can be feeling of giving way, locking, crepitus and stiffness of the knee.

With pain as the principle complaint, information should be elicited about the onset (acute or insidious), location and any antecedent trauma. Mechanism of injury is a key factor. Pivoting injury associated with a "pop" inside the knee and swelling in a sports person suggests ACL injury. A twisting injury to the knee with a history of locking of the knee suggests a meniscal tear. A dashboard injury to proximal tibia pushing it backwards suggests injury to PCL. A valgus and a varus force may lead to MCL and LCL injury respectively.

Location of pain gives a clue about the etiology. Pain over tibial tuberosity in an adolescent suggests Osgood Schlatter's disease while pain over patellar tendon/tibial tuberosity in an adult basketball or volleyball player suggests an overuse syndrome–"jumper's knee". Retropatellar pain or pain on either side of patella which gets worse with prolonged sitting or stair climbing suggests patellofemoral pain. Pain in popliteal fossa is commonly seen in synovitis especially in osteoarthritis patients. Location of pain at specific sites suggests the diagnosis of bursitis or tendinitis.

When a history of swelling is present, its onset, progression, history of waxing /waning and associated symptoms should be inquired about. A progressive swelling in a growing child with sudden history of increase in pain and swelling and inability to walk may suggest pathological fracture.

History of pain and swelling with progressive stiffness and pain on attempted movements suggests inflammatory arthritis of the knee. History of constitutional symptoms, involvement of other joints and history of iritis / iridocyclitis, urethritis, diarrhoea or sexual contact should be enquired about when relevant (as in Reactive Arthritis).

Examination Inspection of the knee must be carried out with both the lower limbs exposed from groin downwards for ready comparison. Gait of the patient should be observed, as should be any swelling in the region of knee. Any muscle wasting (especially in the region of vastus medialis) should be noted. Alignment of the knee should be noted (normally 5°–7° valgus is present). Presence of any flexion deformity or genu recurvatum should be noted.

During palpation, all the bones (patella, distal femur and proximal tibia) and medial and lateral joint line should be palpated for tenderness. Tibial tuberosity and adductor tubercle should also be palpated for tenderness. Palpation should also try to ascertain the presence of any bony swelling (such as exostoses). Palpation should assess the soft tissue status such as synovial hypertrophy (doughy feel), tenderness in region of MCL and LCL attachment, patellar tendon, quadriceps, pes anserinus, biceps femoris, iliotibial tract and peroneal nerve. Menisci can be evaluated for tear by a variety of tests available. Special tests are also available to assess the integrity of ACL, PCL and other supporting structures around the knee.

Range of motion, both active as well as passive, should be carefully tested. Flexion (normal 0°–135°), extension (normal 0°–10° hyperextension) and rotations (normal up to 10° of internal and external rotation from neutral) are tested. Any pain, spasm, crepitus or locking is noted.

A distal neurovascular examination is done in all cases.

Investigations

Radiographic Examination

Normally anteroposterior (AP), lateral and patellar (skyline or sunrise) views (Fig. 18.1a) constitute the standard radiographs of the knee. AP view should be taken in weight bearing position to accurately assess deformity and instability. Special radiographs include intercondylar notch view (AP in Flexion), Rosenberg view (flexion weight-bearing PA for early arthritis) (Fig. 18.1b) and weight bearing lower extremity view on (51") long films to measure mechanical and anatomic axes. In addition stress views can be taken to evaluate the instability or ligamentous injuries.

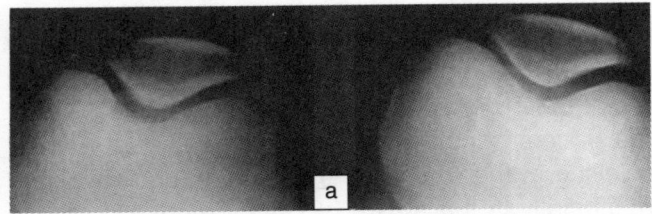

Fig. 18.1a. Skyline view of both patellae

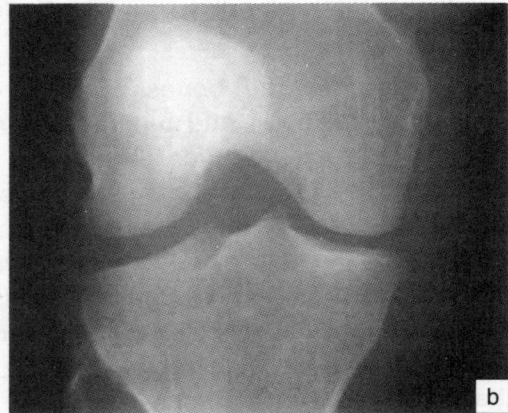

Fig. 18.1b. Rosenberg view (X-ray in flexion)

Computerised tomography is particularly useful for bony pathology, intraarticular fractures and for evaluating patellofemoral disorders.

Bone Scan can detect Osteochondritis, subtle arthritis and document the extent of involvement of the joint by the pathology.

Magnetic Resonance Imaging is an invaluable investigation to evaluate the intra articular structures (ACL, PCL, menisci), MCL, synovial dis-

eases and osteonecrosis. Even small effusion can be diagnosed early with MRI.

Arthroscopy is rarely used for only diagnostic purposes. The advent of arthroscopy has made the diagnosis and treatment of meniscal pathologies, ACL and PCL pathologies, synovial plicae and other synovial pathologies, articular cartilage pathologies and loose bodies within the joint extremely easy.

Congenital and Developmental conditions

1. Bipartite Patella is the result of failure of ossification of the superolateral facet of the patella. It may be seen as a separate fragment superolaterally and may be confused with a fracture. However, it is often an incidental finding without any history of antecedent trauma. It is non-tender clinically, is often bilateral, has smooth margins and the edge is cortical bone unlike a patellar fracture (the edges are irregular and are cortical-cancellous bone).

2. Bow Legs and Genu Varum Normally infants have symmetric bowing of the legs which starts changing to genu valgum or knock knees after the age of 1.5 years and evolves completely into knock knees by 2.5 years. The valgus then gradually reduces to physiological valgus by 4 years.

Thus genu varum in children less than 2 years of age is physiological and needs no treatment.

Pathological conditions which can cause genu varum and/or bow legs include internal tibial torsion, osteogenesis imperfecta, rickets, trauma, osteochondromas and Blount's disease.

3. Internal Tibial Torsion Internal tibial torsion leads to apparent bow legs or genu varum when the child walks with the knees forward and the feet rotated externally. Examination reveals internal tibial torsion. Most cases resolve by 4 years of age. Apparent bowleg deformity disappears with resolution of tibial torsion.

4. Blount's Disease (Tibia Vara) is a disease of unknown etiology that causes progressive bowing of the leg due to a disorder of the posteromedial tibial physis. It is particularly common in blacks and hispanic, obese male children. The disease can occur as early as 2 to 3 years of age. The disorder can be unilateral (in adolescents; less severe variety) or bilateral (in infants; more severe variety). Diagnosis is based on radiographs which show decreased medial tibial physeal growth with resultant metaphyseal–diaphyseal angle abnormality (Fig. 18.2). Drennan's metaphyseal-diaphyseal angle is measured between a line joining metaphyseal beaks and a line perpendicular to the long axis of the tibia. An angle more than 11° is abnormal.

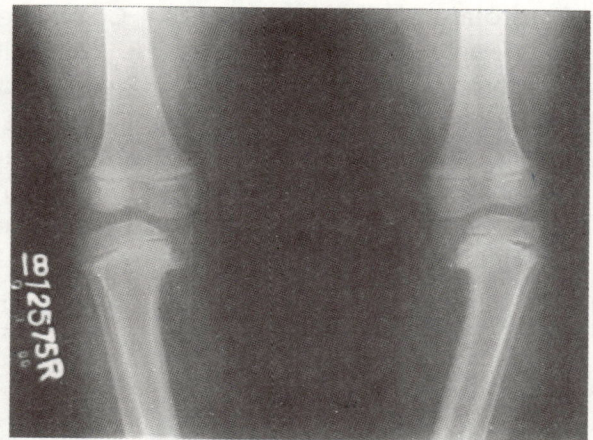

Fig. 18.2. X-rays showing characteristic beaking of proximal medial tibia and increased metaphyseo diaphyseal angle in Blount's disease

Later on, radiographs show distortion of medial articular surface and fusion of the physis. A progressive angular deformity develops as the lateral growth plate continues growing while the medial side is tethered. The characteristic defect on the posteromedial part of tibial articular surface is best shown by *Siffert-Katz sign* (rocking in flexion of knee) and also on arthrography.

Treatment of Blount's disease is based on the age and stage of the disease. Mild cases may spontaneously improve. Severe cases need tibial osteotomy to realign the extremity and reduce the load on medial tibial plateau. Osteotomy can be performed in the metaphyseal areas of tibia, intraepiphyseally or at both the sites. Physisplasty and cartilage autografting are the latest techniques being used.

Rickets may lead to bow legs due to development of soft bones, which bow with the load of weight bearing.

Children with hypophosphatemic rickets (X-linked dominant) are often short and have bilateral symmetric bowing of legs. Treatment is with phosphates and massive doses of vitamin D supplements but it has little effect on bowing. Surgical correction may be required if the bowing is severe.

Treatment of Genu Varum is reassurance in cases with physiological genu varum. Other cases should be investigated for underlying pathology. Bracing (*Mermaid Splints*) was tried in the past but has been given up now. Surgical treatment is needed if the intercondylar distance at the knee is more than 8 cm. A tibial osteotomy below the tibial tubercle with removal of lateral based wedge and fibular osteotomy is the procedure performed.

5. Genu Valgum

Children between 2 to 6 years age can have a valgus angle of up to 15 degrees as a normal physiological phenomenon. Pathological genu valgum is associated with trauma, infection, renal osteodystrophy (most common cause of bilateral genu valgum), and tumours (osteochondromas) It may often be idiopathic (Fig. 18.3). Apparent genu valgum may be caused by external tibial torsion though the latter condition is uncommon. Genu valgum, if severe, may be associated with recurrent dislocations of patella (due to increased Quadriceps–"Q" angle–formed between a line joining ASIS to middle of patella and another line joining middle of patella to tibial tuberosity) and flat foot.

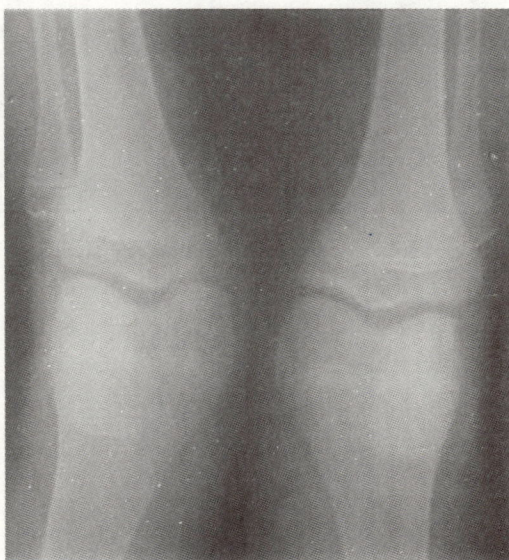

Fig. 18.3. X-rays showing bilateral genu valgum

Conservative treatment with shoe wedges, (mermaid) splints and braces is ineffective. Surgery should be considered if the tibiofemoral angle (angle between the long axis of tibia and the long axis of femur) is more than 15–20 degrees or the inter-malleolar distance is more than 10 cm. Hemiepiphysiodesis or stapling of medial epiphysis can be done for severe deformities before completion of growth. A supracondylar medial close wedge femoral osteotomy can be done at any age to correct the deformity. Care should be taken to avoid injury to common peroneal nerve by stretching while correcting severe genu valgum deformities.

6. Bowing of tibia can be of three types

a) **Posteromedial** (Fig. 18.4a) is commonly associated with calcaneovalgus foot as both arise from abnormal uterine positioning. Spontaneous correction is the rule and tibial osteotomy is not indicated.

b) **Anteromedial** bowing is typically caused by congenital absence of fibula with or without the absence of lateral rays (Fig. 18.4b,c). It is the most common congenital skeletal deformity in the leg. It is commonly associated with ankle instability, equino-varus foot, tarsal coalition and femoral shortening. Significant limb length discrepancy (LLD) is commonly associated with this disorder. A Syme's amputation is often performed in these cases in view of severe LLD.

c) **Anterolateral bowing of tibia** Commonest cause of anterolateral bowing is the congenital pseudarthrosis of the tibia (Fig. 18.4d). About 50% patients have associated neurofibromatosis. Dysplasia, sclerosis and cystic changes are seen in the tibia. Ipsilateral fibula is also commonly affected. Congenital pseudarthrosis is classified into 6 types of Boyd. They are:

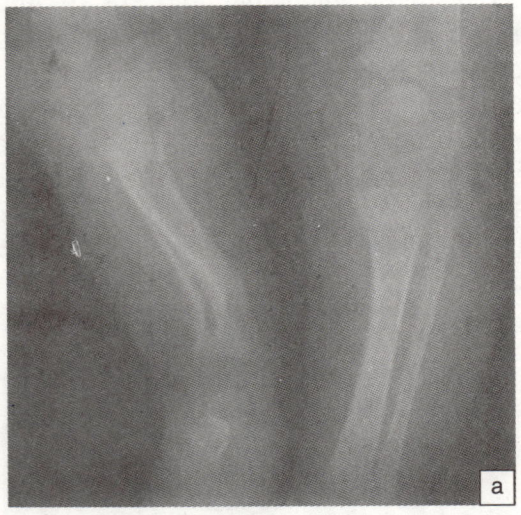

Fig. 18.4a. Posteromedial bowing of tibia

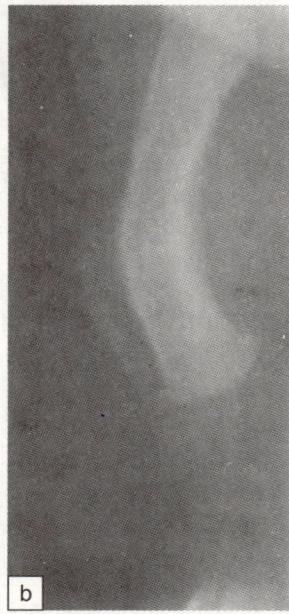

Fig. 18.4b. Antero medial bowing of tibia
(Note absence of fibula)

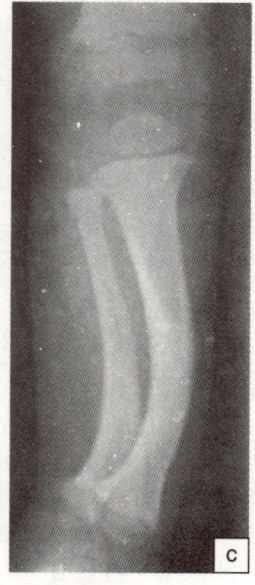

Fig. 18.4c. Antero medial bowing of tibia

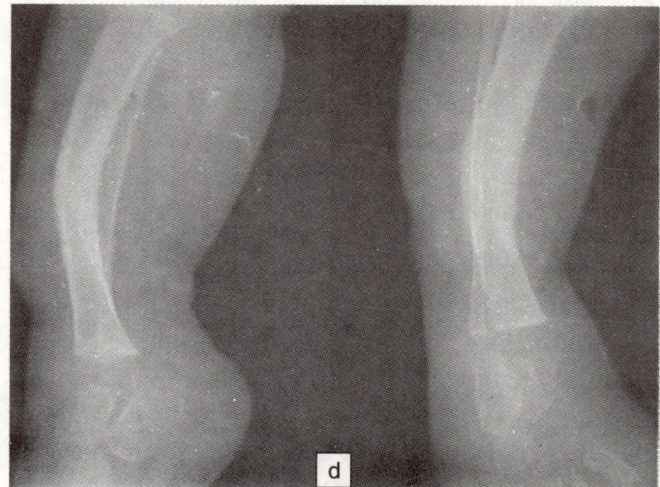

Fig. 18.4d. Anterolateral bowing of tibia

Boyd Classification of congenital pseudarthrosis of tibia

Type I: Anterior bowing and defect in tibia

Type II: Anterior bowing and hourglass constriction of tibia
Fracture develops before 2 years of age.

Type III: Intraosseous cyst gives rise to fracture which occasionally is seen at birth

Type IV: Sclerotic bone leads to stress fracture

Type V: Associated with dysplastic fibula (Fig 18.5a-b)

Type VI: Intraosseous neurofibroma / schwannoma.

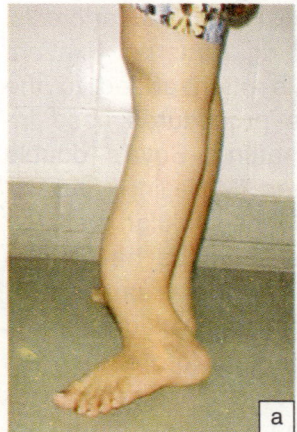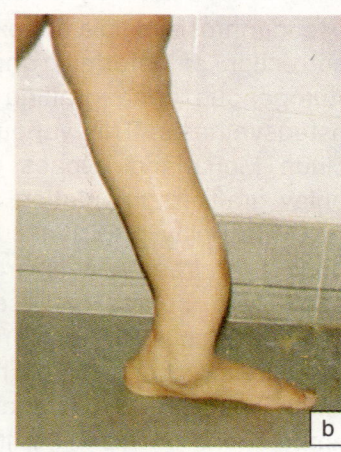

Fig. 18.6a,b. Clinical photographs of a patient with congenital pseudarthrosis of tibia. Note the antero-lateral bowing at the junction of middle and lower thirds of leg

at the junction of middle and lower thirds of the leg (Fig. 18.6c).

All children with any variety of this disorder need treatment. If anterolateral bowing is present without fracture, protective bracing is indicated. Corrective osteotomy of anterolateral bowing should not be done because it often leads to pseudarthrosis. McFarland posterior bypass grafting may be used in high risk patients (sclerotic bone, hourglass constriction of tibia).

Prognosis is worse in children with a fracture at a younger age, especially before 3 years. The tendency to fractures decreases with age. If the first tibial fracture occurs at or after 8 years of age, it may heal following plaster immobilisation with or without bone grafting. Principles of treatment of

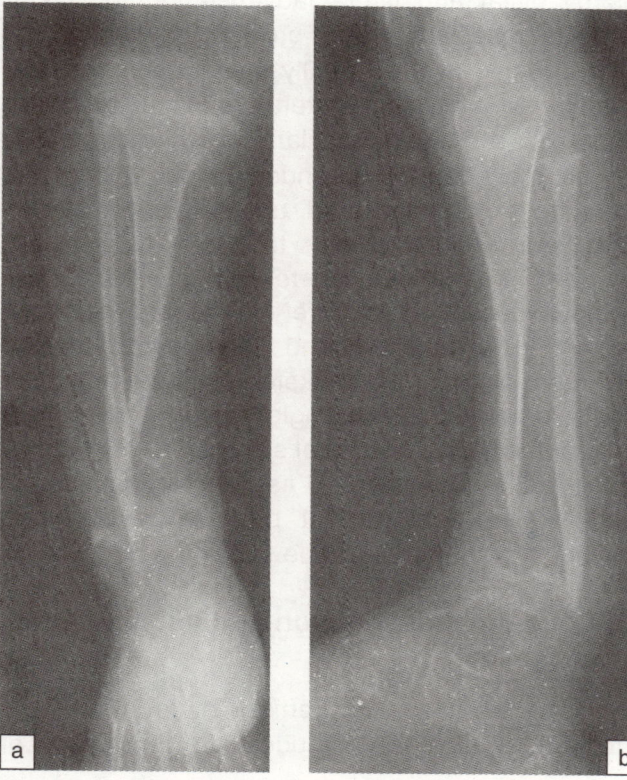

Fig. 18.5a,b. Congenital pseudarthrosis of tibia (Boyd Type V). Note the dysplastic fibula

Clinical features include

- Anterolateral bowing of the tibia ± fibula (Fig. 18.6a,b)

- Patient presents with pseudarthrosis usually by 2 years of age (sometimes at birth)

- Limb length discrepancy (sometimes marked)

- Varus deformity of the ankle

- Characteristic location of the pseudarthrosis is

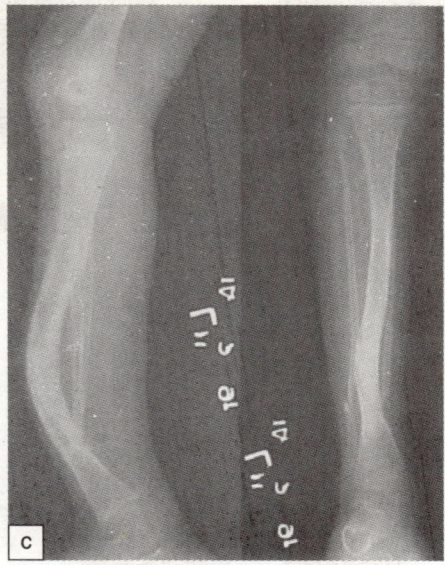

Fig. 18.6c. X-rays of the patient shown in figure 18.6a,b

pseudarthrosis of tibia are excision of pseudarthrosis, correction of deformity and rigid internal fixation. Autogenous bone grafting is often added to the osteosynthesis. The various procedures used include McFarland bypass grafting; Boyd's double onlay graft, fragmentation and IM nailing, and, IM nail with onlay graft. Vascularised fibular graft (on pedicle or free) and Ilizarov methods have been used with some success in the treatment of pseudarthrosis. However, repeated failed attempts at reconstruction and/or marked (more than 18 cms) limb length discrepancy are indications for amputation. Surgical treatment is not often successful in this condition and the parents should be counselled about the ultimate need for an amputation if necessary.

7. Congenital and habitual dislocation of Patella

Congenitally dislocated patella presents at birth. The primary defect lies in the vastus lateralis (muscle and fascia), vastus intermedius and the iliotibial band. These structures are contracted and result in dislocated patella. When the patella stays dislocated, the knee does not extend from the flexed position. The treatment is surgical release of iliotibial band and lateral retinaculum, mobilisation and recession of vastus lateralis from patella along with excision of any fibrotic bands in vastus lateralis or intermedius. Vastus medialis is transferred distally and laterally.

Habitual dislocation of patella is a condition where patella dislocates every time the knee is flexed and reduces with extension. Patients often present with a clicking sensation on flexion and extension of the knee. The child may keep the knee flexed and patella permanently dislocated because of the pain.

Palpation of the patella which is displaced laterally clinches the diagnosis (Fig. 18.7a). An ossified patella in an older child makes the diagnosis straightforward on x-ray of the knee. In cases with severe tightness, the tibia may be subluxed laterally on x-rays (Fig. 18.7b).

Treatment is release of the tight lateral structures and proximal realignment of the extensor apparatus by distal and lateral advancement of vastus medialis muscle. Other procedures, which can be performed in a skeletally immature patient are Campbell's procedure (lateral retinacular release along with a medial capsular flap which is passed around the quadriceps tendon to pull it medially. The flap is then sutured upon itself), Galeazzi procedure (semitendinosus tendon is used to pull the patella and patellar tendon medially), and Roux-Goldthwait procedure (lateral half of patellar tendon is detached and reattached medial to the medial half). In a skeletally mature patient with an increased Q angle, distal realignment procedures (such as Hauser's procedure-osteotomy of the tibial tuberosity and its transfer distally and medially) with or without proximal realignment procedures should be done.

8. Congenital dislocation and subluxation of the knee

The spectrum of congenital dislocation and subluxation of knee includes, in the order of

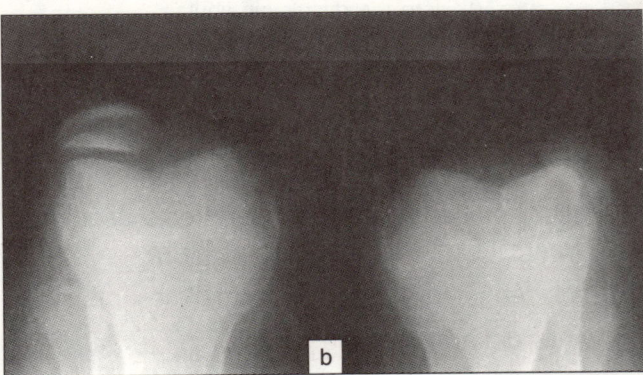

Fig. 18.7.   (a) Bilateral habitual dislocation of patellae showing lateral displacement (b) Skyline view

increasing severity, congenital hyperextension, congenital subluxation and congenital dislocation.

Hyperextension is frequently normally present at birth in breech babies but may also be present along with subluxation and dislocation.

Subluxation is more common than dislocation. Difference from dislocation can be appreciated on x-rays (Fig. 18.8a). The subluxated knee may have up to 20–40 degrees of flexion. The prognosis is better than congenital dislocation.

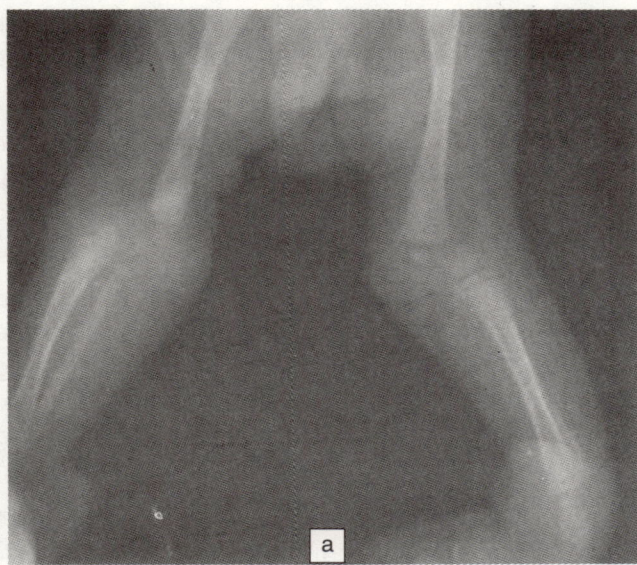

Fig. 18.8a. Bilateral congenital dislocation of the knee

Congenital dislocation is characterised by anterior displacement of tibia on femur with complete loss of contact between the two. The tibia is usually internally rotated and often laterally displaced. Associated congenital anomalies may be present in 60% of patients with congenital dislocation of the knee. Children with Arthrogryposis multiplex congenita often have associated dislocation of knee (Fig. 18.8b).

Children with congenital hyperextension/dislocation of knee should be thoroughly evaluated for congenital dislocation of hip.

Treatment of hyperextension and subluxation should begin soon after birth and consists of manipulation (passive flexion of knee) followed by plaster cast. Casts are changed every week till 90° flexion is achieved. Splintage is continued after that to prevent recurrences.

Dislocated knee is treated by open reduction and release of contracted quadriceps and its lengthening by V-Y plasty. Anterior capsule is released

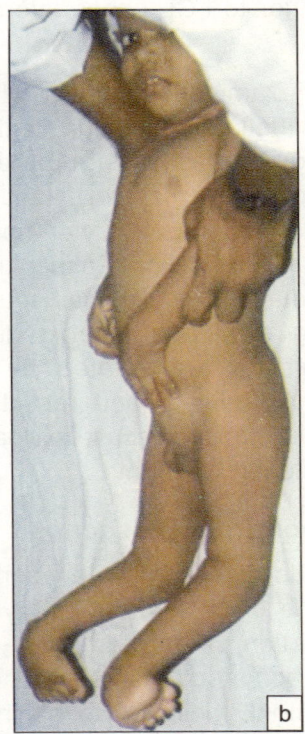

Fig. 18.8b. Child with bilateral congenital knee dislocation. Note the bilateral congenital talipes equinovarus of feet.

and collateral ligaments are freed if required. The knee is reduced and flexed to 90° and immobilised.

Prognosis of knee dislocations which need open reduction is not good and movements more than 90° flexion are seldom obtained.

9. Discoid Meniscus

The normal menisci are semilunar in shape and wedge shaped in cross section. Sometimes the abnormal development of the lateral meniscus (or very rarely medial meniscus) leads to formation of a discoid (or rounded) meniscus. Discoid shape reduces the normal cupping function of the meniscus, may cause instability, results in hypermobility and increased incidence of tear of the menisci. Males and females are equally affected. Usually unilateral, the disorder can sometimes be bilateral.

Clinically, the patient presents with loud clicking over the lateral meniscus during movements of the knee. Usually the clicking is painless but sometimes it may be associated with aching or effusion. The knee may sometimes give way during walking or running. A discoid meniscus may undergo degeneration and form a meniscal cyst, which usually presents along the lateral joint line just anterior to LCL (when lateral meniscus is discoid).

Radiological examination shows widening of the joint space in the lateral compartment (upto 11mm). Other findings are squaring of lateral femoral condyle, cupping of lateral tibial plateau and hypoplastic lateral intercondylar spine. MRI and arthroscopy are diagnostic. Treatment is not indicated for asymptomatic discoid meniscus. Significant and disabling symptoms arising due to tear in discoid meniscus are treated by arthroscopic debridement of the tear and resection of central portion of discoid meniscus to leave behind a roughly semilunar remnant.

10. Osteochondritis Dissecans

Osteochondritis dissecans is a poorly understood disorder of the distal femoral condyle ossification centre. A portion of the articular cartilage and subchondral bone softens, shears or separates. Though commonly believed to be the disorder of young adults, it occurs not infrequently in children between 10 and 15 years of age. It occurs three times more commonly in males as compared to females. It occurs infrequently in adults. The lateral intercondylar portion of the medial femoral condyle is most commonly involved. Lesion may also occur in dome of talus, patella, capitellum and the femoral head. The causes implicated are trauma, ischemia or abnormal epiphyseal ossification.

Clinically the patient presents with activity-related pain, localised tenderness, stiffness and swelling with or without mechanical symptoms.

Radiological examination usually clinches the diagnosis. Plain x-rays show an irregular fragment of the surface outlined by a radiolucent area. Tangential views such as intercondylar notch view can evaluate the condyles and show the lesion well.

MRI can delineate the lesion very well and show whether underlying bone is involved and whether the overlying cartilage has actually separated.

Arthroscopy is an extremely useful tool for diagnosis and is also used for treatment in most cases.

Poor prognostic factors include sclerosis of underlying bone, greater age and lateral condyle lesions.

Treatment Young children with asymptomatic disease need no treatment as in most of these

patients the disease undergoes spontaneous healing. Preadolescent children (< 15 years) with symptoms, where diagnosis is made before the articular cartilage fractures, can be treated in a cylinder cast for 6–12 weeks. The lesion heals in most cases following immobilisation. Conservative treatment is likely to fail in skeletally mature patients and in large lesions especially those associated with cartilage separation or displacement. Surgical treatment in these cases includes drilling with multiple holes, fixation of large fragments and bone grafting of large lesions. Surgical excision of the defect with drilling of the base can be done for separated fragments but the results in these cases are not good.

11. Osgood Schlatter's Disease

11. Osgood Schlatter's Disease is the osteochondritis or fatigue failure of the tibial apophysis of the tubercle in a growing child due to traction by extensor mechanism.

Clinically, it presents typically in a 10 to 15 year old boy. Symptoms vary from mild ache at the tubercle to severe pain. Pain is worse during climbing up or down the stairs, running or jumping. There may be a soft tissue swelling over the tibial tubercle due to the formation of a bursa. Tibial tubercle is tender on palpation.

Radiological examination shows soft tissue swelling anterior to the tubercle and thickening of the patellar tendon. Fragmentation and irregularity of the tibial tubercle apophysis is seen in older children (Fig. 18.9). Often separate free frag-

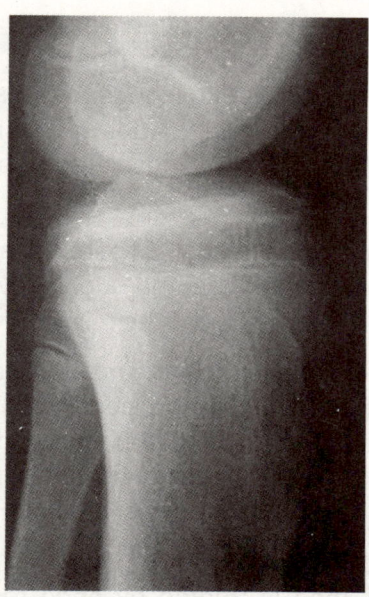

Fig. 18.9. Radiologic appearance of tibial tuberosity in Osgood Schlatter's disease

ments of bone due to heterotopic formation are seen anterior and superior to the tubercle.

Treatment in most cases is expectant, as the disease is self-limiting. Most cases resolve spontaneously around 15 years of age when fusion of the tubercle occurs.

When symptoms are severe and interfere with patient's activities, immobilisation in a cylinder cast for 6–8 weeks may allow the patient to return to the normal activities. Very rarely, late excision of the separate ossicles may be required with peg grafting and therapeutic fusion of the tibial tuberosity apophysis (Bosworth procedure).

12. Popliteal cyst (Baker's cyst)

Popliteal cyst is a synovial cyst which arises from the semimembranosus bursa, from joint capsule or from underneath the medial head of gastrocnemius. In children it most typically arises from semimembranosus bursa, is filled with gelatinous fluid and has a lining of fibrous tissue, synovial cells and/or inflammatory cells. In children the swelling is *always* lateral to the semitendinosus. Popliteal cyst is usually asymptomatic but very large cysts can cause discomfort. The cyst always **transilluminates** unlike a vascular anomaly or a tumour.

In adults, the popliteal cysts are associated with rheumatoid arthritis or osteoarthritis of the joint and are often herniations from the joint.

Treatment of asymptomatic popliteal cysts is observation especially in asymptomatic cysts, which are not increasing in size. Most cysts remain asymptomatic while some may regress.

If a popliteal cyst continues to enlarge or causes symptoms, it can be excised.

13. Quadriceps Contracture

Quadriceps contracture can occur following injections in childhood when the intramuscular drugs are administered in quadriceps. The other causes of quadriceps contracture are congenital, arthrogryposis multiplex congenita, chronic osteomyelitis of femur, fracture shaft of femur and scarring due to surgery.

Clinically, the patient has limitation of flexion and inability to squat. Quadriceps wasting is present in all cases.

Treatment in most cases should begin with physiotherapy. Resistant cases require excision of cicatrised muscle and V-Y plasty of the quadriceps.

Inflammatory Arthritis of Knee

Pyogenic Arthritis

Pyogenic arthritis of the knee can occur by hematogenous route, by contiguous spread from osteomyelitis of distal femur (as distal femoral metaphysis is partly intra-articular) and directly by penetrating injuries. Staphylococcus aureus is the most common pathogen.

Clinically, the patient presents with acute onset of constitutional symptoms and pain and swelling over the affected knee. The diagnosis is easy due to the superficial location of the joint. The affected knee is warm, tender, may be erythematous and all the attempted movements are painfully restricted. The joint assumes an attitude of flexion (to increase the joint capacity to accommodate pus).

Radiological examination may be normal initially. The neglected cases may show areas of destruction in the articulating bones and loss of articular cartilage (seen as narrowing of the joint space). Bony or fibrous ankylosis may occur in advanced cases without treatment.

Laboratory investigations reveal polymorphonuclear leucocytosis with raised erythrocyte sedimentation rate. Blood culture may sometimes isolate the offending organism.

Aspiration of the knee joint should be performed in all the cases where septic arthritis of the knee is suspected. It should be done under full aseptic precautions in the operation theatre. Aspirate should be sent for gram stain and culture and sensitivity studies. Aspiration of pus is an indication for immediate evacuation of pus either by arthrotomy or arthroscopically.

Treatment of suspected septic arthritis of the knee begins with the institution of parenteral antibiotics depending on the most prevalent sensitivity pattern of the likely pathogens.

Evacuation of pus, joint washout and closure of the joint over a drain is done in cases where diagnosis is confirmed on aspiration.

Evacuation of the pus and joint debridement and

lavage can be effectively done arthroscopically with considerably lesser morbidity as compared to arthrotomy.

Drainage of the joint through closed suction drainage is continued till the drainage stops and constitutional symptoms subside. The limb is splinted in plaster cylinder cast for the next 3 to 4 weeks and then mobilised.

In cases where the patient presents late and the joint has already been deformed and/or destroyed, joint debridement and arthrodesis can be done to provide a stable, pain free knee.

Tuberculosis of Knee Joint

Tuberculosis of the knee joint can begin in a juxta-articular (metaphyseal) location, in synovium or in the bones within the joint. It is always secondary to a primary focus elsewhere in the body. Though earlier common in children, it can be seen in adults nowadays with HIV becoming more and more common.

Clinically, the patient presents with pain, swelling and limp. Swelling is gradually progressive. Constitutional symptoms are often present. Night cries may be present.

Examination reveals marked quadriceps wasting, effusion, synovial thickening and marked painful restriction of the movements. Advanced cases may present with complete disorganisation of joint with destruction of ligaments manifested as *triple deformity* i.e. flexion, external rotation and posterior subluxation of tibia on the femur. Valgus deformity of the knee is often superadded.

If disease is not treated, discharging sinuses may form due to superficial location of the joint.

Radiological examination Plain x-rays show generalised osteoporosis and erosions (Fig. 18.10). Joint space gets diminished with progress of the disease and may get completely obliterated. Laboratory investigations reveal raised ESR. ELISA and/or PCR for the tubercular antigen performed on serum or synovial fluid may be positive.

Synovial biopsy is often required in the synovial type of disease where joint movements may be maintained for a long time. It can be done arthroscopically or by a small arthrotomy incision.

Treatment of tuberculosis of the knee begins with institution of antitubercular treatment. In early

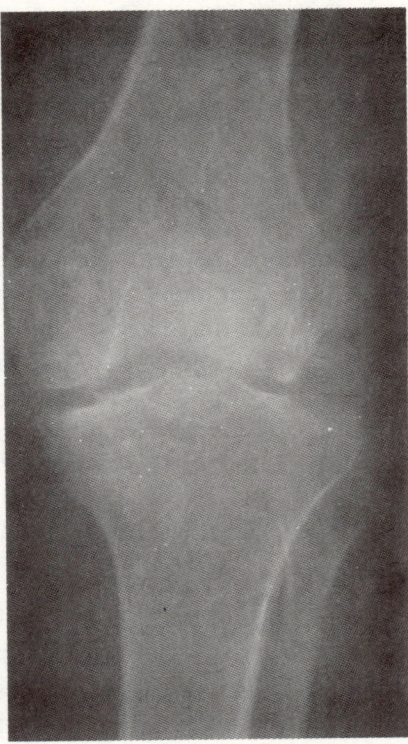

Fig. 18.10. X-rays showing tuberculosis of knee joint

cases with salvageable joints skin traction is applied to relieve pain and muscle spasm and prevent the occurrence of deformity. Once the acute pain and muscle spasm subside gradual mobilisation of the joint can be started. Weight bearing can be permitted gradually.

When the disease has destroyed the joint and useful movements are not expected, the deformity is corrected by traction and the limb is immobilised in cylinder plaster cast to achieve fibrous ankylosis of the knee in acceptable position. If the joint remains painful, deformed or unstable after healing of the disease, *Charnley's compression arthrodesis* is done to achieve painless, stable joint.

Other Inflammatory Arthritides Affecting Knee Joint

Rheumatoid Arthritis commonly affects the knee joints. Usually bilaterally symmetrical involvement occurs and patients are often unable to walk. Joints are swollen, painful and stiff. Wasting of quadriceps muscles is marked. Genu valgum and flexion deformities are common (Fig. 18.11a). Other joints are usually involved.

Radiographs show osteopenia, articular erosions and reduced joint space (Fig. 18.11b).

Treatment should begin with disease modifying anti rheumatic drugs (DMARD) and physiotherapy. Single joint involvement with preserved joint space and failure to respond to conservative treatment for 6 months is indication for synovectomy. Severe, advanced cases with compromised mobility of the patient benefit from total knee replacement.

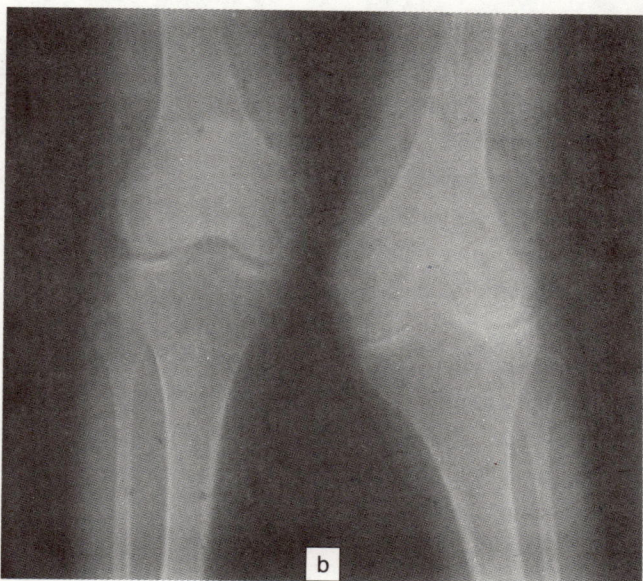

Fig. 18.11b. X-rays showing rheumatoid arthritis involving both knees. Note the bilateral genu valgum.

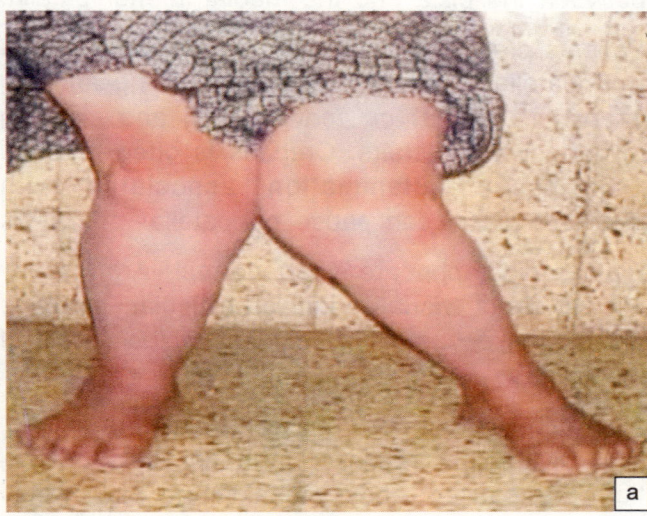

Fig. 18.11a. Clinical photographs of a patient with rheumatoid arthritis showing bilateral genu valgum

Ankylosing spondylitis, reactive arthritis and Reiter's disease often present with synovitis of bilateral knee joints. Treatment is aimed at the management of the underlying disease.

Clutton's Joints Clutton's joints are seen in tertiary syphilis. There is painless symmetrical effusion of both the knee joints. There is full range of knee movements. Patients usually have no complaints.

5 **S's** of Clutton's joints are: Symmetric, Seldom painful, swelling due to Syphylitic Synovitis.

X-rays are normal. Treatment is observation since this is a self-limiting condition.

Avascular Necrosis/Osteonecrosis

Avascular necrosis implies death of bone cells due to ischemia and is associated with vascular injury, fractures, thrombosis or systemic conditions such as alcoholism, steroid therapy or bone marrow disease. However, most cases are idiopathic. Avascular necrosis in the knee involves the medial femoral condyle.

Clinically patients, most commonly females over 50 years of age, present with acute onset of pain in the knee. Stiffness and swelling are often associated.

Radiographs are normal in the early stages. Later the radiographs show a lucent region of the subchondral bone with surrounding sclerosis. Secondary degenerative changes may occur.

MRI is extremely sensitive and picks up these lesions early and also depicts the extent of these lesions.

Bone Scan is also useful for early detection of the lesion in cases where plain radiographs are normal.

Arthroscopy allows direct visualisation of the articular involvement and allows assessment of the extent and severity.

Treatment of osteonecrosis is conservative initially. Restricted weight bearing and NSAIDs are useful in treatment.

Persistent symptoms need treatment by osteotomy or unicompartmental arthroplasty.

Anterior Knee Pain

Young patients often complain of pain in the anterior portion of the knee. The various causes responsible for anterior knee pain are shown in Table 18.1.

Table 18.1. Causes of anterior knee pain

1. Related to extensor mechanism
   Quadriceps tendon rupture
   Patellar tendon rupture
   Patellar tendinitis (Jumper's knee)
   Quadriceps tendinitis
2. Patellofemoral disorders
   Related to altered patellofemoral biomechanics
   Patellar instability
   Chondromalacia
   Excessive lateral pressure syndrome
   Abnormalities of patellar height
       i) patella alta
      ii) patella baja
   Patellofemoral arthritis
3. Bursitis
   Prepatellar bursitis
   Pes anserinus bursitis
4. Synovial plica (esp. medial synovial plica)
5. Anterior fat pad syndrome (Hoffa's syndrome)
6. Neuritis
   Saphenous neuritis

It is extremely important to be specific about the area of pain for accurate diagnosis of the cause of anterior knee pain. Examination for patellar instability and evaluation of extensor apparatus are mandatory. Local examination to rule out bursitis and neuritis are required. Arthroscopy, CT and/or MRI may be required in selected cases for accurate diagnosis.

Excessive Lateral Pressure Syndrome (ELPS)

Excessive lateral pressure syndrome results from tight lateral retinaculum with lateral tilting of the patella. Degeneration develops laterally on the patella and trochlea without any evidence of subluxation. The patient, usually female, presents with lateral knee pain especially while sitting and climbing stairs. Examination reveals lateral patellar tenderness and tightness.

Skyline radiographs of the knee show lateral sclerosis and narrowing of lateral patellofemoral joint space.

Treatment   Non operative treatment includes modification of activities, NSAIDs and strengthening exercises for vastus medialis oblique (VMO) muscle.

Persistent symptoms warrant lateral retinacular release.

Chondromalacia

Chondromalacia implies softening or degeneration of the articular cartilage of the patella. Chondromalacia can occur as a result of direct blow, excessive forces across the patellofemoral joint and patellofemoral instability or by friction between the plica and the medial inferior patella.

Patients present with activity related anterior knee (retropatellar) pain especially with sitting for long interval (*"Cinema" or "movie" sign*) and climbing up or down the stairs. Crepitus is often present. Soft tissue inflammation associated with chondromalacia can cause peripatellar pain.

Plain radiographs are often normal. Arthroscopy allows direct visualisation of articular cartilage and allows accurate assessment of the extent of the disease.

Treatment options for chondromalacia are limited. NSAIDs, weight reduction and activity modification are started early. Recalcitrant cases may need surgical treatment.

Macquet's osteotomy (elevation of tibial tuberosity to reduce pressures across patellofemoral joint), patelloplasty, patellectomy and patellar resurfacing have been described in selected cases.

Osteoarthritis of the knee joint

Osteoarthritis is the most common musculoskeletal problem in people over age of 50. It is the result of mechanical and biologic events, which lead to an imbalance between the degradation and synthesis of articular cartilage and subchondral bone. Unlike the hip, primary osteoarthritis of the knee is more common than secondary osteoarthritis in Indian patients. Osteoarthritis of the knee is common in females, obese patients and in people with over-use as well as under-use of the joint. Secondary osteoarthritis results from degenerative changes in a joint damaged by pre-existent disease such as infection, trauma etc.

Clinically, the patients present with pain, crepitus, swelling and stiffness of the joint. Pain is activity related initially but comes even on rest in the later stages of the disease. Deformities, especially flexion deformity, and genu varum (Fig. 18.12a) occur with progress of the disease (genu valgum

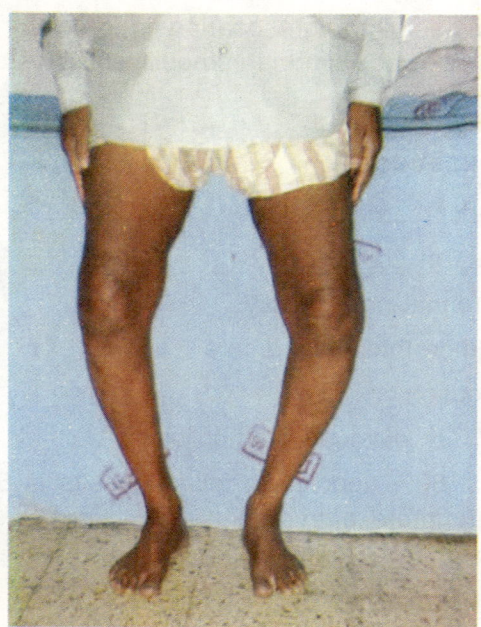

Fig. 18.12a. Clinical photograph of a patient with severe osteoarthritis of both knees with bilateral genu varum

is uncommon is primary osteoarthritis). Crepitations are present in most cases. Tenderness may be present over the joint. Variable degrees of inflammation may be seen in some cases.

Radiological examination reveals narrowing of the joint space, squaring of the condyles, subchondral sclerosis, osteophyte formation and occasionally subchondral cysts (Fig. 18.12b).

Treatment is conservative in early phases. Activity modification, weight reduction, patient education, ambulatory supports such as walking stick and exercises (including aerobic and occupational exercises) are important non pharmacologic mea-

sures. Paracetamol in dose up to 1 gm every 6 hours is the drug of choice. Opiates, NSAIDs, topical analgesics and chondroprotective agents (glucosamine, chondroitin sulphate) are other useful agents, which can be used judiciously. Intra articular injections of hyaluronic acid (5 injections with an interval of one week between two sequential injections) improve lubrication in the joint and benefit many patients.

Operative treatment is indicated for relief of pain, to correct mechanical derangement and to maintain and improve function.

Arthroscopic debridement is used to wash out the joint to remove products of cartilage degeneration, which cause chemical synovitis. In addition, torn menisci and degenerated articular cartilage can be debrided. The limitation of this procedure is that the relief is only short lasting and symptoms recur.

Osteotomy is done in proximal tibia (in genu varum) or distal femur (in genu valgum) to correct malalignment and relieve intraosseous hypertension (which causes rest pain). Osteotomy is best used in cases where only one compartment of the knee is mainly involved (e.g. medial compartment in the presence of genu varum deformity). The operation, by correcting malalignment unloads the arthritic compartment and allows redistribution of weight bearing forces to larger area of the joint surface. However, the relief after osteotomy may last for a variable period (7–8 years).

Arthrodesis is used to provide a painless, stable joint but at the cost of knee movements. It may be unacceptable to the patient as it is a significant disability in our society. At present, it can only be advised as salvage procedure for failed arthroplasty or when the patient is too poor to afford replacement arthroplasty.

Arthroplasty Total knee replacement (TKR) has yielded remarkably good results for relief of pain in patients with osteoarthritis. The main reason for performing TKR is relief of pain though it improves alignment and range of motion. The most commonly used knee joint designs nowadays are semiconstrained and rely on *both* the prosthetic design and the surrounding soft tissue envelope for stability. Contraindications to TKR are sepsis, neuropathic knee joint and non-functioning quadriceps.

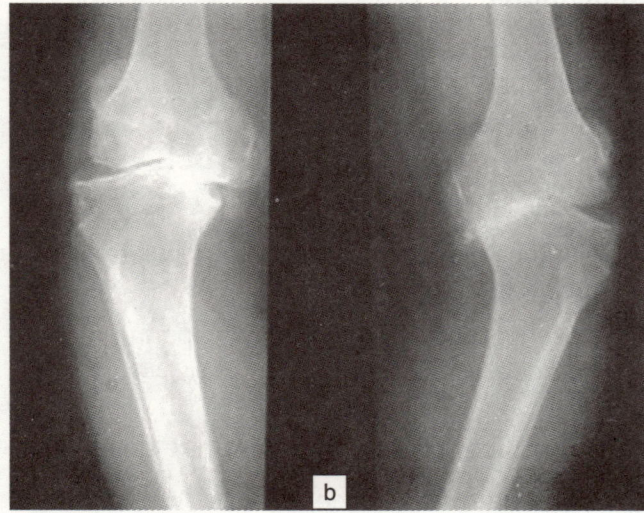

Fig. 18.12b. X-rays of patient with osteoarthritis both knees

Important Surgical Procedures on Knee

High Tibial Osteotomy (HTO)

Indications

1. Unicompartmental disease in an active patient less than 65 years of age
2. Stable knee ligaments
3. Flexion deformity less than 15°; at least 100° flexion possible
4. Patient motivated to undergo rigorous physiotherapy
5. Varus deformity less than 12°, valgus less than 15°
6. Radiographic evidence of joint space of at least 2mm of the involved compartment

Contraindications

1. Obese patient
2. Rheumatoid arthritis
3. Varus/Valgus deformity >15°
4. Patient not likely to participate in rehabilitation

Presence of patellofemoral arthritis is not a contraindication

Done proximal to tibial tuberosity.

Attempt is made to overcorrect the deformity to normal valgus of 5°–7°.

Technique

1. Coventry: lateral close wedge (1-mm resection equals 1° correction).
2. Macquet (Dome osteotomy) (Fig. 18.13)

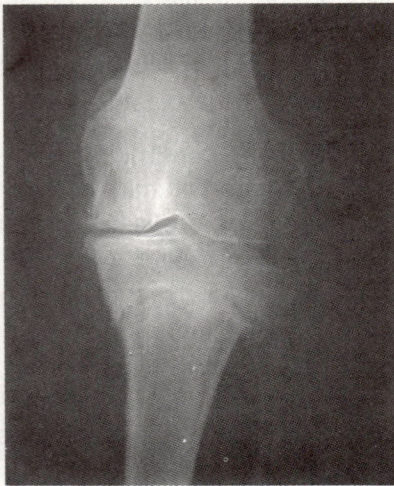

Fig. 18.13.   X-ray showing Dome high tibial osteotomy

Immediate full weight bearing in cylinder plaster cast is allowed. Limb is immobilised till osteotomy unites.

Complications

1. Under correction
2. Loss of correction
3. Peroneal nerve palsy
4. Compartment syndrome
5. Infection
6. DVT or pulmonary embolism

Results: 80% good to excellent results at 5 years but deteriorate after that.

Distal Femoral Osteotomy

Indications

1. Young, active patient with isolated lateral compartment arthritis.
2. Valgus 10°–15° or varus > 15°.

Technique

Medial close wedge supracondylar osteotomy (for valgus deformity)

Complications

1. Under/over correction
2. Peroneal nerve palsy
3. DVT or pulmonary thromboembolism

Arthrodesis

Indications

1. Most commonly for infected total knee arthroplasty in developed countries (Fig. 18.14).
2. Tubercular arthritis is the commonest indication in our country.
3. Septic arthritis
4. Neuropathic joint (though it is difficult to achieve fusion in these cases)
5. Absence of functioning quadriceps in any painful knee condition.

Contraindications

1. Ipsilateral hip or ankle disease
2. Not preferred for bilateral disease

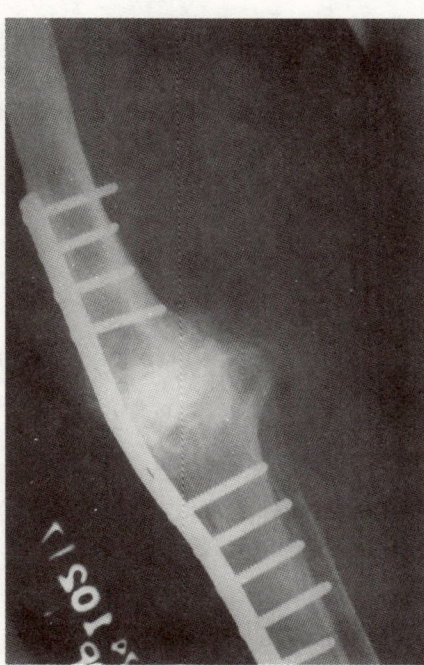

Fig. 18.14. Arthrodesis of the knee using compression plating

Technique

➤ Charnley's compression arthrodesis using Charnley's clamps

➤ Knee should be fused in 5°–10° flexion to allow ground clearance

➤ Healing takes 10–12 weeks.

Complications

1. Shortening

2. Malalignment

3. Pseudarthrosis

4. Strain on ipsilateral hip, ankle and on the spine

Knee Replacement

1. Unicompartmental

Indications Unicompartmental disease (alternative to H.T.O. in osteoarthritis).

Contraindications

• Deformities >10° varus or >15° valgus

• Incompetent cruciates

• Torn lateral meniscus (for medial compartment replacement)

• Rheumatoid arthritis.

Technique

• Femoral and tibial articulating surfaces in one compartment are resurfaced

• Both the cruciates are preserved

• Can be changed to tricompartmental TKR subsequently.

Complications

Under-correction and over-correction are associated with increased wear of component and accelerated degeneration of opposite (unresurfaced) compartment respectively.

2. Tricompartmental

Indications

To relieve pain and restore function in an arthritic knee (Fig, 18.15a,b).

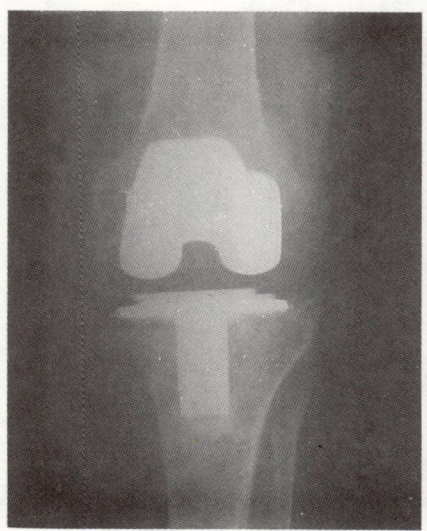 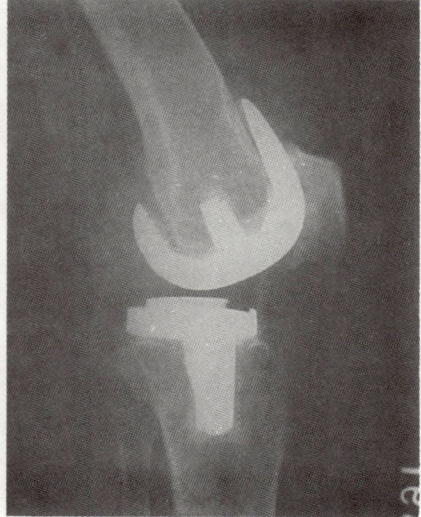

Fig.18.15a,b. AP and lateral X-rays following total knee arthroplasty

Contraindications

- Active Sepsis
- Absence of functional quadriceps
- Neuropathic joint.

Prosthesis design

- Commonly Bicondylar semiconstrained design
- Both Posterior cruciate ligament (PCL) retention and sacrificing designs are available.
- Metallic femoral component (with trochlear flange to articulate with patella) and a UHMW (ultra high molecular weight) polyethylene (PE) tibial component (usually with a metallic tibial tray) and UHMW PE patellar component.
- Present day most designs use bone cement (Polymethylmethacrylate) for fixation of all the components.
- Cementless femoral components have also been used with some success.

Complications

1. Infection
2. Neurovascular injury
3. DVT and Pulmonary thromboembolism
4. Femoral or tibial fractures
5. Patellar complications:

   maltracking, patella baja, fracture, loosening of patellar component.
6. Loosening of femoral or tibial component

Ankle

Relevant Anatomy

Ankle is a hinge joint between the box like frame, the "mortise", made by distal tibia and fibula and the dome of the talus, which fits like tenon into the mortise.

Osteology

Distal Tibia participates in the formation of ankle joint through the inferior quadrilateral surface, which articulates with the talus, and a pyramid shaped medial malleolus. Distal tibia is joined to the distal fibula through the tibio fibular syndesmosis, a ligamentous complex made of the anterior and posterior inferior tibiofibular ligaments, the interosseous ligament and the inferior transverse ligament.

The ossification centre for the medial malleolus appears at 7–8 years of age.

Talus Dome of talus articulates with distal tibia and fibula while its head articulates with navicular. Talus also articulates with calcaneus at the subtalar joint. Posteriorly, it has medial and lateral tubercle with the intervening groove for the flexor hallucis longus (FHL). The talar dome is wider anteriorly than posteriorly; hence the ankle is more stable in dorsiflexion than plantar flexion. No muscles are

attached to the talus; hence it has precarious blood supply.

Ossification centre for the talus appears in 7th fetal month.

Lateral Malleolus/Fibula Lateral malleolus extends distal to the medial malleolus. It gives attachment to the lateral ligament complex of the ankle. The ossification centre for the fibula appears at 18 months.

Joint The ankle is a hinge joint and allows only flexion and extension movements. The ankle has several important stabilising ligaments.

Ligaments

Deltoid Ligament is a strong fan-shaped ligament medially. It has a superficial (tibionavicular, tibiocalcaneal) and a deep part. The deep (tibiotalar) part is most important for stability.

Lateral Ligaments are three:

(i) Anterior talofibular ligament: is the key lateral ligamentous stabiliser and is the structure injured in ankle sprain,

(ii) Calcaneofibular; and

(iii) Posterior talofibular ligament.

Syndesmotic ligaments maintain the stability of

the distal tibiofibular joint and the width of the mortise. When these ligaments get injured, the fibula gets separated from the tibia, and the mortise widens with instability of the talus.

Muscles

Dorsiflexors are tibialis anterior, extensor hallucis longus, extensor digitorum longus and peroneus tertius. They are all in the anterior compartment of the leg and are innervated by the deep peroneal nerve.

Plantarflexors are the gastrocnemius, soleus, plantaris (all three in superficial posterior compartment of leg and supplied by tibial nerve), tibialis posterior, flexor hallucis longus and flexor digitorum longus (all three in deep posterior compartment of leg and supplied by tibial nerve); and, peroneus longus and peroneus brevis (both in lateral compartment and supplied by the superficial peroneal nerve).

Nerves

Tibial nerve (L_5, S_1, and S_2) passes behind the medial malleolus between the posterior tibial artery and flexor hallucis longus. It courses deep to flexor retinaculum and divides into medial (L_5) and lateral (L_5, S_1) plantar nerves and the medial calcaneal branches (S_1, S_2).

Deep peroneal nerve (L_4, L_5) crosses under the extensor retinaculum between the dorsalis pedis artery and extensor digitorum longus and innervates extensor digitorum brevis and supplies sensations to the first web space on the dorsum of the foot.

Superficial peroneal nerve (L_5, S_1) passes superficial to the extensor retinaculum to supply sensations to the dorsum of foot except over first web space (deep peroneal), lateral border of foot (sural) and lateral one and half toes (lateral plantar).

Sural nerve (S_1, S_2) is located halfway between lateral malleolus and lateral edge of tendo achilles and supplies sensation to lateral part of foot and heel.

Vessels

Anterior tibial artery along with deep peroneal nerve courses deep to extensor hallucis longus and becomes dorsalis pedis as it crosses in front of the ankle under extensor retinaculum.

Posterior tibial artery along with tibial nerve passes behind medial malleolus between flexor digitorum longus and flexor hallucis longus and divides into medial and lateral plantar arteries.

Evaluation of Patient with Ankle Disorder

Evaluation of patient with ankle disorder should take into account the age of the patient. Arthritis is more common in elderly people while ankle sprains and overuse syndromes are more common in younger patients. Tendo achilles disorders including rupture are typically common in middle aged patients.

The occupation of the patient is important with respect to the ligament and tendon disorders. Attempt should be made to elicit in the history the onset, chronicity, progression and waxing and waning, if any, of the symptoms. Localisation of pain and / or swelling is important for the diagnosis of the likely cause. In case of injury, the mechanism can provide a clue about the structures that might have been injured.

A past history of ankle sprain may provide a clue about the osteo-chondral lesion of the talar dome. History of catching or locking suggests peroneal tendon subluxation or dislocation or osteo-chondral injuries of the talus. History of loss of active movements following a bout of pain may suggest tendon disruptions while stiffness indicates the inflammatory (rheumatoid) or degenerative (osteoarthritis) disorder of the joint. Recurrent history of giving way suggests instability and detailed history should be taken to rule out ankle sprain, Charcot joint or fracture / dislocation of the ankle as a cause.

History of any neurological disorder and diabetes should be elicited in case of suspected neuropathic joint. Presence of burning sensation along with pain can suggest nerve entrapment or reflex sympathetic dystrophy.

On examination, gait of the patient should be carefully observed. Swelling, skin changes and any abnormal contours are looked for and recorded. Too many toes may be visible on inspection from behind in case of a tibialis posterior tendon rupture. Palpation of the malleoli as well as ligaments, tendons, anterior aspect of ankle joint and retrocalcaneal bursa is done to elicit tenderness.

Ankle movements are tested and recorded. Both dorsiflexion (normal 0°–20°) and plantarflexion (normal 0°–50°) are tested actively and passively.

A detailed neurovascular examination should be performed including the strength testing of the ankle dorsiflexors and plantarflexors.

Special Tests

1. Tests for integrity of lateral ligaments of ankle.

   a) *Talar tilt test* Performed by applying inversion stress to the ankle. Talus tilts abnormally (>10°, or 5° more than opposite side) in cases where both anterior talofibular and calcaneofibular ligaments are torn.

   b) *Anterior drawer's test* is used for testing integrity of anterior talofibular ligament. Anteriorly directed force is applied to the heel with ankle in plantar flexion (to relax calcaneofibular ligament) and abnormal anterior translation is noted. A comparison with opposite ankle is helpful.

2. Tests for integrity of syndesmotic ligaments

   a) Squeezing the calf causes pain at ankle (squeeze test) in case of disruption of syndesmosis.

   b) Abduction and external rotation of the ankle causes pain in case of syndesmosis disruption.

3. Tests for integrity of achilles tendon:

   Thompson's test Squeezing the calf (with the patient lying prone and feet beyond the edge of the table) does not cause plantar flexion in cases with tendo achilles rupture.

   Imaging Studies Standard ankle radiographs include the AP, lateral and the mortise view. Anteroposterior view is useful for evaluation of malleolar fractures and osteo-chondral fractures. Lateral view in useful to evaluate ankle subluxation or dislocation, talar neck fractures, fractures of anterior or posterior tibial margin and fibular fractures. Mortise view is done with the ankle in 15° internal rotation and it clearly shows the mortise. Mortise view is also useful to evaluate for disruption of the inferior tibiofibular syndesmosis. The following features suggest disruption of syndesmosis:

   a) Asymmetry of spaces on medial and lateral sides of talar dome (normally both are less than 4 mm and equal.)

   b) Less than 1 mm overlap between lateral edge of tibia and medial edge of fibula; and,

   c) A distance greater than 5 mm between tibia and fibula measured 1 cm above the tibial plafond (Tibiofibular clear space).

Stress Radiographs

Stress radiographs are useful for evaluation of the lateral ligaments. Stress anteroposterior x-ray is done while giving an inversion stress to the ankle. Talar tilt angle is measured between the tibial plafond and the talar dome. A comparison with the opposite ankle should also be done.

Anterior drawer stress radiograph is lateral radiograph of the ankle taken while applying a forward-directed force to talus. Anterior talar displacement is noted; comparison with the opposite ankle is helpful.

Bone scan can help in the diagnosis of reflex sympathetic dystrophy, infections and osteochondritis.

CT Scan can delineate bony pathology and is useful for plafond fractures, osteo-chondral fractures of talus, osteochondroma of talus and for evaluation of area of destruction in case of infection.

MRI is useful for early diagnosis of infection, tumor, synovial lesions and osteo-chondral fractures.

Arthroscopy is an extremely useful diagnostic and therapeutic tool. It is invaluable for diagnosis and treatment of osteo-chondral lesions of the talus, synovitis (synovial biopsy and synovectomy), intra-articular loose bodies and in cases of osteoarthritis of the ankle.

Common Disorders of the Ankle

Tendon disorders

1. Tendinitis/Tenosynovitis

Tendinitis/Tenosynovitis is the inflammation of the tendon/synovial sheath of the tendons resulting from irritation (of prolonged repetitive movements) where they pass under the retinacula at the ankle. Sometimes localised tenosynovitis may be the manifestation of a systemic disease such as rheumatoid arthritis.

Clinically the patient presents with pain over the affected tendon as shown in Table 19.1.

Table 19.1. Location of pain in tenosynovitis of tendons around ankle

Tendon involved in tenosynovitis	Location of pain and tenderness
1. Tibialis anterior	anteromedial aspect of ankle
2. Tibialis posterior	posteromedial aspect of the ankle
3. Peroneus longus/ Peroneus brevis	posterolateral aspect of the ankle

Pain is activity related. There may be fullness, crepitation and tenderness over the tendon. Passive stretching as well as active function of the inflamed tendon causes pain (active eversion and passive inversion at ankle reproduces pain in tendinitis/tenosynovitis of peroneal tendons).

Plain radiographs are normal. MRI can demonstrate inflammatory changes in the tendon sheath.

Treatment is most often conservative with NSAIDs, orthotic shoe inserts and physical therapy. Activity should be reduced in the acute phase. Immobilisation in a cast or splint can be done in cases with severe symptoms making ambulation difficult. Operative decompression is indicated rarely for recalcitrant cases.

2. Rupture of tendons

Rupture of a tendon represents the end stage of tendinitis or tenosynovitis. Mechanical attrition of the tendon in the presence of the tenuous blood supply predisposes the tendon to rupture. Achilles tendon, tibialis posterior and peroneal tendons are most commonly affected.

Rupture of tibialis posterior tendon is common in females in or after the 5th decade. It presents as acquired flat foot as the tibialis posterior tendon normally supports the arch. Inspection from behind shows more toes laterally on the involved side ("*too many toes*" *sign*) because of collapse of the medial arch. When the patient is asked to rise on the toes, normal hind foot inversion is not seen in patients with rupture of tibialis posterior tendon. Inversion strength is reduced and tenderness can be elicited along the course of tendon. Treatment is repair and augmentation with flexor digitorum longus tendon. Avulsion from navicular

can be treated by direct repair with drill holes through the bone. Orthosis can be tried in old ruptures. Persistently symptomatic feet need triple arthrodesis.

Rupture of tibialis anterior tendon Tibialis anterior tendon undergoes degeneration less commonly than the tibialis posterior and its disruption is caused more commonly by laceration. In cases of laceration, the diagnosis is made at the time of evaluation of laceration. Patient has weakness of active ankle dorsiflexion. A gap may be felt along the course of the tendon. A bulbous swelling may be felt beneath the extensor retinaculum (retracted proximal end of the tendon). Chronic degenerative tears present with history of vague ankle pain in the past. The patient has a painless, high stepping (slapping) gait. Chronic tears can be treated by tibialis anterior sliding graft, or, extensor hallucis longus graft.

Rupture of peroneus longus tendon is uncommon. The rupture most commonly occurs through os peroneum(cartilaginous or fibrocartilaginous mass in the tendon over lateral aspect of calcaneus).The patient presents with weakness or inability to evert the foot actively. A gap may sometimes be palpable along the course of the tendon. Treatment of ruptured peroneus longus tendon is by operative repair. Attaching the proximal stump of the peroneus longus tendon to the peroneus brevis tendon can treat old ruptures.

Subluxation/dislocation of peroneus brevis tendon (Subluxation or dislocation of peroneal tendons from their fibro-osseous tendon sheath). Instability of the peroneal tendons commonly results from violent dorsiflexion of the ankle when the foot is everted. It can happen during certain sports, especially skiing. The patient presents with pain and swelling (when acute) or a snapping sensation (when chronic) from the posterolateral aspect of the ankle joint. Plain radiographs may show a thin cortical fracture of the posterior lateral malleolus. The treatment in acute injuries is by immobilising the ankle in plantar flexion (to reduce the tendons) in a plaster cast for 4–6 weeks. Chronic cases need operative reconstruction using part of achilles tendon or calcaneofibular ligament.

Posterior heel and ankle pain

Three distinct areas give rise to posterior heel or ankle pain. These are:

1. Tendo Achilles
   (a) Tendinitis
   (b) Paratendinitis
   (c) Intrinsic degeneration
   (d) Rupture of tendo achilles
2. Retrocalcaneal area
   (a) Retrocalcaneal bursitis
   (b) Haglund's disease
3. Posterior calcaneal area
   (a) Insertional achilles tendinitis
   (b) Calcific insertional achilles tendinitis
   (c) Posterior calcaneal bursitis (Pump Bumps)
   (d) Sever's disease (in children)

Heel Pain Apart from the pain on posterior aspect of heel and ankle, heel pain can also be caused by plantar fascitis, heel pad injury, fractures of calcaneus, diseases of calcaneus such as infections and tumors, subtalar arthritis, and foreign body.

Disorders of Tendo Achilles

Achilles tendinitis is inflammation of achilles tendon and the paratenon surrounding the tendon. The inflammation is commonly seen in association with tight hamstrings, tibia vara, tight heel cord, valgus heel and flat foot patients with hyperpronating feet. Running on hills and low-heel shoes predispose the runners to achilles tendinitis.

Clinically patients present with posterior ankle pain, soft tissue swelling or crepitus. Palpation and passive stretching of tendo achilles aggravates the pain. Tenderness and swelling is noted approximately 3 to 4 cm proximal to the insertion of tendo achilles on the calcaneus. Dorsiflexion of the ankle may be restricted. Partial tears of the achilles tendon and intrinsic degeneration may present as achilles tendinitis. MRI can help in diagnosis of the partial tear in chronic cases of tendinitis not responding to conservative treatment.

Treatment of achilles tendinitis is NSAIDs, heel raise and heel cord stretching exercises. Severely symptomatic cases can be immobilised in a cast or splint for 7–10 days. A soft orthotic with navicular pad and 1/8" medial wedge can be prescribed in patients with hyperpronating feet. Local injections of hydrocortisone are contraindicated as they can lead to rupture of the tendon.

In chronic cases where MRI reveals partial tear of tendo achilles or areas of degeneration, surgical treatment to excise those areas is helpful.

Retrocalcaneal bursitis is the inflammation of the retrocalcaneal bursa. The retrocalcaneal bursa is located between the upper one third of calcaneus and the achilles tendon. Inflammation occurs following repetitive ankle dorsiflexion and plantarflexion or in cases where the heel counter rubs against the posterolateral prominence of the calcaneus (Fig. 19.1). Pain in the retrocalcaneal area can

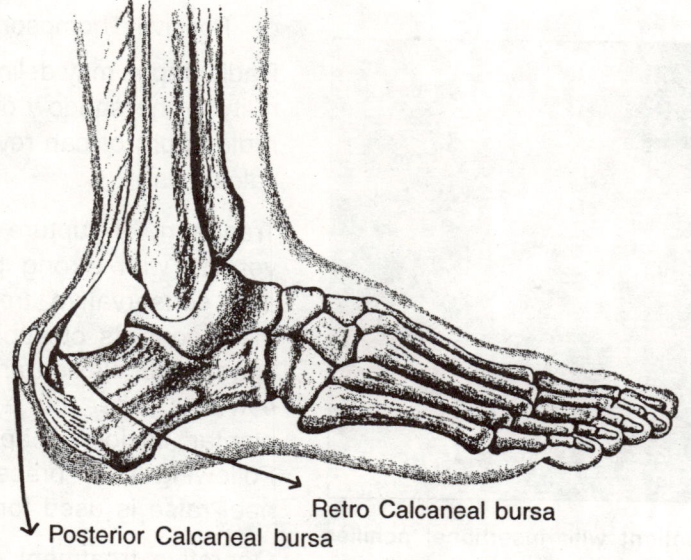

Retro Calcaneal bursa

Posterior Calcaneal bursa

Fig. 19.1. Pathology of Retrocalcaneal bursitis (Posterolateral prominence of calcaneum)

also occur due to Haglund's disease, which is the prominence of the posterior superior aspect of the calcaneus. This prominence may impinge on the achilles tendon during dorsiflexion.

Clinically the patient with retrocalcaneal bursitis has heel pain, which gets worse with dorsiflexion. Swelling, tenderness and redness may be present just anterior and superior to the insertion of tendo achilles on the calcaneus.

Treatment consists of 1/4 to 1/2 inch elevation of heel to relax the tendo achilles and to elevate heel above the counter. In order to remove pressure on calcaneus, the heel counter may be removed. Hot or cold compresses, NSAID's and steroid injections in the bursa may expedite the recovery.

Surgical treatment is rarely indicated. Persistent symptoms are treated by excision of the retrocalcaneal bursa and the posterolateral bony prominence of the calcaneus.

Insertional Tendinitis of tendo achilles: Insertional achilles tendinitis presents as pain, tenderness and swelling posteriorly at the insertion of tendo achilles. Calcific insertional tendinitis presents with more redness and swelling, and a bony prominence in the region of insertion of tendo achilles (Fig. 19.2). These conditions arise as a result of friction of the upper border of the heel counter of the shoe.

Radiographs show bony spur at the insertion of the achilles tendon.

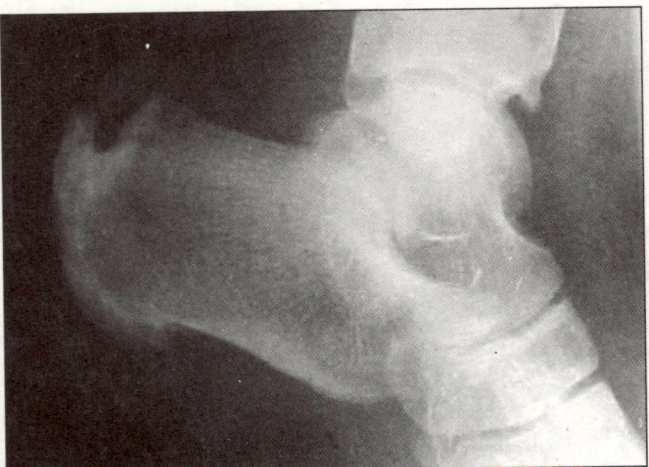

Fig. 19.2. X-ray of a patient with insertional achilles tendinitis. Note the bony prominence in the region of tendon insertion

Treatment is with rest, NSAIDs and open heeled shoes. A U-shaped pad can be placed between the heel and the counter to reduce irritation. Local hydrocortisone injections may lead to rupture of the tendon. Chronic and recalcitrant cases may need surgery in the form of osteotomy of prominent tubercle of calcaneus, resection of spur or osteotomy of the calcaneus.

Posterior calcaneal bursitis (PUMP BUMP) Posterior calcaneal bursitis is an inflammation of the subcutaneous bursa superficial to the insertion of tendo achilles. It is caused by friction of the heel counter against the posterior heel. Treatment includes taking the pressure of counter off the heel, NSAIDs and heel raise. Local injections of hydrocortisone are not advised. Recalcitrant painful bursae can be excised.

Rupture of Tendo Achilles Rupture of tendo achilles most commonly results from the forced dorsiflexion against a plantar flexed foot. Clinically the patient presents with a history of sudden pop and pain in the posterior ankle region along with swelling. Often patient feels as if he has been struck with a stick on the back of the ankle or lower leg. This injury occurs most commonly in basket ball, diving and racquet sports. On examination, there are three diagnostic signs:

a) A palpable defect 2 to 6 cm above the insertion of tendo achilles.

b) Weak plantar flexion against resistance or failure to perform tip toe standing.

c) Positive Thompson's squeeze test (vide supra)

Radiographs may delineate tendon rupture (discontinuity in the shadow of tendo achilles in the lateral radiograph) or can reveal a bony avulsion from the calcaneus.

Treatment of rupture of tendo achilles is controversial, with strong proponents of both surgical and conservative treatment. Conservative treatment consists of application of long leg cast with knee in 45° flexion and ankle in plantar flexion for 4 weeks. After this a short leg cast with ankle in plantar flexion is applied for another 4 weeks. Following this, brace with gradually decreasing heel raise is used for the next 4 weeks.

Operative treatment consists of surgical approximation of the ruptured tendon. Postoperatively the repair is protected in a POP cast just like the conservative treatment. Surgical treatment has reportedly slightly decreased rate of rerupture and results in more fatigue tolerance of tendon. However, the problems of wound healing and infection can spoil the surgical results.

Inflammatory Conditions

Rheumatoid Arthritis (RA) (Fig. 19.3a,b)

Ankle is uncommonly involved in patients with RA and the involvement in usually mild. It usually presents with boggy, painful synovitis of the ankle. Stiffness is a common feature. Tenosynovitis is commonly present. Treatment initially is conservative with shoe and brace. Synovectomy may be useful in cases without extensive destruction of articular cartilage. Arthrodesis may rarely be indicated. Total ankle arthroplasty has been performed with limited success in these patients.

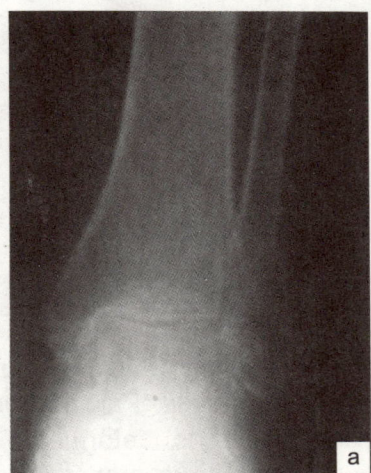

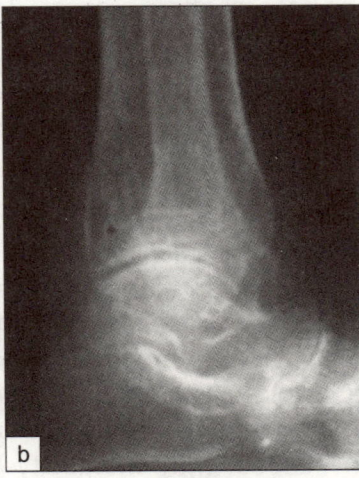

Fig. 19.3a,b. AP and lateral radiographs of a patient with Rheumatoid arthritis of the ankle

Tuberculosis

Tuberculosis of ankle joint is uncommon. The disease spreads from a remote focus by hematogenous route. The disease can be synovial or bony. Patient presents with pain, swelling, increased temperature over ankle, stiffness and limp. Multiple discharging sinuses may form in chronic untreated cases. Radiographs show osteopenia, lytic lesions in the bone and diminished joint space (Fig. 19.4).

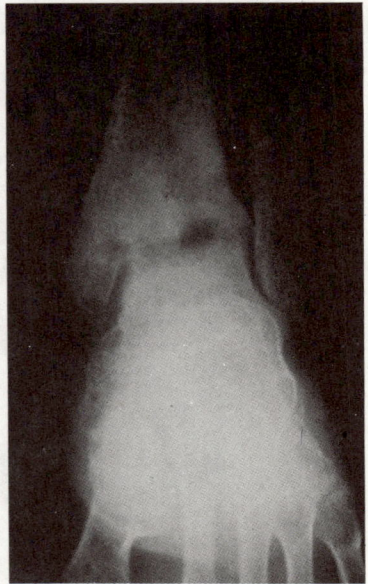

Fig. 19.4. Tubercular Ankle Joint

Treatment is institution of antitubercular drugs. Early movements of the joint are encouraged in cases where disease is synovial and good range of movements is expected. Cases with articular damage are immobilized in a plaster to achieve stiff ankle in functional position. Painful and /or deformed ankle following healing of the disease is best treated by ankle arthrodesis.

Osteoarthritis of Ankle Joint

Primary osteoarthritis of the ankle is rare. Secondary osteoarthritis may occur following trauma (ankle fracture or dislocation) (Fig. 19.5a-c), synovial chondromatosis, rheumatoid arthritis, osteochondritis dissecans and avascular necrosis.

Clinically the patients present with ankle pain and stiffness, often bilateral.

Radiographs reveal joint space narrowing, subchondral sclerosis and osteophytes (Fig. 19.5d).

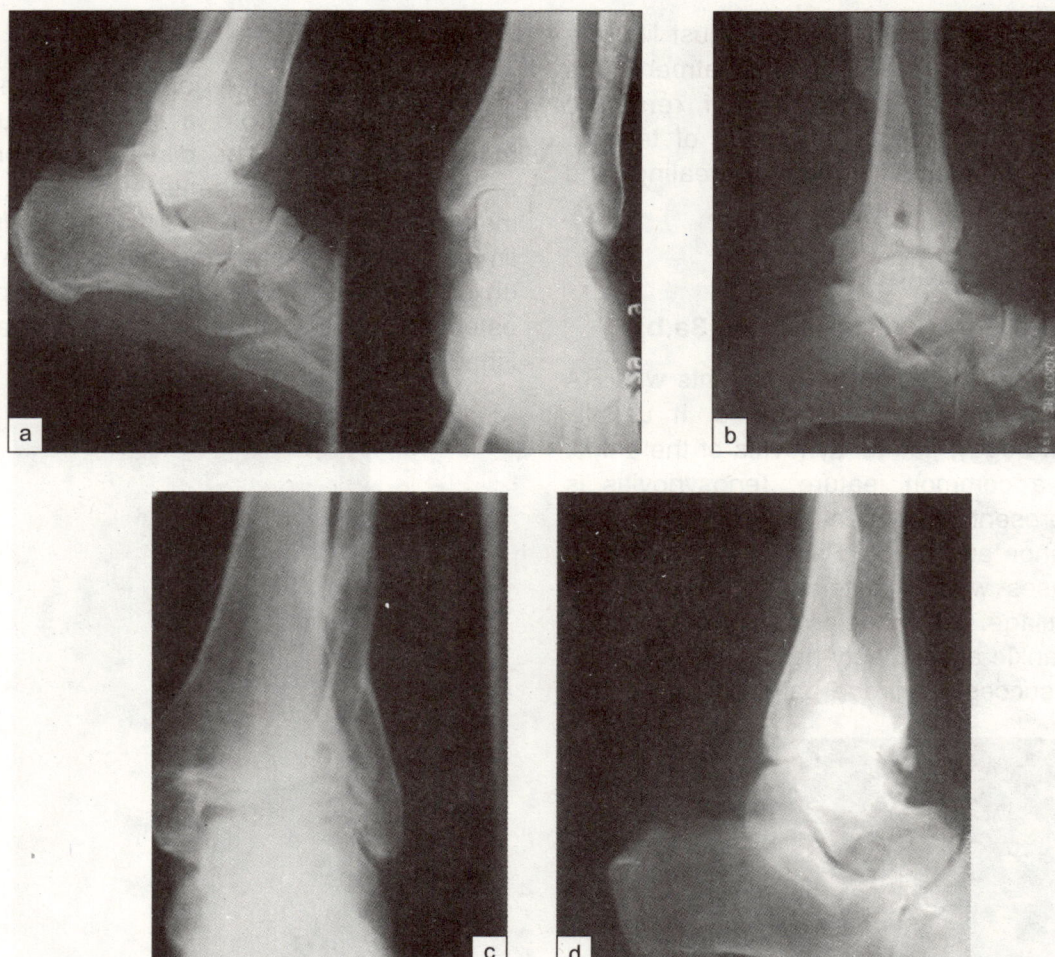

Fig. 19.5a-d. Post traumatic osteoarthritis of ankle joint following malunited bimalleolar fracture
Note the joint space narrowing and osteophyte formation

Deformity is often present. Treatment is conservative initially with NSAIDs, orthosis (Ankle Foot Orthosis – AFO) and shoe modification. Surgical treatment can be in the form of synovectomy, loose bodies removal (both arthroscopically) and excision of osteophytes from the tibia and talus in cases where disease is limited to anterior joint.

Arthrodesis is a sound option to achieve a pain free stable joint in cases with severe pain with or without deformity.

Total ankle arthroplasty has been tried in the treatment with limited success and the results are not very good.

Charcot Joint (Neuropathic joint)

Neuropathic or charcot joints are seen in diabetes mellitus, syphilis, syringomyelia and other neuropathic conditions.

Clinically patients present with swelling, redness and warmth over the ankle. Pain is conspicuous by its absence. Ankle is deformed-most commonly a valgus deformity is present. Crepitations and loose bodies are often present. The joint is grossly unstable in advanced cases.

X-rays show severe joint destruction, evidence of instability and multiple bony loose bodies in the joint.

Treatment consists of long term plaster or orthotic protection (from 4 months to even up to 18 months). Surgical treatment is associated with high incidence of infection and should be chosen reluctantly. Arthrodesis is not predictable (as the bony fusion is difficult to achieve in these cases) but is the only treatment of late resistant cases with instability and / or deformity.

Surgical Procedures for Ankle Joint

Arthrodesis

Indications

Painful stiff ankle due to

- Osteoarthritis
- Rheumatoid Arthritis
- Post traumatic Arthritis
- Neuropathic joint

Contraindication

- Poor bone stock.

Position of Arthrodesis

Neutral with respect to plantar/dorsiflexion

5°–7° valgus (No Varus)

0°–5° external rotation (No Internal Rotation)

Technique

➢ Anteromedial and anterolateral approach used

➢ Attempt made to achieve maximum bony contact

➢ Fixation methods
  – Internal fixation - Compression screw
  – External fixator - Calandruccio apparatus
  – Anterior tibial graft slide followed by plaster immobilization (Fig. 19.6a-c)

Total Ankle Arthroplasty

Indications

- Osteoarthritis
- Rheumatoid Arthritis
- Post traumatic arthritis

Should be used only in older and less active patients.

Contraindications

- Active sepsis
- Significant laxity
- Poor bone stock
- Osteonecrosis of talus

Complication rate in total ankle arthroplasty is high and the results are poor.

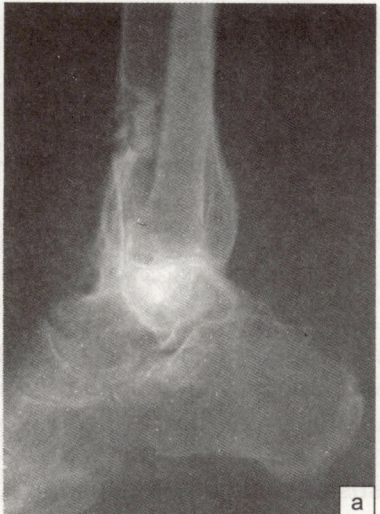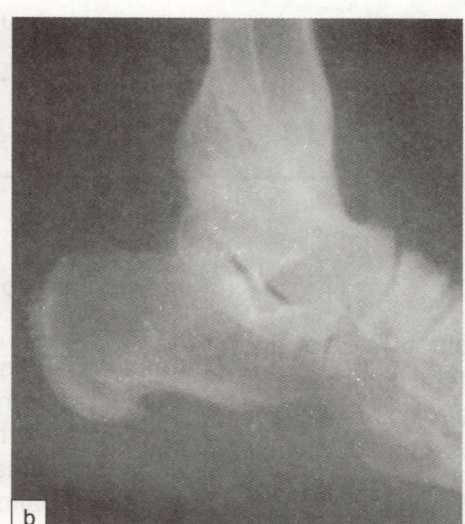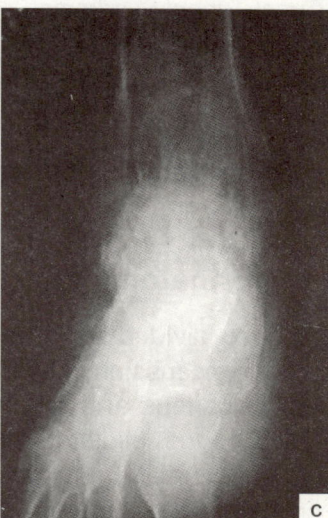

Fig. 19.6a-c. Ankle arthrodesis using anterior tibial graft slide

CHAPTER 20

Foot

Relevant Anatomy

Foot is often divided into the hindfoot, midfoot and forefoot for discussion. The hindfoot comprises of talucas, calcaneus and the subtalar joint between these two bones. Midfoot includes cuboid, navicular and the cuneiforms. Metatarsals and phalanges constitute the forefoot.

Osteology

The foot has seven tarsals, five metatarsals and fourteen phalanges.

Tarsals

Tarsal bones are calcaneus, talus, navicular, cuboid, lateral cuneiform, middle cuneiform and medial cuneiform.

Calcaneus is the largest bone of the foot. It articulates with talus above and cuboid in front. A large posterior tuberosity of the calcaneus provides attachment for the achilles tendon. A medial shelf, called sustentaculum tali supports head of talus superiorly and has a groove for flexor hallucis longus inferiorly. Medial and lateral plantar tubercles give attachment to ligaments and muscles of the sole.

The ossification center for the calcaneus appears in the 6th fetal month.

Talus has a large posterior body and rounded anterior end called head. The neck of the talus joins the two. Main blood supply to talus enters through the neck, hence fractures of the neck of the talus may cause avascularity of the talus. Talus has no attachment of any muscles and is largely covered with articular cartilage. It articulates with distal tibia superiorly to form ankle joint, with calcaneus inferiorly to form subtalar joint and with navicular anteriorly.

The ossification center for the talus appears in the 7th fetal month. Navicular has a proximal cup-shaped surface to articulate with head of the talus. Distally it articulates with the three cuneiform bones. Navicular is at the apex of the medial longitudinal arch which is maintained by the posterior tibial tendon (which attaches to tuberosity of the navicular) and the calcaneonavicular (spring) ligament.

The ossification center for navicular is not present at birth and appears in the fourth year.

Cuboid articulates with anterior end of calcaneus proximally and with the bases of the fourth and fifth metatarsals distally.

Cuboid has a plantar groove for peroneus longus.

The ossification center for the cuboid appears in the 9th fetal month.

The *three cuneiforms* are called the medial (articulates with 1st metatarsal distally), middle (articulates with 2nd M.T.) and lateral (articulates with 3rd M.T.) cuneiforms. Proximally, they all articulate with navicular.

Lateral cuneiform ossifies in the first year, the middle in the fourth year and the medial in the third year of life.

Joints

Subtalar joint is a stable articulation (gliding joint) and has three facets (posterior, middle and anterior) for articulation between talus and calcaneus. The joint has anterior, posterior, medial and lateral talocalcaneal ligaments as well as the strong talocalcaneal interosseous ligament (also called cervical ligament).

Talocalcaneonavicular joint is also arthrodial joint allowing gliding and rotation. It is supported by a dorsal talonavicular ligament and plantar calcaneocuboid ligaments, which support the head of the talus.

Calcaneocuboid joint is also arthrodial joint allowing gliding and rotation and is supported by the dorsal and plantar calcaneocuboid ligaments, the bifurcate ligament (calcaneocuboidnavicular) and the long plantar ligament.

The calcaneoucuboid joint and the talonavicular joint together constitute the transverse tarsal joint or the *Chopart's joints*. There is an obliquity between the subtalar joint and the transverse tarsal joint due to which the midfoot is flexible in pronation and becomes rigid in supination.

Tarsometatarsal joints (*Lisfranc's joints*) are relatively transverse gliding joints which are quite stable because of their bony architecture and supporting dorsal, plantar and interosseous ligaments. Intrinsic bony stability of this joint complex is due to the fact that the second metatarsal base extends more proximally than the remaining metatarsal bases. This "key stone" effect provides bony stability. In addition, all the metatarsal bases are trapezoid shaped like a roman arch - a fact which considerably adds to the bony stability. Strong transverse metatarsal ligaments (between the metatarsal heads and the four lateral metatarsal bases) and Lisfranc's ligament (connecting the second metatarsal base to the medial cuneiform) provide ligamentous stability at Lisfranc's joints and between metatarsals.

Metatarsophalangeal joints are condyloid joints and permit flexion, extension and abduction and are stabilized by the collateral (two) and plantar ligaments.

Interphalangeal joints are ginglymus joints and permit flexion and extension and are stabilized by the collateral (two) and plantar ligaments.

Muscles

There are 19 intrinsic muscles of the foot and all except extensor digitorum brevis and dorsal interossei (4 in number) are plantar.

The plantar muscles are considered in four layers:

a) *Superficial layer* Abductor hallucis, flexor digitorum brevis (both medial plantar nerve) and abductor digiti minimi (lateral plantar nerve).

b) *2nd layer* Quadratus plantae (innervated by lateral plantar nerve) flexes toes. Lumbricals arise from medial aspect of long flexors to phalanges and extend distal phalanges. Lumbricals are innervated by medial plantar nerve (first lumbrical) and lateral plantar nerve (second, third and fourth).

Tendons of FDL and FHL are also in this layer.

c) *3rd layer* Flexor hallucis brevis (medial plantar nerve), Adductor hallucis and flexor digiti minimi brevis (both innervated by lateral plantar nerve).

d) *4th layer* Plantar interossei (three in number – supplied by lateral plantar nerve).

Tendons of tibialis posterior and peroneus longus are in this layer. (The four dorsal interossei are also supplied by lateral plantar nerve).

Vessels

Dorsalis pedis passes between EHL and EDL into dorsum of foot and terminates as first dorsal metatarsal artery and the deep plantar branch, which supplies the plantar arch of the foot.

Posterior tibial artery divides into medial and lateral plantar arteries. Medial plantar artery joins deep branch of dorsalis pedis to form the plantar arch. Lateral plantar artery is the main contributor to the plantar arch.

Nerves

Tibial nerve divides into medial and lateral plantar nerves and the medial calcaneal branches (purely sensory).

Medial plantar nerve provides plantar sensation to medial 3½ toes and provides motor innervation to flexor hallucis brevis, abductor hallucis, flexor digitorum brevis and first lumbrical.

Lateral plantar nerve provides plantar sensation to lateral 1½ digits and provides motor innervation to abductor digiti minimi, quadratus plantae, lumbricals (2nd to 4th), adductor hallucis, flexor digiti minimi brevis and all the seven interossei.

Deep peroneal nerve provides sensations to the first web space. Rest of the dorsum receives sensory innervation from superficial peroneal nerve (through dorsal digital nerves).

Sural nerve is dorsal lateral cutaneous nerve of the foot and innervates lateral border of the foot.

Saphenous nerve provides sensory innervation to the medial border of the foot.

Evaluation of a Patient with Disorder of Foot

History of the complaints pertaining to foot should take into account the age of the patient. In infants, toddlers and preschool children, intoeing (*Pigeon toeing*) and flat feet are common complaints. In adolescents, accessory navicular and prehallux, tarsal coalition and *Sever's disease* are common underlying diseases giving rise to symptoms in the foot. Adults commonly complain of heel pain (usually plantar fascitis; spondyloarthropathy should be ruled out), pain over big toe (due to gout) and referred pain in the foot due to spinal disorders. Middle aged and elderly patients have complaints due to foot strain, degenerative arthritis (e.g. Hallus rigidus) or due to hallux valgus. Infections and trauma can occur at all ages. The duration and chronicity of the symptoms are important facts to elicit. In case of pain, the exact location of the pain, activities aggravating and relieving the pain and its relation to exertion should be enquired. Recurrent sprains and apprehension to walk on uneven surfaces suggest instability. History of involvement of opposite foot, other joints of the body and any systemic involvement (e.g. as in Rheumatoid Arthritis) is very important.

The examination of the foot should be performed in standing, walking and non-weight bearing (sitting) positions.

Inspection is performed with the patient sitting. Swelling, color change, arches of the foot, deformities and any scars / sinuses are noted.

Palpation of the bones and soft tissues is performed carefully to accurately localize the area of tenderness. Temperature changes, if any, are noted. Movements at the ankle, subtalar joint (inversion/eversion normal 0°–5° each), midtarsal joints (forefoot adduction – normal 0°–20°; forefoot abduction-normal 0°–10°), 1st metatarsophalangeal joint (flexion–normal 0°–45°; extension – normal 0°–70°) and toes are evaluated. Patient is then asked to stand and alignment of lower limbs, heel varus or valgus and arches of the foot are noted. Correctability of hind foot deformities is noted. The patient is asked to rise on toes and normal heel varus and supination of foot on rising are noted.

The gait of the patient is observed for any limp,

torsional abnormalities and pattern of the gait.

Patient's shoes should be evaluated for unusual pattern of wear, which results from the foot deformities.

Detailed neurovascular examination including motor, sensory and deep tendon reflex examination and palpation of peripheral pulses is performed.

Imaging for foot disorders

Plain radiographs are satisfactory for evaluation of most of the common foot disorders and include anteroposterior (AP), lateral and oblique views. Special views such as standing AP and lateral radiographs provide useful information about the flat feet, hallux valgus and certain congenital abnormalities. Axial view of the heel is useful for diseases of calcaneus (trauma, tumour, infection) and talocalcaneal tarsal coalition.

Technetium Bone Scan is useful to evaluate osteomyelitis or stress fractures when plain x-rays are normal. Three phase bone scan is extremely valuable in diagnosis of reflex sympathetic dystrophy.

Computerised Tomography (CT) provides useful information about the hindfoot. Calcaneus, talus, ankle joint and subtalar joint are evaluated much better with CT scan than with plain x-rays.

Magnetic Resonance Imaging (MRI) is useful for evaluating soft tissue disorders such as tendinitis or tendon rupture, bone and soft tissue tumours, and osteomyelitis.

Arthroscopy is a relatively new tool for investigation and treatment of the foot disorders. Subtalar joint and the first metatarsophalangeal joints are being scoped at many centers in the world but it will be some time before it is routinely practiced everywhere. Plantar release for fascitis is being done endoscopically at some centers.

Congenital and Developmental Disorders

1. Metatarsus Adductus

Metatarsus adductus is a common cause of intoeing seen in infants during the first year of life. The forefoot is adducted and supinated at tarsometatarsal joints and the deformity is present at birth. Metatarsus adductus is believed to be a disorder of

uterine packing and is associated with hip dysplasia, internal tibial torsion and torticollis.

Clinically the patients have adduction and supination of the forefoot with convex lateral border (normally the lateral border of foot forms a straight line from the heel to fifth toe) and frequently wide space between the first and second toes. A line bisecting heel (on examining the foot from the bottom) points to the second toe normally but in metatarsus adductus, it points to third (mild deformity), fourth (moderate deformity) or fifth toe (severe deformity). The deformity can be flexible, partially flexible or rigid.

Radiographic examination reveals medial angulation at the tarsometatarsal joints and there may be increased talocalcaneal angle due to hindfoot valgus.

Differential Diagnosis

Metatarsus adductus should be differentiated from clubfoot (CTEV) deformity by the presence of TA contracture, hindfoot varus, and small heel in CTEV.

Other *causes of intoeing* should be differentiated:

Internal tibial torsion presents as intoeing in second year of life. Transmalleolar axis (and therefore, the foot) is internally rotated compared to the thigh. This is best measured as the thigh foot angle with the child prone.

Normally, up to 20° of internal tibial torsion is normal in infants. It may be associated with physiological genu varum and may apparently exaggerate the deformity.

Transmalleolar axis normally rotates externally in childhood and results in 15°–20° of external tibial torsion by the adolescence.

A persistent internal tibial torsion results in internally rotated ankles (compared with the knee) and intoeing results. In a child with internal tibial torsion, though the feet turn in, *the patellae face forwards.*

Most cases improve spontaneously. Only for severe persistent internal tibial torsion deformity, supramalleolar osteotomy is indicated.

Femoral anteversion leads to intoeing in children between 3 to 6 years of age. Normal infants have up to 45° of anteversion, which gradually reduces to an average of 15° during adolescence. Exaggerated femoral anteversion leads to increased internal rotation (>70°) at the hip, decreased external rotation (30°) and internal rotation of the entire leg during gait, thus resulting in intoeing. During gait, in the child with in toeing due to femoral anterversion, both the *patellae are turned inward* towards each other.

Most cases resolve spontaneously. Severe persistent femoral anterversion in late childhood is indication for derotation osteotomies.

Treatment of Metatarsus Adductus

Most cases correct spontaneously with growth and stretching. Rigid deformities at birth need serial casting between 1 to 8 months age. Casting is ineffective after 8 months of age. Surgery is needed for painful, severe, rigid foot and for cosmetic reasons. In children less than 2 years, abductor hallucis tenotomy with or without first cuneiform–metatarsal release is done.

Heyman-Herndon tarsometatarsal release is done between 3 and 7 years. Older children need metatarsal osteotomy.

2. Clubfoot

Clubfoot (Congenital Talipes Equino – Varus, CTEV) is a congenital foot deformity of unknown etiology. Multiple factors are implicated such as genetic (polygenic inheritance), persistence of fetal positioning, primary germ plasm defects, neuromuscular factors, mechanical factors (twins, malposition in utero) and drugs.

The disorder occurs in 1/1000 live births and affects males twice as commonly as females. Half the cases are bilateral. It is the commonest congenital deformity.

Pathology The foot is small and the calf is hypotrophied. The equinus deformity occurs at the ankle, the inversion at the subtalar joint and adduction and supination of the forefoot occurs at the midtarsal joints. Deformities are due to underdeveloped and contracted soft tissues on the medial, posterior and plantar aspect of the foot.

The calcaneus is small and rotates through the subtalar joint in a medial direction and inverts (varus tilt). Anterior part of the talus is deviated medially and in plantar direction. Talonavicular joint is dislocated and navicular is displaced medially. Cuboid is often subluxated medially.

Clinically the deformity is present at birth. The typical equinus, varus and adduction deformities are present in varying severity and flexibility. It is not possible to manipulate the foot into normal position. A simple test for equinus is based on the observation that in normal newborns, the dorsum of the foot can be brought up to touch the skin. Failure to achieve this suggests the presence of the equinus deformity.

Two types of deformities are identified. An *extrinsic* foot is flexible, the deformity is not very severe and the foot has sparse subcutaneous tissues. An *intrinsic* foot has plenty of subcutaneous tissue, well marked deep skin creases on concavity of the deformity, rigid and severe deformities and a small heel. An extrinsic foot is likely to respond to conservative treatment while an intrinsic foot is difficult to correct and maintain in a plaster and often needs surgery.

A child who starts walking on the clubfoot deformity (neglected clubfoot) develops callosities on the lateral border of the foot. Genu valgum and genu recurvatum deformities may be associated in these patients.

Associated congenital abnormalities such as spina bifida should be ruled out in these patients.

Radiological examination reveals increased lateral tibiocalcaneal angle (>120° due to equinus), decreased lateral talocalcaneal angle (<35°; normal 35°–50°) and anteroposterior talocalcaneal angle (<20°: normal 20°–40°) – both due to hindfoot varus. Talo – first metatarsal angle on AP film (normally zero) suggests talo-navicular dislocation. (Fig. 20.1a,b)

Treatment

Treatment of the clubfoot deformity should be started immediately after diagnosis. Treatment in postnatal period consists of corrective manipulation and casting. The order of manipulation for correction of deformities is adduction, heel varus and lastly, equinus. Failure to do so will lead to rocker-bottom foot. Casts are changed every one to two weeks for 3 months. The corrected foot is

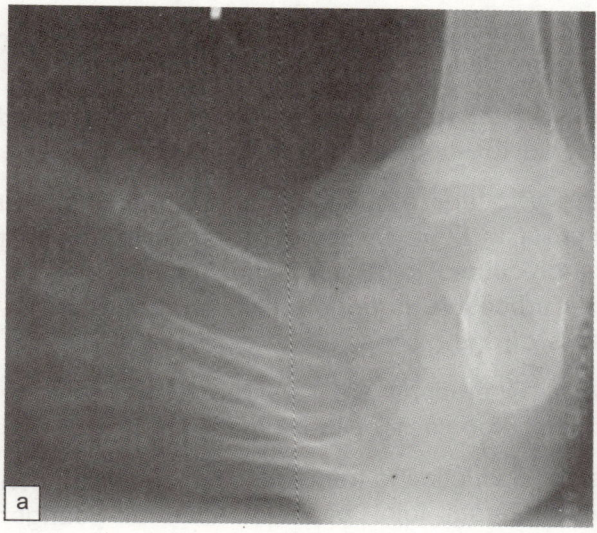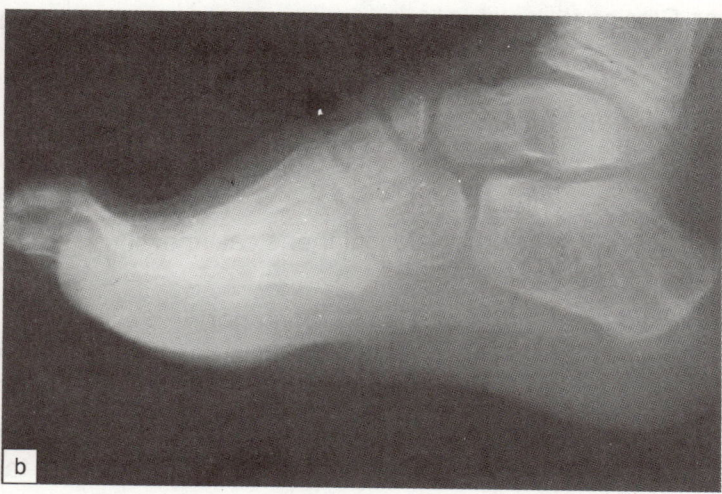

Fig. 20.1a,b. Antero posterior and lateral radiographs of a patient with congenital talipes equino varus

then held in a cast or brace (*Denis Browne splint*) till the child starts walking when he is advised to wear CTEV shoes.

Surgical treatment is required if the deformity does not respond to conservative treatment or if the CTEV has been neglected (A neglected CTEV is said to exist when the child starts walking on the deformity without any prior treatment). (Fig. 20.2a,b)

The most commonly done surgery for CTEV is Postero Medial Soft Tissue Release (PMSTR). It can be done as early as 4 months of age but is often recommended at 8–9 months of age because of the following reasons:

a) Release in a very small foot in a very young child is technically quite difficult, as the structures in the foot are very small.

b) A very small foot may be difficult to hold in a plaster after surgery so maintenance of correction may be difficult.

c) A child who is close to the age of standing and weight bearing at the time of surgery can start walking soon afterwards. The walking on a corrected foot stimulates the near normal growth of foot bones and soft tissues.

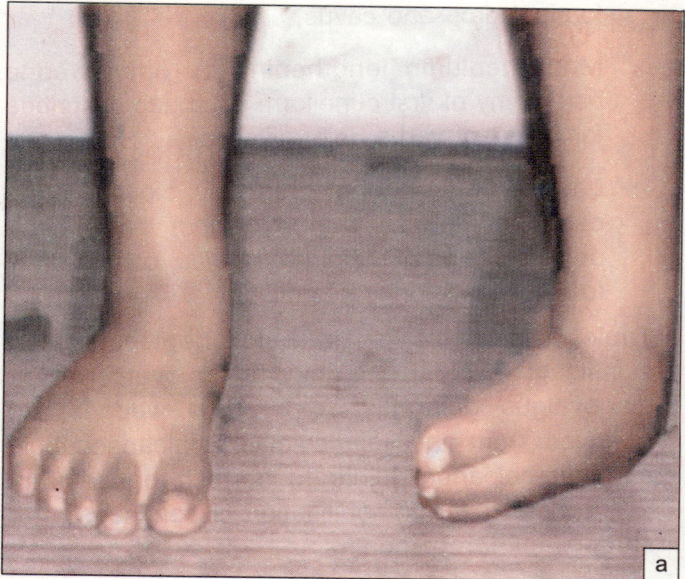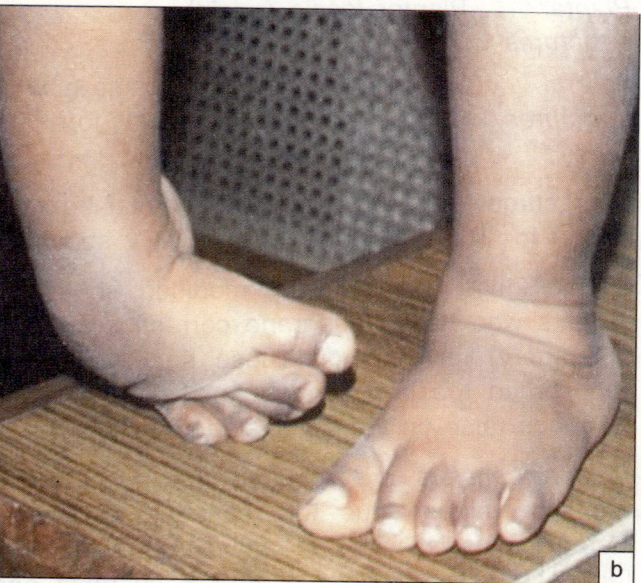

Fig. 20.2a,b. Clinical photographs of children with neglected club foot

PMSTR can be done by a posteromedial (Turco) or Cincinnati incision

Following structures are released:

Posteriorly Tendo achilles (Z – plasty)

Capsule of ankle joint and subtalar joint

Posterior talofibular and calcaneofibular ligaments

Medially Tendons: Tibialis posterior
abductor hallucis muscle
Sometimes FDL & FHL

Superficial medial release of the subtalar joint

Superficial deltoid (calcaneo-tibial and tibionavicular)

Calcaneonavicular (spring) ligament talonavicular ligament dorsally

Deep medial release

Bifurcate ligament (Cal-caneonavicular and calcane-ocuboid)

Talocalcaneal interosseous ligament

Capsule of talonavicular (medial, dorsal and plantar), naviculocunei-form, cuneiform–first meta-tarsal and medial side of subtalar joint.

Plantar structures Plantar fascia (origin)

Lateral structures Lateral talonavicular capsule and dorsal calcaneo-cuboid joint (if required).

After surgery, the correction is maintained in a plaster for 3 months followed by CTEV shoes.

CTEV Shoes are specially modified shoes for patients who have undergone correction (casting or surgery) for clubfoot. These shoes have no heel, broad toe box, straight medial border and 3/16 inch raise on the outer side of sole.

Tendon transfers are required for cases which occur or relapse due to weakness of evertor (peroneii) muscles with resultant invertor overaction. Tendon transfers are done after 5 years of age (when the patient can comply with muscle re-

education program) in a supple foot that is other-wise corrected.

Tibialis anterior or posterior tendon is transferred to cuboid to supplement evertor action.

Evan's Procedure aims to shorten the lateral column of the foot by a wedge resection done at calcaneo-cuboid joint in addition to the PMSTR. Evan's procedure is done for children between 4–8 years of age.

Salvage Operations are required for resistant or residual deformities of the foot.

Forefoot Adduction is treated by Heyman–Herndon tarsometatarsal joint capsulotomies in younger children and by metatarsal osteotomies when the deformity becomes rigid in older children.

Heel varus

Dwyer's osteotomy is open wedge osteotomy on the medial side of calcaneus. Bone grafts are packed at the osteotomy site. The skin healing may be a problem in this procedure.

A modified operation is close wedge osteotomy on lateral aspect of calcaneus but it has a disad-vantage of further reducing the size of an already small calcaneus.

Mid foot deformities

➢ Midtarsal osteotomies (Japas) can be modified to correct supination of forefoot as well as the forefoot drop and cavus.

➢ Medial column lengthening by open wedge osteotomy of first cuneiform has been described for resistant varus deformities.

➢ Lateral column shortening by close wedge osteotomy of calcaneus (*Simon*) or cuboid;– decancellation of cuboid (*Litchblau*) can be done for resistant bony deformities.

Triple arthrodesis is done for neglected feet, significant residual deformity or for overcorrected planovalgus deformity. Appropriate wedges are removed from the talonavicular, calcaneocuboid and talo-calcaneal joints to correct the deformi-ties. Plaster cast immobilisation is continued after surgery for three months.

Triple arthrodesis is not done before twelve years of age because

(a) In the younger patient the bones are mainly cartilaginous and excessive resection may have to be done down to bone.

(b) Tarsal bones are cartilaginous, hence fusion is difficult to achieve.

(c) Growth of the foot is markedly impaired and an already small foot becomes smaller.

External Fixator

Correction of rigid, recurrent, residual and/ or multiply operated scarred clubfoot or club foot with poor overlying skin (or unstable scars) is possible by external fixator. Both Ilizarov (Fig. 20.2c) as well as JESS (Joshi's External Stabilising System) fixators can be used. The principle of correction by these devices is one of differential distraction (both sides of the deformity are distracted-concave more than convex) to correct the deformities. After correction the foot should be immobilised in corrected position for 8–12 weeks.

3. Calcaneovalgus deformity

Calcaneovalgus deformity presents at birth with dorsiflexion and eversion of the foot. The condition is often bilateral.

This is an innocuous condition and most cases resolve spontaneously by the end of first year. Calcaneovalgus should be differentiated from congenital vertical talus. In the latter condition the calcaneum is in equinus and the hindfoot is rigid. In calcaneovalgus, the calcaneum is dorsiflexed (i.e. in calcaneus) and the hindfoot is supple. Parents can be reassured and told to gently manipulate the foot into corrected position.

4. Congenital Vertical Talus (Congenital convex pes valgus)

Congenital vertical talus presents with rocker bottom foot deformity at birth. The deformity is usually associated with other anomalies, syndromes (Nail–patella syndrome, multiple pterygium syndrome, Marfan's syndrome, arthrogryposis), chromosomal abnormalities (trisomy 13–15 or 18) or with neuromuscular problems (e.g. spina bifida).

Pathology

Calcaneus is in equinus and rotated posterolaterally. Talus is plantarflexed and rotated medially. Head of the talus is palpable medially. Navicular is dislocated dorsolaterally. Cuboid is subluxed dorsally and laterally on calcaneus. Soft tissues on the posterior, anterior and lateral aspect of ankle are contracted.

Clinically the patient has equinus and valgus at the hindfoot while the forefoot is dorsiflexed and abducted.

Differential diagnosis of congenital vertical talus is calcaneovalgus deformity of the foot.

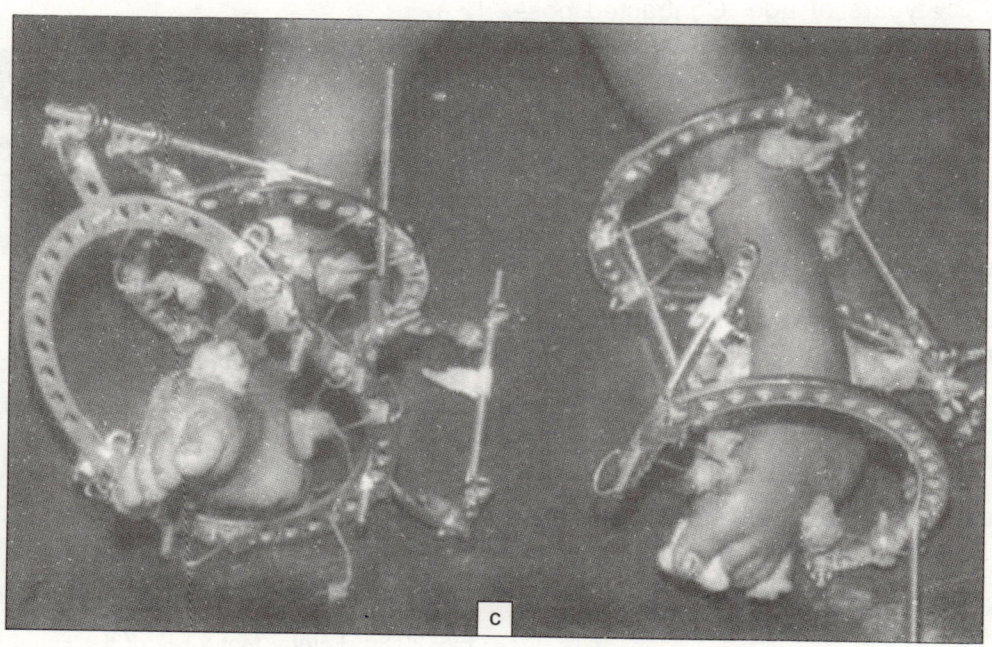

Fig. 20.2c.   Ilizarov correction of bilateral club foot

Radiologically, there is increased talocalcaneal angle on AP and lateral x-rays. On lateral film, calcaneus is in equinus and talus is plantarflexed (Fig. 20.3a-c). A stress lateral view with forced plantar flexion differentiates congenital vertical talus from flexible hindfoot valgus. Talometatarsal alignment is restored in flexible deformity while it remains disturbed in congenital vertical talus as navicular remains dislocated.

nous or fibrous fusion between the tarsal bones leading to pronated rigid flat foot and spasm of peroneal muscles on inversion. It is present since birth though it presents only during 8–16 years of age. Some cases may be familial with autosomal dominant inheritance.

The commonest coalition is calcaneonavicular followed by talocalcaneal (where middle facet is

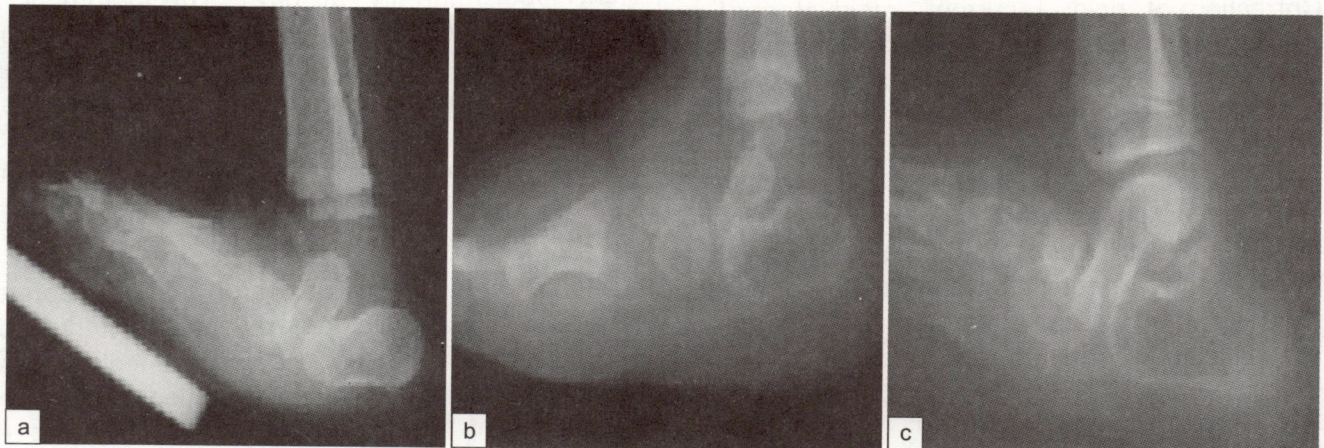

Fig. 20.3a-c. Radiographs of a patient with bilateral congenital vertical talus

Treatment during the first 3–4 months is stretching of dorsolateral soft tissue by manipulation followed by casting (Plaster is applied in the position of clubfoot deformity).

Surgery is done for children over 4 months of age and consists of one stage soft tissue release in children up to 2½ years of age. Contracted posterior, anterior and lateral structures are released. Talonavicular joint and calcaneocuboid joints (if dislocated) are reduced and fixed with K-wire (Fig. 20.3d). Tibialis anterior is transferred to the neck of the talus if neurogenic imbalance is present.

Other procedures

➤ Grice Green extra-articular subtalar arthrodesis can be done in children who are 4–6 years old.

➤ Children over 3 years of age with severe deformities due to neuromuscular causes may need excision of navicular.

➤ Triple arthrodesis is required in patients who are over 12 years old.

5. Tarsal Coalition (Peroneal Spastic Flatfoot)

Tarsal coalition is characterized by bony, cartilagi-

more commonly fused than anterior facet). Talonavicular coalition is rare.

Clinically the patient presents with rigid flatfoot, peroneal spasm on stretching, local tenderness, increased incidence of ankle sprains and reduced subtalar motion.

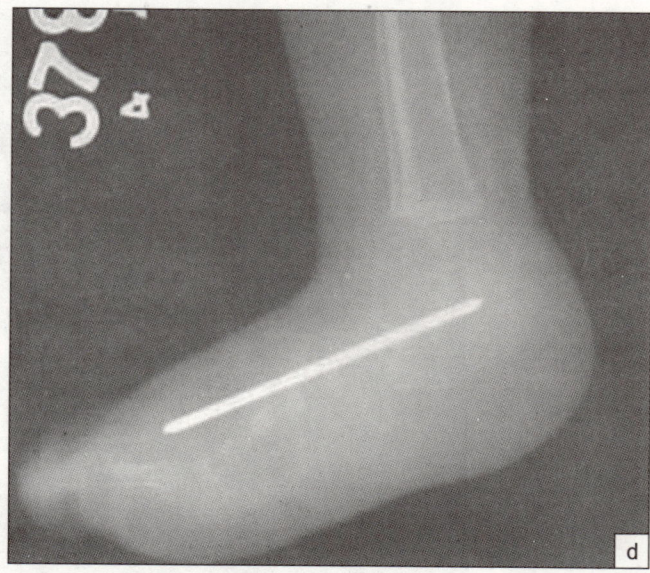

Fig. 20.3d. Lateral foot x-ray of the same patient following surgical correction

Radiologically the routine views may be normal and special views such as 45° oblique view (for calcaneonavicular coalition) and 45° axial view of the calcaneus (for talocalcaneal coalition) are often required.

CT is ideal investigation for demonstrating the bony bar while MRI is useful in fibrous or cartilaginous coalitions. Tarsal coalition should be differentiated from other causes of peroneal spasm such as Juvenile Rheumatoid Arthritis, osteoid osteoma, trauma and infection.

Treatment

Initial treatment is always conservative. Analgesics, rest and local heat provide relief in most cases. A below knee cast applied for a few weeks can relieve symptoms if pain is not controlled. If symptoms recur frequently, surgical treatment is indicated.

If there are no arthritic changes in the involved joint, then the resection of the bar and interposition of fat can be tried. Triple arthrodesis is indicated in cases of arthritic changes or failed resection cases.

6. Pes Planus (Flat foot)

Pes planus is the condition when the longitudinal arch of the foot is low or non existent. The foot is pronated, the navicular is prominent and the heel is in valgus. Flatfoot can be flexible or rigid. The rigid flatfoot remains flat in sitting, standing and in tiptoe standing positions of the foot. The flexible flatfoot, on the other hand, is flat only on standing. Etiology of the flatfoot is unknown but following pathologies are associated with flat foot:

a) Congenital

b) Ligament laxity (Down's syndrome, Marfan's syndrome)

c) Muscle imbalance (as in poliomyelitis)

d) Tendo achilles contracture

e) Residual of calcalcaneovalgus foot

f) Congenital vertical talus (Rocker bottom foot)

g) Accessory navicular (Prehallux syndrome)

h) Tarsal coalition

Rheumatoid arthritis and rupture of tibialis posterior tendon can lead to flat foot in later life.

Infantile flat foot

All infants have flat foot and this is because of several reasons:

a) Normal longitudinal arch develops usually by 3–5 years.

b) Infants have ligamentous laxity thus, their arches collapse on weight bearing.

c) Infants have baby fat in the sole, which disappears by the age of 3–5 years. Hence, before 3–5 years, the arch may look flat even if it does not ultimately turn out to be flat foot.

Congenital hypermobile flatfoot is no longer considered an abnormality but a normal variant.

This is a genetic trait and is not considered to be an indication for treatment.

Accessory navicular syndrome is caused by a separate ossicle in the posterior tibial tendon adjacent to the navicular. The prominence of this bone may cause symptoms (Fig. 20.4a). Sometimes, this accessory bone receives anomalous insertion of tibialis posterior tendon along with the flattening of the longitudinal arch – the *"Prehallux Syndrome"*. The treatment is by padding and foot exercises. Occasionally excision of the accessory navicular may be required.

Clinically the patient may be asymptomatic or may present with pain. Arch pain results from foot

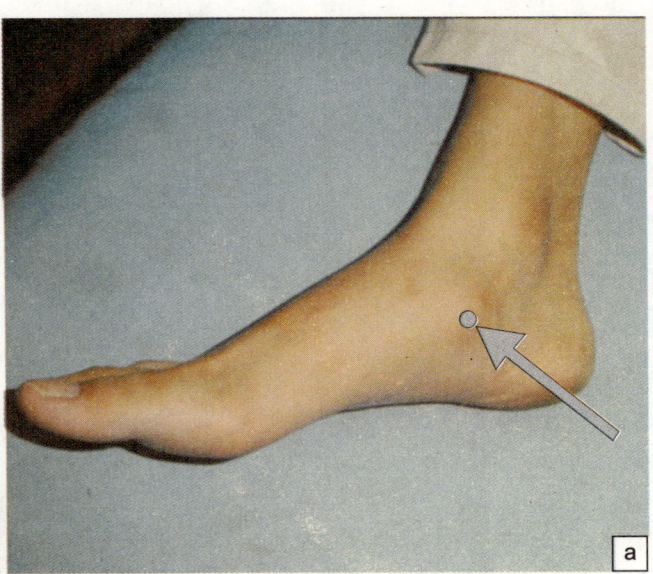

Fig. 20.4a. Clinical photograph of a patient with accessory navicular. Arrow marks the site of accessory navicular

strain in severe cases with excessive use. Calf pain is typically caused by tight heel cords.

The patients with flatfeet also often present with uneven wear of the shoes ; the inner side of sole wears more.

Radiologically on the weight bearing lateral view of the foot, loss of arch is seen. The sagging can be at the talonavicular or naviculocuneiform joint. On the AP view the talocalcaneal angle is increased. Accessory navicular may sometimes be seen on radiographs (Fig. 20.4b).

Treatment of the pes planus is required only for the symptomatic feet. Shoes with good arch support and stretching for the tendo achilles contractures are useful measures. Medial navicular pad, Thomas heel (C&E: Crooked and Elongated Heel) consisting of medial heel wedge and longitudinal arch support is often used. Surgery is required for persistent pain, excessive shoe wear problems or to address specific underlying condition (such as tendon transfer for paralytic conditions, triple arthrodesis for tarsal coalition or excision of accessory navicular).

Surgical procedures for treatment of flatfoot can be soft tissue procedures (distal advancement of plantar calcaneonavicular ligament and posterior tibial tendon) or bony procedures (talonavicular fusion, naviculocuneiform fusion, subtalar arthrodesis or triple arthrodesis).

7. Pes Cavus

Pes cavus is fixed equinus deformity of the forefoot on the hindfoot ("forefoot drop" for those who believe equinus can occur only at ankle) leading to accentuated longitudinal arch and contracture of the plantar soft tissues. Pes cavus is frequently associated with hindfoot varus and claw toes. Both calcaneus (calcaneocavus) and equinus (equinocavus) may be associated with pes cavus. Pes cavus can be idiopathic, familial or congenital. It can be caused by muscle imbalance (e.g. weak tibialis anterior with strong peroneus longus, paralysis of intrinsics, paralysis of triceps surae with strong long toe flexors) or by neuromuscular diseases (such as muscle dystrophy, peripheral neuropathies, myelomeningocele, diastematomyelia, Friedrich's ataxia etc).

Clinically position of hindfoot, appearance of toes, flexibility of foot, and muscle imbalance should be assessed. The patient has accentuated longitudinal arch and callosities under the metatarsal heads. Toes are curled and develop callosities on the dorsal aspect due to rubbing against the shoes.

Investigations for pes cavus must include muscle power examination, EMG/NCV, X-rays of the spine and the opinion of the neurologist.

Treatment is conservative in mild cases in the form of stretching, metatarsal pads and lateral

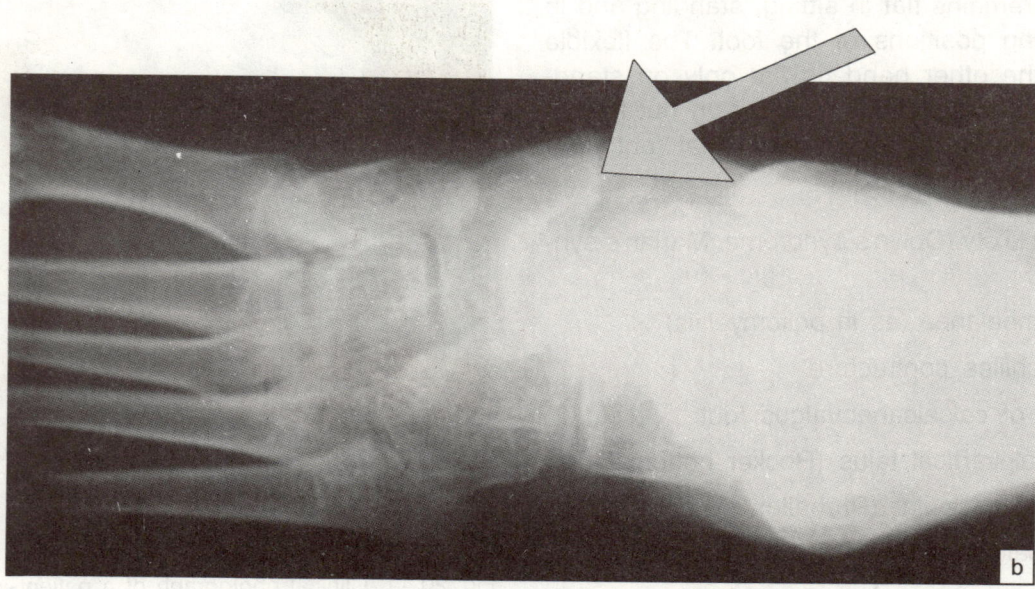

Fig. 20.4b.   Radiographs of a patient with accessory navicular (arrow)

wedge for the heel varus. Surgical treatment consists of Steindler's plantar release (release of contracted plantar fascia, muscles and ligaments), tendon transfer (long toe extensors to necks of metatarsals), dorsal wedge resection or Japa's V osteotomy of the tarsus, osteotomy of the calcaneus (Dwyer's lateral closing wedge) or triple arthrodesis.

Osteochondrosis

Osteochondritis can affect calcaneal apophysis (*Sever's*), navicular (*Kohler's*) or second metatarsal head (*Freiberg's*).

Clinically, the patient is an adolescent who complains of pain. X-rays show irregularity and fragmentation of the epiphysis/apophysis (Fig. 20.4c). Treatment is conservative and symptomatic with rest, NSAIDs and plaster cast if required.

Soft tissue conditions of the foot

Morton's metatarsalgia (Plantar digital neuroma)

Morton's metatarsalgia is due to a painful neuroma at the level of metatarsal heads due to degeneration and proliferation of the plantar digital nerve. It is commonly caused by nerve compression or microtrauma. It is much more common in males (4:1) than females, in the fourth to sixth decades. The commonest site is just proximal to the division of nerve usually in the third web space (85%), followed by the second web space (15%). Predisposing factors are high heeled shoes, and prolonged standing on inflexible surfaces.

Clinically, it presents as burning or shooting type of pain in the third web space radiating distally to the affected digit. Pain increases on weight bearing. Patient may have paraesthesiae of third and fourth toes. The condition is most commonly painful when wearing shoe with a narrow toe box.

Physical examination reveals tenderness at third web space. Lateral compression on metatarsal heads causes pain.

Treatment

Conservative treatment consists of NSAIDs, wider shoes, metatarsal pad or local steroid injections. If symptoms do not respond, then excision of the neuroma through a plantar approach (proximal to the intermetatarsal ligament) relieves the symptoms.

Plantar Fascitis

Inflammation of the plantar fascia leads to pain on the plantar aspect of the heel. The pain is typically most severe after getting up in the morning when the patient is unable to walk even a few steps initially.

The patients are often overweight, wear faulty

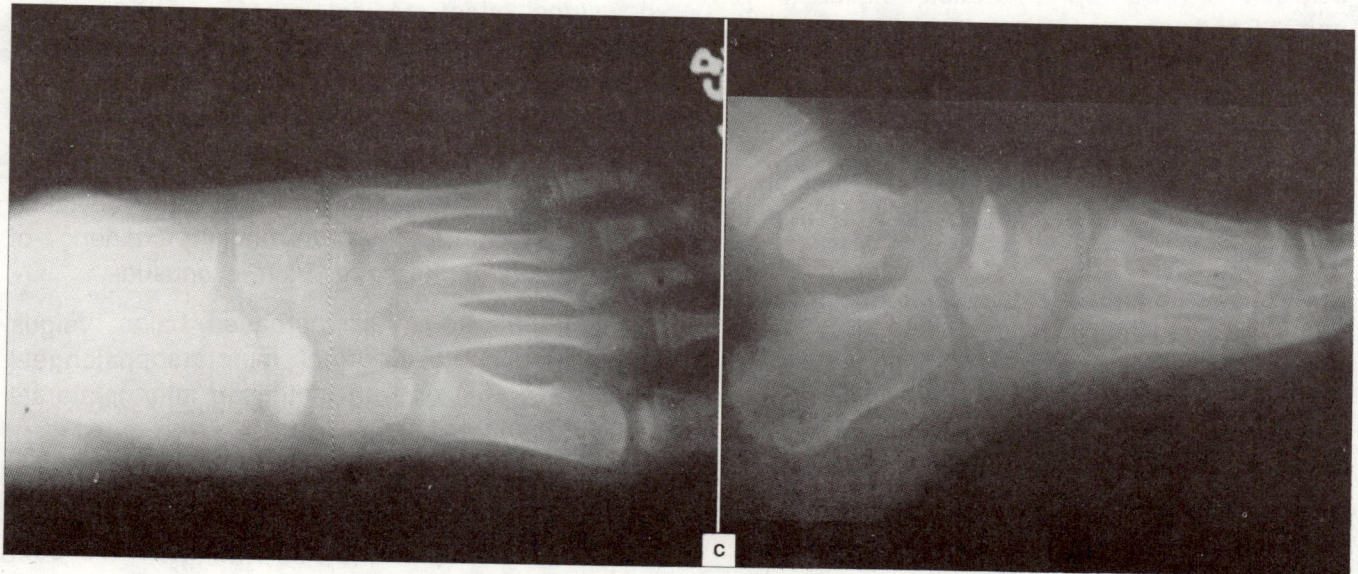

Fig. 20.4c. Radiographs of a patient with Kohler's disease

shoes (i.e. rigid sole shoes), stand for long hours, often run long distances or have a cavus foot.

Examination reveals tenderness most commonly over the medial subcalcaneal region.

Radiographs often reveal a calcaneal spur (calcification at the origin of flexor digitorum brevis) in the lateral view of the foot but no causal relationship has been proved.

The condition should be differentiated from other causes of heel pain such as infalmmation of the plantar heel pad, tarsal tunnel syndrome, stress fracture of the calcaneus or the disorders of the achilles tendon.

Treatment includes rest, heel cushions, NSAIDs and stretching exercises for the tendo achilles and plantar fascia. Local injection of hydrocortisone acetate at the site of tenderness affords relief frequently. Rarely plantar fasciotomy may be needed to treat unremitting pain refractory to other treatments.

Hyperkeratotic disorders (corns)

Localized areas of keratosis are caused by pressure due to bony prominence. Treatment consists of shoe modification and/or surgical removal of the offending bone.

Tarsal Tunnel Syndrome is caused by entrapment of posterior tibial nerve or one of its branches due to ganglion, lipoma, exostosis, scar, tarsal coalition or hypertrophic abductor hallus (in runners). Condition presents with chronic heel pain increased by running. Pain radiates from the medial aspect of the heel into the medial ankle area and can radiate laterally across the foot.

Diagnosis is by tenderness over the first branch of lateral plantar nerve deep to the abductor hallucis muscle.

EMG shows abnormal findings in abductor hallucis and/or abductor digiti minimi.

Treatment Conservative treatment consists of orthosis, NSAIDs and injection.

Surgery involves release of the tarsal tunnel to decompress tibial nerve and resection of flexor retinaculum.

Sinus Tarsi Syndrome presents as pain on the lateral side of the foot on walking seen in pes cavus or pes planus, arthritides (such as rheumatoid arthritis, gout and seronegative spondyloarthropathies) or trauma (fibula fracture, ankle sprain, calcaneal or talar neck fracture). Diagnosis is by sharp pain when palpating the sinus tarsi.

Treatment consists of injection of local anaesthetic steroid in the sinus tarsi, NSAIDs, immobilisation and physiotherapy.

Recalcitrant cases may need surgical decompression of sinus tarsi.

Bony Lesions of the Foot (Big toe disorders)

Hallux valgus (bunion) develops most often due to abnormal foot pressure creating a valgus thrust on the great toe. It is more common in females and is often associated with deformities such as metatarsus primus varus, pronated hallux, hammered second toe and arthritis of the first metatarsophalangeal joint.

Common causes are congenital, hereditary, flat foot, short first metatarsal, trauma, inflammation and high-heeled shoes with narrow toe box.

Patho-anatomy

Abductor hallucis is laterally displaced and rotated plantarwards. Adductor hallucis pulls the proximal phalanx and sesamoid in valgus position and aggravates the deformity. Flexor hallucis brevis and flexor hallucis longus aggravate the deformity by bowstring effect. Medial capsule stretches and the lateral capsule contracts with worsening of the deformity. A bursa (bunion) forms over the prominent metatarsal head medially.

Clinically the chief complaint is deformity at the first metatarsophalangeal joint with lateral deviation of the great toe and a large medial prominence of the first metatarsal head. Pain is unusual.

Radiographs show an increased hallux valgus angle (Fig. 20.5) (normal metatarsophalangeal angle is $\leq 15°$) and an increased intermetatarsal angle (normal $\leq 9°$).

Treatment Non operative treatment option includes shoe modification to relieve pressure over the medial prominence e.g. high wide toe box, rubber wedge soles, intertoe spacers and soft leather uppers.

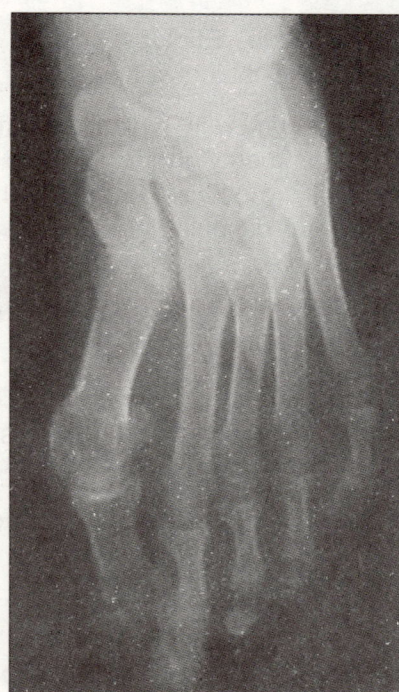

Fig. 20.5. Radiographs of a patient with hallux valgus showing metatarsophalangeal angle more than 15°

Surgery Many types of surgical treatments are available for the treatment of severe deformity. Procedures are broadly divided into soft tissue procedures, bony procedures or combined. Bunionectomy, that is, excision of prominent medial eminence is the most commonly performed procedure when the bunion impinges against the toe box of shoe. Soft tissue procedures and osteotomies (distal metatarsal, proximal metatarsal or proximal phalangeal) are done in younger patients while in elderly patients with osteoarthritic changes, resection arthroplasty (Keller) or arthrodesis of the first metatarsophalangeal joint is done.

Bunionette (*Tailor's Bunion*) is prominence of the fifth metatarsal head. Bunionette is associated with hallux valgus, splay foot or lateral deviation of metatarsal. Abnormal alignment of the metatarsal leads to lateral bowing of the diaphysis of the fifth metatarsal and a painful prominence of the lateral condyle of the fifth metatarsal head.

Clinically it presents with painful prominence and lateral or plantar keratosis.

Radiographs reveal lateral bowing of the fifth metatarsal.

Treatment Conservative treatment consists of shoe modification. Surgical treatment involves excision of lateral portion of head with or without lateral condyle of the proximal phalanx; or alternatively, osteotomy of the neck, shaft or base if lateral deviation of the metatarsal shaft is the underlying cause.

Hallux Rigidus is the degenerative arthritis of metatarsophalangeal (MTP) joint of the great toe characterized by pain and stiffness (especially restriction of dorsiflexion). Etiology can be repetitive trauma, metabolic disease (gout), arthritides (osteoarthritis, psoriatic arthritis) or surgery.

Clinically patient presents with painful MTP joint, prominent bony spur on dorsal aspect of the first metatarsal head and stiffness of the joint. Physical examination reveals tenderness and decreased dorsiflexion of the MTP joint.

Radiographs reveal MTP joint narrowing and dorsal bony spur over metatarsal head.

Treatment Non operative treatment consists of NSAIDs and orthoses (rigid sole or rocker sole).

Surgical treatment consists of chielectomy (removal of bone spur and up to one third of metatarsal head to allow 60–80° dorsiflexion) in relatively younger patients. Older patients with advanced osteoarthritis are treated by arthrodesis or excision of proximal third of the base of proximal phalanx (Keller).

Hallux varus can be congenital or arises as iatrogenic deformity following operative treatment of hallux valgus.

Clinically, it presents with pain along the medial side of the great toe and discomfort while wearing shoes. Great toe looks adducted.

Treatment Non operative treatment consists of valgus strapping and splinting. Operative correction of deformity can be done for recalcitrant cases.

Lesser toes disorders

Hammer toe

Hammer toe is characterized by contracture of the FDL tendon leading to plantarflexion of the PIP joint with dorsiflexion of the MTP joint. It can result from trauma, poorly fitting shoes, muscle imbalance in association with neuromuscular disorders, inflammation or can be idiopathic.

Clinically the patient has bony prominence on the dorsum of PIP joint. Tender corns overlie the prominence. Longer digits are typically affected more often. Patient has pain, discomfort and difficulty fitting the shoes. Deformities can be fixed or flexible.

Radiographs reveal dorsiflexion of the proximal phalanx with plantarflexion of the middle and/or distal phalanges.

Treatment can be conservative in form of treatment of corns, splinting devices and high wide toe box shoes.

Surgery for flexible deformity consists of flexor to extensor transfer. Rigid deformities are treated by resection of distal portion of the proximal phalanx.

Clawed toes

Clawed toes are characterized by hyperextension of MTP joint and hyperflexion at PIP and DIP joints. There is simultaneous contracture of the long extensors and long flexors of the toe. The condition also reflects an imbalance between the intrinsic and extrinsic muscles of the foot.

Etiology may be familial, traumatic, inflammatory, neuromuscular, shoe wear (high heel or short narrow toe box) or idiopathic.

Clinically it affects multiple toes and is typically bilateral.

There are bony prominences and corns on the dorsum of the PIP joint. Typical deformities are differentiated from hammer toe by hyperextension at MTP joint.

Radiographs reveal dorsiflexed position of the proximal phalanges and a plantarflexed position of the middle and distal phalanges.

Treatment Conservative treatment consists of high wide toe box shoe and splintage.

Surgical treatment consists of tendon transfer (flexor to extensor) for flexible deformity.

Fixed deformities can be treated by distal hemiphalangectomy or diaphysectomy of proximal phalanx.

Mallet toe is defined as flexion deformity of the DIP joint of the toe. Etiology can be traumatic, idiopathic or poorly fitting shoes.

Clinically, it presents with typical deformity, which occurs most commonly in the second toe. Pain occurs when the tip of the toe strikes the ground. Distal tip corn and difficulty in fitting the shoes are common.

Radiographs show a flexion contracture at the DIP joint.

Treatment Non operative treatment consists of padding to prevent the tip of toe from striking the ground.

Surgical treatment consists of release of tight FDL tendon or partial/complete resection of middle phalanx.

Inflammatory Disorders of the Foot

Rheumatoid Foot

Rheumatoid arthritis may involve the foot in about 15–20% cases and involvement is usually symmetric. Forefoot changes occur early and commonly and consist of hallux valgus, claw or hammer toes, hyperextension at MTP joints and prominent metatarsal heads (Fig. 20.6a). Synovitis of MTP joints leads to subluxation and dislocation of the joints.) Chronic synovitis of the joints and ligament laxity lead to splaying of forefoot.

Midfoot (tarsal and tarsometatarsal joints) are typically not severely involved in rheumatoid foot. Chronic synovitis and loss of joint space lead to fibrous and bony ankylosis.

Loss of longitudinal arch occurs due to sagging of the metatarsocuneiform or naviculocuneiform joints (Fig. 20.6b).

Hindfoot changes in rheumatoid arthritis occur late and are related to destruction of tissues around subtalar joint. Hindfoot valgus, rupture of tibialis posterior tendon, loss of longitudinal arch and ankylosis of subtalar joint can occur.

Clinically, the patients have pain and erythema over the involved joints with involvement of the PIP and MTP joints. Typical deformities occur later in the course.

Radiographs show only soft tissue swelling in early stages. Later on typical deformities, disorganization of MTP joint and ankylosis of tarsal joints is evident (Fig. 20.6c,d).

Treatment: Non operative treatment is drug therapy, physical therapy and orthotic devices. Surgical treatment consists of resection of metatarsal heads with or without resection of bases of phalanges for toe deformities. Hindfoot deformities are treated with subtalar or triple arthrodesis.

Tuberculosis of foot bones

Tubercular infection of small bones of the foot is not very common. Tubercular dactylitis (*SPINA VENTOSA*) leads to expansion and thickening of the phalanx. The changes are most marked near the center where the nutrient artery enters the phalanx (as the infection is hematogenous). Patient presents with pain, swelling and stiffness of foot joints. Multiple discharging sinuses may be present. Radiographs show osteoporosis, lytic areas in foot bones and diminished joint space. Treatment consists of antitubercular treatment, splintage in plaster slab and rest (Fig. 20.7).

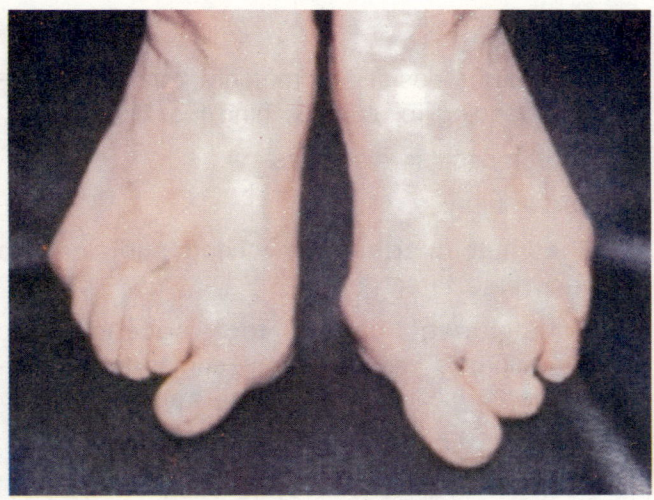

Fig. 20.6a. Rheumatoid foot with Bilateral hallux valgus and clawing of all four toes

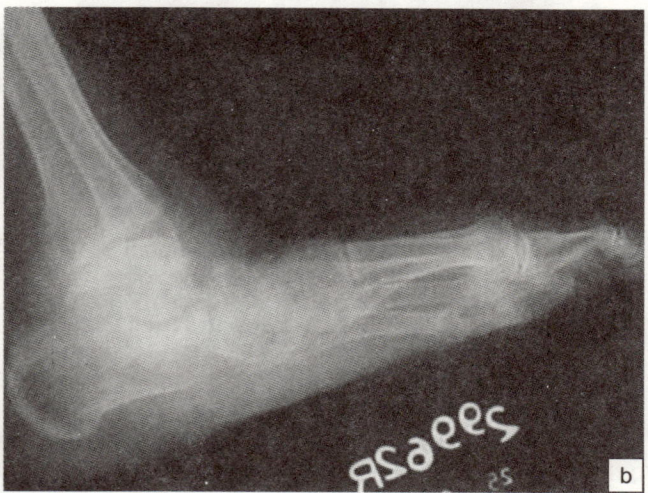

Fig. 20.6b. Radiographs of a patient with RA showing flat foot

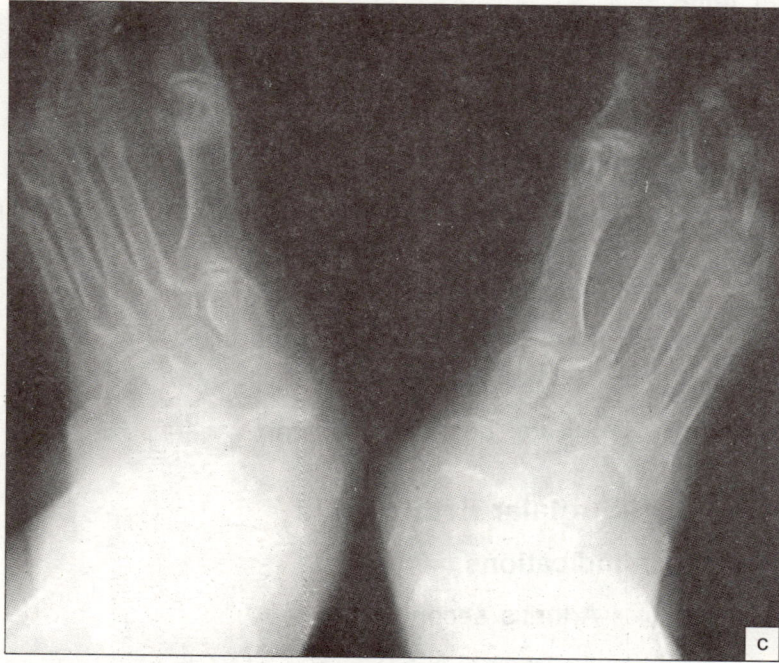

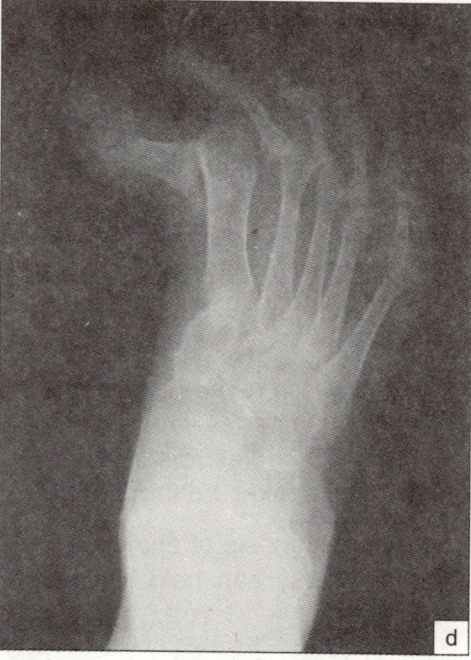

Fig. 20.6c,d. Radiographs showing disorganization of MTP joints in RA

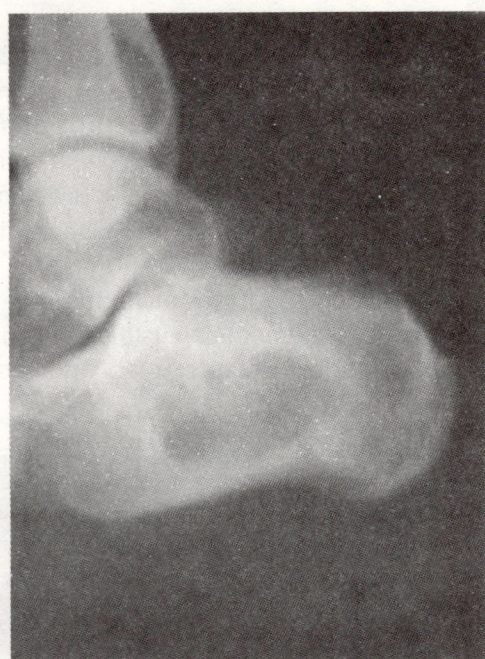

Fig. 20.7.   Tuberculosis of the calcaneum
Note the osteolytic lesion

Other disorders of the foot

Charcot's joint

Charcot's joints are caused by diabetes, spina bifida, syringomyelia and other neurological disorders associated with diminished sensations. The damage to the bones and joints of the foot arises from mechanical trauma in an insensate foot as well as from a neurally stimulated vascular reflex causing bone resorption.

Charcot's joints affect males and females equally. Almost one-third cases are bilateral.

Clinically patient presents with swelling of the ankle and foot with increased temperature. In later stages the joint gets completely disorganized and may have crepitus due to plenty of osteocartilaginous bodies arising out of synovial metaplasia.

Radiologically X-rays initially show soft tissue swelling. Later stages are characterized by loose osteochondral bodies, disorganization of joint, deformities like rocker bottom foot, and splay foot.

Differential diagnosis of charcot's joint is low grade infection. Biopsy can help reach the diagnosis in difficult cases.

Treatment of charcot's joints is avoidance of trauma and bracing of the ankle and foot. Surgical proce-

dures should be generally avoided. Arthrodesis of the joint is the only useful procedure if needed. However, difficulty to achieve fusion and high incidence of infection remain the serious problems with bony procedures in charcot's joints.

Arthrodesis of the Foot Joints

Triple Arthrodesis

Triple arthrodesis refers to the fusion of subtalar (talocalcaneal), talonavicular and calcaneocuboid joints.

Indications

*   Triple arthrodesis is commonly done for conditions leading to unstable hind foot like:
*   Neuromuscular disorders
*   Nerve injury
*   Rheumatoid arthritis involving subtalar and transverse tarsal joints
*   Malalignment of the foot secondary to arthrofibrosis resulting from compartment syndrome, crush injury or severe trauma
*   Symptomatic calcaneo-navicular coalition
*   Posterior tibial tendon dysfunction

Position of Arthrodesis

Hindfoot in 5° valgus

Transverse tarsal joints in 0-5° abduction

Forefoot in less than 10° varus

Complications

➢ Pseudarthrosis most commonly of the talonavicular joint
➢ Degenerative arthritis of the ankle
➢ Avascular necrosis of the talus
➢ Malalignment
➢ Sural nerve entrapment

Subtalar Arthrodesis

Indications

• Arthritis secondary to

    Trauma (most commonly following calcaneal fractures)

Rheumatoid arthritis

Talocalcaneal coalition

- Muscle imbalance

- Posterior tibial dysfunction

Neuromuscular disorders: Poliomyelitis (Fig. 20.8), Charcot-Marie-Tooth disease

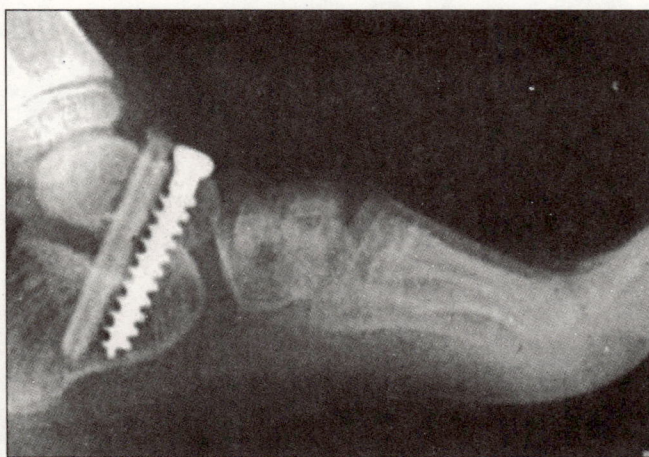

Fig. 20.8. Extraarticular subtalar arthrodesis in a patient with poliomyelitis

Position

5° valgus

Complications

➢ Nonunion

➢ Malalignment

Metatarsophalangeal Joint Arthrodesis

Indications

- Severe Hallux valgus

- Rheumatoid arthritis

- Hallux rigidus

- Posttraumatic arthritis

Hallux valgus deformity after CVA, head injury or cerebral palsy

Contraindications

- Arthritis of the interphalangeal joint

- Insensate foot

- Arthritis of first metatarsocuneiform joint

Complications

➢ Nonunion

➢ Malalignment

➢ Arthritis of interphalangeal joint of great toe

Interphalangeal joint arthrodesis of great toe

Indications

- Posttraumatic arthritis

- Fixed flexion contracture after trauma

Part of modified Jones procedure (after transfer of EHL to the neck of first metatarsal)

Position

Neutral valgus with 5–10° of plantar flexion

Complications

➢ Nonunion and malunion

1st Metatarsophalangeal Joint Arthroplasty

It was recommended in the past for severely deformed rheumatoid forefoot and hallux rigidus. Silastic and metal implants were used. The procedure became unpopular due to short-term and long-term complications like weakened support for great toe, osteolysis of the proximal phalanx and fragmentation, synovitis, collapse and bone overgrowth.

SECTION III
Trauma

General Characteristics of Fractures

A fracture is defined as a complete or incomplete break in the continuity of a bone. The strength of bone is about 1/10 that of steel. A dominant quality of bone is its brittleness; bone behaves more like glass than like rubber. The hydroxyapatite structure (inorganic element) is responsible for its compressive strength and the collagen fibre (organic matrix) provides for its tensile strength. Normal bone is capable of withstanding the stresses it is generally subjected to, in routine everyday use. Only when these stresses are exceeded or if for any reason bone is weakened (pathological), its structure fails.

Fractures may be classified based on location (proximal, middle, distal thirds), direction (transverse, spiral, oblique, complex) and associated features (e.g. open fractures, blood vessel/nerve injury, dislocations). A classification is useful as it serves as a basis for treatment decisions and for evaluation of the results (Fig. 21.1).

Location Each long bone is divided into segments-two epiphyseal, two metaphyseal and one diaphyseal segment. The metaphysis and epiphysis are considered as one segment in adults because the morphology of the metaphyseal fracture influences the treatment and prognosis of the epiphyseal (articular) fracture. A diaphyseal fracture extending into the joint is considered an

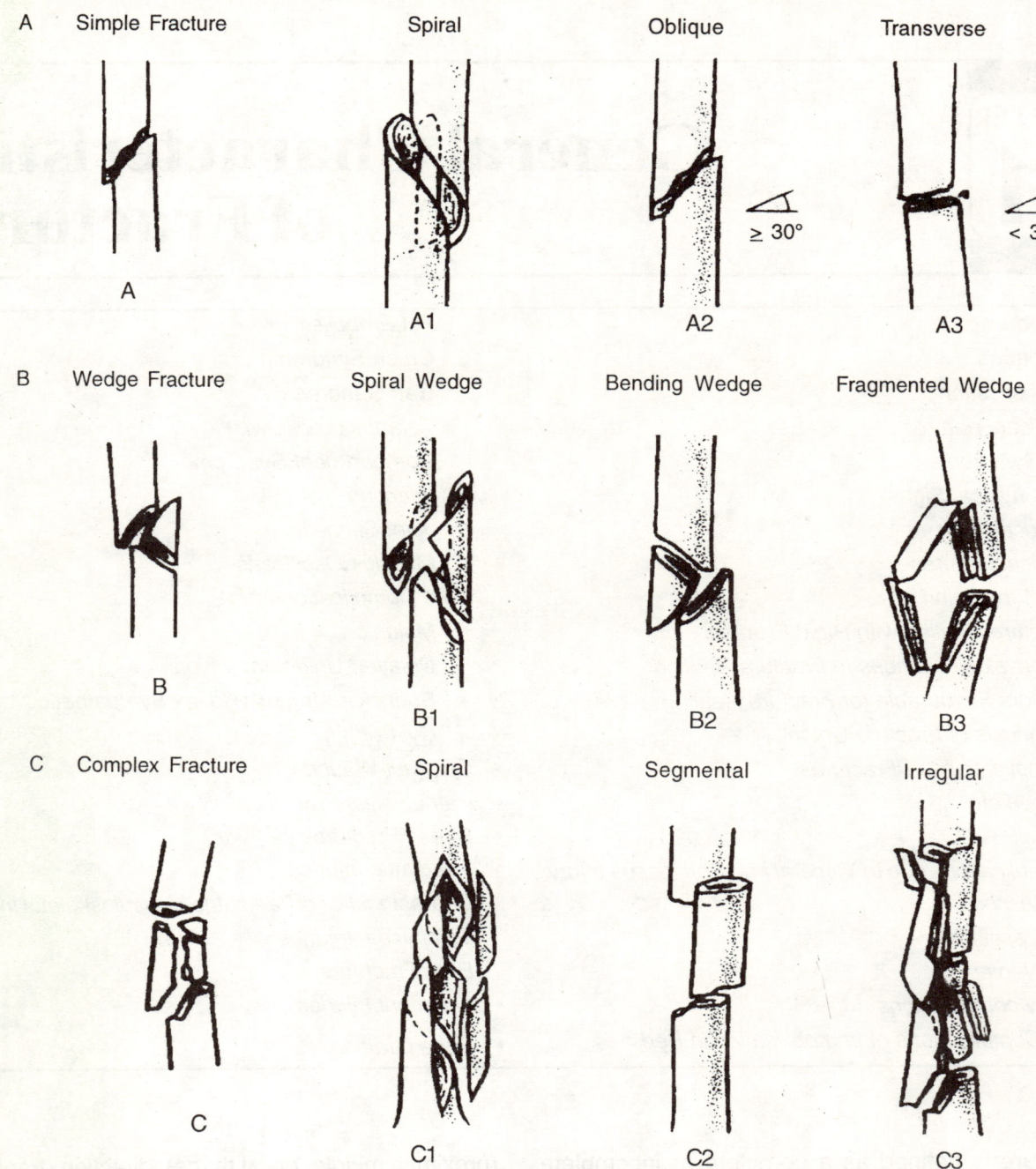

A	Simple Fracture	Spiral	Oblique	Transverse
	A	A1	A2 ≥ 30°	A3 < 30°

B	Wedge Fracture	Spiral Wedge	Bending Wedge	Fragmented Wedge
	B	B1	B2	B3

C	Complex Fracture	Spiral	Segmental	Irregular
	C	C1	C2	C3

Fig. 21.1. AO Classification of Diaphyseal fractures

articular fracture. Some complex fractures may, however, not be classifiable by segment localisation.

Pattern/Direction Depending on the orientation of the fracture line, the fracture may be simple or multifragmentary.

Simple Fracture There is a single circumferential disruption of the diaphysis or metaphysis or a single disruption of an articular surface. Simple fractures may be further categorised as:

Transverse The fracture line is transverse. It is caused by an angulatory force. Following accurate reduction this fracture is stable due to the interdigitation of spikes.

Oblique The fracture line is oblique. The fracture is caused by a rotational (twisting) force. The reduction is not stable, as the fracture fragments tend to slip over each other.

Spiral The fracture line runs a long spiral. These

fractures are also caused by a rotational (twisting) force. The reduction is not stable. However due to a wider surface area union is rapid.

Impacted This is a stable fracture of the metaphysis or epiphysis in which the fragments are driven one into the other.

Multifragmentary Fracture The fracture has one or more completely separated intermediate fragment(s). This includes the wedge and complex fractures.

Wedge A fracture with one or more intermediate fragments in which, after reduction, there is some contact between the main fragments.

Complex A fracture with one or more intermediate fragment(s) in, which after reduction, there is no contact between the proximal and distal fragments.

The term comminuted is vague and imprecise and should not be used.

Articular Fracture The fracture involves the articular surface. They are subdivided into partial and complete.

Partial Articular Fracture The fracture involves only part of the articular surface, while the rest of the surface remains attached to the diaphysis. They are further categorised as :

1. **Pure Split** The direction of the fracture is usually vertical.

2. **Pure Depression** There is pure depression of the articular surface without a split. The depression may be central or peripheral.

3. **Split-Depression** A combination of split and depression in which, the fragments are usually separated.

4. **Multifragmentary Depression** The joint surface is depressed and the fragments are completely separated.

Complete Articular Fracture The articular surface is disrupted and completely separated from the diaphysis.

Note Extra-articular fractures do not involve the articular surface, although they may be intra-capsular e.g. fracture neck of femur, avulsion of the ACL.

Miscellaneous

Greenstick Fracture This injury is seen only in children when the bones are soft and resilient. It is caused by a bending force. It is an incomplete fracture in which the cortex is broken on the convex side while continuity remains on the concave side. The fracture is stable and unless further violence is applied, it is unlikely to displace.

Torus Fracture There is buckling of the cortex without any break. It is caused by a compressive force e.g. torus fracture of distal radius caused by fall on the outstretched hand. The fracture is seen at the metaphyseo-diaphyseal junction of long bone where there is transition from cancellous to cortical bone.

Avulsion Fracture These fractures are caused by traction–a ligament, tendon or muscle tearing off a fragment of bone e.g. fracture of the patella due to pull of the quadriceps. When the fragment is avulsed by a ligament, joint instability may result.

Compression Fracture This fracture occurs in cancellous bones like the vertebral body and calcaneum. Due to the compressive stress, the bone mass is compressed into itself. If the compressive forces are great the bone appears to explode-the fracture fragments are driven outwards-the so-called 'burst' fracture.

Diagnosis The diagnosis of fractures and dislocation should be considered to be essentially clinical. However radiography is required to confirm the diagnosis and help classify the fracture or dislocation. Occasionally special investigations (CT scan, bone scan) may be needed to confirm a fracture.

Clinical Features

Symptoms

1. History of injury

2. Pain is the commonest symptom. In a multiply injured patient, however, pain may not be a prominent feature or it may be concentrated at one site, masking an injury elsewhere.

3. *Loss of function* The patient is usually reluctant to use the limb and supports it with the hand or clothing or indigenous splints e.g. wooden stick, foot ruler. In some cases, e.g. compression fracture of the spine, impacted femur neck fracture, there may not be complete loss of

function and the patient may stand or walk, but usually does so with difficulty.

Physical Signs

1. *External appearance* There may be a deformity and the limb may be swollen or bruised. The limb may be shortened or bent at an awkward angle or there may be a step in alignment, e.g. acute kyphus at the dorso-lumbar junction in fracture of the spine.

2. *Tenderness* This is the most constant and consistent physical sign. Careful and gentle palpation over the injured area is required to detect the tenderness.

3. *Swelling* When the fracture is first seen the swelling may be minimal but it usually increases with time for the first 24 hours. This is partly due to the fracture hematoma, and partly due to the inflammatory exudate. A rapidly progressive swelling should arouse suspicion of vascular injury. Strong clinical suspicion of a fracture but absence of swelling should make one wary of an external or internal communication.

4. *Abnormal mobility and crepitation of the fracture ends* This feature is mentioned here for the sake of completion only and should never be attempted in clinical practice so as to avoid further injury to the soft tissues especially the neurovascular structures.

Note In addition to eliciting the signs of fracture, the following points should also routinely be ascertained and recorded at the time of clinical examination.

a) Presence of skin wound which denotes that the fracture is probably compound.

b) Evidence of vascular compromise and nerve injury, distal to the fracture.

c) Examination of adjoining bones and joints for presence of concomitant injury:

   (i) fracture of the calcaneum classically occurs in fall from height and may be associated with femur neck fracture, spinal compression injury

   (ii) fracture of the upper third of ulna may be associated with dislocation of the radius head (Monteggia fracture-dislocation).

Radiological Examination Whenever a fracture is suspected, x-rays must be obtained for confirmation. Standard anteroposterior (AP) and lateral radiographs,

including the joint above and below the fracture level, are the minimal requirement for most fractures. The films must be of good quality. Poor quality radiographs should be repeated. Radiographs provide the following additional information.

1. Localisation of the fracture or dislocation accurately and determining the classification of the fracture.

2. Direction and degree of fragment(s) displacement.

3. Evidence of pre-existing pathology in the bone.

4. Presence of an opaque foreign body.

5. Diagnosis of an unsuspected injury.

6. It may show air in the soft tissues suggesting a penetrating injury.

In some cases the fracture line may not be visible for a few weeks and in these cases the fracture may have to be treated on clinical suspicion, e.g. fracture scaphoid, where repeat radiographs are taken after an interval of two weeks, to confirm the presence of the fracture.

Dislocation A dislocation is complete disruption of the joint so that the articular surfaces are no longer in contact. Subluxation is minor disruption of the joint where articular contact still remains. Most subluxations are associated with fractures of the joint.

Clinical features

1. *Pain* As with other injuries, there is severe pain that persists till the dislocation is reduced.

2. *Loss of motion* In all dislocations, active and passive motion is grossly limited.

3. *Attitude* The position in which the limb is held may be diagnostic e.g. flexion, adduction, internal rotation at hip-posterior dislocation; flexion, abduction, external rotation at hip-anterior dislocation.

4. *Neurovascular injury* The incidence of neurologic damage is much higher in dislocation than with fractures (Table 21.1).

Distal vascularity must always be recorded at the initial examination e.g. There is a high risk of popliteal artery damage (50%) with dislocation of the knee.

Radiological Examination X-rays are indispensable part of the work up of the patient with

Table 21.1. Nerve injuries associated with dislocations

Dislocation	Nerve Injury
Shoulder	Axillary, brachial plexus
Elbow	Ulnar
Radial head	Posterior interosseous
Hip (posterior)	Sciatic (common peroneal division).
Knee	Common peroneal

suspected dislocation or subluxation. X-rays complement a good clinical examination but cannot substitute for it e.g. posterior shoulder dislocation may be missed on radiography if clinically, limitation of motion (zero external rotation) is not elicited. Associated fractures can be detected, by radiological examination.

Fracture Union

Besides liver, bone is one of the few tissues of the body, which can undergo spontaneous regeneration to restore the anatomy to the condition, which existed prior to the injury. The moment the fracture occurs, repair processes start. There are still many gaps in our knowledge regarding fracture union. The ultimate end point of fracture healing is cortex to cortex union.

The repair process occurs continuously but certain stages can be recognised. All the stages occur simultaneously at any given time, at different places in the fracture hematoma. The different stages are so labelled only because that particular process is predominant at that given moment. For the sake of simplicity and since it includes all the stages of fracture healing, fracture union in a long bone is taken into consideration. The pathological changes of bone healing (Fig. 21.2) described below take place when the fractured bone ends are firmly (not rigidly) held together so that some micro-movement between the bone ends is possible.

Stage 1 (*Impact*)   This stage includes the interval from the first application of force to bone until the energy of the force is completely   dissipated. Depending on the amount of energy absorbed and the rate, at which it is applied, bone fractures into a specific pattern.

Stage 2 (Stage of *hematoma*)   With the interruption in continuity of bone, the periosteum is torn and bleeding occurs forming a clot in and around the fracture site. Vessels in the Haversian system (Haversian vessels run logitudinally; Volkmann's canals are oriented horizontally) are disrupted for a variable distance from the fracture site. The bone immediately adjacent to and for a variable distance from the fracture site becomes necrotic. The exact function of the hematoma is not known but it is believed to provide a latticework of fibrin upon which the cellular elements can proliferate i.e. osteoconduction.

Stage 3 (Stage of *inflammation/cellular proliferation*) Within a few hours of the fracture, inflammatory cells arrive at the injured site and this is associated with dilatation of capillaries, exudation of fluid and white cells and cellular proliferation. Dead tissue and clot are removed by phagocytes and there is migration of osteoblasts from the cambium layer of the periosteum (primarily) and the endosteum (to a small extent) into the hematoma. This proliferation of osteogenic cells continues from both fragments of the fractured bone until they meet and blend together restoring cellular continuity between the bone ends. In the early stages, cellular proliferation exceeds the rate of vascular ingrowth.

Stage 4 (Stage of *callus formation*)   Vascular proliferation starts from budding of pre-existing blood vessels in the vicinity of bone ends, from the medullary cavity and from the surrounding soft tissues. With increasing vascularity, cells differentiate into osteoblasts, which start to lay down collagen matrix. This matrix becomes impregnated with calcium salts to form immature bone (woven bone) of fracture callus. Callus formed from the periosteal cells is the external callus, and that arising from the endosteum is the internal callus. At the end of this stage the bone is firmly united, callus is clinically palpable and visible on x-rays. In some areas of reduced vascularity, the cells differentiate into chondroblasts and chondrocytes, which lay down cartilage. Cartilage in callus has temporary existence and is eventually replaced by bone by endochondral ossification.

Stage 5 (Stage of *consolidation*)   During this stage the woven cancellous bone of the callus is gradually replaced by the lamellar compact bone.

Stage 6   (Stage of *Remodelling*)   During this stage bone forms along the lines of stress and the surplus bone outside the line of stress is gradually resorbed. The medullary canal is restored and bone assumes its normal shape and size.

Stage I: Stage of Impact (from time of application to dissipation of force)

Stage II: Stage of Hematoma (First few hours)

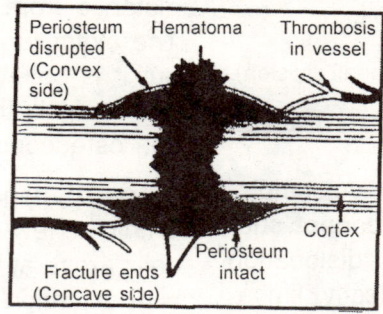

Stage III: State of Inflammation (2-12 days)

Early: Cellular Proliferation   Late: Vascular ingrowth

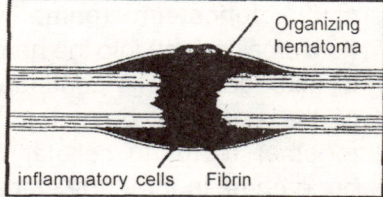
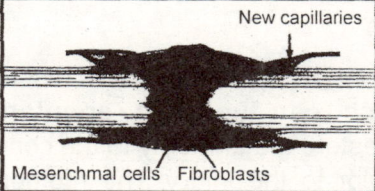

Stage IV/V: Stage of Callus formation/Consolidation (Conversion of lamellar
(upto 6 months)

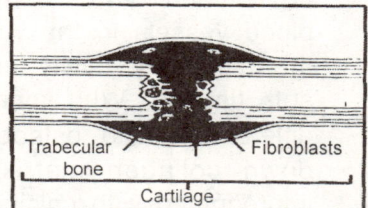
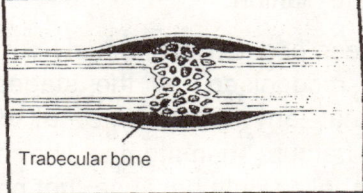

Stage VI: State of remodelling (Orientation of callus along lines of stress)

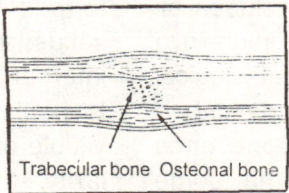

Fig. 21.2. Stages of Fracture healing

Remodelling follows the *Wolff's law* (*form follows function*)

Fracture healing with rigid fixation

When the fracture ends are accurately approximated and securely fixed under compression e.g. plate and screws, little or no external callus forms. Repair depends to a great extent on the formation of internal callus. The fracture hematoma no longer remains since it is removed at the time of surgery while fixing the plate with screws. No periosteal (external) callus is visible radiologically. Fragment end resorption (gap at the fracture site due to bone death) does not occur. The process of internal remodelling of the haversian system, uniting the fracture ends in the only process that occurs. An organelle composed of osteoclasts, osteoblasts and capillaries, referred to as '*cutting cone or cutting head*' has been described (Fig. 21.3). Osteoclasts migrate along the empty

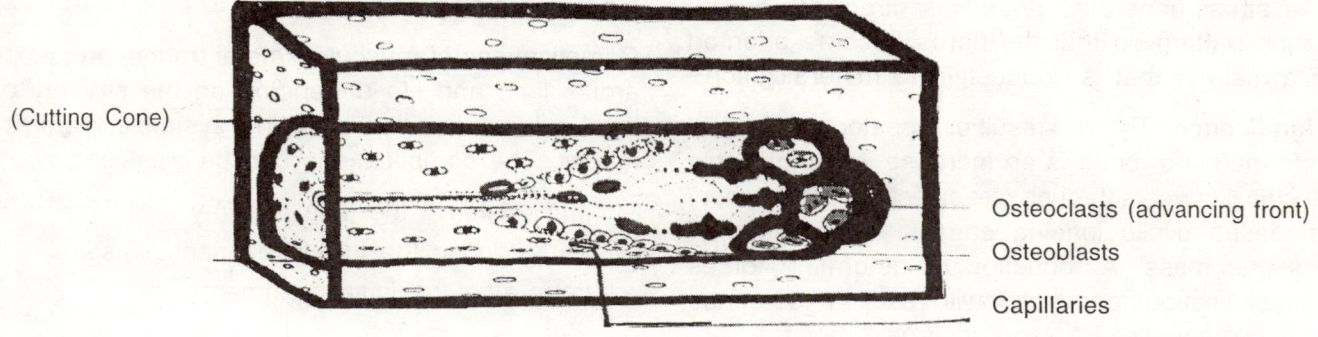

(Cutting Cone)

Osteoclasts (advancing front)

Osteoblasts

Capillaries

Fig. 21.3. Cutting Cone

haversian canals resorbing necrotic bone, cross the fracture site and enter the empty haversian canals of the opposite fragment. Osteoblasts follow close behind laying down collagen matrix, which then mineralises. The bone fragments thus unite and require no later remodelling. Direct bone healing does not lead to faster union.

Note Fracture union with callus by the classic stages of fracture healing is referred to as *'indirect bone healing'* because bone formation progresses through several different tissue types to restore the normal lamellar bone structure. Bone healing after intra-medullary nailing occurs by large amounts of periosteal callus formation.

Biophysical Changes In Fracture Healing

Induction of fracture healing processes, their maintenance and cessation following fracture union remain a mystery. The process of remodelling of a healed fracture shows a peculiar phenomenon resulting in straightening of angulation at the fracture site with passage of time. Of the various physical forces that act on bone cells to induce their genetically determined response, electric potentials are the most extensively researched.

Electric phenomena are integral features of biologic processes in all tissues. Electromechanical interactions are thought to regulate cellular phenomenon such as proliferation, differentiation and metabolism. The source of electric energy may reside within the bone (standing potential) or may result from stress (stress-generated potential).

Standing Potential Living bone tissue exhibits a steady resting potential recorded in the range of microvolts. This resting potential depends on cell viability and may be influenced by mechanical stress and exogenous electric stimulation. In normal bone the metaphysis is strongly **electronegative** with respect to the epiphysis, with decreasing electronegative voltage towards the diaphysis which may be isopolar (neutral) or slightly electropositive.

Stress-Generated Potential When bone is mechanically stressed, it deforms. Area of bone under compression (concave aspect) becomes electronegative while the tension side (convex aspect) becomes electropositive. New bone is deposited around the electronegative area and resorbed from the positive region. This is one of the postulated mechanisms of remodelling.

When a fracture occurs in the diaphysis, almost the entire surface of the bone becomes electronegative with a large peak of electronegativity at the fracture site. This electric phenomenon persists till fracture union. These bioelectric potentials probably induce and maintain healing process in a fracture since active areas of bone growth and repair are electronegative and the less active areas are electrically neutral or electropositive.

Piezoelectrical Property of Collagen

Piezoelectricity is defined as electricity resulting from deformation of crystals. When a structure is stressed and deformed, the separation in the centres of positive and negative charges produces a net polarisation.

Collagen, the main organic component of extracellular matrix carries a net positive charge, with the head end of the macromolecule being more positive with respect to the tail. The collagen units are arranged into fibrils, fibres and bundles in an orderly array so that the charges are additive. Unmineralized collagen fibres are positively charged, deformable elements that lie in close proximity to the negatively charged surfaces or osteoblasts.

The stress-generated potentials direct the aggregation pattern so that the fibres become oriented in a manner that is conductive to mineralization.

Significance The end result of repeated mechanical deformation of bone is an increase in the pulsatile electrical currents through piezoelectric phenomenon. Increased cyclic loading causes an increase of osseous mass. A reduction of deforming forces (immobilisation, paralysis) will result in decrease of bone mass and osteoporosis will result.

Factors Favourable for Fracture Healing

1. Minimal soft tissue trauma at the time of fracture i.e. fractures due to less severe violence.
2. Fracture through cancellous bone, i.e. fracture near ends of long bones where vascularity is rich e.g. distal radius, proximal tibia.
3. Adequate blood supply to both the fragments.
4. Well-contained hematoma under the muscles, i.e. closed fractures heal faster than open injuries.
5. Impacted, oblique and spiral fractures heal faster.
6. Absence of infection at fracture site.
7. Good nutrition.

Diagnosis of fracture union

Clinical union is complete when –

1. There is no tenderness over the fracture site.
2. No mobility at the fracture site.
3. No pain on applying angulatory stress to bone.
4. Transmission of rotation across the fracture site.

Clinical union usually precedes radiologic union.

Radiological features of union are:

1. Visible external callus is present and bridges the fracture fragments.
   Note Primary bone healing which occurs following rigid immobilisation is associated with no visible callus.
2. Bony trabeculae are seen crossing from one fragment to another.
   Note The impacted fracture and the overlapping fragments can give an erroneous impression of trabeculae crossing the fracture site on x-rays.

Complications of Fractures

Complications of musculoskeletal trauma can jeopardize limb and life depending on the severity of local trauma and the resulting systemic manifestations. The complications can be classified as:

– Immediate: at the time of injury
– Early: during the initial treatment phase.
– Late: after the initial treatment.

Immediate

Shock

Shock is defined as a clinical state in which there is inadequate tissue perfusion with resultant tissue hypoxia, threatening irreversible damage to the vital organs. There are four categories of shock:

– Hypovolemic
– Neurogenic
– Cardiogenic
– Septicemic

Hypovolemic (hemorrhagic) shock is by far the most common type of shock occurring in the multiply injured patients. The blood loss may be external (compound fracture) or internal. Internal hemorrhage sufficient to cause shock can be intra-thoracic (hemothorax), intra-peritoneal (spleen injury), retro-peritoneal (pelvic ring disruption) or into muscles in long bone fractures (closed fracture femur can conceal up to one litre of blood). Shock is clinically manifested by tachycardia, low volume pulse, tachypnoea, falling systolic blood pressure, cold and moist extremities and cyanosis of ears, nails and mucous membranes. Shock must be treated before the definitive treatment of the fracture. Severe shock persisting even for a few minutes can cause irreversible cerebral and renal damage.

Acute hemorhage is classified into 4 categories (Table 21.2).

Treatment

The treatment of shock is the first priority in the management of the patient.

The goal of treatment is to safely restore adequate intravascular volume and oxygen-carrying capacity. The following measures are used in the treatment of shock:

Table 21.2. Classes of Acute Hemorrhage

	Class I	Class II	Class III	Class IV
Blood loss (ml)	750	1000-1,250	1,500-1,800	2000-2500
Blood loss* (%)	15	20-25	30-35	40-50
Pulse rate (bears / min)	72-84	> 100	> 120	>140
Blood pressure+ (mmHg)	120/80	110/80	70-90/50-60	<50-60 systolic
Pulse pressure (mmHg)	40	30	20-30	10-20
Respiratory rate	14-20	20-30	30-40	>35
Capillary blanch test	Normal	Delayed	Delayed	Delayed
Urinary output (ml/hr)	30-35	25-30	5-15	Negligible
Mental status	Slightly anxious	Mildly anxious	Anxious, confused and restless	Confused + lethargic
Fluid replacement	Crystalloids	Crystalloids+ Blood	Crystalloids+ Blood	Crystalloids+ Blood

* % blood volume in a standard 70 Kg male.

+ assume normal B.P. 120/80 mmHg.

1. A: Ensure clear Airway

2. B: Ensure adequate Breathing

3. C: Restore Circulatory volume. Obtain immediate i.v. access with at least two, 16 G cannulas. Prior to starting the infusion collect 5–10 cc of blood for investigations, grouping and cross-matching.

4. Start infusion with crystalloids: Ringer lactate or normal saline up to 3–4 litres can be rapidly and safely infused (remember: Up to 95% of the infused crystalloid leaks into the interstitial space). Colloids (Haemaccel, Dextran) raise the intravascular volume for 3–4 hours and help buy precious time prior to blood transfusion.

5. Stop external bleeding. Pressure and slight elevation above the level of the heart can check bleeding in the majority. Use of tourniquet is contraindicated.

6. Relieve pain by splinting the fracture(s) and administration of analgesics. If head injury is excluded intravenous pethidine is the best analgesic. In a patient with shock, the peripheral circulation is depressed and drugs given intra-muscularly are not adequately distributed.

7. Infection should be prevented by:

    – washing the wound with normal saline prior to bandaging,

    – tetanus toxoid: 0.5 mg

    – broad spectrum antibiotics-intravenous crystalline penicillin, gentamycin and cephazolin is the ideal combination.

8. Catheterize the bladder to record urinary output. In a normal adult 20–30 ml/hour indicates adequate renal function.

Monitoring the Patient in Shock   In the patient being resuscitated, blood pressure (especially pulse pressure), urinary output and central venous pressure (CVP) must be closely monitored. These are all indirect measurements to help ascertain the patients' intravascular volume. More accurate monitoring of the intravascular volume and cardiac output can be obtained from a Swan-Ganz catheter.

In a patient with shock, *Do Not*:

1. Blame head injury as cause of shock

2. Use a tourniquet

3. Forget tetanus prophylaxis

4. Move the patient till the vitals are stable and an orthopaedic surgeon has evaluated the spine.

5. Use uncross-matched blood.

6. Use vasopressin to raise the blood pressure.

Hydrocortisone is of questionable value in the treatment of hemorrhagic shock.

Complications due to visceral and soft tissue injury

Visceral   The soft tissue damage, which accompanies certain fractures, may be of greater importance than the fracture itself. Sometimes, the management of the soft tissue injury will frequently take precedence over that of the fracture.

e.g. Bladder and urethral injury associated with pelvic fractures

Splenic rupture with fracture of lower left ribs

Laceration of the lung with rib fractures

Knowledge of the likely association between certain fractures and corresponding soft tissue injury is likely to lead to an early diagnosis and appropriate referral.

Soft tissue injury

Varying degrees of soft tissue injury may be associated with fractures and influence the ultimate outcome. Compounding of fractures and neurovascular injuries are the important components of soft tissue injury.

Open Fractures

Open fractures are those with communication to the external environment due to breach in the continuity of the skin and soft tissues. Classification of open fractures is important to plan the treatment and in the prediction of prognosis. The most widely used classification system is that of Gustilo-Anderson. This system divides open fractures into 3 types.

Type I clean, <1 cm wound, caused by low energy injury, compound from inside out, with minimal soft tissue damage.

Type II minimally contaminated wound, >1 cm/<10 cm in size caused by low energy trauma with moderate soft tissue damage, compound from outside in. Fractures may be comminuted.

Type III

A: usually >10 cm long, highly contaminated wound caused by high velocity trauma associated with severe soft tissue injury and varying amounts of comminution. However soft tissue coverage of bone is possible.

B: is similar to type A, the difference being that the amount of soft tissue damage is severe with crushing and loss of coverage leading to exposed bone ends.

C: wounds of any size (usually >10 cm), caused due to high velocity trauma where there is a vascular injury requiring repair.

Wounds caused by shot-gun, high velocity gun shot, or crushing force from fast moving automobile, those associated with a segmental fracture with displacement, diaphyseal bone loss, with major vascular injury requiring repair or occurring in farm yard are always classified as Group III.

Vascular Injury to blood vessels especially large arteries

e.g. subclavian artery-scapulothoracic dissociation

brachial artery-surpacondylar fracture humerus

popliteal artery-knee dislocation

internal iliac artery-sacroiliac disruption

is potentially life-threatening. Vascular injury must be suspected and clinically assessed by the internist while examining the limbs for fractures. The most important sign of vascular injury is the absence of a peripheral pulse. Presence of capillary circulation and seemingly adequate venous return in the superficial veins in not an assurance of adequate circulation. Arterial spasm must never be blamed for absence of arterial pulsations. Sometimes the effects of vascular injury can develop insidiously. In general, elevation of the limb and avoidance of tight constricting bandages and plaster casts will avoid ischemic consequences. If there is doubt of major vessel injury an angiogram must be done immediately (when facilities are available) to establish the diagnosis and level of arterial damage. Else it is safer to explore the vessels to confirm the diagnosis, remove extraneous compression on vessels, if any, and repair or graft the vessels when injured. Along with repair of the artery, the accompanying vein must also be repaired.

Nerve Majority of the nerve injuries associated with closed fractures are due to stretching or contusion of the nerve (neuropraxia or axonotmesis) and there is potential for spontaneous recovery. Immediate exploration of damaged nerves, except in compound injuries (where suspicion of complete transection is high) is rarely justified.

Examples of nerve injuries associated with trauma

1. Spinal cord-spine fracture

2. Axillary nerve-shoulder dislocations

3. Radial nerve-humerus fracture

4. Ulnar nerve-medial epicondyle fracture of humerus

5. Median nerve-supracondylar fracture humerus

6. Sciatic nerve-Posterior dislocation of hip

7. Common peroneal nerve-lateral knee injury.

Early complications

Immediate complications occur at the time of trauma and are unavoidable, except by preventive measures. However, many of the complications arising during the early phase of fracture management are avoidable with good management. They may be classified as local and systemic.

Systemic	Local
1. Fat embolism	1. Compartment syndrome
2. Crush syndrome	2. Infection
3. Complications due to immobilisation	3. Joint stiffness
-hypostatic pneumonia	
-Pressure sores	
-Deep vein thrombosis	
-Urinary tract infection	
-Constipation	
4. Gas gangrene	4. Myositis ossificans
5. Tetanus.	

Complications of immobilisation in bed

Sometimes the patient has to be kept for long periods in bed for management of fractures, e.g. pelvic fractures, polytrauma. In this situation, elderly patients are quite prone to develop the following complications, any of, which may be deleterious to the well being of the patient. Every attempt should be made to prevent them.

1. Hypostatic pneumonia can be prevented by deep breathing exercises and allowing the patient to sit up if possible.

2. Pressure sores over back and heels can be prevented by:

   – regular skin care and cleaning

   – an inflatable water or air mattress should be used.

   – bed clothes should have no wrinkles.

   – patient should be turned to the sides every two hours to avoid prolonged pressure over bony prominences.

3. Deep venous thrombosis and pulmonary embolism: This can be prevented by

   – keeping the calf free from compression

   – regular active ankle and calf muscle exercises

   – low molecular weight heparin

   – early mobilisation of the patient, where possible

4. Urinary retention and infection can be avoided by ensuring adequate fluid intake. Urinary tract infection is the most common nosocomial infection (6–8%).

5. Constipation can be quite troublesome. This can be prevented by a diet rich in roughage and use of mild laxatives. Occasional enema may be required.

Fat Embolism is a major cause of morbidity and mortality following multiple trauma. It is one of the most important causes of adult respiratory distress syndrome (ARDS). Its exact incidence is difficult to determine. Fat embolism, as a subclinical event, however, occurs with nearly all fractures of long bones. Clinical symptoms and signs are evident in 0.5-2% of patients with long bone fractures and upto 10% of patients with unstable pelvic fractures. It is a curious fact that it is rarely seen in children and old age. The incidence of fat embolism syndrome (FES) is considerably less in open fractures.

Pathogenesis The pathogenesis of FES is a subject of conjecture and controversy. Most investigators however agree that bone marrow is the source of embolic fat. Tissue thromboplastin released along with the marrow elements activates the complement system and extrinsic coagulation cascade via factor VII. Intravascular coagulation by-products such as fibrin and fibrinogen degradation products are then produced. These substances along with leukocytes, platelets and fat globules are filtered by the lungs where they increase pulmonary vascular permeability (pulmonary oedema) by direct action on the endothelial lining.

Clinical picture Early diagnosis is extremely important in the management of fat embolism. The diagnosis of FES is often missed and the most important factor in the diagnosis is awareness of the occurrence of this complication. Early literature had placed emphasis on a lucid interval; this is more apparent than real. In fact the onset may be immediate but it classically presents 24–72 hours after injury. The clinical presentation includes:

1. Shortness of breath, which begins relatively suddenly, followed by restlessness.

2. A striking feature is rapidly changing neurologic status, sudden onset of restlessness, disorientation, followed by confusion, stupor and coma.

3. Tachycardia.

4. Tachypnoea

5. Flat temperature elevation to 39-40°C.

6. The blood pressure does not vary and remains within normal limits.

7. A petechial rash may be seen which is characteristically located across the chest, axilla, root of the neck and conjunctiva. Retinal lesions can be identified by fundoscopic examination and appear as microinfarcts at the end of the retinal arterioles.

Laboratory findings

1. *Arterial blood gas analysis* (*ABG*) Arterial hypoxemia is the hallmark of FES. A pO_2 of <60 mmHg indicates significant pulmonary hypoxemia. Serial determination of arterial pO_2 can provide an index of effectiveness of therapy.

2. *Thrombocytopenia* (< 1,50,000 platelets/cu mm) in the early stages.

3. *Serial chest X-rays* should be obtained. They may demonstrate progressive snow-storm like pulmonary infiltrations. These changes are characteristic but not specific.

4. *Analysis of urine* for fat can be done but is not accurate.

Management FES can be prevented to some extent by early immobilisation of fractures in splints or plaster and by gentle handling of the patient. Once the signs appear there is no specific treatment but the following measures are used:

General

1. Airway must be maintained.

2. Circulatory volume and oxygen carrying capacity must be restored.

3. Fluid and electrolyte balance must be maintained.

4. Immobilise fractures as they are and defer any manipulative or operative intervention.

5. CVP and urine output should be monitored.

Specific

1. Oxygen must be administered to all trauma patients. The arterial oxygen content should be maintained over 90 mmHg. ABG monitoring is mandatory for all adult polytrauma patients.

2. If hypoxemia is severe, ventilatory support should be considered.

3. Heparin is sometimes useful and is given in dose of 10,000 IU 12 hourly. It probably helps by reducing platelet aggregation and by emulsifying the fat globules thereby reducing obstruction in arterioles and capillaries. However the therapeutic value has not been unequivocally demonstrated.

4. Corticosteroids: Recent studies support the use of methylprednisolone in the treatment of FES. The anti-inflammatory action is hypothesised to protect the capillary endothelium, reduce complement activity, retard platelet aggregation and minimise transudation of interstitial oedema.

Crush Syndrome

Crush syndrome generally refers to the systemic symptoms and signs resulting from the products of devitalised tissue entering the circulation. The primary problems are:

1. Sudden severe hyperkalemia with possibility of arrhythmia

2. Acute oliguric renal failure secondary to pigment nephropathy. With ischemia or blunt trauma to a large muscle mass, myoglobin is released into the circulation. This pigment is filtered from blood at the glomerulus and reabsorbed by the tubule. Although myoglobin is not directly nephrotoxic, in presence of aciduria, it is converted to ferrihemate, which is toxic to renal cells. Hypovolemia compounds the damage.

Management Maintenance of a high urinary output of at least 100 and preferably 200 ml/hour for 48–72 hours will help prevent renal failure. Maintaining an alkaline urine by infusing sodium bicarbonate intravenously (1-2 meq/kg/hour) reduces the likelihood of myoglobin precipitating and occluding renal tubules.

Gas Gangrene

Gas gangrene is a life threatening complication of open wounds, particularly those contaminated by soil. This is a clostridial infection caused not by the extra virulence of the organism but rather by unique local conditions. Clostridial species capable of producing gas gangrene are ;

Clostridium perfringens (Cl. welchii): (Most important)

Cl. Septicum

Cl. histolyticum

Cl. bifermentans

Cl. fallax

Clostridia are obligate anaerobes that cannot multiply in healthy living tissue. Clostridium perfringens in a non-motile, gram-positive bacillus without spores. It is a saprophytic commensal of the alimentary tract and can be isolated from skin in approximately 20% of the patients. It is a universal organism found in the operating room, emergency department, hospital wards and shoes. The factors predisposing to clostridial myonecrosis are:

1. Deep penetrating wounds of the buttocks and thighs

2. Tight plaster casts

3. Loss of blood supply to otherwise intact muscles e.g. arterial injury

4. Delay in surgical debridement of open wounds

Clinical findings: The incubation period is about 24 hours. The initial symptom in the affected area is throbbing pain, associated with oedema and a serosanguinous exudate from the wound. Initially, there is a dissociation between tachycardia and temperature elevation (the pulse rate is significantly elevated but the temperature is not high). Progress of myonecrosis is rapid. With systemic absorption of the toxins (Table 21.3), the blood pressure falls, the pulse rate increases and profound shock may occur. Examination of the wound will show it to be tense and indurated ; the skin shiny and bronze coloured with a sickly sweet odour and slight amount of gas. The muscle involvement is invariably greater than the skin changes.

Table 21.3. Histotoxins

Lecithinase (α-toxin)
Collagenase
Hyaluronidase
Leukocidin
Deoxyribonuclease
Protease
Lipase

Treatment

Diagnosis of gas gangrene is clinical. Radiographic interpretation of gas in soft tissue is not pathognomonic of gas gangrene (Table 21.4). Bacteriologic demonstration of clostridia in the exudate is of limited significance as the organisms are commensals with universal presence.

Management

Early recognition (a high index of suspicion in penetrating thigh and buttock wounds) with immediate and aggressive surgical debridement significantly reduces the morbidity and mortality. Management includes the following measures:

1. Fluid and electrolyte replacement (CVP and urinary output monitoring aid in the fluid replacement).

2. Blood transfusion is important, since severe anemia develops rapidly.

Table 21.4. Causes of crepitant non clostridial lesions

1.	Bacterial	
	A.	Aerobic aerogenic infections
		- Coliforms
		- Mixed
	B.	Hemolytic staphylococcal fascitis
	C.	Hemolytic streptococcal cellulitis
	D.	Anaerobic streptococcal infections
	E.	Infection with bacteroides organism
2.	Non bacterial	
	A.	Irrigation of wound with hydrogen peroxide
	B.	Mechanical effect of trauma
	C.	Gun shot injury
	D.	Air hose injury
	E.	Subcutaneous emphysema due to lung/airway injury

3. Wound exploration remains the cornerstone of treatment. All tissue planes are widely opened and decompressed.

4. Extensive debridement of necrotic muscles should be done. This may require excision of whole muscle, muscle groups or even removal of the whole compartment. Wound is left open.

5. Vigorous antibiotic therapy is an important adjunct to operative treatment. The drugs preferred are:

   a) Crystalline penicillin 1,00,000 to 2,00,000-IU/kg body weight in 6 divided doses per day for five days.

   b) Gentamicin is added because open injuries have mixed flora. In patients allergic to penicillin, clindamycin is effective. The adult dose is 20mg/kg/day. The use of antitoxins for passive immunisation has been abandoned.

6. Amputation: Gas gangrene is confined to an individual muscle or group of muscles at least in the early stages. Amputation is required in:

   – Massive gangrene with involvement of most muscles of the injured segment of the limb.

   – Serious impairment of blood supply to the injured part of the limb when the main artery has been damaged.

   – Cases who present late for treatment and are severely toxic.

   The amputation must be sufficiently high to allow all infected muscles to be excised. The wound should never be closed. Secondary suture or re-amputation at a higher level is performed when the infection is under control and the patient's general condition has improved.

7. Hyperbaric oxygen: Oxygen is given at three times the atmospheric pressure for 60–90 minutes and repeated 8–12 hourly for seven sittings. Oxygen tension in the tissues rises upto 15 times and in some cases the detoxification is dramatic.

   Note This is merely an adjunct to surgery, as it alone will not cure the condition.

Tetanus (Lockjaw)

Tetanus is a potentially fatal disease that is entirely preventable by appropriate immunisation.

Clostridium tetani is a large gram-positive motile bacillus, strictly anaerobic. The spores are extremely resistant and can remain dormant for years. Tetanus can occur in a patient with a superficial wound or no demonstrable wound unlike gas gangrene (Clostridial myonecrosis).

Clostridium tetani bacilli and spores are found widespread in faecal matter of both animals and human beings. Three factors favour progression of infection:

1. Deep wound without exposure to air

2. Wounds with dead tissue

3. Wounds infected with other organisms. (The bacteria consume oxygen-making conditions favourable for germination of spores)

The bacillus produces two exotoxins-tetanospasmin (neurotoxin) and tetanolysin (hemolysin). Tetanospasmin is carried by way of peripheral nerves to the CNS and is bound with high affinity to the gangliosides. The toxin causes a presynaptic blockade of neuromuscular transmission and functional denervation of muscles. Voluntary muscles are more sensitive than involuntary muscles.

Clinical Picture The incubation period is about one week. Shorter period is associated with graver prognosis.

1. *Trismus* is due to spasm of muscles of mastication.

2. *Risus sardonicus* (risus-grin; sardonic-scornful): This is a sneering grin on the face of the patient due to sustained spasm of the facial muscles in which the corners of the mouth are drawn back.

3. Difficulty in swallowing (lockjaw) is due to spasm of pharyngeal muscles.

4. *Opisthotonus* extreme arching backwards of the spine and due to spasm of the muscles in that region.

5. *Convulsions* occur secondary to minimal stimuli.

6. *Death* occurs due to asphyxia associated with unremitting spasm of laryngeal and pharyngeal muscles.

Diagnosis The diagnosis is purely clinical.

Prophylaxis Active immunisation with tetanus

toxoid is highly effective and provides excellent protection. All children should receive primary immunisation. Following initial immunisation, one dose of adult tetanus toxoid should be given every 10 years. However, the success of prophylaxis also depends on prompt surgical wound management. Wounds should not be closed primarily if doubt exists about anaerobic conditions within the wound.

A guide to the use of tetanus toxoid and immunoglobulin is shown in Table 21.5.

Full Course Tetanus toxoid-3 doses

First dose   –0.5 ml
Second dose –0.5ml after 6–8 weeks
Third dose   –0.5 ml at 6–12 months.

Antibiotics have no effect against the toxin produced. Penicillin, given immediately after injury however has a deterrent action against clostridium tetani infection by taking care of the organisms not removed surgically.

Note In patients sensitive to penicillin, tetracycline should be used.

Treatment   Successful treatment for established tetanus requires intensive care facilities. The patient is paralysed and given ventilatory support through tracheostomy. Wound debridement is essential. All devitalised tissues should be excised. This is supported by mega-doses of crystalline penicillin (6 million units every 6 hours). Intensive care may be required for several weeks till the effects of the toxin wear off.

Compartment Syndrome This is one of the most devastating complications that can occur after limb trauma. It was first described by Richard Von Volkmann in 1881. Compartment syndrome is defined as a condition in which circulation and function of tissues within a closed space are compromised by an increased pressure within that space. Normal pressure in a closed osseofascial compartment is 0 ± 4 mm Hg. Pressures exceeding 30 mm Hg or within 10–30 mm Hg of the diastolic pressure are highly suggestive of the diagnosis.

Pathophysiology Increase in tissue pressure in a closed osseofascial space leads to collapse of the thin-walled veins. Further increase in pressure leads to decrease in transmural pressure difference (i.e. arteriolar pressure minus tissue pressure) and finally the arterioles collapse. The net effect is reduced microcirculation, anaerobic metabolism and increased capillary permeability. A vicious cycle is set up that can be broken only by an adequate decompression (Fig. 21.4).

Diagnosis 5 'P' s.

1. *Pain* is the earliest and most consistent symptom. It is typically deep, poorly localised, progressive and increases on passive stretch of the involved muscles (Volkmann's sign).

2. *Pallor* may or may not be present. In fact, the extremity may appear cyanotic early in the course due to venous obstruction.

3. *Paraesthesia* occurs in the cutaneous distribution of a peripheral nerve that courses through the affected compartment. This is an early sign of impending, yet reversible, compartment syndrome. eg. tingling in the radial three fingers suggestive

Table 21.5. Immunisation protocol in tetanus

Patient immunity status	Type of wound	
	Recent, clear wound	Wound >6hr old, contamination present or deep wound
Immunised, booster within one year	Nil	Nil
Immunised, Booster within 10 years	Nil	TT Booster
Immunised, no booster within 10 years	TT* Booster	Ig# + TT Booster
Status unknown	TT Booster+ full course	Ig + TT Booster + full course

* Tetanus Toxoid
# Immunoglobulin

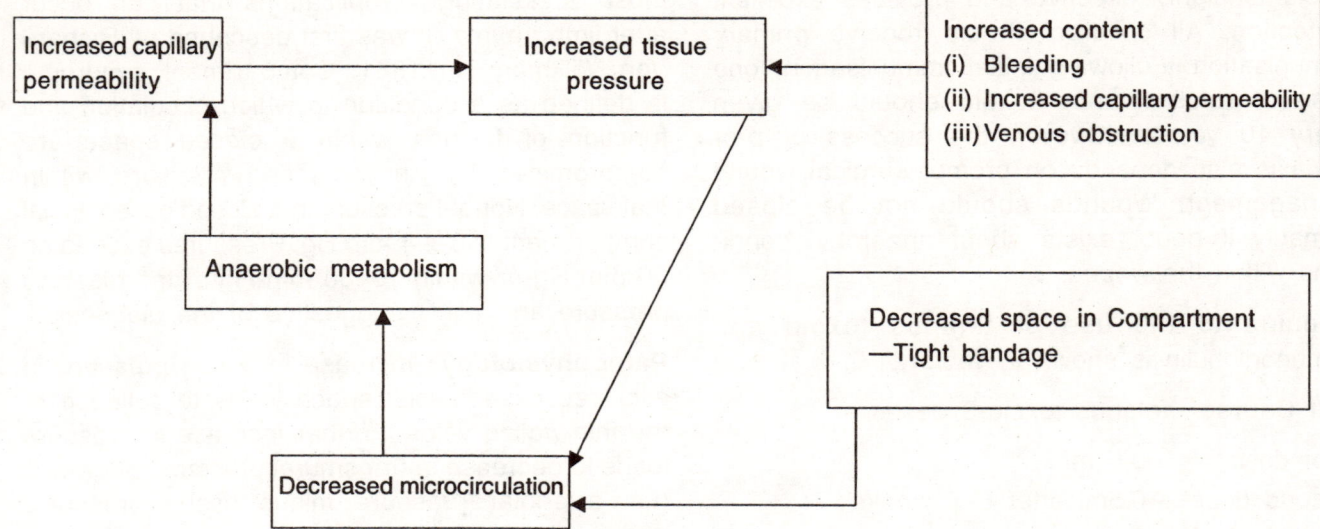

Fig. 21.4. Vicious cycle leading to compartment syndrome

of median nerve ischemia in the forearm compartment syndrome.

4. *Paralysis* Sensory disturbances precede motor dysfunction. Impairment of two-point discrimination is the earliest sign of impending compartment syndrome.

By the time motor paralysis occurs, compartment syndrome is well established. Irreversible function loss is inevitable despite adequate decompression.

5. *Pulselessness* Loss of pulse occurs late and sometimes not at all in the course of compartment syndrome. Irreversible tissue damage can occur in a patient with a palpable pulse. The only exception to this is when the absent pulse is due to arterial injury rather than high compartment pressure. (Absent pulse is an indication for arteriography).

Note Irreversible muscle damage occurs after 4 hours and nerve damage after 12 hours following onset of ischemia. Symptoms and signs are confusing and may be difficult to interpret. A high index of suspicion is therefore mandatory when dealing with traumatised limbs. Isolated vascular/nerve injuries must be differentiated from neurovascular involvement due to compartment syndrome (Table 21.6). An open fracture does not prevent the development of an acute compartment syndrome. The more extensive the wound, the better protected the compartment is against

Table 21.6. Features of compartment syndrome, arterial and nerve injury

Symptom/sign	Compartment syndrome	Arterial injury	Nerve injury
Pain on passive stretching	Present	Present	Absent
Sensory dysfunction	Present	Present	Present
Motor dysfunction	Present	Present	Present
Peripheral pulse	Palpable	Not palpable	Palpable
Compartment pressure	Increased	Increased (late)	Normal

increased pressure, but compartments that are not open are still at risk.

A technique of objective assessment of the intra-compartmental pressure advocated by Whitesides is shown (Fig. 21.5)

Treatment Generous skin incisions should be utilised as skin is a potentially limiting structure. All compartments must be decompressed.

Concomitant muscle debridement is necessary for any ischemic muscle. Ischemic muscle lacks normal colour, consistency, contractility and capacity to bleed.

Infection Infection of a closed fracture or dislocation is extremely uncommon, but all open fractures are at high risk of contamination and subsequent infection. Infection delays union; in fact it may actively prevent it leading to non-union.

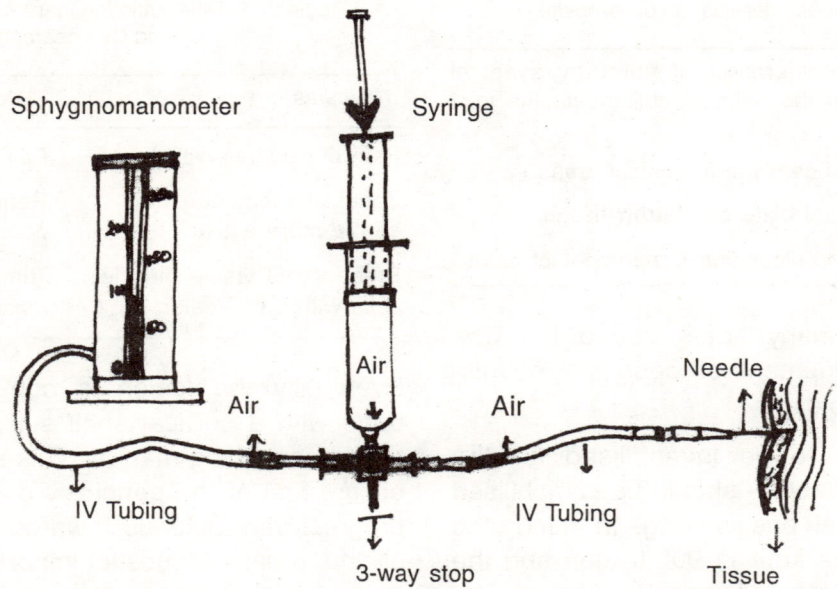

Fig. 21.5. Whitesides method of measuring intra-compartmental pressure

Pathophysiology The pathophysiology of post-traumatic osteomyelitis (i.e. osteomyelitis from direct inoculation of bacteria) is different from that of acute hematogenous osteomyelitis. The hematoma formed after injury acts as a fertile culture medium for the bacteria during the period of contamination. The initial six hours is the golden period as after this period, there is an exponential increase in the number of bacteria. As bacteria multiply, an inflammatory response is evoked. The bacteria spread through the hematoma and along vascular planes to reach the bone. Hematoma is converted to necrotic debris.

Management Despite advances in antibiotic therapy, the treatment of osteomyelitis remains a great challenge to the orthopaedic surgeon. Prevention remains the cornerstone. Adequate wound cleaning and debridement contribute significantly to reduce this risk. Broad-spectrum antibiotics are a useful adjunct. The principles of antibiotic therapy are shown in Table 21.7. Once infection is established, its treatment is along the same lines as those of chronic osteomyelitis. The following measures are required:

1. Removal of all dead bone
2. Adequate drainage of the infected area
3. Continued immobilisation of the fracture till union
4. Systemic antibiotics depending on culture report

Table 21.7. Principles of antibacterial therapy.

1. Select the drug most likely to be effective with the least side effects.
2. Administer the drug by an appropriate route for sufficient time to eradicate or control infection.
3. Monitor the patient closely for clinical and bacteriologic response and tolerance of the drug.
4. Modify the dosage when circumstances indicate.
5. Discontinue the drug when infection is eradicated or controlled, when resistance emerges in vitro or in vivo or when intolerance (side-effects) develops.
6. Use adjunctive therapeutic measures, surgical debridement, drainage or removal of foreign material, whenever necessary.

Internal fixation should be avoided in infected area.

Joint stiffness

Fractures near joints, intra-articular fractures and inappropriate immobilisation quite frequently lead to stiffness. Certain joints like shoulder, finger and knees are more prone to develop stiffness. Effects of stress deprivation on synovial joints are shown in Table 21.8.

These complications can be prevented to a great extent by the following measures:

1. Active exercises of muscles and joints (when not splinted) of the affected limb should be

Table 21.8. Effects of stress deprivation on synovial joints

1. Time dependent proliferation of fibrofatty synovial connective tissue to the point of obliterating the joint space.

2. Pressure necrosis of cartilage in contact areas.

3. Breach of subchondral plate by marrow tissue.

4. Cartilage erosion and ulceration in non-contact areas.

Table 21.9. Differentiating features between Myositis and Osteosarcoma

Myositis	Osteosarcoma
Pain diminishes with time.	Pain progressively increases
Zonal phenomenon with centre more active	Random arrangement with periphery most active
Presence of viable muscle cells within the lesion	Tumour tends to destroy muscle as it advances.

practised regularly many times during the day. This prevents development of oedema and disuse atrophy of muscles.

2. Joints that have to be immobilised for the management of the fracture should be immobilised in optimum functional position e.g. in hand, the MCP joints should be kept in 90° flexion and the IP joints in full extension (*James Position*).

3. Following removal of plaster an elastic bandage should be used to prevent development of persistent and recurrent oedema.

4. Passive mobilisation/manipulation of the joint should be done to increase the range of movement on removal of plaster.

5. Displaced intraarticular fractures should be operated and the joints mobilised at the earliest possible opportunity.

Myositis ossificans is heterotopic bone formation in soft tissues (skeletal muscle, tendon, ligament) and at times, near bone and periosteum. The propensity for development of myositis ossificans is related to the severity of the initial injury and the occurrence of repeated injury during the recovery period. The muscles most often involved are brachialis, gluteus minimus and piriformis.

The cause is unknown. Trauma appears to trigger the subsequent cascade of events. Hematoma formation occurs following injury. This is followed by an oedematous inflammatory reaction. The cellular elements (collagenoblasts) lay down large masses of collagen, which has the tendency to mineralise (dystrophic calcification). This is followed by metaplasia of the collagenoblasts to osteoblasts and chondroblasts. When osteoblastic activity is florid, distinction from osteosarcoma on microscopy may be difficult. Features that help differentiate myositis from osteosarcoma are shown in Table 21.9.

Eventually the lesion is converted into mature bone with a cortical shell surrounding cancellous tissue containing marrow. This sequence of events occurs first at the periphery of the hematoma and progressively extends towards the centre. This is of the great diagnostic importance and referred to as the "*Zone phenomenon*".

Three zones are seen:

Central Highly cellular.

Intermediate Fibroblastic tissue.

Peripheral Mature, well-oriented new bone.

Radiologically three stages are seen:

Stage 1 Fine amorphous flakes of calcium (*Cotton-Candy Appearance*) appear in the vicinity of bone two to three weeks after injury.

Stage 2 These calcific areas coalesce, ossification progresses and the whole extent of the lesion is delineated.

Stage 3 The ossified mass shrinks and becomes dense.

The diagnosis of post-traumatic ossification should be suspected when after immobilisation is discontinued the joint movements do not improve or the movements already gained are lost. It is quite likely to form after massage and passive manipulation, which is commonly used with the hope of mobilising stiff joints after trauma. This complication is most commonly seen in injuries around the elbow. Myositis is also seen in patients with head injuries and paraplegics.

Treatment consists of the following measures:

1. Complete rest to the injured part to minimise hemorrhage and inflammation.

2. Immobilisation is discontinued when local

warmth has subsided. This takes approximately two to three weeks. Range of movement exercises are commenced within the tolerance of pain.

3. After full range of movements is attained, strengthening exercises are begun.

4. Excision of the bony mass should only be performed after the mass has matured and is well delineated. If excision is done before maturation, ossification will recur over a wider area. Usually the maturation of the myositic mass takes one to two years.

Late Complications These problems occur after the period of initial treatment and may be delayed by months. They are usually related to the fracture itself and are restricted to the involved bone or limb.

The late complications include:

1. Malunion
2. Delayed union
3. Non-union
4. Avascular necrosis
5. Osteoarthritis
6. Sudeck's atrophy

Malunion is defined as union in a clinically significant imperfect position. Function is impaired in several ways.

1. An abnormal joint surface may cause irregular weight transfer leading to osteoarthritis especially in the lower limbs.
2. Overriding of fracture fragments or bone loss can cause shortening.
3. Rotation or angulation may interfere with gait in the lower limb and positioning of the upper extremities.
4. Movements of neighbouring joints may be blocked.
5. Change in arc of motion.

Initial fracture care is critical to avoid this. Malunion is caused by inaccurate reduction, slipping of reduction or ineffective/inadequate immobilisation during healing. Sometimes, however, malunion may occur despite expert treatment, e.g. Type V epiphyseal injury. Surgery is indicated only when function is impaired. It is rarely justified for cosmetic reasons alone (exception: cubitus varus following malunited supracondylar fracture humerus).

Delayed union/non-union: The differences between delayed union and non-union are mostly of degree and the distinction is not always clear. A fracture that allows free movement of the bone ends at 3-4 months after injury is considered to have delayed union and if it persists for >6 months a diagnosis of non-union can be made. By this time there is evidence, clinical and radiologic, that healing has ceased and union is highly improbable. These problems are more common with high-energy injuries.

Causes of delayed union/non-union:

1. **Inadequate immobilisation** If there is significant motion between the fracture ends, the process of union stops at the stage of fibrocartilage formation and progresses to non-union.

2. **Interposition of soft tissues** In a fracture where the bone ends are widely displaced, muscle, tendon, periosteum and sometimes nerve, get entrapped between the fracture surfaces. As the bone ends are not in direct contact union may not occur.

3. **Inadequate bony contact** Inadequate bony contact interferes with the fracture union. Excessive traction, distraction, inadequate reduction and comminuted open fracture with bone loss are some important causes of inadequate bony contact.

Separation of the fracture ends by traction has deleterious effects on bone healing. The newly formed vascular channels are torn apart and cannot bridge the gap. Distraction is seen most commonly in the fractures of the shaft of humerus treated in a hanging cast where gravity causes distraction at the fracture site.

4. **Inadequate blood supply to one or both fragments** Both the fracture fragments should have adequate blood supply to support vascular ingrowth into the fracture hematoma for union to proceed. Impairment of the blood supply (wide separation of fracture ends, peculiarity of bone, soft tissue disruption) delays/prevents union.

Examples :

(a) *Femur neck fracture* The femoral head becomes avascular as the main source of blood supply to head is through the metaphyseal vessels, which are disrupted when the fracture occurs.

(b) *Fracture of the distal third tibia* The distal half of tibia is relatively avascular as it is in a subcutaneous situation without muscle attachments and, the nutrient artery enters the tibia at the junction of the middle and the lower one third and passes upwards.

(c) *Fracture of scaphoid/talus* The proximal fragment becomes avascular as the blood supply to bone enters through the distal fragment. The proximal fragment does not have any direct blood supply since it is circumferentially covered by articular cartilage.

(d) Blood supply to bone may be substantially damaged during open reduction. Periosteal and muscle attachments are important sources of blood supply to bone after fracture, and during operative treatment stripping of these tissues should be kept to a minimum.

5. **Infection** Presence of infection retards the process of union.

6. **Intraarticular fractures** can undergo nonunion as the fracture hematoma gets washed away by the synovial fluid in these cases.

7. **Ill advised attempts at internal fixation** leading to compromise of vascularity, loss of fracture hematoma, and possibly infection. In addition, the internal fixation device (such as plate) can keep the bone ends distracted after the resorption of the bone ends occurs.

8. **Intact fellow bone** In isolated fractures of tibia with intact fibula and in fractures of both bones of the leg where fibular union is always faster, fibula can occur as a strut and keep the tibial fragments apart and result in non union.

9. **Pathological fractures** occur secondary to weakened bones, as in metastasis, primary malignant bone tumour etc., will not unite until the primary disease is dealt with.

10. **Repeated manipulation** Frequent attempts to restore alignment destroy the vascular channels. Such attempts are particularly harmful after 2 weeks of injury, when neo vascularisation is at its peak.

Note Sometimes more than one of the above factors may be present in the same patient.

Features of non-union

1. Painless, abnormal mobility at the fracture site.

2. Absence of local tenderness.

3. Radiological signs:

   – Sclerosis of the fracture ends/resorption.

   – Smoothening (rounding-off) of bone ends

   – Obliteration of medullary canal.

   – Callus formation is minimal/absent.

Serial x-rays best show the gradual development of non-union. Stress films may sometimes be necessary to detect mobility if it is not clinically obvious.

Sudeck's Atrophy

(Reflex Sympathetic Dystrophy)

RSD is a condition characterised by pain, stiffness and swelling out of proportion to the degree of trauma, that initiated the event. Functional recovery is delayed and the residual disability may be permanent.

Pathogenesis Three major factors must be present at the same time to produce RSD: (Fig. 21.6).

– A persistent painful stimulus

– Diathesis (patient susceptibility)

– Abnormal sympathetic reflex.

Symptoms and signs RSD is characterised by 4 cardinal features:

1. **Pain** is the most outstanding feature. It can be searing, burning or lancinating and is aggravated by movement, light touch, weather changes and emotion.

2 **Swelling** is the most consistent physical finding and may extend with time.

3. **Stiffness** is the most disabling sign.

4. **Discoloration**, depending on the stage of the disease, may vary from redness to cyanosis.

Secondary Signs

1. Osteoporosis (classically juxta – articular)

2. Hyperhidrosis (excessive sweating) in the early stages. Late in the disease dryness develops.

3. Trophic changes in the skin – shiny appearance, disappearance of wrinkles.

4. Temperature changes: The affected extremity is initially warm but later becomes cooler compared to the contralateral limb.

5. Vasomotor instability

Diagnosis All four cardinal signs and one or more secondary features are necessary to diagnose RSD clinically. Clinical classification of RSD was given by Langford & Evans (Table 21.10). The confirmatory test is symptomatic relief, irrespective of degree, objective or subjective, after interruption of the sympathetic reflex, e.g. stellate ganglion block for RSD of hand.

Management

The best results can be expected only with early diagnosis and treatment.

1. Pain relief is of paramount importance. In most cases it is due to the injury but may be due to secondary factors, e.g. tight plaster or uncomfortable position such as marked wrist flexion. Heat massage and gentle active exercises also help relieve pain and oedema. Patience, persistence and encouragement are required because recovery is slow and takes months. Great care should be taken during physical therapy to avoid pain.

2. Sympathetic block: Pain relief is best achieved by interruption of the abnormal sympathetic reflex. The modalities are:

a) Regional blocks: Stellate ganglion block
   Epidural blocks
   Peripheral nerve block
   Intravenous regional blocks

b) Oral medication: Sympatholytic drugs
   Centrally acting
   1. Clonidine
   2. Methydopa
   Alpha adrenergic blockers
   1. Phenoxybenzamine
   2. Prazosin

Gunshot Wounds

The mechanism of tissue damage and management of gun shot wounds have certain peculiarities that

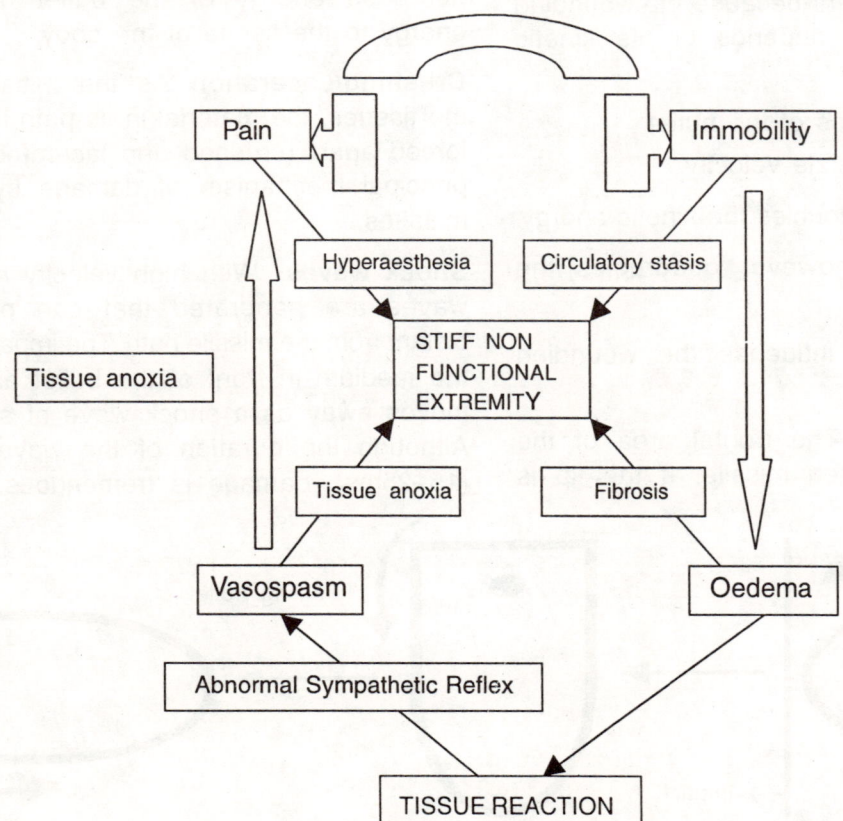

Fig. 21.6. Vicious cycle leading to RSD

Table 21.10. Stages of RSD (Langford and Evans)

Stage	Period (mths)	Findings
I (Early)	0-3	Pain, swelling, warmth, decreased ROM, normal radiograph
II (Dystrophy)	3-6	Pain, cool and glossy skin, mild contracture and patchy osteoporosis
III (Atrophy)	6->12	Tight skin, flexion contractures, cool limb, diffuse osteoporosis

should be understood and borne in mind while treating these injuries. Depending on the speed with which a bullet exits the firearm the muzzle velocity of the missile may be low, medium or high (Table 21.11).

Table 21.11. Muzzle Velocity of Missile

Velocity (feet/sec)	Class
< 1000	low
1000-2000	medium
>2,000	high

This distinction is important because the wounding capacity of the missile depends on its kinetic energy (KE).

$$KE = 1/2 \, mv^2 \quad m : \text{mass of the bullet}$$
$$v : \text{muzzle velocity}$$

Doubling the mass only doubles the kinetic energy.

Doubling the velocity however quadruples the kinetic energy.

The other factors that influence the wounding capacity are:

Profile of the bullet The frontal area of the bullet is that of a pointed missile. If the tip is deformed, the impact of the missile is dispersed over a wider tissue area producing greater energy exchange and more damage.

Tumble The centre of gravity of a bullet is closer to its base. Spin and yaw are bullet movements that occur after the gun is fired. After impact, momentum tends to carry the base of the bullet forwards and the centre of gravity then becomes the leading point, causing the bullet to tumble (Fig. 21.7).

Pathophysiology

Energy can neither be created nor destroyed. Interaction between the bullet and the tissue will decrease energy of the bullet by transfer of energy to the tissue of the body.

Crushing/Laceration As the missile penetrates the tissues, the material in its path is crushed and forced apart (crushed and lacerated). This is the principal mechanism of damage by low velocity missiles.

Shock waves With high velocity missiles shock waves are generated that can produce injury distant from the missile path. The impact compresses the medium in front of the bullet and this region moves away as a shock wave of spherical form. Although the duration of the wave is negligible (15–25ms), damage is tremendous.

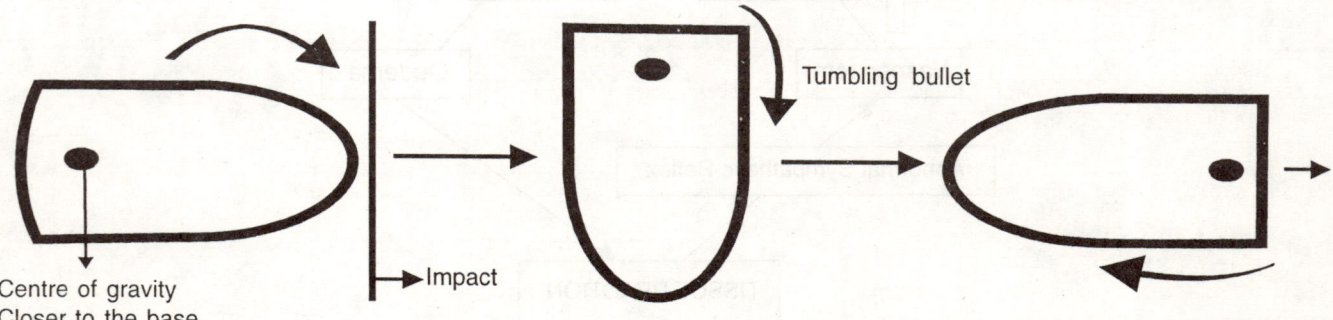

Centre of gravity
Closer to the base

Impact

Tumbling bullet

Fig. 21.7. Tumble of a Bullet

Cavitation This is seen with high velocity missiles. The missile accelerates the medium forwards and sideways away from its path with such force that the particles, due to inertia, continue to move after the missile has passed and expand the track of the missile into a cavity (temporary cavity). This cavity is at sub atmospheric pressure and sucks in air, bacteria and clothing from both ends of the wound. This cavity may expand and close several times leaving a permanent cavity wider than the missile track. The size of the cavity depends on the velocity of the bullet and is inversely proportional to the expandability of the tissue, i.e. muscle damage is less compared to liver, kidney, bone (Fig. 21.8).

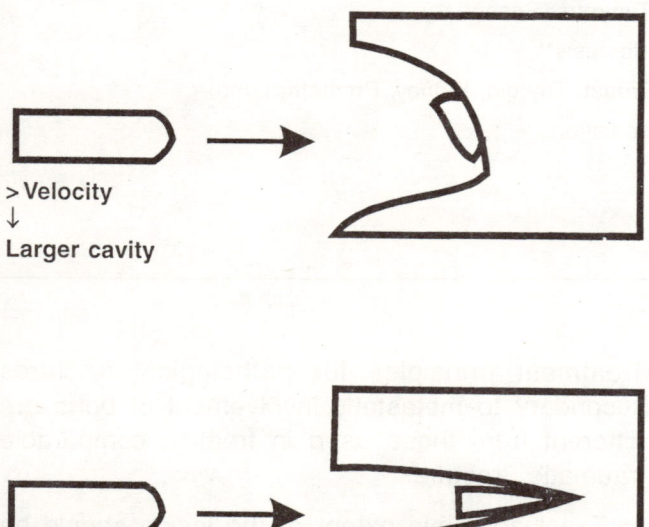

> Velocity
↓
Larger cavity

< Velocity
↓
Smallar cavity

Fig. 21.8. Size of cavity is proportional to velocity of the bullet

Secondary missiles Fragments of bone resulting from the fracture may tumble around in tissues adding to the injury. Pieces of bullet (which breaks after hitting bone) may also become secondary missiles.

Shotgun injury The injuries sustained by shot gun missiles are different from single gun shot wounds. The muzzle velocity is 1100–1300 ft/sec (medium) but the weight is significant. Therefore, kinetic energy at the muzzle is very great. However this dissipates as the distance increases. Most human injuries occur at close range. Tissue destruction is massive. In addition, shot gun shells have wadding made of plastic, cork and felt placed between the powder and shot. At close range this wadding becomes embedded in the wound that adds to the complications.

Principles of management

The principles of management of the gunshot wounds are:

1. The general principles of resuscitation remain the same.

2. Meticulous search for entry and exit wounds gives an idea of:

   (a) number of missiles

   (b) direction of the bullet

   (c) what organs are likely to have been injured, and,

   (d) whether the bullet has crossed the midline.

3. Peripheral circulation and neurological status: Diminished or absent pulse, rapidly increasing hematoma or a pulsatile mass are absolute indications for emergency angiography and surgery. Prognosis for neurological recovery is generally poor. A mixed pattern of nerve injuries is seen. Another significant problem is causalgia when a mixed nerve is partially damaged.

4. X-rays: A minimum of two views, with the joint above and below the fractured bone is mandatory.

5. Culture swabs from the entry and exit wounds.

6. Debridement, wound irrigation is the most important step. All the devitalised tissues up to fresh bleeding muscle margins should be excised. Non-metallic foreign body/bodies especially in shot gun injury must be removed but small pellets need not be searched extensively. The resulting wound should never be closed. Systemic antibiotics should be administered. Treatment of soft tissue destruction must be given priority over treatment of the fracture.

7. The fracture is treated with traction or by an external fixator.

Pathological Fractures

Pathological fracture is defined as fracture in an abnormal bone following subnormal stress. The causes of pathological fractures are listed in Table 21.12.

Table 21.12. Causes of Pathological fractures

Generalised bone disorder	Localized disorder
A. Congenital : Osteogenesis imperfecta Osteopetrosis Dyschondroplasia	A. Infection : Pyogenic osteomyelitis* Tuberculosis
B. Metabolic** : Osteoporosis Osteomalacia Rickets Scurvy	B. Bone Tumours : Primary 1. Solitary bone cyst 2. Aneurysmal bone cyst 3. Fibrous dysplasia 4. Giant Cell tumor 5. Osteosarcoma 6. Ewings sarcoma
C. Blood disorders : Hemophilia Lymphoma Leukemia	C. Bone Tumours: Secondary 1. Metastasis** (Breast, Thyroid, Kidney, Prostate, Lung)
D. Drugs : Corticosteroids Anti-convulsants	D. Post irradiation
E. Malignancy : Multiple myeloma*	
F. Immunological disorders : Rheumatoid arthritis	

* Common causes   ** Commonest cause

Management

The underlying cause of weakening of the bone should always be determined and whenever possible, treatment of the disease should be started concurrently with treatment of the fracture. Osteoporosis is one of the commonest cause of pathological fractures and it is essentially a "diagnosis by exclusion" (Fig. 21.9). The work-up should proceed in a logical fashion.

Metastasis   Bone is the third most common site of metastatic disease after the lungs and liver. More than three fourths of skeletal metastases come from the breast, prostate, thyroid, lung and kidneys. Bony metastases can be lytic, blastic or mixed pattern (commonest). Spine is the most common site for skeletal metastasis. In 15 % of patients with metastasis, the site of the primary tumour is unknown. In 20% of patients with bony metastasis, the skeletal lesion is the first manifestation of disease. Patients with skeletal metastasis should be carefully examined and thoroughly investigated to find the source of the primary (Fig. 21.10).

Treatment principles for pathological fractures secondary to metastatic involvement of bone are different from those used in treating comparable traumatic fractures.

1. Exact anatomic extent of the lesion should be defined. Skip lesions in the involved bone should be meticulously looked for.

2. Assess bone stock

3. Reconstruction and fixation should be such that fracture healing is not a necessary component to achieve full weight bearing or allow mobilisation.

4. Bone cement should be used to augment internal fixation. Conservative management of pathological fractures is associated with increased morbidity. Pain control is poor and union rate is low.

The advantages of surgical stabilisation of the impending fracture of long bone are:

1. Pain relief

2. Improved limb function

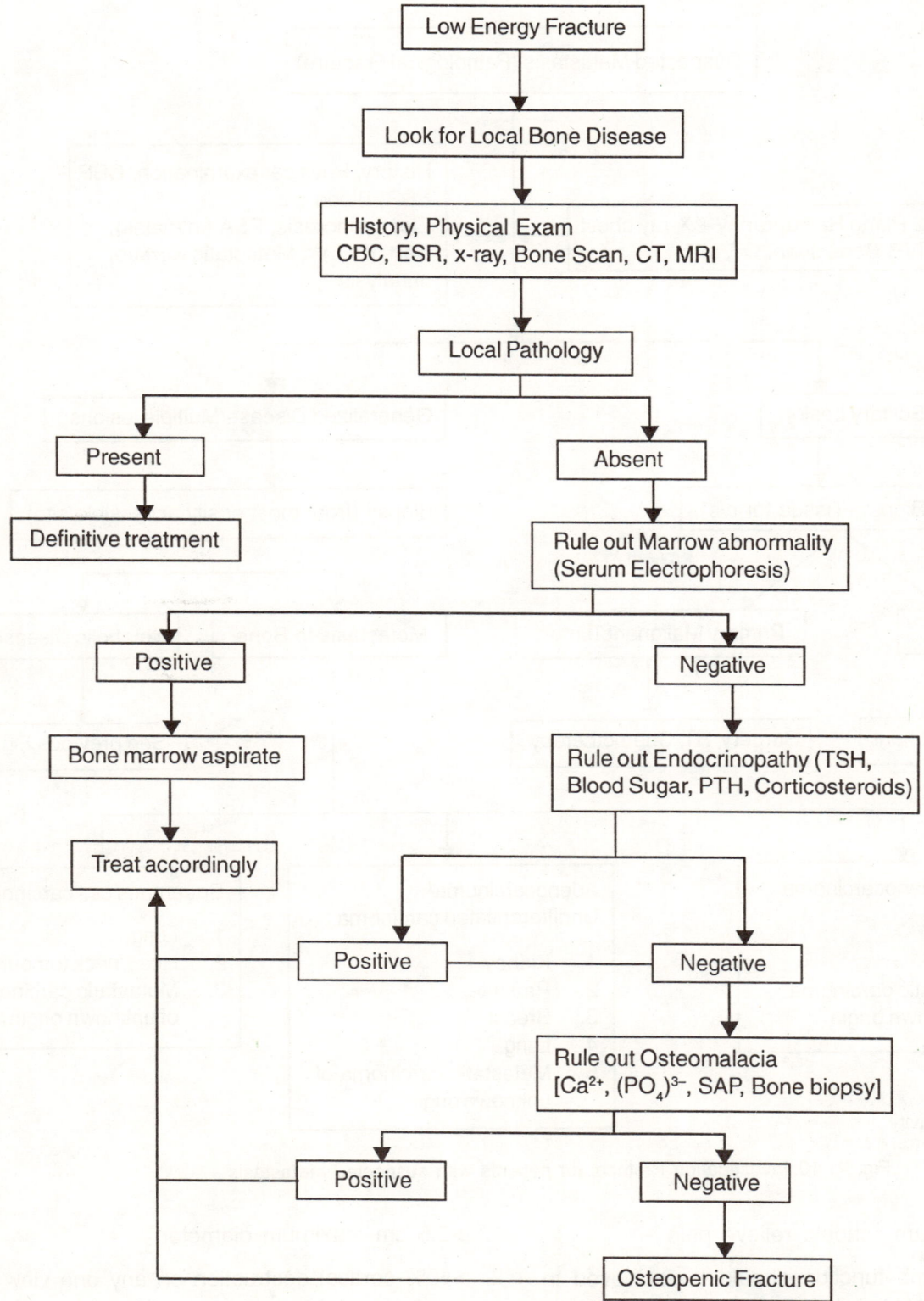

Fig. 21.9. Work-up of an insufficiency fracture

3. Tissue diagnosis

Pre-requisites for surgical stabilisation are:

1. Reasonable projected life expectancy (more than 12 weeks)

2. The patient should be able to withstand anaesthesia and surgical stress.

3. The quality of bone proximal and distal to the fracture must be sufficient to support fixation.

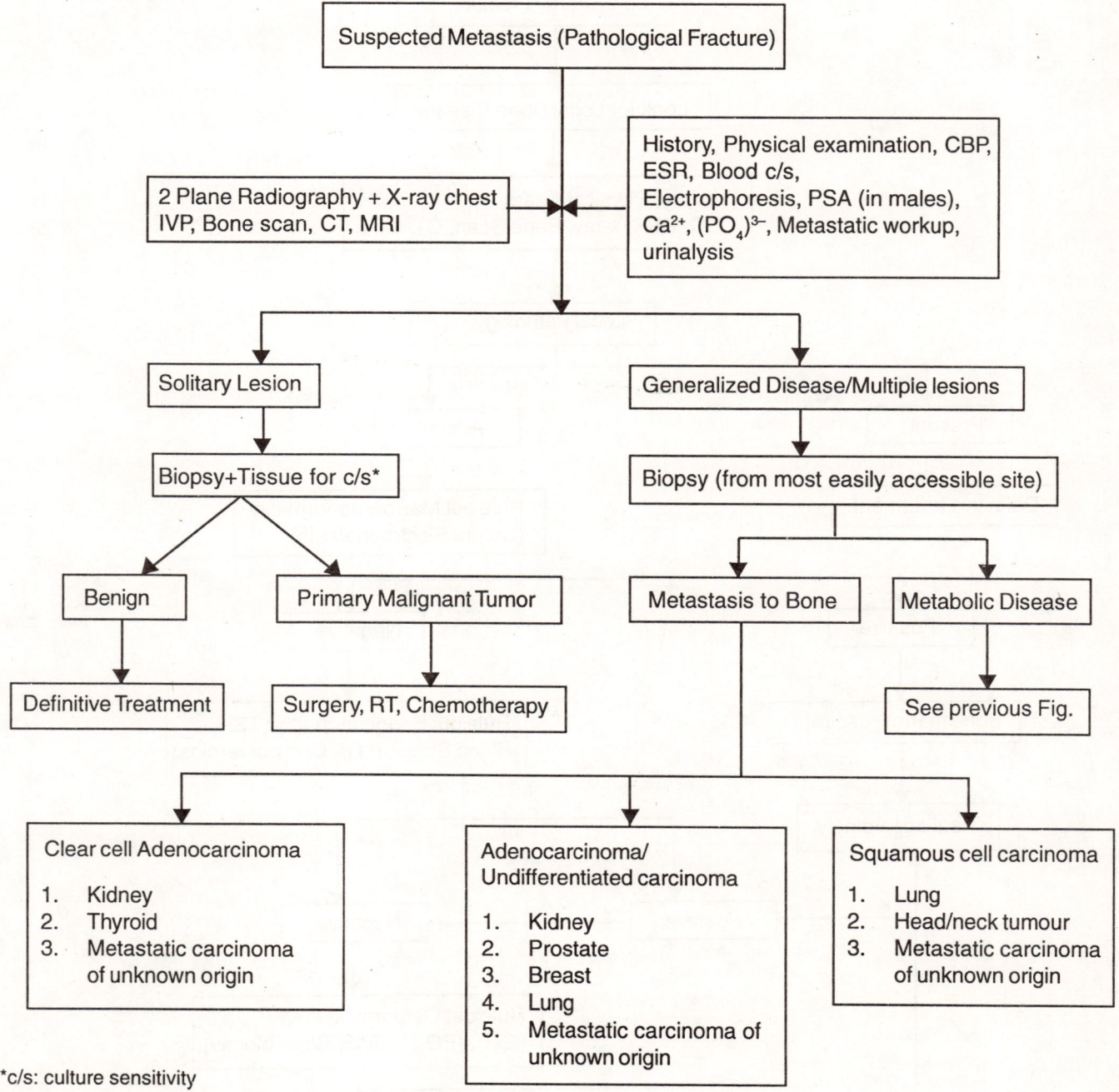

*c/s: culture sensitivity

Fig. 21.10. Investigation Protocol for patients with suspected metastasis

4. The procedure should relieve pain

5. Improved limb function should be achieved in the immediate post-operative period because of the short life expectancy.

Prophylactic fixation: In a long bone with metastasis, prophylactic internal fixation is a useful procedure and may save the patient from pain and disability.

Criteria for prophylactic fixation of a lytic lesion are:

1. >2.5 cm maximum diameter

2. >50% cortical destruction on any one view

3. Persistence of pain despite radiation therapy >2 weeks ago.

Many of these patients have microfractures that will progress to complete displacement.

In permeative and osteoblastic lesions there are as yet no definite guidelines.

Stress Fractures

A stress fracture is a partial or complete fracture of a bone resulting from its inability to withstand non-violent forces that are applied in a rhythmic and repeated sub threshold manner. No single traumatic episode is identifiable. They are commonly seen in army recruits, long distance runners, ballet dancers and in the eager athlete at the beginning of the season.

Stress fracture should be differentiated from insufficiency fracture (fracture that occurs when normal stress is applied to abnormal bone, i.e. rheumatoid arthritis, osteoporosis) and pathological fracture (fracture due to subnormal stress in abnormal bone, i.e. fracture through cyst).

Pathogenesis Two theories have been set forth.

1. *Muscle fatigue* Muscle fatigue secondary to stress overload leads to a reduction in its shock absorption function and allows excessive force to be transmitted to the underlying bone.
2. *Muscle pull* Repeated muscular contractions acting on bone can produce a stress fracture.

Bone responds to stress via Wolff's Law. During normal remodelling, resorption (osteoclastic activity) is followed by replacement (osteoblastic activity). Replacement is slow while resorption is relatively rapid producing a stage of temporarily weakened cortex. If stress is applied during this phase, remodelling is accelerated and a stress fracture can occur.

Clinical Picture

Stress fractures can occur at all ages but are most frequent in young adults (18–28 years age). Stress fracture should be thought of in terms of a process (rather than a single event) where the exact starting moment is impossible to decide.

Pain is the presenting complaint. Because of lack of specific trauma the pain is initially ignored and 2–3 weeks pass before medical advice is sought. Pain is aggravated by activity and relieved by rest. Generally pain is sharply localised within a circumscribed area, which is also tender on palpation. Certain sports have higher risk for specific stress fractures (Table 21.13).

When the fracture occurs near a joint, passive

Table 21.13. Sports likely to give rise to Stress Fractures

Sport	Site
1. Running, Tennis	Metatarsals-midshaft, anatomical neck (3 > 2 > 4 in order of frequency)
2. Soccer	Lateral 3 metatarsals. The 5th MT base is prone to non-union
3. Basket ball	Metatarsals – midshaft, anatomical neck and tibia
4. Dance	Metatarsal – base of 2nd MT and midshaft tibia

joint movement at extremes of range causes discomfort in the region of the fracture. Effusion rarely develops.

Swelling occasionally to the point of pitting oedema is present, e.g. dorsum of foot in metatarsal stress fracture. The swelling is diffuse and does not entirely disappear after elevation. The affected area may be erythematous and warm. Stress fractures are commonest in metatarsals, followed by tibia. The other bones frequently affected are shown in Table 21.14.

In the skeletally immature patient, stress fracture is a manifestation of overuse injury. Almost every bone in the lower extremity and pelvis is susceptible to stress fracture. Important differential diagnoses are osteomyelitis and osteosarcoma.

Investigation

X-rays taken shortly after the onset of symptoms may not show any abnormality. Changes usually take 3–4 weeks to appear. Subperiosteal and endosteal callus formation with or without a small cortical crack may be seen. Subsequently callus formation slowly progresses to a fusiform area of maturing callus. Serial x-rays and regular follow up is required.

Bone scans are valuable in early diagnosis of stress fractures since the isotope accumulates in areas of high metabolic activity and blood flow. Technetium 99^m labelled phosphate is the most commonly used isotope. It is highly sensitive but non-specific.

CT Scan can demonstrate subtle callus and fracture lines. However it is not practical to use it routinely.

MRI is highly sensitive and specific. Subtle bony abnormalities can be defined. The age of the lesion can also be estimated.

Treatment Stress fracture is explainable as an incomplete attempt by bone to remodel itself, whereby bone is deposited in sites subjected to stress and resorbed from sites where there is no excessive stress. Being a living tissue capable of repair, bone can adapt to tremendous stress, given time.

Treatment is conservative and consists of reduced physical activity, rest and at times immobilisation in plaster. Cross-training emphasising non-weight bearing activity (swimming, cycling) is recommended to avoid muscle atrophy. This applies to the common stress fractures like those of the metatarsals, fibula, calcaneum. Fractures of the anterior tibial cortex, and femur neck, however, require careful observation and regular follow-up because of their propensity to progress to a complete fracture. Prolonged immobilisation is therefore necessary in these cases. There is increasing use of prophylactic pinning in the treatment of stress fractures of the femoral neck.

Paediatric Injuries—An Overview

Characteristics of paediatric musculoskeletal injuries

Fractures and dislocations in children are unique and several features of these injuries are not seen in adults. The differences are most striking in the infant and toddler and as the age increases, the differences become less obvious.

1. **Fractures are more common** The incidence of fractures is higher in children and more likely to occur after seemingly insignificant trauma. Also children, in general are more injury prone.

2. **Periosteum** The periosteum is thicker, stronger and loosely attached to bone. As it is stronger and easily separates from bone there is less likelihood of its complete circumferential rupture. This intact periosteal sleeve, usually on the concave (compression) side (as in a green-stick fracture) prevents wide displacement and is useful in achieving and maintaining reduction. The young periosteum also exhibits greater osteogenic potential. In fact, complete loss of bone with reasonably intact periosteal sleeve may be followed by 'regeneration of missing bone'.

3. **Joint injuries, dislocation, and ligament injury** Ligaments in the growing child exhibit a greater degree of laxity compared to adults. Yet ligament injuries and dislocations are uncommon because the joint capsule and ligaments are more resistant to stress than the underlying bone where they attach. Tension on the ligament produces epiphyseal separation through the growth plate, rather than ligament tear.

4. **Rapid bone healing** Bone healing is relatively rapid in childhood due to the extremely osteogenic periosteum and rich blood supply. The younger the child, more rapid the union. Age is the most important factor influencing the rate of bone healing in children. The other factor is location of the fracture. Growth plate (physis) injuries take half the time to unite compared to metaphyseal and diaphyseal fractures. Non-union is rare in children.

Table 21.14. Bones affected by Stress Fractures

Bone	Location
Metatarsals 2nd, 3rd, (most common)	Base, midshaft, anatomical neck
Tibia	Posteromedial cortex at junction of M/3 and D/3
	Anterior cortex-midshaft (Notorious for nonunion)
	Medial tibial condyle (rare) (Fracture can extend intra-articularly)
Fibula	Lateral cortex just proximal to ankle joint
Calcaneum	Junction of posterior body of calcaneum with mid aspect
Femur	Neck *Tension aspect(superior; high propensity to progress to complete fracture)
	*Compression aspect (inferior margin; do not displace)
	Shaft-junction of M/3 and D/3 at medial cortex

5. **Growth plate at the ends of bone** Growth plates at the end of bones are areas where longitudinal and latitudinal growth occurs. Injury may damage the physis and cause chronic growth disturbance. Therefore it is necessary to warn the parents of potential late growth abnormality.

6. **Correction of deformity** The normal process of remodelling in a growing child will correct certain degree of malalignment and therefore accurate anatomical reduction of the fracture, though desirable, is not necessary in children. The younger the child and closer the fracture to the growth plate, the greater is the potential for correction of malalignment. Angular deformity in plane of motion of an adjacent joint corrects readily, while correction is minimal in angular deformities in other directions, e.g. anterior/posterior angulation of a supracondylar fracture humerus corrects spontaneously unlike cubitus varus. Rotational deformities do not remodel.

7. **Role of open reduction** As a general principle, open reduction and internal fixation is rarely indicated as this may affect the normal healing pattern. However, exceptions occur.

– intraarticular fractures: type III, IV physeal fracture
– fracture neck femur

8. **Comminution** Bone modelling and remodelling is so active that bone is relatively porous in children compared to adults. This porosity impedes fracture propagation and comminution is uncommon.

9. **Bowing** is a peculiar phenomenon seen in the resilient immature bone. The bone is deformed beyond full elastic recoil into a phase of permanent *plastic deformation*. The younger the child, the more it is likely that this type of skeletal injury may occur. Commonly seen in the ulna and fibula, it can limit reduction of the fractured bone of the pair.

10. **Growth stimulation** Fractures may stimulate longitudinal growth by increasing the blood supply to metaphysis, physis and epiphysis (repair is associated with neovascularisation). Therefore, some degree of over-riding with bayonet (side to side) apposition may be desirable in long bone fractures of the lower limb.

11. **Diagnostic dilemma** The epiphyses are variably radiolucent, making radiographic interpretation difficult. Mistaking the normal epiphyseal line for fracture is not uncommon. This problem can be overcome to a great extent by comparing the x-ray of the opposite limb. The commonest site for such problems is the elbow.

12. **Blood loss** The total blood volume is proportionately smaller in a child than an adult. Loss of a certain amount of blood in an adult may be 10% of his blood volume and can be well tolerated but the same amount of blood loss in a child will be 30% of his blood volume and has serious consequences if not replenished quickly. Circulating blood volume by weight in adults: 65–75 ml/kg: children 80–85 ml/kg.

13. **Common complications** of paediatric fractures are:

1. Growth disturbance-due to physeal injury

2. Extensive osteomyelitis likely due to increased porosity and loosely attached periosteum.

3. Volkmann's ischemia

4. Myositis ossificans

Uncommon complications include:

1. Joint stiffness following immobilisation-due to ligament laxity.

2. Fat embolism is extremely rare.

Epiphyseal Injuries

The growth plate (physis) (Fig. 21.11) is more susceptible to fracture than is injury to attached ligaments; therefore if there is any question, one must assume that there is an injury of the physis until proved otherwise. Potentially significant complications are associated with these injuries. E.g. limb length discrepancy, progressive deformity. An understanding of the physeal architecture is of paramount importance to any physician concerned with treatment of these injuries (see Fig. 21.11).

Architecture of growth plate

Zone of Growth (*Zone of resting cartilage, Zone of proliferation*) Longitudinal growth occurs only in this region. This zone makes up about one-half of the height of the growth plate. The columnar pattern is maintained by the formation of longitu-

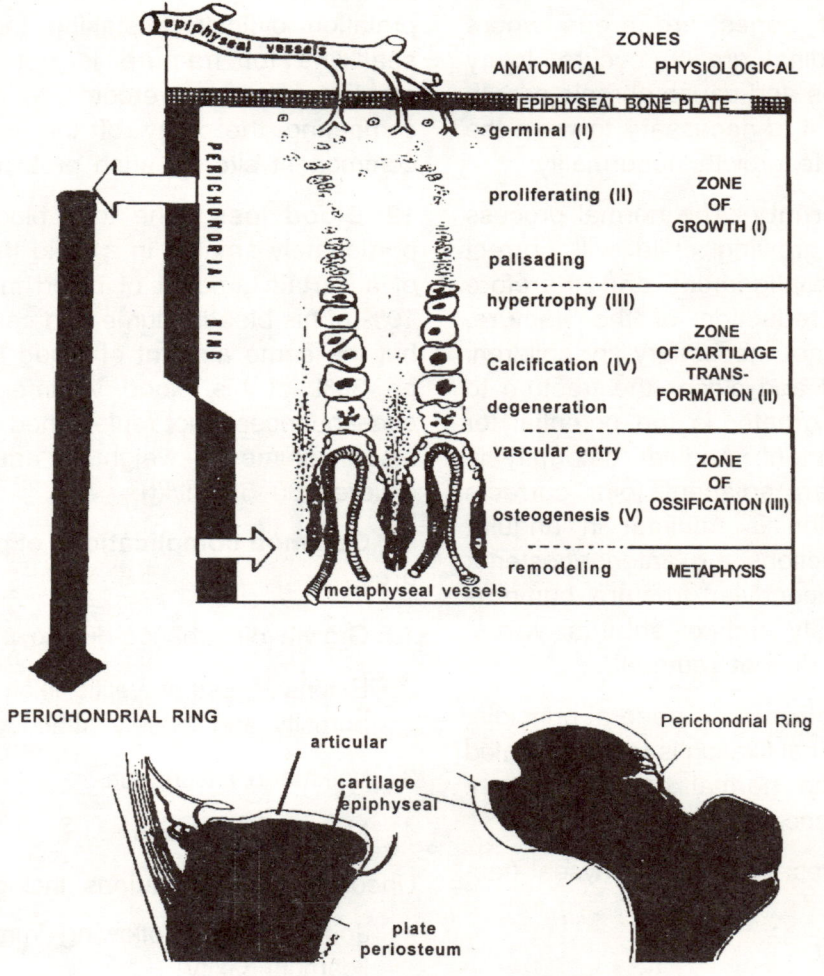

Fig. 21.11. Architecture of growth plate

dinally oriented bundles of collagen fibres in the intercellular matrix.

Zone of cartilage transformation (*Zone of maturation*) This consists of Zone of hypertrophy and Zone of provisional calcification. The chondrocytes undergo progressive degeneration. Calcification of the matrix begins. The weakest portion of the physis is the zone of hypertrophy. Strength is provided by the intercellular matrix. As the cells hypertrophy, the collagen fibre bundles thin out and make this area prone to shearing, bending and tension stress. Resistance to compression remains unaltered.

Zone of ossification Blood vessels penetrate the calcified cartilage matrix. Bone-forming osteoblasts appear and lay down osteoid (unmineralised bone matrix) which subsequently mineralises. There is no distinction between medulla and cortex. During remodelling a cortex and medulla appear and the diameter of bone diminishes.

Blood supply Blood supply to the growth plate arises from 3 sources: (Fig. 21.12).

1. *Epiphyseal vessels* These vessels enter the epiphyses between the articular cartilage and growth plate. They penetrate the growth plate and terminate at the zone of growth. Further nutrition occurs by diffusion.

2. *Metaphyseal vessels* These are branches of the nutrient vessel and penetrate upto the zone of ossification. Interruption of these vessels has no effect on chondrogenesis; the growth plate height increases as cartilage does not transform into bone.

3. *Perichondrial vessels* These vessels supply only the perichondrial cells, which are responsible for latitudinal growth. Interruption may upset external remodelling leading to exostosis or failure of narrowing of the metaphysis.

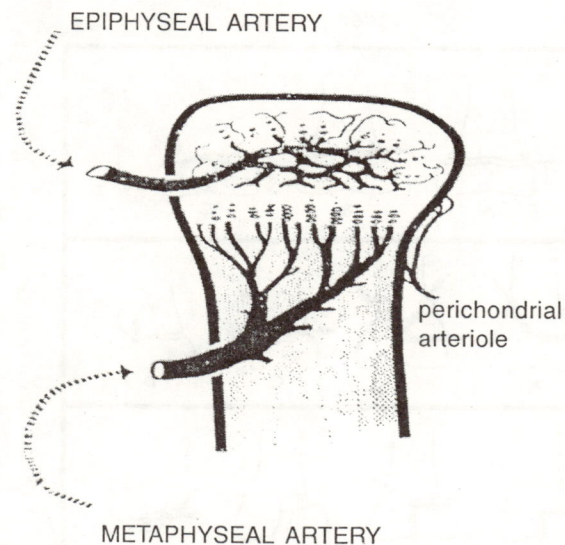

EPIPHYSEAL ARTERY

perichondrial
arteriole

METAPHYSEAL ARTERY

Fig. 21.12. Blood supply to the Growth Plate

Blood supply reaches the epiphysis by one of two different patterns:

1. Epiphyses like femoral head that are completely covered by articular cartilage: The blood vessel (epiphyseal) passes along the neck of the bone and crosses the growth plate before entering the epiphysis. Epiphyseal separation carries a high risk of damaging blood supply to the epiphysis with subsequent avascular necrosis.

2. Epiphyses partially covered by articular cartilage: The epiphyseal blood vessel enters the epiphysis directly. Epiphyseal separation here does not jeopardise blood supply.

Classification of Epiphyseal Injuries

The classification proposed by *Salter-Harris* is the most extensively accepted as it correlates well to the mechanism of injury, treatment and prognosis. Other classifications were proposed by Poland, Ogden etc. The classifications of Poland and Salter-Harris are shown in Fig. 21.13.

Type I is complete separation of the epiphyses without any fracture through bone. The germinal cells remain with the epiphyses as separation occurs through the zone of hypertrophy. The periosteal attachment remains intact and displacement is minimal. This type of injury occurs most frequently in the new born and infants. Reduction is generally not required. Growth disturbance is seldom seen unless there is risk of AVN.

Type II is the commonest type of injury. The fracture line extends along the epiphyseal plate for a variable distance and then out through a portion of the metaphysis producing a triangular shaped metaphyseal fragment (*Thurston-Holland sign*). The germinal cells remain with the epiphysis. Periosteum is torn in the convex side and remains intact on the metaphyseal fragment side. Closed reduction is easy and the intact periosteum prevents over-reduction. Growth is not disturbed.

Type III fracture is intra-articular and extends from the joint surface to the epiphyseal plate and then along the epiphyseal plate to the periphery. This is an uncommon injury and occurs most commonly at the distal tibial epiphysis (*Railing Fracture*). Open reduction is necessary to restore articular congruity. Risk of growth disturbance is minimal provided the blood supply has not been damaged.

Type IV fracture line begins at the articular surface and extends through the epiphyses, the physis and then through a segment of the metaphysis. This type of injury is seen most frequently in the lateral condyle fracture of the humerus. Open reduction is mandatory to restore articular congruity and growth plate apposition. Prognosis is guarded after surgery and poor if perfect reduction is not achieved and maintained.

Type V is an uncommon type of injury, diagnosed retrospectively. It occurs due to compression across the growth plate. Because the epiphysis is not displaced and no fracture line is seen on the x-ray, the diagnosis is difficult. Crushing of the germinal cells causes premature growth arrest. Prognosis is poor.

Management of epiphyseal injuries

1. Reduction should be gentle, as forcible manipulation is likely to damage the delicate physeal cells and epiphyseal vascularity.

2. Reduction is urgent and each day of delay makes atraumatic reduction difficult. Reduction should be attempted within 3 days of injury and definitely not after 5 days in Type I and II injuries.

3. Type III and IV injuries are best managed by an accurate open reduction an internal fixation.

4. Patients should be followed up for at least 1 year for possible development of growth disturbance.

Type	Poland	Salter-Harris	Ogden
I			
II			
III			
IV			
V			
VI			
VII			

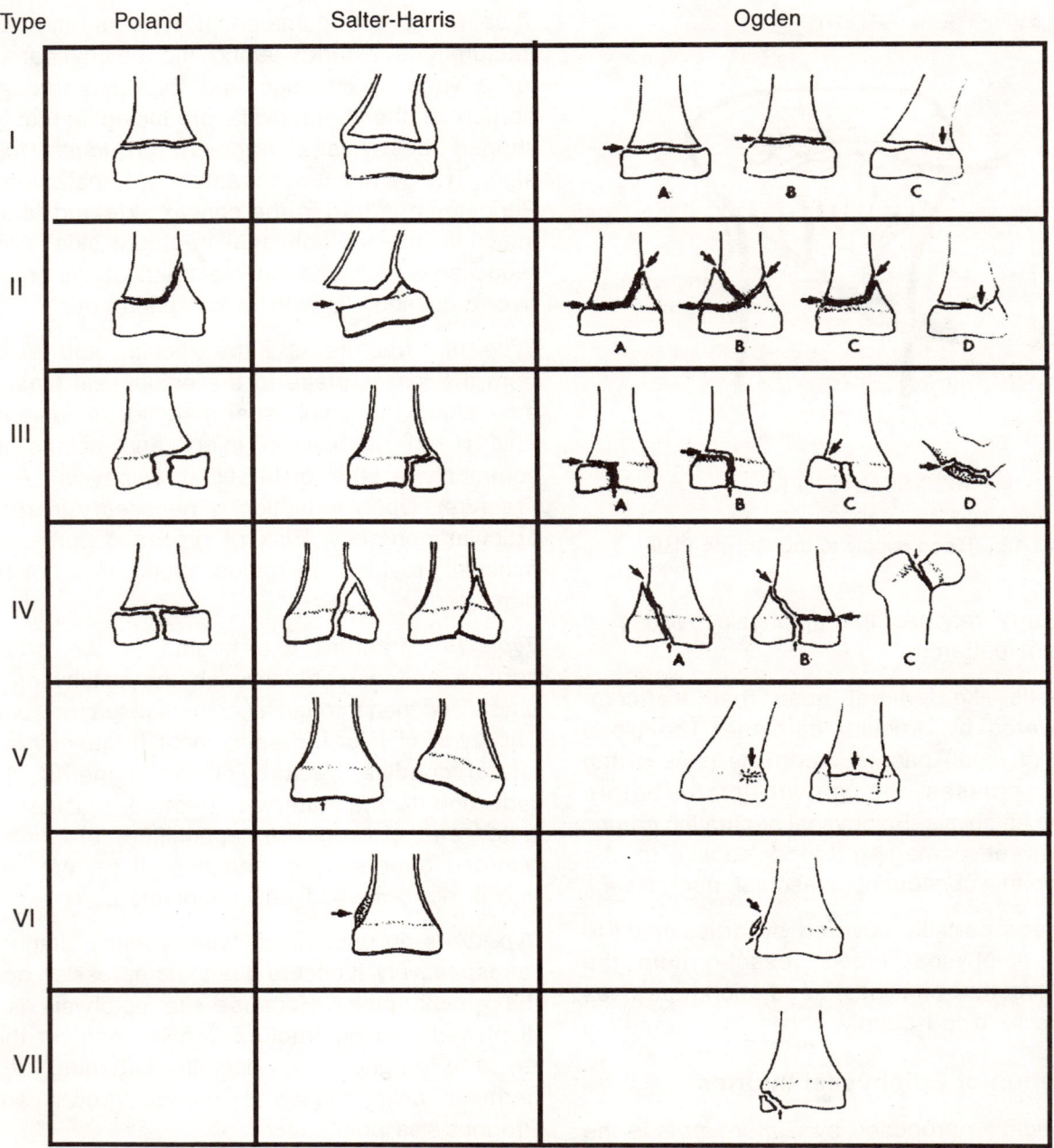

Fig. 21.13. Classification of Epiphyseal injuries (Poland, Salter Harris and Ogden). Note the 3 classifications are similar but with increasing complexity from left to right. Salter-Harris classification is a modification of Poland's classification while Ogden classification adds more sub-classes to the simpler systems.

Parents should be warned of this potential complication, as it is difficult to estimate damage to the germinal cells in any injury.

5. Adequate immobilisation is mandatory. Risk of joint stiffness is negligible in children even after intra-articular fractures.

Prognostic Factors

1. Type of injury

2. Age of child: The younger the child at the time of injury, the more serious any growth disturbance is likely to become since growth remaining at the epiphysis is more (Fig. 21.14).

3. Open/closed injury: Open injuries have risk of infection that can destroy the physis and lead to growth arrest. Prognosis is generally guarded in open injuries.

Birth trauma is an uncommon occurrence but a

cause of great concern among the parents and the physician. Clinical examination is equivocal and interpretation of plain x-rays of unossified ends of long bones difficult. Most of the fractures occur in infants of primiparous women, with a significantly high incidence among breech deliveries. The most common sites of fracture in descending order are clavicle (90%) > humerus > femur. The most common sites of epiphyseal injury in descending frequency are: proximal humerus > distal femur > distal humerus > proximal femur > distal tibia. These are Salter-Harris Type I and are particularly difficult to identify on x-rays. An important differential diagnosis is septic arthritis or osteomyelitis. Needle aspiration of the involved joint may help establish the diagnosis. In contrast, shaft fractures are readily identifiable.

Birth Fractures

Clavicle   It is the most common bone to be fractured during birth. The fractures are usually seen in the midshaft. Predisposing factors are:

1. High birth weight

2. Primipara

3. Breech delivery

4. Shoulder dystocia.

Clinically the neonate presents with pseudo-paralysis of the extremity.

Differential diagnosis of pseudoparalysis of the upper extremity includes:

1. Fracture of the proximal humerus

2. Septic arthritis of shoulder

3. Osteomyelitis

4. Brachial plexus injury

5. Congenital pseudarthrosis.

Note Brachial plexus injury may co-exist with fracture clavicle.

Treatment   These fractures seldom require active treatment. Most heal within 2 weeks with abundant callus formation.

Humerus   Proximal epiphyseal injuries are more frequent than shaft fractures and are the second most common birth injury.

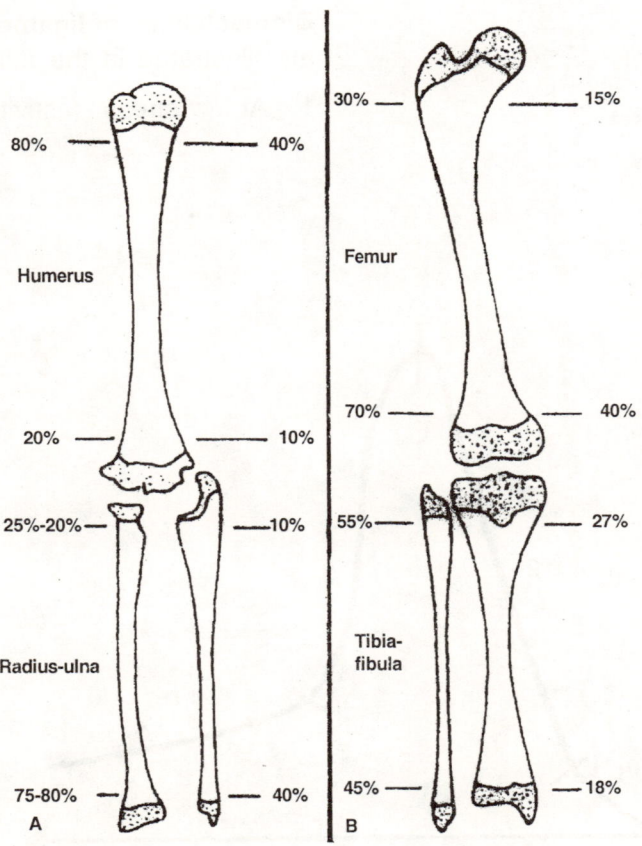

Fig. 21.14. Growth contributions of physes of (a) upper, and (b) lower extremities

Clinically the neonate presents with pseudoparalysis of the extremity and swelling of the shoulder. To confuse matters, Erb's palsy may co-exist. The differential diagnoses are similar to clavicular fracture. The arm should be bandaged to the chest with special care to prevent skin maceration. Most fractures unite within 3 weeks.

Femur Birth fractures tend to be midshaft and transverse. Its presence should alert the physician to the possibility of other pathologic conditions, such as osteogenesis imperfecta. Most fractures unite in four weeks – Bryant's traction for 2 weeks followed by spica for 2 weeks. Up to 1 cm of over riding and 30° angulation will remodel.

Ligament Injuries

Bony injuries are easy to diagnose, but ligament injuries are often missed as they are not visible on x-rays and the two essential steps of careful history and a meticulous physical examination are usually forgotten. Disability from ligament injury most frequently affects the knee and the reasons are:

– Wide range of motion;

– Lack of osseous stability;

– Weight bearing function.

To appreciate the importance of ligaments and the disability due to injury a working knowledge of their structure, biomechanics and function is essential.

Structure

Water comprises about 60–80% of the total weight of ligaments. 70% of the dry weight consists of collagen Type I arranged in parallel bundles. This is the primary tensile resistant substance. Proteoglycans account for 1% of the dry weight. They bind strongly to water and together provide lubrication for gliding and confer viscoelastic property. The rest of the ligament is made up of elastin, reticulum and mesenchymal cells. Ligament vascularity is tenuous.

Ligaments receive blood supply from the periarticular arterial plexuses. Intraligamentous vessels are sparse and diffusion is necessary for mid-substance nutrition. Insertion of ligaments progress from fibres to fibrocartilage to mineralised fibrocartilage and finally to bone. Some fibres insert directly into bone through periosteum. This serves to dissipate force and minimise failures.

Biomechanics of ligament Ligament biomechanics are illustrated in the following figure (Fig. 21.15)

1. At low stress (activities of daily routine) a con-

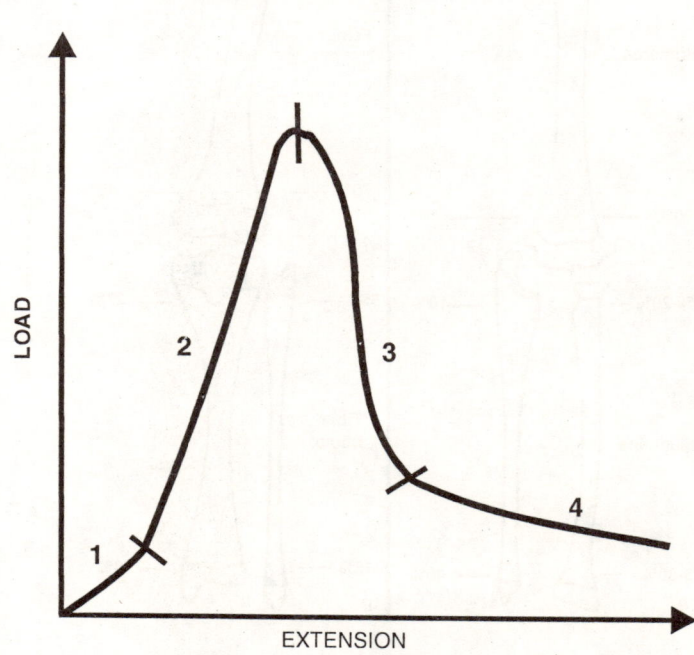

Fig. 21.15. Biomechanical properties of a ligament with increasing load

cave upward slope is seen. The wavy collagen fibres are straightened and the increase in length is not proportional to the load.

2. At moderate to high stress (sports), a linear increase is seen and the ligament remains elastic.

3. At the higher end, microfailures occur in the collagen fibrils and with increased loading progressive failure occurs. Despite the fact that the ligament now becomes functionally useless, it may grossly appear intact.

4. With further extension the fibres start to slide apart at low load.

During slow rate of loading, avulsion failure at ligament insertion to bone is common whereas during rapid rate of loading, mid-substance tear is common.

Function of ligament

1. **Lateral stability of joints** Many joints act in a hinge like manner with movement predominantly in a particular arc e.g. knee, elbow, metacarpophalangeal joints. If motion is confined to one arc (flexion-extension) then ligaments are needed to provide control over other movements i.e. varus /valgus.

2. **Limitation of motion** is the function of capsular ligaments that are found in the front and back of hinge joints and circumferentially in spherical joints.

3. **Progressive control of motion** The ligament origin does not coincide with the axis of joint motion. Due to eccentric location tension arises with movement.

e.g. with metacarpophalangeal joints in extension-abduction, adduction is possible. As flexion increases, sideward movements reduce, and eventually disappear at 90° flexion.

4. **Torque transmission** Ligaments help in transmitting rotational forces along the long axis of bone across joints, without the bone ends having to "climb out" of a closed/ packed arrangement.

Effects of immobilisation Stress deprivation causes qualitative and quantitative alterations in ligament substance.

– Loss of parallelism of collagen fibres.

– Distorted cellular organisation

– Decrease in number of collagen fibres

– Reduced thickness of fibres

– Decrease in water content

– Decreased strength of bone-ligament interface.

It may take the ligament several months to regain normal compliance and normal tensile failure load after being immobilised for only 8 weeks.

Types of Ligament Injury

Incomplete

1. **Simple sprain** The ligament fibres are stretched but the ligament as a whole remains in continuity.

2. **Partial tear** The length of the ligament remains unaltered but a few fibres are ruptured.

Incomplete tears are more painful than complete tears.

Complete

3. **Complete tear** The torn ends of the ligament retract with no continuity between them. Complete tears produce marked instability/dislocation of the neighbouring joint.

Associated injuries Ligament injuries occur due to significant angulatory and rotational stress on the joint and this force can simultaneously produce associated injuries to the neighbouring joint.

1. **Injury to articular cartilage** Cellular damage, fibrillation or macroscopic splits may occur. Significant damage has potential for progressing to osteoarthritis later on. These injuries are difficult to detect at the time of injury.

2. **Synovial membrane damage** This can cause hemarthrosis or effusion. Swelling developing within 4 hours of injury is due to hemarthrosis while effusion takes longer to appear.

3. **Injury to bone** The ligament may fail through its bony attachment. Usually the bone fragment is small and no deleterious effects occur, but sometimes a large fragment may detach and displace into the joint. Prompt surgical intervention becomes imperative.

4. **Injury to nerve** Nerves in relation to the ligament are prone to injury. Risk is higher with complete tears. The nerve injury is of the traction-type, e.g. lateral popliteal nerve injury with fibular

collateral ligament tear. Prognosis is generally grave.

Diagnosis The most important factor in diagnosis is to be aware of the possibility of ligament damage. If after a definite injury no bony damage is detected, a thought should be given to ligament injury. Majorities of the injuries in clinical practice are sprains or partial tears. Few objective physical signs are seen. As a result ligament injuries are frequently misdiagnosed and poorly managed.

Careful clinical examination may show

1. Surface bruising,

2. Local tenderness,

3. Local swelling,

4. Effusion/hemarthrosis in the joint, or

5. Marked pain on stressing the ligament. With complete tears joint instability may be obvious on examination but at times protective muscle spasm can prevent joint movement and thus mask joint instability. In this situation it is necessary to overcome this with local anaesthetic injection at the site of ligament damage or by examination under anaesthesia. Stress x-rays may be obtained for objective documentation.

Treatment Three important factors should be borne in mind when considering treatment of ligament injuries.

1. Amount of scar tissue laid down in partial and complete ligament tears is inversely proportional to the degree of immobilisation of the affected ligament.

2. Accurate apposition of divided ligament fibrils plays a significant role in the quality of the repair process; the greater the gap between the ligament ends the greater the scar tissue, with ensuing laxity and reduced tensile strength.

3. Associated damage to the neighbouring joint.

Majority of ligament injuries heal adequately with conservative treatment; only the complete tears benefit from surgical repair. The objectives of treatment are:

- relief of pain.

- minimise soft tissue swelling and associated joint effusion.

- prevention of adhesions.

Modalities R.I.C.E. is most often used.

Rest This provides pains relief and reduces further trauma.

Ice This is of great value in early treatment. It provides pain relief by sensory numbing and vasoconstriction of local blood vessels. This reduces bleeding into the affected area and decreases swelling and inflammation in the neighbouring joint.

Compression This reduces the soft tissue oedema and helps in faster recovery.

Elevation Elevating the affected limb above the level of the heart reduces soft tissue oedema by facilitating faster venous outflow.

Anti-Inflammatory agents They dampen the inflammatory reaction and reduce pain and joint effusion.

Heat This is beneficial only after danger of bleeding into affected region has passed (approximately one week after injury). The increased blood flow helps in faster healing.

Ultrasound Vibrations generated in bone helps disperse the hematoma. The heat produced promotes local blood flow and healing.

Mobilisation

Simple sprain Gentle mobilisation should be encouraged as soon as pain and swelling subside to avoid adhesions and joint stiffness.

Partial/ complete tear Six weeks of adequate immobilisation is minimum. This should be followed by active physiotherapy.

BONE GRAFTING

Removing bone from one site and transplanting it to another site or individual is a common surgical procedure. It has been in use for a very long time but only in recent decades its biological and pathological aspects have been understood.

Indications for employing bone grafts are:

1. To fill cavities or defects resulting from cyst, tumours, trauma

2. To bridge joints for arthrodesis

3. To bridge major defects and restore continuity of a long bone

4. To provide bone block to limit motion at a joint (arthrorisis)

5. To promote union in a case of non-union (pseudarthrosis)

6. To promote union or fill defects in delayed union, malunion, fresh fractures or osteotomies

The genetic relation between the donor and the recipient defines four types (sources) of bone graft:

(a) **Autografts** Grafts transferred from a donor site to another site in the same individual.

(b) **Isografts** Grafts transferred between people who have identical histocompatibility antigens, i.e. identical twins.

(c) **Allografts** Grafts transferred between genetically dissimilar members of the same species, e.g. mother to child.

(d) **Xenografts** Grafts transferred from a member of one species to a member of another species, i.e. bovine, porcine bone to man.

1. **Autologous (Autogenous) graft** This graft is taken from the patient's own bones. Common sites for obtaining graft are the iliac crest, fibula, tibia and distal femur. The graft may be cancellous, cortical or cortico-cancellous. Cancellous bone is the most commonly used graft in non-unions or cavitary defects because it is quickly remodelled and incorporated. Cortical bone is slower in turnover than cancellous bone and is used for structural defects.

2. **Allogenic (Homologous) graft** At times it may not be possible to obtain enough autologous bone to meet the demands of the surgical procedure, e.g. children with cavitary defect. In such circumstances bone from another individual or cadaveric bone can be used. All allografts must be harvested with sterile technique and donors must be screened for potential transmissible diseases. Allogenic bone graft can be:

Fresh This is highly immunogenic and often excites a florid rejection within a week of implantation.

Fresh Frozen This bone is less immunogenic and the rejection response is delayed. Bone morphogenic protein (BMP), a protein that promotes osteoinduction is however preserved to some extent.

Freeze-dried (*lyophilized*) Bone in bone bank is stored in this form (croutons). Structural integrity is lost, BMP is depleted but it is the least immunogenic of all allografts.

The success of bone grafting leading to absorption, osteogenesis, remodelling and eventual obliteration and healing of a defect by bone graft mainly depends on eliminating immunological reactions.

3. **Xenograft (Heterogenous) graft** Because of the undesirable features of autologous and allogenic grafts, heterogenous bone was tried in early days. The results were unsatisfactory. These grafts incited severe and undesirable foreign body reaction. Consistently satisfactory heterogenous graft material is not commercially available and its use is not recommended in present times.

Pathology of graft incorporation Five stages of graft healing have been recognised.

Stage 1 Inflammation On removal from the donor site the bone graft loses its blood supply and is now an ischemic piece of bone. In the recipient site the graft is surrounded by blood and inflammatory cells. Only the surface cells of the graft survive by obtaining nutrition from its surroundings while the deeper and inner cells die. Necrosis stimulates chemotaxis and macrophages appear. This is followed by capillaries and mesenchymal cells.

Stage 2 Osteoblast differentiation The pleuripotent mesenchymal cells differentiate into pre-osteoblasts and osteoblasts.

Stage 3 Osteoinduction The osteoblasts lay down bone under the influence of osteoinductive proteins, namely Bone Morphogenic Protein, Transforming growth factor ß, platelet derived growth factor.

Stage 2 and 3 begin a week after inflammation of surgical trauma subsides.

Stage 4 Osteoconduction This stage is spread over months. The graft acts as a scaffold over which new bone forms from the recipient bed. Compression between the graft and host bone promotes new bone formation.

Stage 5 Remodelling This stage occurs slowly over many years. The graft eventually becomes enmeshed in the structure of the host bone.

In cancellous bone the mesenchymal cells differentiate into osteoblasts, which then lay down a seam of osteoid (unmineralised bone matrix) along with dead trabeculae of the graft, which are gradually resorbed by the osteoclasts. The gross anatomical structure of the graft remains unchanged and the old necrotic trabeculae and matrix are gradually replaced by living bone. This process is referred to as "creeping substitution". Lastly old marrow spaces are replaced by active new marrow cells.

In cortical bone graft, the process of incorporation is essentially similar but takes a very long time. The graft is replaced through slow remodelling of the existing haversian systems via a process of resorption (this weakens the grafts). Union between the transplant and the host bone occurs from 6 to 12 months, and it is only after union takes place that resorption and porosity and susceptibility to stress fracture become apparent. Resorption is followed by deposition of new bone. The grafted bone regains its normal radiological density and resistance to torsional stress by 1 year. By this time only 60% of the graft is resorbed and replaced. Restoration of mechanical strength requires about 2 years.

Survival of harvested graft

The following physical factors are important while removing and implanting bone grafts to ensure optimum survival of donor cells and osteoinductive elements:

1. Thickness of the graft: Cancellous bone graft should not be more than 5 mm thick. This thickness ensures maximum exposure of superficial cells to host bed and allows rapid incorporation.

2. After removal, graft should be kept wrapped in a sponge soaked with patient's own blood. This prevents desiccation and eliminates adverse effects of high intensity theatre lights. The graft should never be immersed or washed in saline or antibiotic solution. This reduces the osteoinductive substances.

3. Bone graft should preferably be placed in the recipient site as soon as possible as the percentage of viable cells decreases exponentially with time.

4. Grafts placed under compression heal better. Compression between the cortical graft and host favours differentiation of the pleuripotent mesen-chymal cell to form osteoblasts ; tension favours formation of osteoclasts and fibroblasts.

Techniques of bone grafting

1. Onlay bone graft In this method cortical graft is placed on one side of bone (single onlay) or on both sides of bone (dual onlay) and fixed to the host bone with screws. It is meant primarily to provide support. This technique was commonly used before development of inert metallic plates, which provide superior mechanical stability.

2. Inlay bone graft In this method a slot or rectangular defect is created in the cortex of the host bone and an exactly matching size cortical graft is fitted into the space. This technique is simpler and equally efficacious. The inlay method is used in arthrodesis, particularly at the ankle.

3. Dowel graft In this technique the dowel shaped graft is inserted into the osseous substance of the bone. The graft must pass into both fragments and across the fracture site. This is classically used in Cloward's technique of anterior cervical fusion.

4. Strut graft This type of graft is taken from the ribs or fibula and is used in cases of pathological fractures or tuberculosis of the vertebral body. After excision of the diseased bone the graft is placed to span the length of the defect and extend into the vertebral body above and below. It provides immediate stability and being under compression, heals well.

5. H-graft (Clothespin graft) This technique is used in posterior fusion of the cervical and lumbar spine. A full-thickness rectangular graft is harvested from the iliac crest and slots are cut in the proximal and distal portions which give it 'H' shape so that it can be wedged in place between the spinous processes.

6. Structural grafts Allografts with specific structure can be used to replace proximal or distal femur or any other bone for difficult revision joint replacements and tumour surgery.

7. Whole bone transplant The fibula provides the most practical whole bone transplant graft for bridging long defects in the diaphyseal portion of bones of the upper extremity. The shape of the upper end of the fibula makes it a satisfactory substitute for the distal end of the radius. Although the upper limit of the length of the fibular graft that can be harvested is not yet established, the distal ankle mortise must be preserved.

8. **Multiple cancellous chip graft** This is the most widely used grafting technique. Slivers of autologous cancellous bone (iliac crest, proximal tibial metaphysis, distal femoral metaphysis, and greater trochanter) are the best osteogenic material available. Being soft and friable, this bone can be packed into every nook and crevice. It is also useful for filling up defects. In most of the bone graft techniques currently performed, supplementary cancellous bone is used to hasten healing.

9. **Phemister grafting** This is a specialised form of bone grafting technique mainly used for non union/delayed union of tibia. Osteoperiosteal flaps are elevated proximal and distal to the fracture and cancellous bone chips are placed under the flap, bridging across the non-union site. Bone pieces left attached to the periosteum (shingles) and the bone (petals) increase the surface area for union while retaining the vascularity. Prerequisites for Phemister grafting are a fibrous union in an acceptable alignment and mobility at the neighbouring joints. The procedure can be performed in the presence of low-grade infection.

10. **Vascularized bone graft** This is the ideal bone graft. It is an autogenous bone graft that remains alive, resists resorption and maintains its physical characteristics. The donor sites are fibula, iliac crest (common), ribs, and 1st metatarsal (uncommon). A surgical team familiar with microsurgery is essential for the implementation of this technique. Pre-operative arteriograms of both the donor and recipient site must be obtained.

Bone Morphogenetic Proteins (BMPs) Ability of devitalised bone, when reimplanted, to induce formation of cartilage and bone at the ectopic site stimulated search for the osteoinductive substance that lead to the isolation of BMPs. BMP* is the generic name for proteins, extracted from bone matrix capable of osteoinduction. The therapeutic potential is unlimited. They may provide an alternative to bone grafts and their associated problems. While the quantity of autogenous bone is limited, there is a definite risk of transmission of infection with allografts. With use of recombinant DNA technology, BMP can be made in unlimited quantity. When combined with synthetic grafts, BMP should be useful in procedures where bone grafts are currently being used.

*Note Morphogens: These are gene-activating factors that initiate development of tissues and organs.

Synthetic grafts Autografts are the best source for bone grafting because of their superior efficacy and zero risk of infection transmission. However the amount is limited and it necessitates a second surgery with possibility of complications. Allografts are often used. However the greatest risk is that of transmission of infection and an immunological defense reaction by the host cannot be avoided. Synthetic bone grafts provide a useful alternative. They are based on the principle of osteoconduction (support osseous tissue ingrowth). Synthetic grafts available are derived from corals, which have an exoskeleton rich in tricalcium phosphate. The commonly used synthetic grafts consist of a mixture of tricalcium phosphate and hydroxyapatite. BMP and bone marrow can be mixed with the synthetic grafts to increase the osteoinductive potential.

Advantages

The synthetic grafts have the advantage of being

1. Sterile
2. Available in unlimited quantity
3. Free from antigens

Also, they can be combined with autologous bone graft or BMP.

Limitations

1. They are not capable of osteoinduction. Therefore, they should be placed in a bed with regenerative capacity.
2. Poor mechanical strength
3. Contraindicated in infection

Injuries of Shoulder and Arm

Injuries of the shoulder region

Clavicle Fractures

Clavicle is the most often fractured bone in the body. Fortunately due to its intramembranous ossification origin, union is not a problem. Malunion, however, is quite common, as it is quite difficult to control the fracture fragments.

Clavicle fractures often occur in patients with other serious skeletal and extra-skeletal injuries.

Mechanism of Injury

Fractures of the clavicle are caused most often by an indirect injury as fall on the point of the shoulder or on the outstretched hand. However, fractures of the clavicle may also result from the direct impact on the clavicle.

Classification

The fractures of clavicle are classified most commonly according to the location viz. fractures of the middle third (85% – including the fractures at the junction of the middle and the lateral thirds which is the commonest location), lateral third (10%) and medial third (5%) of the clavicle. Fractures of the clavicle can also be classified as post-traumatic or pathologic (following radiation necrosis in patients with breast carcinoma); another way to classify these fractures would be displaced, undisplaced or greenstick (in children).

Evaluation of a patient with clavicular fracture

Patient with clavicular injuries should be assessed for vital functions and associated injuries. Usually patients with displaced fractures present with pain, deformity and shortening of the clavicle. The patient often supports the injured limb with the other hand. Patient resists any attempts to move the shoulder. Tenderness may be the only elicitable sign in patients with undisplaced fractures.

Local bruising appears in cases that present a few days after the injury. A careful neurovascular examination must be done in all cases.

Imaging A single anteroposterior projection of the shoulder is usually adequate imaging study in adults. However, superimposition of scapula and ribs may not allow adequate visualization of the clavicle. Cephalic angled view gets rid of the superimposition. Cephalad angulation of 15° visualizes lateral two thirds of the clavicle while the x-ray beam may have to be angulated 40° cephalad to visualize the medial third of the clavicle. X-rays confirm the diagnosis and reveal the location of the fracture and the degree of displacement of the fragments. The distal fragment typically sags downwards, forwards and medially while proximal end gets elevated (due to the pull of sternocleidomastoid) (Fig. 22.1). Fractures of the distal (or lateral) third of the clavicle are mostly undisplaced as the

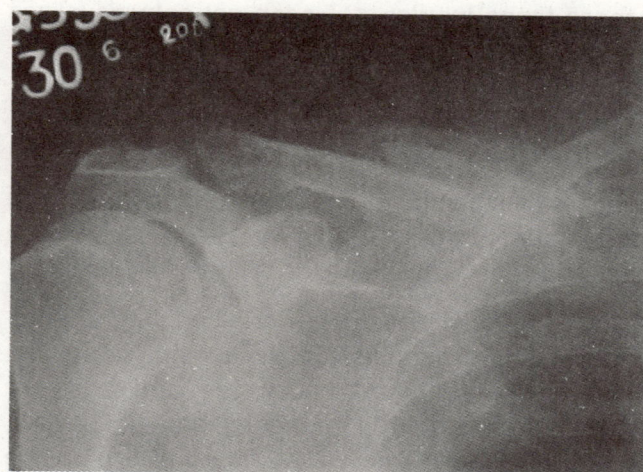

Fig. 22.1. Fracture right clavicle

coraco-clavicular (especially trapezoid) ligaments remain attached to the proximal fragment and prevent its displacement while the acromioclavicular and conoid (lateral part of coraco-clavicular ligament) ligaments remain attached to the distal fragment.

In children the fractures of the clavicle may be very subtle and are difficult to diagnose. Any kinking of the cortical contour should raise the suspicion of clavicle fracture. Including both the shoulders on one film may help in comparison with the normal side.

Associated vascular injuries are rare but when present need angiography.

Management

Any associated injury takes precedence over clavicle fracture for management. The treatment for clavicle fracture is primarily conservative. For undisplaced fractures in children and in elderly, support is provided for the weight of the arm using a sling and these fractures unite readily. Displaced fractures are treated with a figure of 8 bandage or commercially available braces applied with the shoulders braced backwards. A triangular sling is given to the arm in addition. The aim of these methods is to reduce the overlap of fragments and anterior drift of the scapula around the chest wall as well as to relieve pain. Brace or the bandage has to be re-tightened every few days as it keeps on getting loose. Supports are discontinued as soon as the fracture site becomes non tender.

Surgical treatment of clavicle fracture is indicated for associated vascular injuries, compound fractures or the displaced fractures of the lateral third of the clavicle with disruption of coraco-clavicular ligaments. Implants used for internal fixation of the clavicle include intramedullary pins or 3.5-mm reconstruction plate with screws. External fixator may be applied for compound fractures.

Complications

Injury to the neurovascular structures (such as brachial plexus or the subclavian vessels) may occur rarely. Vascular injuries are managed by angiography, repair of the vascular injuries and internal fixation of the clavicle fracture. Closed neural injuries are treated expectantly while open injuries need exploration and repair.

Pneumothorax, other thoracic injuries or thoracic outlet syndrome can occur.

Malunion is the commonest complication. Off–ending and excessive callus may give rise to appearance of a bump under the skin. Some remodeling occurs with time and there is no functional disability.

Non union is rare and reported in 1% to 5% cases. High energy fractures, widely displaced fractures, open fractures and inadequate immobilization are commonly implicated causes. Only symptomatic non unions need management with internal fixation and bone grafting (Fig. 22.2). Shoulder joint stiffness may occur in the elderly. It is managed by physiotherapy to mobilize the joint.

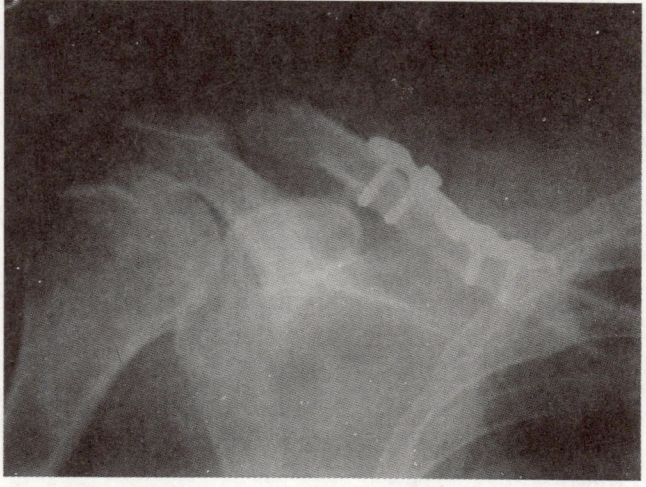

Fig. 22.2. Painful non union of fracture clavicle treated by plating and bone grafting

Dislocation of Sternoclavicular joint

Sternoclavicular joint does not have inherent osseous stability since the articular surfaces are incongruent. Ligaments of the sternoclavicular joint (costo-clavicular, interclavicular and anterior, superior and posterior capsular ligaments) are strong and provide stability to the joint. Epiphyseal injuries of the medial clavicular epiphysis may occur in late second decade of life and may mimic the dislocation of sternocavicular joint.

Mechanism of Injury

Dislocations of sternoclavicular joint occur following a fall on the point of the shoulder, fall on outstretched hand or following a blow on the front of the shoulder. These dislocations may sometimes be seen without any history of trauma or following trivial trauma.

Classification

Sternoclavicular dislocations are divided into anterior (95%) and posterior (5%) depending on the direction of displacement of the medial end of the clavicle out of the joint.

Evaluation of patient with sternoclavicular dislocation

Sternoclavicular dislocations are usually diagnosed clinically. Asymmetry of the medial ends of the clavicle with reduced distance between acromion and the sternoclavicular joint on the affected side are quite obvious. Anterior dislocations have tender prominence of medial end of the clavicle under the skin. Local tenderness is present. Subtle subluxations, however, can sometimes be missed

Posterior dislocations may present more dramatically with dyspnea or dysphagia due to the compression of trachea or the esophagus respectively. Compression of the great vessels may occur in posterior dislocations.

Imaging

Anteroposterior and oblique views when used to diagnose sternoclavicular dislocations are difficult to interpret. *"Serendipity view"*, an AP view taken with 40° cephalic tilt, centered on the manubrium can help in determining the direction of the dislocation.

Tomograms or CT scan are extremely useful to assess these injuries. CT scan not only visualizes the dislocated joint but also the underlying vascular structures and airway.

Treatment

Minor subluxations of the joint are ignored. The limb is supported in a sling for 15–20 days till the pain subsides. The shoulder is then mobilized.

Acute anterior dislocation is reduced with a sandbag under the shoulders with the patient supine. Shoulders are braced backwards and posterior pressure applied on the medial end of clavicle. Immobilization is done with a figure of 8 bandage or clavicular brace with a broad arm sling for 4–5 weeks. Reductions are frequently unstable in which case they can just be ignored with good functional outcome.

Acute posterior dislocation is a serious condition and thoracic surgeons must be available to tackle any complication Closed reduction is attempted with shoulder abduction and pull on the dislocated medial end of clavicle anteriorly with a percutaneous towel clip.

Irreducible dislocations need open reduction, which is fraught with risks and complications.

Complications are mainly due to injury to the neurovascular structures. Superior vena cava injury, pneumothorax and subcutaneous emphysema may occur. Posttraumatic arthritis of the joint may occur.

Persistent, recurrent or irreducible anterior dislocations are common and usually do not interfere with function. Persistently symptomatic chronic dislocations can be managed by resection of the medial end of the clavicle.

Dislocation of the Acromio–clavicular joint

Acromioclavicular joint is extremely stable and is supported by strong coraco-clavicular and acromio-clavicular ligaments. Trapezius and deltoid muscles also contribute to the stability of the acromio-clavicular joint.

Mechanism of Injury

Acromioclvicular dislocations usually result from both the direct and indirect forces. Most commonly the injury occurs due to a fall on the shoulder.

Classification

Neer and Rockwood have classified these injuries into 6 types :

Type I Acromioclavicular ligament sprain

Type II Acromioclavicular ligament tear with sprain of coracoclavicular ligament

Type III Acromioclavicular ligament tear with coracoclavicular ligament tear (25% to 100% subluxation of the joint occurs).

Type IV Complete ligament tears with posterior dislocation of clavicle through the trapezius muscle.

Type V Complete ligament tears with detachment of deltoid and trapezius and clavicle elevated > 100%.

Type VI Complete ligament tears with clavicle displaced inferior to the coracoid.

Assessment of patient with acromioclavicular joint disruption

The acromioclavicular joint must be assessed with the patients standing. Both shoulders should be exposed for comparison. These measures reduce the likelihood of missing acromioclavicular joint injuries as the latter often reduce spontaneously in recumbency.

The outer end of the clavicle is prominent in patients with the acromioclavicular joint injuries. Pain and tenderness over the joint are common.

Imaging

Anteroposterior radiographs of the both the shoulders should be taken with the patient standing (Fig. 22.3). Another commonly used method is to ask the patient to hold weights in both the hands and then take anteroposterior x-ray of both the shoulders. Rupture of coraco-clavicular (conoid and trapezoid) ligaments is suggested by displacement of the clavicle by a diameter or more relative to the acromion. Axillary views of the shoulder also show the acromio-clavicular joint quite well.

Treatment

Treatment of acromio-clavicular ligament sprains (Type I and II injuries) is by a broad arm sling, NSAIDs and early range of motion exercises. Type III injuries are managed conservatively in most

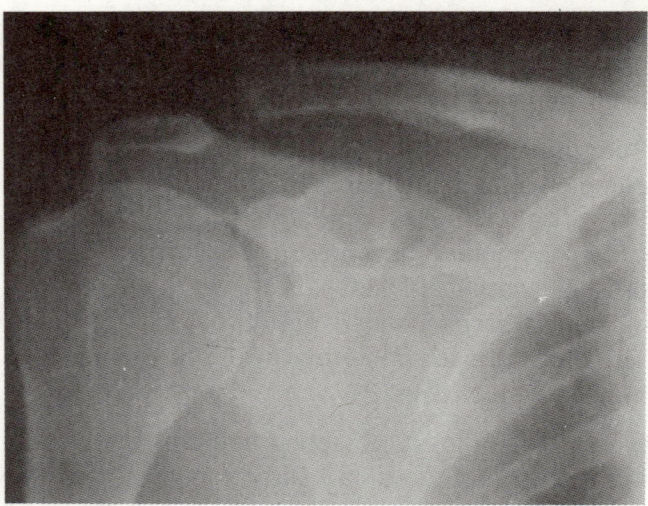

Fig. 22.3. Acromio-clavicular joint dislocation

cases but some cases especially high performance athletes and heavy laborers may need operative stabilization. Types IV, V, VI are treated surgically with open reduction with repair of coraco-clavicular ligament (with or without a screw from the clavicle into the coracoid process). Repair of the acromio-clavicular joint by transarticular absorbable sutures can also be performed in addition. Any tears in trapezius or deltoid are repaired. Many people like to combine this procedure with resection of distal clavicle to minimize symptoms due to acromioclavicular arthritis later in life. All internal fixation devices are removed two months after the surgery.

It must be remembered that even in cases with gross instability, good results are seen following conservative treatments. This fact, along with the high complication rate following surgery, makes conservative treatment method of choice for most cases except in patients who are involved in heavy work or who have to work with prolonged elevation of the arms.

Complications

Acromioclavicular arthritis may occur following the injury to the joint. Persistent symptoms are alleviated by excision arthroplasty of the joint.

Gross instability is rarely symptomatic but when so, can be managed by fascial reconstruction of the coraco-clavicular ligaments.

Hardware related complications such as breakage or migration of screw (clavicle to coracoid transfixion screw), migration of transarticular kirschner wires, loss of fixation and infection are commonly seen following the surgery for acromio-clavicular dislocation.

Scapular Fracture Scapular fractures are uncommon and constitute 1% of all fractures and 5% of all shoulder fractures. Almost half the scapular fractures involve the body and the spine of the scapula. These fractures have a high incidence of associated life threatening injuries. Therefore these fractures are often diagnosed late.

Mechanism of Injury: Scapular fractures are caused by high-energy trauma. Direct injuries are the commonest cause though indirect trauma such as fall on the outstretched hand can also cause scapular fractures especially those of the glenoid cavity.

Classification

Thompson in 1985 divided the scapular fractures (Fig. 22.4a) into class I (coracoid (Fig. 22.4b), acromion (Fig. 22.4c) and small body fractures (Fig. 22.4d), Class II (Glenoid and neck fractures) and Class III (major scapular body fractures). Type II and III have high incidence of associated injuries.

Evaluation of patient with scapular fracture

Patients with scapular fractures must be resuscitated and assessed for associated injuries. These patients sustain high-energy trauma and there is

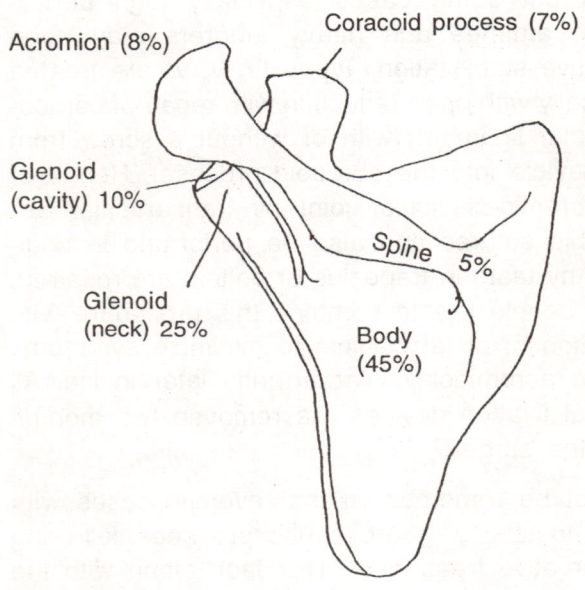

Fig. 22.4a. Location of various scapular fractures

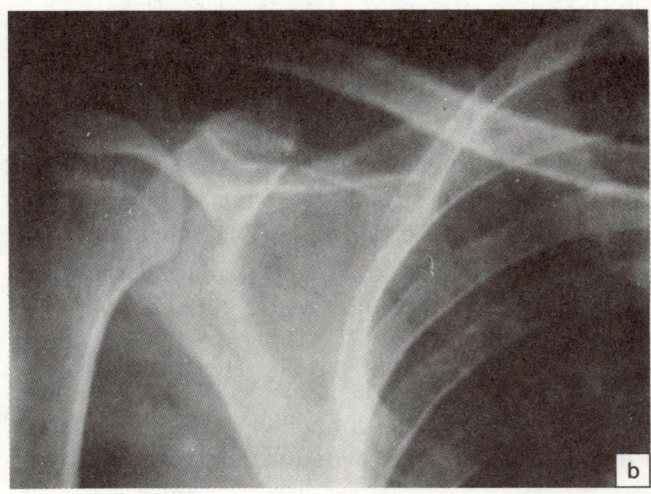

Fig. 22.4b. Coracoid process fracture

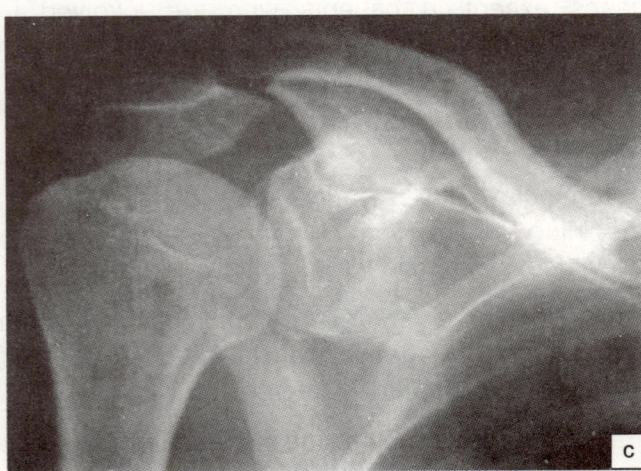

Fig. 22.4c. Acromion fracture

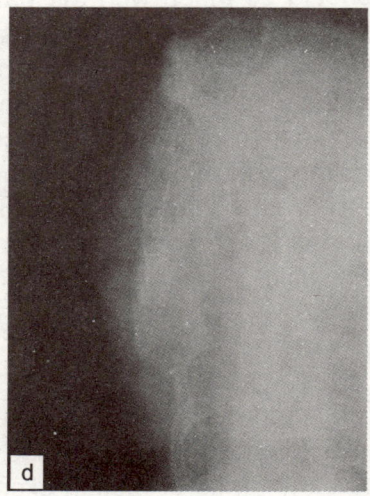

Fig. 22.4d. Scapular body fractures

a high incidence of associated injuries such as head injury, vascular injuries, brachial plexus injuries, clavicle fracture, rib fracture with haemo/pneumo thorax and lung contusion.

Local examination reveals pain, swelling and bruising over the scapula.

Local tenderness is marked and attempted movements at the shoulder are quite painful.

Imaging of scapular fractures

"Scapula trauma series" x-rays include a true anteroposterior of the scapula, a true lateral projection of the scapula, scapular Y x-rays (Fig. 22.4e) and a true axillary projection of the glenohumeral joint (Fig. 22.4f) and the scapula.

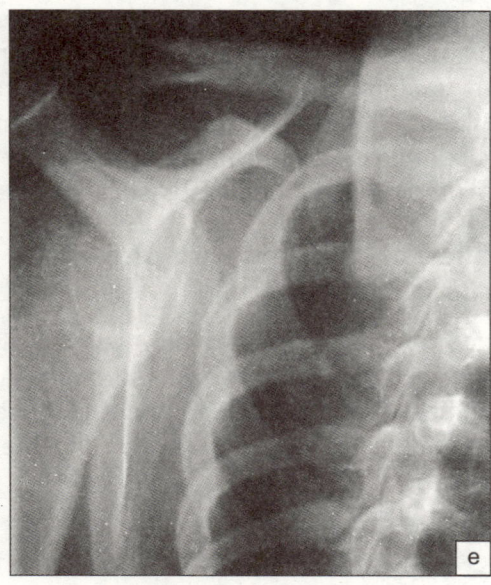

Fig. 22.4e. Scapular Y view

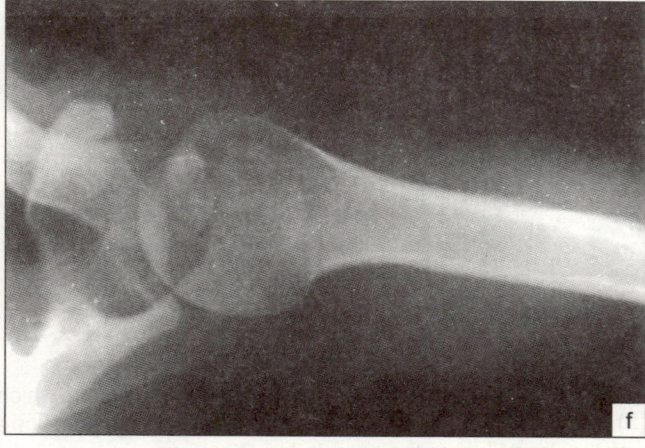

Fig. 22.4f. Axillary view

The orthopedist must be able to adequately visualize and assess the body and spine of scapula and its three processes, acromion, coracoid and glenoid. Anteroposterior view shows the acromion, the glenoid fossa, and the neck of the scapula. Axillary view shows the glenoid fossa, coracoid and the glenoid neck. Tangential scapular Y (true lateral) view taken tangentially shows the coracoid, scapular spine and the scapular body in profile. All the three joints formed with scapula (acromio-clavicular, scapulothoracic and glenohumeral) must also be evaluated.

CT should be obtained and is helpful for the assessment of complex scapular fractures. 3-D reconstruction further helps in visualization – elimination of the proximal humerus allows adequate visualization of the glenoid cavity.

Treatment

Over 90% of scapular fractures and all the fractures involving the body and the spine of the scapula can be treated conservatively. Limb is supported in a broad arm sling for a short period. As soon as the pain subsides, progressive range of motion is encouraged. Healing is usually complete in six weeks without any functional limitation.

Surgical treatment of scapular fractures is indicated for neck and glenoid fractures such as intraarticular fractures with intraarticular step >5 mm, fractures involving more than 25% of glenoid fossa with subluxation of humerus, or scapular neck fractures with angulation of more than 40°. Either anterior or posterior approach may be used depending on position of major fragments. Devices used for fixation include cannulated interfragmentary screws, malleable reconstruction plates and kirschner wires. Postoperatively early range of motion is encouraged depending on rigidity of fixation. Less rigidly fixed fractures are protected in a sling and swathe immobilizer for 3–6 weeks.

Complications of scapular fractures include the high incidence of associated injuries especially clavicle and rib fractures, axillary artery injuries, brachial plexus injuries and pneumothorax. Stiffness of the glenohumeral joint may occur.

Scapulothoracic dissociation is a rare condition where separation of scapulothoracic articulation occurs. It is also called closed traumatic amputation of the upper limb as vascular (subclavian) and brachial plexus and cervical nerve root injuries occur in all the cases. Anteroposterior chest radiographs show increased distance between the medial border of scapula to the midline on the affected side. The condition is treated by closed reduction and vascular repair. Complex reconstruction of the nerve injuries is performed later. The prognosis is poor.

Intrathoracic dislocation also known as *locked scapula* is characterized by the lower angle of scapula being locked between the ribs. Pulmonary injuries are common. Treatment is closed reduction and management of the pulmonary injury.

Fractures of proximal humerus

Proximal humerus fractures represent about 5% of all fractures and account for three fourth of all humeral fractures in patients older than 40 years of age. Elderly patients with these fractures often have poor bone quality and medical comorbidities. These facts make the treatment of these fractures challenges to meet.

Mechanism of injury

Elderly people with osteoporotic bones sustain these fractures most commonly following a fall on the side or on the outstretched hand. Young patients sustain these injuries due to high-energy trauma, which can lead to the severe disruption of the soft tissues such as labrum, capsule, rotator cuff, brachial plexus and neurovascular structures.

Classification

Fractures of the proximal humerus can be undisplaced or displaced. Neer's classification is the most often used system to classify these fractures. It is based on the displacement of the four parts distinguished on the proximal humerus namely, greater tuberosity, lesser tuberosity, humeral head and shaft fragment (Fig. 22.5). Any fragment separated by 1 cm or angulated more than 45° from the anatomic position is considered displaced. Classification is then according to the number of the displaced fragments i.e. one part fractures (undisplaced), 2 part fracture, 3 part fracture and four part fracture. In addition, there can be fracture dislocations with any of the above mentioned fracture patterns and fractures of the articular surface (impression fracture or split fractures)

Evaluation of a patient with proximal humerus fracture

It is important to elicit the history especially with reference to the mechanism of the injury. Associated injuries must be looked for and assessed. Patient complains of pain in the shoulder and

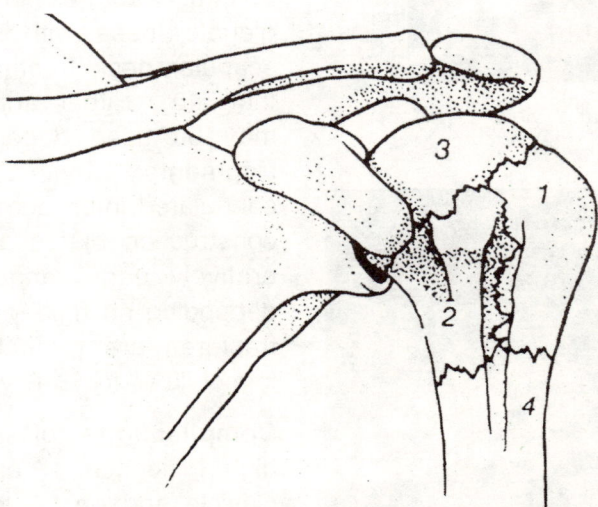

Fig. 22.5. The four parts of the proximal humerus referred to in the Neer classification of fractures of this region, which include the greater tuberosity (1), lesser tuberosity (2), anatomic neck (3), and surgical neck (4). Fractures are classified according to displacement of one or more of the "parts" from the remainder. Displacement is defined as separation of greater than 1 cm from the humerus or angulation of the part greater than 45 degrees.

often is seen supporting the injured arm with the other hand. Swelling and tenderness are present at the upper end of the humerus. Patient resists movements at the shoulder due to pain. Local bruising is common and often stains distal arm by gravitating down if the patient presents late. Distal neurovascular examination must be performed especially for the axillary nerve.

Imaging Anteroposterior and good trans-lateral view of the shoulder allow the diagnosis and the understanding of the fracture pattern. Complex fractures can be evaluated by CT scan, which allows three-dimensional reconstruction of images. In children the physis is often mistaken as fracture line. In case of doubt x-rays of the opposite shoulder should be obtained.

Management

Most fractures of the proximal humerus (nearly 80%) are undisplaced or impacted and can be treated symptomatically in a cuff and collar sling for a few days till the pain subsides. Mobilization should then be started to avoid stiffness of the shoulder. Table 22.1 delineates the principles of treatment of the proximal humeral fractures.

Epiphyseal injury of proximal humeral epiphysis (Type II Salter Harris) occurs in adolescents (13–15 years of age) and is often displaced. Closed reduction is performed by abduction, flexion and external rotation of the arm (*salute* position). Open reduction and stabilization with K-wires is indicated in irreducible cases. Immobilization is continued for 4–6 weeks.

Complications

- Neurovascular compromise due to injury to axillary artery and nerve or brachial plexus may occur due to traction in these cases.

- Stiffness of the shoulder is very common after proximal humeral fractures and can be minimised by early mobilization of the joint.

- Non union of the proximal humeral fractures is treated by internal fixation and bone grafting.

- Malunion is a common complication of proximal humeral fractures and is seen frequently after conservative treatment. Most cases of malunion manage with minimal functional disability but impingement can be quite troublesome following malunited fracture of the greater tuberosity.

- Associated dislocations especially anterior dislocations may be associated with fractures of greater tuberosity and are frequently missed. Dislocation should be diagnosed early and reduced and fracture of the greater tuberosity is reassessed. Often the greater tuberosity falls back in acceptable position. Persistent displacement is treated with ORIF.

- Avascular necrosis can occur with any fracture pattern but is more common with 3-part and 4-part fractures. Persistently symptomatic cases warrant replacement arthroplasty.

- Tears of the rotator cuff are frequently associated and need repair if large.

- Myositis ossificans can occur following proximal humeral fracture.

- Hardware related complications (loosening, breakage, infection) are common especially in elderly osteoporotic patient.

Dislocation of the Shoulder

Shoulder joint depends on the surrounding soft tissues for stability. The articular surfaces are incongruent. Whereas the shallow glenoid and limited contact between the glenoid and humeral head allows wide range of movements it also makes the joint extremely unstable. The dislocations of the shoulder are classified according to the direction of displacement of the humeral head with respect to glenoid and can be anterior, posterior, or inferior.

Anterior dislocation of the shoulder

Anterior dislocation is the commonest type of shoulder dislocation. Anterior dislocation occurs commonly in adults due to vehicular and athletic injuries and in elderly due to falls. It is rare in children.

Mechanism of Injury Anterior dislocation of the shoulder is caused by abduction and external rotation. Most commonly a fall on the hand which internally rotates the trunk over the fixed hand leads to external rotation and dislocation of the shoulder. Anterior dislocation leads to extensive damage to the anterior soft tissues. Anterior capsule is often avulsed from its glenoid attachment (*Bankart lesion*) and may take glenoid labrum with it. Avulsion fractures of the glenoid rim, greater

Table 22.1. Treatment of Proximal Humeral Fractures

Classification	Type	Treatment	Complications
One-part	**Undisplaced # (all types)** **Impacted**	Conservative	Shoulder stiffness
Two-part	**Displaced #** (Separation> 1cm; Angulation > 45°) Surgical neck	Closed reduction: Stable: conservative Unstable: ORIF (Rush pin/ Enders nail/ T- buttress plate), Percutaneous pinning	Shoulder stiffness
	Greater tuberosity	ORIF + Tension band Repair of rotator cuff	Associated with ant. dislocation of shoulder/rotator cuff tear
	Lesser tuberosity	Small fragments: Excise + repair subscapularis tendon Large fragment: ORIF	Associated with post. dislocation of shoulder/subscapularis tear
	Anatomic neck	Closed reduction; if fails, ORIF (with screw)	Avascular necrosis of head fragment

135° Normal angle

Three-part

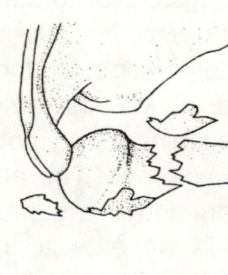

Greater tuberosity +Surgical neck	Elderly: conservative Young: ORIF (Screw + TBW)	Nonunion, malunion, shoulder stiffness
Lesser tuberosity +Surgical neck		

Four-part

All four fragments	Young: ORIF Elderly: conservative/ Hemiarthroplasty with reattachment of tuberosities and cuff repair	Avascular necrosis, Shoulder stiffness

Fracture—Dislocation

Anterior 2/3-part	Closed reduction/ ORIF for displaced fragments	Avascular necrosis, Shoulder stiffness
4-part	Prosthetic replacement	
Posterior 2-part	Closed reduction	
3-part	ORIF	
4-part	Prosthetic replacement	

Posterior fracture dislocation

Anterior fracture dislocation

tuberosity or impaction fractures over superolateral aspect of the head (*Hill–Sach's lesions* (Fig. 22.6a) may occur. Rotator cuff, axillary artery, axillary nerve or brachial plexus may be injured.

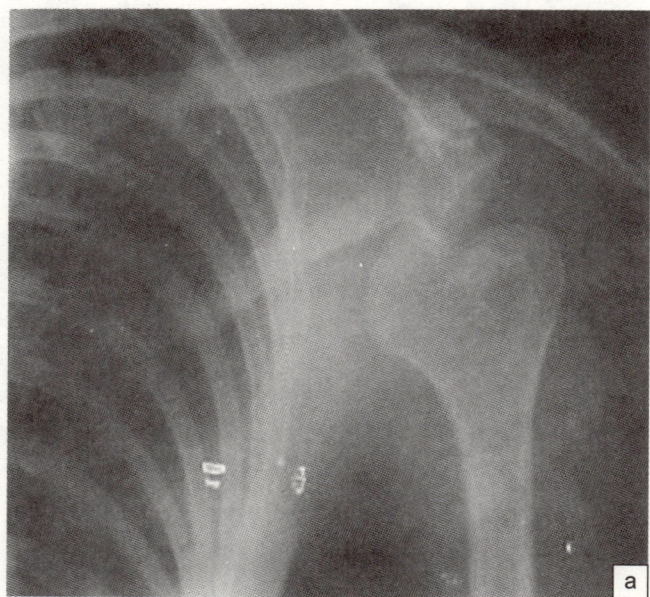

Fig. 22.6a. Anterior dislocation of shoulder with Hill Sach's lesion on superolateral aspect of humeral head

Classification Anterior dislocation of the shoulder is classified according to the position which the humeral head occupies after dislocating namely subcoracoid, subglenoid and subclavicular. Subcoracoid dislocation is the commonest type.

Evaluation of a patient with anterior dislocation of the shoulder

Patient presents with history of trauma and severe pain in the shoulder and inability to move the shoulder. Arm is held in slight abduction and the patient often supports it with the other hand. The patient should be examined with both the shoulders exposed for comparison. The affected shoulder appears flattened and the supero-inferior dimension of the axilla appears to be increased (*Callaway's sign*). Patient is unable to touch the contralateral shoulder with his hand (*Duga's Test*). Palpation distal to edge of the acromion reveals loss of the resistance usually offered by the humeral head. Displaced humeral head is often palpable anteriorly. Attempted movements at the shoulder are painful and resisted by the patient.

Careful neurovascular examination must be done in all cases of anterior dislocation of the shoulder. The most commonly injured nerve is axillary nerve and is tested by assessing sensations in "*regimental badge*" (C_5) area. While shoulder abduction cannot be tested due to pain, deltoid function can be evaluated by asking the patient to try to abduct and feeling the deltoid contraction.

Imaging Routine radiographic evaluation includes the anteroposterior (AP) and lateral (scapular Y) view in all cases. Axillary view can show avulsion of the glenoid rim and confirms dislocation and its direction but may be difficult to obtain due to pain. An apical oblique view can be taken to assess glenohumeral relationship in case it is difficult to take axillary view due to pain. *Westpoint* view (prone axillary lateral with 25° lateral and posterior tilt) evaluates the fractures of the anterior glenoid margin. Hill Sach's lesions can be evaluated by 60° internal rotation anteroposterior view or by *Stryker Notch* view (Fig. 22.6b) taken in supine position with hand on head and 10° cephalic tilt of the beam.

Ultrasonography can detect associated rotator cuff tears. MRI can evaluate the capsular and labral tear where young patients and athletes with high demand shoulders are being considered for repair. Associated rotator cuff tears can also be diagnosed.

Arthroscopy can be used to diagnose, assess and treat the acute as well as chronic instabilities of the shoulder.

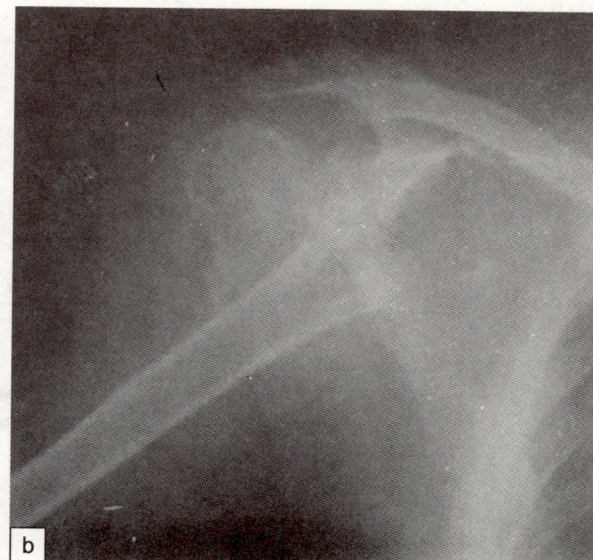

Fig. 22.6b. Stryker Notch View for Hill Sach's lesion

Treatment Treatment of anterior dislocation of the shoulder is by closed reduction under adequate relaxation and immobilization for 4 weeks. Progressive range of motion exercises are started after that.

Reduction manoeuvres

i) **Kocher's method** (TEA : Traction-External rotation – Adduction)

Longitudinal traction is applied along the axis of the arm and the arm is gradually externally rotated to 90°. If the shoulder is not reduced at this stage, gently adduct and finally internally rotate the shoulder.

ii) **Hippocratic method** Traction is applied along the axis of the arm and the surgeon puts his stockinged heel against the chest to act as a fulcrum. The arm is gradually adducted and reduction achieved.

iii) **Stimson's gravity method** Patient is put prone with sandbag under the clavicle and his arm is allowed to hang over the side. The shoulder may reduce spontaneously if relaxation is adequate.

After reduction the position is checked with x-rays and the arm is immobilized with adduction and internal rotation at the shoulder in an arm chest bandage (External rotation must be prevented). In older people the immobilization is discarded at two weeks (instead of four) to prevent shoulder stiffness.

Complications

Injury to neurovascular structures

Injury to axillary nerve is usually in continuity and often recovers. These patients are treated expectantly with physiotherapy. Musculocutaneous is the next most commonly injured nerve. Suprascapular nerve may be injured and has excellent prognosis for recovery. Radial portion of the posterior cord of brachial plexus may be injured and is again treated expectantly. Exploration or tendon transfers may be required if the lesion fails to recover.

Brachial artery is injured in elderly patients where it has undergone atherosclerotic changes. Urgent angiography and vascular repair are indicated.

Associated fractures

Fractures of greater tuberosity, surgical neck of humerus or the glenoid rim can occur along with the shoulder dislocation. In cases with fracture of greater tuberosity or glenoid rim, the fracture is ignored and the dislocation is reduced. The fracture is again assessed radiologically after reduction of dislocation. Persistently displaced fracture needs ORIF.

Associated fractures of surgical neck of humerus are serious as they make closed reduction of the dislocation very difficult. Open reduction of the dislocation with internal fixation of the neck humerus fracture is required. The elderly people with this injury often do well just with mobilization. Therefore major surgery should be avoided.

Associated Rotator Cuff Tears are common in elderly patients (over 40 years). They should be diagnosed early and treated based on their merits.

Missed anterior dislocation of the shoulder

The anterior dislocation may be missed especially in multiply injured patients. Closed reduction may be attempted preceded by traction in injuries less than 6 weeks old. If it fails, open reduction may be attempted. The procedure is risky and fraught with complications and the patient may end up with a stiff shoulder. Often mobilizing these patients, when diagnosed late, alone can help them regain useful function without any intervention.

Recurrent dislocations are common in younger patients (almost 50% dislocations in patients younger than 20 years recur) and are uncommon in patients more than 40 years. Length of immobilization does not affect the risk of recurrence. Various causes implicated in the causation of recurrent dislocations are Bankart lesion, capsular and/or subscapularis laxity and posterior lateral defect (Hill Sach's lesion–"*Hatchet*" *head*) on the humeral head. Dislocations occur with progressively minor degree of trauma. Hill Sach's lesions can be visualized on axillary and internal rotation views. CT scan and arthroscopy can diagnose the Bankart lesions. Treatment is surgical and Putti Platt (double breasting of subscapularis to limit external rotation) and Bankart repair (reattachment of the capsule to the glenoid edge–

open or arthroscopic) are most commonly performed operations. Other options are bone block (Bristow using coracoid process with attached tendons) and osteotomies of proximal humerus or scapular neck (glenoplasty).

Posterior Dislocation of Shoulder

Posterior dislocation of shoulder constitutes less than 5% cases of shoulder dislocation. Its importance lies in the fact that it is often missed clinically and radiologically. Posterior dislocations are especially missed when they occur in association with Erb's palsy and obstetric palsies.

Mechanism of Injury

Posterior dislocation of shoulder occurs following forced internal rotation of the shoulder or a blow directly on the front of the shoulder. This injury is common after electric shocks and epileptic seizures. Posterior dislocations may be bilateral in these cases.

Posterior dislocation leads to damage to the posteriors capsular structures (Posterior Bankart). Lesser tuberosity fractures may be seen. Impaction fractures of the humeral head over anteromedial aspect may be seen.

Classification Posterior shoulder dislocations are classified into subacromial and subcoracoid types depending on the location of the humeral head on the anteroposterior and axillary x-rays.

Evaluation of patient with posterior dislocation of the shoulder

Patient presents with history of severe trauma or electric shock or may not remember anything when he has had an epileptic convulsion. Patient complains of pain and inability to move the shoulder. Pain, however, may not be a prominent feature when posterior dislocation occurs as a complication of a neurologic disorder. The bruising over anterior aspect of shoulder may suggest direct injury leading to dislocation. The arm is held in slight adduction and is internally rotated at the shoulder. The patient is unable to externally rotate the shoulder. Careful neurovascular examination must be performed in all cases.

Imaging

Anteroposterior and axillary views should be ob-

tained in all cases. Anteroposterior view shows empty glenoid (*vacant glenoid sign*), gap between glenoid and head (*daylight sign*) and cystic and hollow appearance of the humeral head due to internal rotation (appearance of the head is similar to the appearance of humeral head seen in antero posterior check x-ray of the shoulder after reduction of the anterior dislocation).

CT scan and arthroscopy can diagnose the labral lesions.

Treatment is by closed reduction followed by immobilization for four weeks. Gradual progressive range of motion exercises are started after that.

Reduction manoeuvre

Traction is applied to the arm in 90° abduction and the arm is then gently externally rotated. Reduction is achieved easily and the arm immobilized in a sling.

Complications

Associated fractures Fracture of the lesser tuberosity, posterior glenoid and humeral head may be associated. The dislocation is reduced and the fractures reassessed radiologically. Persistently displaced fragments need ORIF.

Irreducible dislocation can be ignored and shoulder mobilized in elderly or an open reduction is performed in young patients with high demand shoulders.

Unreduced dislocation

Posterior shoulder dislocation is often missed. Attempt to reduce are advised upto one year after injury by many workers. Failure of reduction warrants open reduction by posterior approach in young patients.

Recurrent dislocations

Bankart (open or arthroscopic) or reverse Putti Platt using a posterior approach are recommended procedures for managing recurrent posterior dislocations.

Inferior Dislocation of Shoulder (*luxatio erecta*)

Inferior dislocation of the shoulder is a rare injury. It is associated with high incidence of injury to neurovascular structures and the rotator cuff.

Mechanism of injury

Luxatio erecta is caused by a hyperextension injury.

Evaluation

Patient presents with the arm held in abduction and inability to adduct or lower the arm. Pain and deformity are obvious. Humeral head can be palpated in the axilla. Detailed neurovascular examination must be performed as compressive neuropathy or axillary artery thrombosis can occur in almost 60% patients.

Imaging A single anteroposterior radiograph of the shoulder is adequate to diagnose luxatio erecta.

Treatment Urgent reduction must be done to prevent further damage to the neurovascular structures. Reduction is achieved by applying the traction with the limb in abduction (the position of deformity) and gently adducting the shoulder. The shoulder is immobilized in a sling for 4 weeks and then gradually mobilized.

Complications

The most fearsome and the commonest complication of luxatio erecta is the injury to neurovascular structures. These injuries must be diagnosed and treated early to prevent permanent disability.

Injuries of the Arm

Fractures of the Humeral Shaft

Fractures of the shaft of the humerus comprise of 1% of all the fractures. These fractures have a bimodal incidence pattern. The first peak is in young adults where these fractures occur due to violent high-energy trauma. Associated injuries are very commonly seen in these patients. The second peak occurs in elderly patients with osteoporotic bones.

Mechanism of injury

Shaft of humerus fractures can be caused by direct injury (fall on the side or direct impact on the arm) as well as by indirect injury (such as fall on the outstretched hand).

Classification

Classification of humeral shaft fractures is de-

scriptive such as transverse, short oblique, spiral and comminuted.

Evaluation of a patient with humeral shaft fracture

Initial evaluation includes assessment of vital functions and search for associated injuries. Patient complains of pain and inability to move the arm. Patient often prefers to support the injured arm with the other hand. Deformity is often quite obvious and swelling and bruising at the fracture site are commonly seen. Radial nerve must be tested in all cases. Radial nerve is particularly vulnerable in middle third fractures or laterally angulated fractures at junction of middle third and distal third (*Holstein-Lewis fracture*), gunshot wounds to arm and in open fractures.

Imaging Plain radiographs – Anteroposterior and lateral are adequate for confirmation of diagnosis and assessment of fracture configuration, comminution and displacement (Fig. 22.7a,b). In the proximal third fractures, the proximal fragment is adducted due to unopposed action of pectoralis major while the proximal fragment is abducted in the mid third fractures due to the pull of the deltoid. Persistent gap at the fracture site

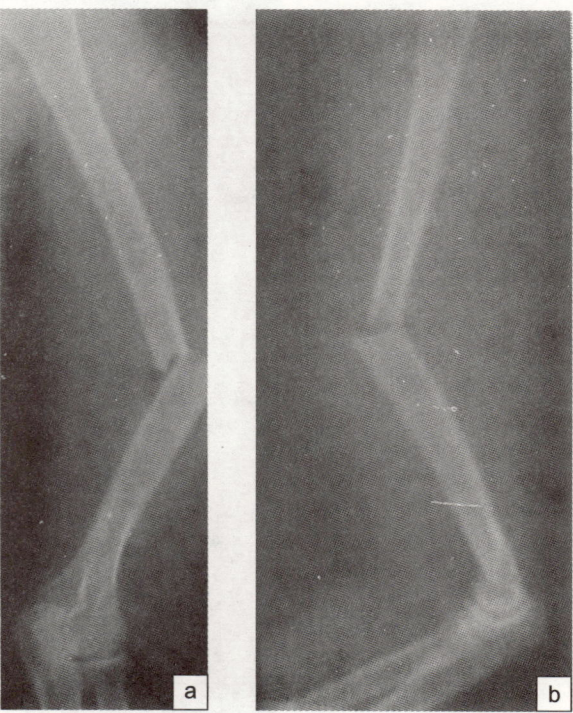

Fig. 22.7a,b. AP and lateral x-rays showing fracture of the humeral shaft

suggests soft tissue interposition or over-distraction (as with the weight of hanging cast). Gap at the fracture site in the post manipulation check x-ray with radial nerve palsy, which appears after manipulation, strongly suggests entrapment of the radial nerve at the fracture site.

Treatment

The treatment of closed humeral shaft fractures is non-operative. Conservative treatment is associated with high union rate (95%) and satisfactory functional results. The acceptable reduction (associated with good function and cosmesis) includes less than 20° anterior angulation, less than 30° of varus/valgus angulation and upto 1 inch shortening (Fig. 22.7c,d). The conservative treatment of shaft of humerus fracture includes closed reduction (if alignment of fragments is not acceptable) and immobilization in a slab or a hanging cast and collar and cuff sling in ambulant patients. The gravity acting through weight of the limb aligns the fragments and patients who are not ambulatory cannot be treated satisfactorily by non-operative method. Fractures usually unite in 8 to 12 weeks.

Functional bracing is a widely used method of treating humeral shaft fractures non-operatively. Stabilization of the fracture fragments is achieved by compression of the rigid wall of brace against the soft tissue while the exercises are permitted at the elbow and the shoulder joints. Satisfactory alignment of fragments occurs when patient is erect and stiffness at the neighbouring joints is prevented. Anatomical reduction is neither possible nor intended in this method but the final angulatory deformities are cosmetically acceptable and functionally satisfactory. Obese patients, patients with spastic disorders, patients with large breasts, patients with injury to neurovascular structures, patients with compound fractures and polytraumatized patients are difficult to manage by non operative treatment.

Surgical treatment is indicated in polytrauma patients (with injuries to multiple extremities), vascular injuries, open fracture, head or spinal cord injuries, inadequate reduction after closed treatment, radial nerve injury following manipulation and pathologic fractures.

Open reduction and internal fixation when

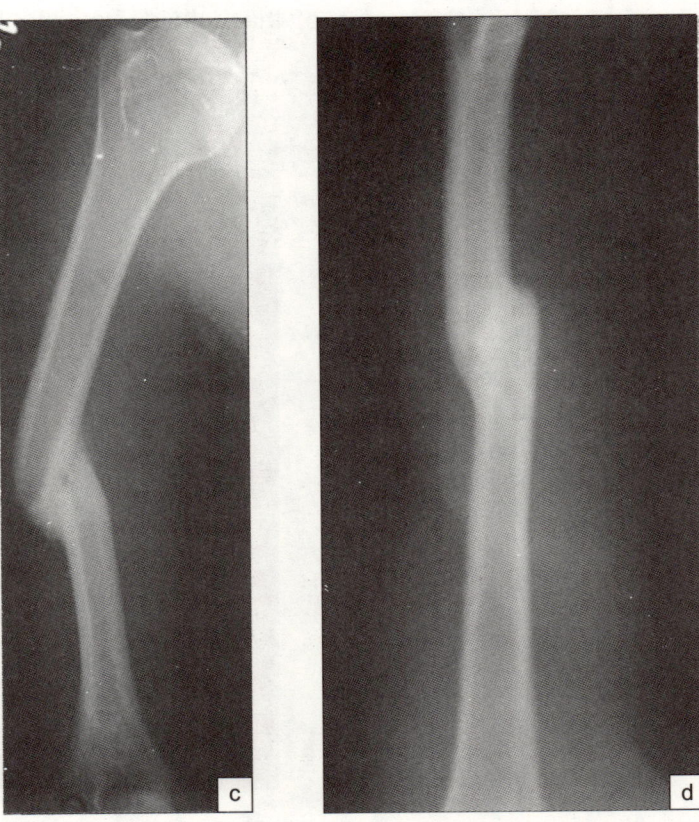

Fig. 22.7c,d. Malunited fracture of humeral shaft. Note the lateral angulation and overriding; however, this is acceptable

indicated can be performed using plate and screws, intramedullary devices and external fixation.

Plates and screws provide rigid fixation (Fig. 22.7e,f) and are especially useful for distal shaft fractures (where the shaft becomes triangular in cross section and intramedullary nailing becomes difficult). Union rates with plating for humeral shaft fractures are high and functional outcome excellent. Iatrogenic radial nerve palsy, infection and failure of fixation in osteoporotic bones are the main problems with this method of treatment.

Intramedullary devices

Intramedullary devices can be both rigid and flexible. Flexible solid nails (such as Ender pins, Rush pins) are passed in unreamed fashion either in a crossed fashion through either side of elbow or as "stacked" nails to pack the medullary canal through an entry portal just proximal to the olecranon fossa. This method provides only limited axial and rotational control and therefore, external support is necessary. However this method is associated with high incidence of malunion, delayed union and non-union. Nail migration, discomfort due to hardware and adhesive capsulitis of shoulder are other common complications.

Interlocking nails (e.g. Russell-Taylor nail) have been used to treat humeral shaft fractures with excellent results. Nails can be inserted using antegrade technique through the greater tuberosity at the lateral edge of the rotator cuff or retrograde from just proximal (1.7 cm) to the olecranon fossa. Locking reduces the incidence of nail migration, malunion and nonunion. Common complications of this method are shoulder discomfort, compromised shoulder function and iatrogenic comminution.

Intramedullary nailing with or without bone cement is the treatment of choice for pathologic fractures.

External Fixator for humeral shaft fractures is indicated for open fractures (especially due to gunshot wounds or those associated with vascular injury or in multiply injured patient). External fixation allows rapid skeletal stabilization so that vascular repair or soft tissue management can be undertaken quickly.

Problems of external fixators include pin tract infection, patient discomfort, stiffness of neighbouring joints due to transfixation of muscles and radial nerve injuries.

Complications

Radial nerve palsy occurs in 5–10% cases and recovers spontaneously in most cases. Exploration

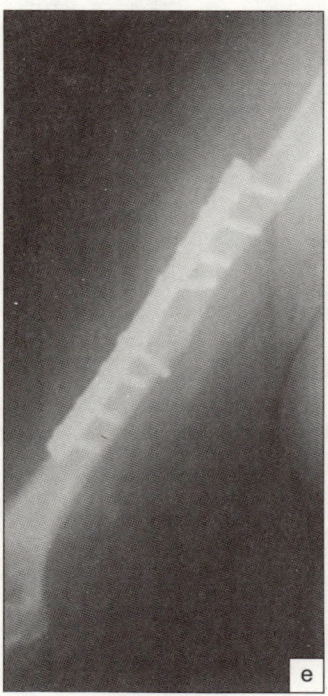 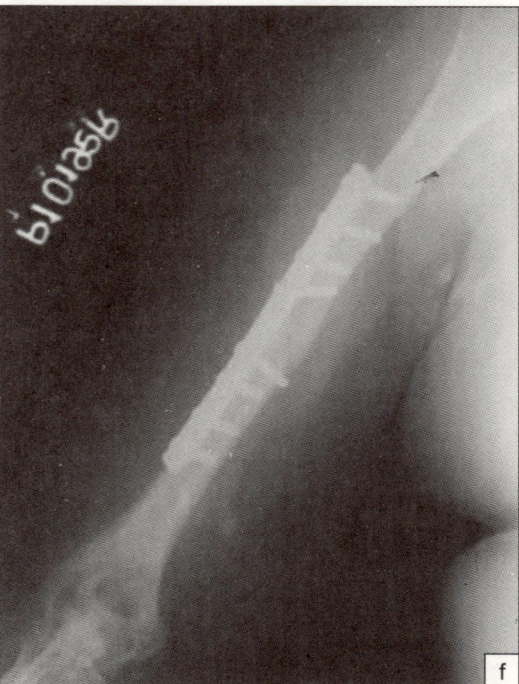

Fig. 22.7e,f.   Fracture shaft humerus treated by ORIF with dynamic compression plating

is indicated in open fractures with radial nerve palsy, palsy occuring after closed manipulation or ORIF and no clinical or electromyographic evidence of recovery 3 months after injury.

Vascular injuries should be managed by rapid stabilization of fracture (ORIF with plating or external fixator) followed by vascular repair.

Non Union is unusual in humeral shaft fractures and occurs most commonly due to distraction at the fracture site, soft tissue interposition or due to infection or inadequate stabilization in operated cases. Bone grafting and ORIF with plate and screws or intramedullary nailing is the method of choice.

Malunion is common but needs treatment only if deformity is more than accepted norms as described above and is associated with unsatisfactory cosmesis and function.

Stiffness of the shoulder is a common complication and is managed with physiotherapy.

Hardware related complications include infection and loss of fixation.

Injuries Around Elbow

Fractures and Dislocations of Adult Elbow

Fractures of Distal Humerus

Distal end of humerus consists of two columns, a medial and a lateral, linked together by trochlea and creating a triangular construct. On the dorsal side, olecranon fossa lies within the triangle. Proximal tip of the olecranon occupies the olecranon fossa in full extension. The distal humerus tilts forward 30 degrees with respect to the shaft. The distal humerus participates in the formation of two functionally independent joints the humero-ulnar and the radio-capitellar. Neurovascular structures travel in close association with the distal humerus. Fractures of the distal end of humerus account for one third of the fractures around elbow. The most important aspect of the treatment of all these injuries is early mobilization to prevent the stiffness of the elbow joint.

Mechanism of injury

These fractures can be caused by both direct as well as indirect injuries. Direct injuries can be blunt (as in fall on the point of elbow, direct blow from a bat) or penetrating (as in gunshot wounds). Indirect injuries with torsional force on the distal humerus can lead to supracondylar or intercondylar fractures. Capitellum fractures are caused by a shear stress from the radial head.

Classification

There are multiple classification systems but none of them is comprehensive. These fractures are often classified on the basis of columnar concept of the distal humerus or on the basis of anatomy and severity of fracture (AO group: Type A extra-articular; Type B partially articular; and, Type C: completely articular).

Columnar concept divides the fractures of distal humerus in 3 main groups.

1. *Extra capsular* isolated (usually avulsion) injuries to epicondyles (medial and lateral).

2. *Extra-articular/intra capsular* supracondylar (high) and transcondylar (low).

3. *Intra-articular*

- single column (medial or lateral) often subdivided into:

  Type I: lateral trochlear ridge intact;

  Type II: fracture through lateral trochlear ridge.

- Both columns (T fractures, Y fractures, H fractures, medial or lateral lambda fractures depending on configuration of fractures)

Capitellum Fractures

Type I: coronal plane fracture (*Hahn Steinthal*);

Type II: sleeve fracture of articular surface with minimal bone; and,

Type III: comminuted.

Evaluation of patient with distal humerus fractures

Patient with distal humerus fracture presents with pain and swelling at the elbow. Elbow looks deformed and may have overlying ecchymosis. Palpation reveals severe tenderness. Attempts to move the elbow are extremely painful. Associated neurovascular injuries must be looked for (especially in open and/or comminuted fractures) in view of the close proximity of neurovascular structures to the distal humerus.

Imaging

Plain radiographs including anteroposterior and lateral views form the standard examination of the elbow. Plain radiographs confirm the fracture and divulge the fracture configuration and comminution. Undisplaced fractures may be suspected when the joint effusion is present as evident by visualization of anterior fat pad or elevation of the anterior fat pad. Minimally displaced fractures of the distal end of humerus can be diagnosed by extending distally a line along the anterior cortex of the humerus on lateral view. Normally one third of the distal articular surface should lie anterior to it. Even minimally posteriorly titled distal articular fractures can be diagnosed by this sign. If capitellum fracture is suspected but not visualized on the standard views, a capitellum view (modified lateral view of elbow taken with x-ray beam angled 45° towards the patient) may be obtained.

Treatment

Fractures of the distal humerus are often quite complex and present the treating surgeon with big challenge.

Treatment is aimed at stable reduction and early active range of motion.

Conservative treatment is indicated with undisplaced stable fractures, which can be put to early range of motion exercises.

Skeletal traction through an olecranon pin or skin traction to forearm are used sometimes in cases with severe comminution (especially when expertise and facilities for complex reconstruction are not available) or in cases where surgery or anesthesia are contraindicated because of medical reasons. Conservative treatment is also chosen sometimes in elderly patients with severely comminuted fractures in osteopenic bones. These patients are immobilized in plaster for 2–3 weeks and once pain subsides, are encouraged to perform the range of motion exercises.

ORIF is indicated in unstable fractures and in intra-articular fractures where anatomical reduction and stable fixation of articular fragments is mandatory.

1. **Extracapsular fractures** are rare in adults and occur in children. Medial Epicondylar fractures are more common than lateral. Minimally displaced fractures are treated with immobilization and early range of motion exercises. Displacements more than 1 cm are indication for ORIF.

2. **Extra-articular-Intra-capsular** (supracondylar/transcondylar) fractures are trans columnar fractures extending across both columns and sparing the articular surface. Undisplaced and minimally displaced fractures are treated with immobilization in above elbow plaster slab for 1–2 weeks and then gentle range of motion exercises. ORIF is indicated for inability to obtain reduction, fractures with associated vascular injury or for multiple fractures in the same extremity. Internal fixation is done using AO plate with screw (for high fractures) or crossed Rush pins / kirschner wires for low fractures. Early mobilization is recommended.

Unlike pediatric age group closed reduction and percutaneous pinning is not a widely used method in adults.

3. **Intra-articular fractures** Single condyle fractures which are unstable (can be displaced on stress as shown on stress x-rays) or widely displaced fractures (usually Type II) are treated by ORIF using one or two lag screws. Undisplaced or minimally displaced fractures (usually type I with lateral trochlear ridge intact) are treated in plaster slab for 4–5 weeks followed by exercises.

(a) Intercondylar fractures (Fig. 23.1a,b) with separation of fragments in adults are treated by ORIF.

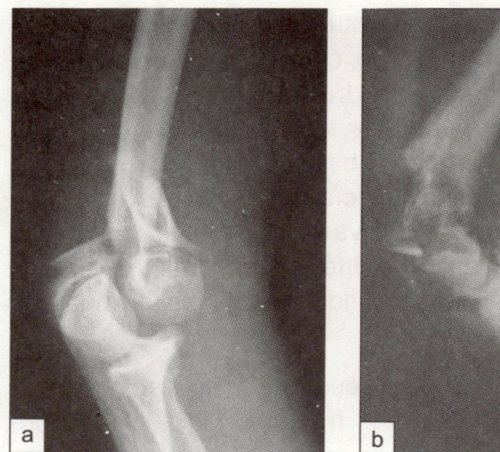

Fig. 23.1a,b. Comminuted intercondylar fracture of the humerus following side swipe injury

A posterior triceps splitting or transolecranon (through olecranon after performing its osteotomy) approach is used. The articular surface is first reconstructed using screws (without compression of the fragment to avoid constricting articular surface of trochlea). The articular surface is then fixed to columns most commonly using two plates at 90° to each other, a reconstruction plate posterolaterally and a 1/3rd tubular plate medially fixed with 3.5 mm cortical screws. Less severe fractures can be fixed with plate on one column and cancellous screw for the other column. Post-operatively elbow is immobilized for short duration followed by early range of motion exercises.

(b) Fractures of capitellum are caused by a shear stress from the radial head, which usually displaces the fracture fragment anteriorly and proximally (Fig. 23.2a,b). Undisplaced fractures are

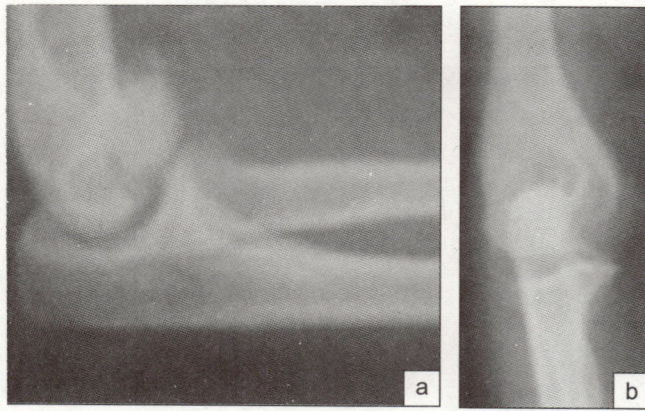

Fig. 23.2a,b. Pre-operative X-rays of a patient with fracture capitellum Type I

treated with posterior splint with elbow flexed and pronated for 2–3 weeks.

Displaced (more than 2 mm) fragments are treated surgically. Large fragments are fixed with screw(s) passed from posterior to anterior direction to fix the fragment without injuring the overlying articular cartilage. Special (Herbert) screws can also be used to fix the fracture (Fig. 23.2c,d). If the fragments are small, they are excised and elbow mobilized early.

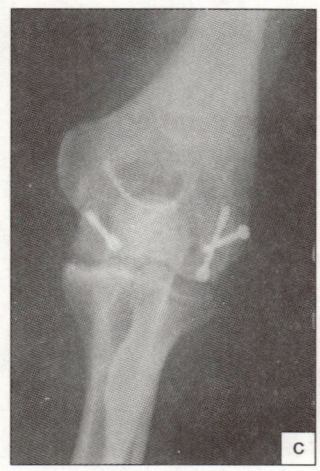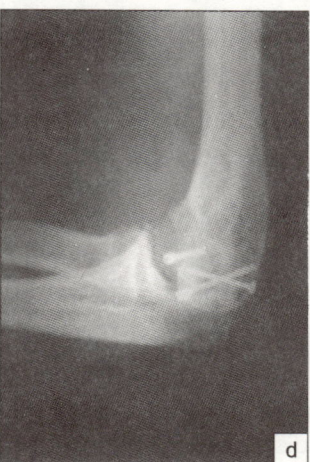

Fig. 23.2c,d. Post-operative X-rays of the same patient following ORIF with Herbert's screw. Note coexistent trochlear fracture fixed with Herbert screw

(c) Fractures of the trochlea (*Laugier's fracture*) are very uncommon and are treated by ORIF and early movements. Small fragment or inability to reduce and fix the fragment is an indication for excision of the fragment.

Complications

Stiffness of the elbow is the commonest complication. Anatomic reduction, stable fixation and early mobilization for operated cases are best preventive measures.

Injury to neurovascular structures is commonly associated. Ulnar nerve may be damaged during surgery. Ulnar neuropathy may also occur with deformities or non-union and is treated with anterior transposition. Non-union occurs in operated cases when fragments are not adequately fixed. ORIF and bone grafting are indicated for treatment.

Heterotopic ossification occurs in almost 5% cases treated with surgery and indomethacin can be given orally for prophylaxis. Mature heterotopic bone interfering with function can be treated with late excision.

Malunion is common after these fractures and should be treated on its merits. Hardware related complications are common and include breakage or loosening of implants, infection, non-union and painful bursa especially over tension band wiring of olecranon osteotomy.

Fractures of the Olecranon

Fractures of olecranon are common in adults but may uncommonly occur in children.

Mechanism of injury Olecranon can be fractured as a result of direct injury, (direct blow or fall on the point of elbow) or indirect injury due to violent contraction of triceps muscle. Fall on the out stretched hand with elbow flexed and contraction of triceps results in avulsion of the olecranon.

Classification No universally accepted classification system is available. However olecranon fractures are often categorized as undisplaced or displaced. Displaced fractures can be further classification as avulsion fractures, transverse, oblique, comminuted or fracture dislocations.

Evaluation Patient presents with pain, swelling and hemarthrosis of the elbow. Tenderness can be elicited over olecranon and patient is unable to extend the elbow. Defect may be palpable between the fragments in widely displaced fractures. Occasionally ulnar nerve injury may occur so ulnar nerve must always be examined.

Imaging Plain anteroposterior and lateral radiographs are adequate to confirm the diagnosis and displacement of the fracture fragments (Fig. 23.3a). However, one must be careful in diagnosing olecranon fracture in children as normal epiphyseal line may be mistaken for fracture. An x-ray of opposite elbow and absence of tenderness will solve the problem. Olecranon epiphysis may also show developmental variations (bifid epiphysis, *patella cubiti* which is due to ossification in triceps tendon) in growing children and these must be kept in mind.

Management Undisplaced (<2 mm displacement, no further opening of fracture with 90° flexion) fractures of olecranon are uncommon and are treated in plaster slab with elbow in 45°–90° flexion, close radiologic follow up and early range of motion exercises at 3 weeks after injury. In flail elderly persons mild to moderate displacement can be accepted and fractures treated conservatively.

Displaced fractures are treated by ORIF to restore the extensor mechanism of the elbow.

Transverse fractures are treated by tension band wiring technique with 2 parallel kirschner wires or an intramedullary screw and cerclage wire (Fig. 23.3b). Oblique fractures are treated with inter fragmentary screw and supplemental fixation with plating or tension band wiring.

Small avulsion fractures are treated with excision of fragment and repair of triceps tendon.

Comminuted fractures are stabilized with plate and screws. Severely comminuted fractures are treated with excision of the fragment and repair of triceps. However excision of olecranon in the presence of associated coronoid fracture or excision

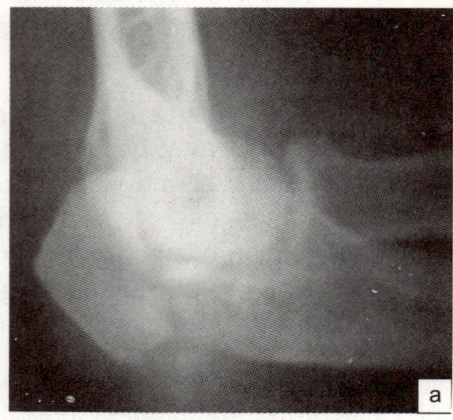 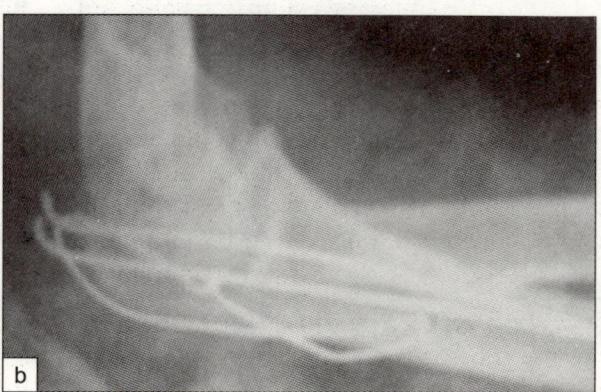

Fig. 23.3.   (a) Fracture of the Olecranon;   (b) Treated by tension band wiring

of more than 50% of olecranon can lead to instability of the elbow.

Fracture-dislocations are treated by ORIF with screws or intramedullary device with or without tension band wiring.

Complications

Complications of olecranon fracture include stiffness of the elbow, malunion, posttraumatic degenerative arthritis, non-union and hardware related complications such as infection, breakage of implants, loss of fixation or painful bursa over tension band wiring.

Fractures of the coronoid

Coronoid process is extremely important for anterior stability of the elbow. Coronoid process fractures rarely occur in isolation. About 10% cases of elbow dislocation have associated coronoid fracture.

Coronoid fractures are classified into three types:

1. Type I is avulsion of the coronoid tip

2. Type II is fractures involving half or less than half of the coronoid and

3. Type III when the fracture involves more than 50% of the coronoid.

Diagnosis is made on radiograph.

Treatment in type I and type II is conservative. Associated elbow dislocation is reduced and coronoid usually falls back in place. Exercises are started after 3 weeks of immobilization. Large fragments (type III fractures; fragment representing greater than one sixth of the circumference of the trochlear notch) are fixed with a small screw, a wire or stout braided non absorbable suture passed through drill holes.

Complications of coronoid fracture include non-union, malunion and recurrent dislocation. Latter needs bone block reconstruction of the coronoid.

Fractures of Radial Head

Radial head fractures are common injuries in adults and account for one third of elbow fractures. Radial head and neck fractures are seen in 50% to 60% of elbow dislocations.

Mechanism of injury Radial head fractures most frequently result from indirect violence most commonly due to an axial load on a pronated forearm. Radial head strikes the capitellum and articular damage to latter is a frequently associated injury. Sometimes, radial head fracture may be caused by a direct injury such as a fall or blow to the side of the elbow.

In cases where axial load is very severe, comminuted fractures of radial head occur and interosseous membrane may be torn resulting in proximal migration of the radius and subluxation of the inferior radio-ulnar joint (*Essex-Lopresti* fracture dislocation).

Classification

Most commonly used classification is modified *Mason's*, which also reflects management options.

Type I includes undisplaced or minimally displaced (<2 mm) fracture that do not restrict forearm rotation, type II includes larger, displaced (>2 mm) two part fractures, fractures which restrict forearm rotation or simple comminuted fractures which can be operatively fixed. Type III fractures are so comminuted that operative fixation is not possible. Type IV fractures are radial head fractures associated with dislocation of the elbow (Fig. 23.4a,b).

Evaluation Patient presents with pain in the elbow. There may be associated local swelling and bruising. Tenderness over the fractures may be elicited by placing the thumb over the radial head and gently rotating the forearm into pronation and supination. Rotations may be restricted.

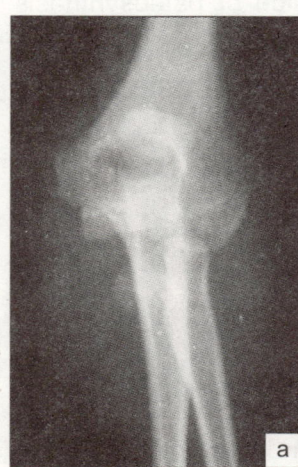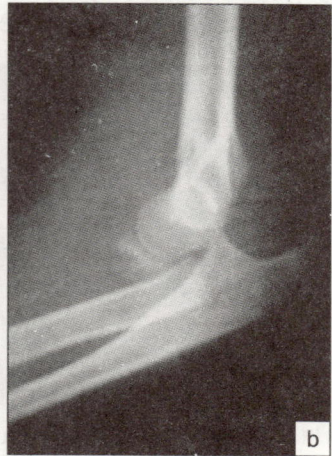

Fig. 23.4a,b. Type IV fracture of radial head with dislocation of the elbow

Elbow extension is almost always restricted. Wrist and forearm should always be examined to exclude Essex-Lopresti fracture-dislocation.

Imaging Plain anteroposterior and lateral radiographs of the elbow reveal the radial head fracture in most cases. However, if radiographs are negative in the presence of strong clinical suspicion, additional anteroposterior x-rays in different rotations and/or a capitellum view can reveal the fractures. Wrist and forearm should be x-rayed in cases with severely comminuted radial head fracture when proximal migration of radius is suspected.

Management

Type I fractures can be treated conservatively with good results. Elbow is immobilized in a sling for 2–3 weeks and then mobilized. If type I fracture involves more than one third of the radial head, close radiographic monitoring is required to detect displacement of the fracture.

Type II fractures with large fragments are treated with ORIF using 1.5 or 2.7 mm screws or special (Herbert) screws. Small, displaced fragments are treated with excision. Some people recommend trial of conservative treatment with early movements for three weeks and assessment of rotations. Symptomatic patients or functional limitation can be addressed by late excision of the radial head.

Type III fracture (comminuted) are treated by early excision of the radial head (preferably within 48 hours to avoid myositis ossificans). The time for surgery is within 48 hours or after 3 months.

Type IV fractures are treated with reduction of the dislocation followed by excision or osteosynthesis of the radial head (Fig. 23.4c).

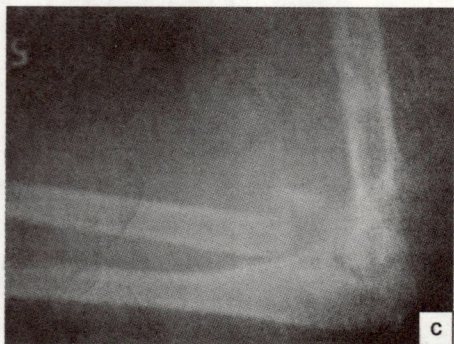

Fig. 23.4c. Fracture dislocation of elbow shown in fig. 23.4a,b following closed reduction of dislocation. Radial head excision was done subsequently

Prosthetic replacement of the radial head is indicated when lateral columnar support of the elbow is required or when radial head excision is contraindicated as in

a) Essex-Lopresti fracture dislocation

b) Comminuted radial head fracture with medial collateral ligament injury

c) Posterior dislocation of the elbow with radial head comminution and coronoid process fracture (*Terrible triad*)

Silastic radial head prostheses were used initially but were associated with problems of breakage and particulate synovitis. Metallic prostheses are now being evaluated at present for replacing radial head.

Radial head replacement with osteoarticular allograft is also being studied especially in cases where comminution extends to radial neck and currently available prostheses do not provide sufficient length in this situation.

Complications of radial head fractures include restriction of elbow extension (commonest) and forearm rotations, myositis ossificans, elbow instability (when associated with injury to medial collateral ligament or posterior dislocation of the elbow) and wrist instability (inferior radio ulnar joint subluxation in *Essex-Lopresti* fracture dislocation).

Dislocation of Elbow

Elbow is the third commonest joint to dislocate after shoulder and finger. Elbow dislocations can occur in both adults as well as children.

Mechanism of injury

Elbow dislocation is caused by fall on the outstretched hand. The forearm bones are pushed backwards, side-wards and proximally out of the elbow articulation. Severe injury to stabilizing soft tissues (ligaments, capsule, muscles and periosteum) and neighbouring neurovascular structures may occur. A forward directed direct blow on the dorsum of proximal ulna can lead to fracture of olecranon and anterior fracture dislocation of the elbow. A complex type of anterior dislocation is seen in side swipe injury so called "*baby car fracture*" (in cases where the flexed elbow of the driver resting on the window ledge of the car is struck by another vehicle). This injury results in fracture olecranon with anterior dislocation of elbow, fracture of distal humerus, fracture of ulna and sometimes fracture of the radius.

Classification Elbow dislocations are classified according to the direction of the dislocation. Most common dislocation is posterolateral, which accounts for 80% of all dislocations (Fig. 23.5a,b). Other types are anterior (associated with fracture of olecranon), medial, lateral and *divergent*. In the *divergent* variety distal humerus may displace radius and ulna into divergence either anteroposteriorly or mediolaterally by displacing between them.

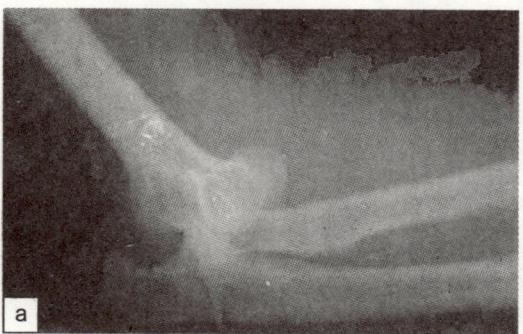

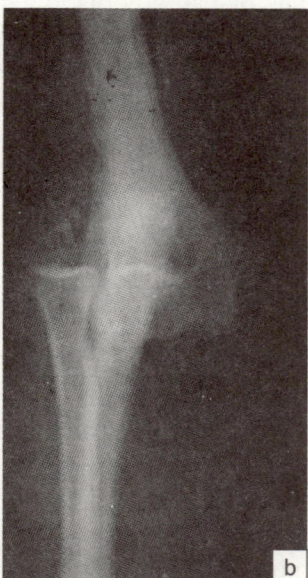

Fig. 23.5a,b. Posterolateral dislocation of the elbow

Evaluation Patient presents with pain, swelling and deformity around the elbow. Patient resists any movements of the elbow. Triceps appears taut. The three bony point relationship on posterior aspect of elbow is reversed-tip of olecranon which is normally most distal becomes most proximal. This is the most important differentiating feature from supracondylar fracture of humerus where 3 bony point relationship is not altered.

Assessment must include evaluation for damage to median nerve, ulnar nerve or brachial artery.

Imaging

Plain anteroposterior and lateral radiographs confirm the diagnosis and evaluate direction and degree of displacement of forearm bones. Associated fractures (coronoid, radial head, radial neck, lateral condyle, medial epicondyle) are looked for. Intra-articular entrapment of medial epicondylar fragment must be looked for.

Management

Initial management for all elbow dislocations is reduction under anesthesia, using traction in slight extension with distraction and pressure on olecranon. Range of motion and stability is checked after reduction. Stable reductions are splinted in a pop slab in 90° for one week and then mobilized. Unstable reductions are immobilized for 3 weeks followed by range of motion exercises. In dislocations with fractures, the dislocation is reduced and fracture reassessed radiologically. In most cases the fractures are reduced to an acceptable position. Persistently displaced fragments are treated surgically.

Other indications for surgical treatment are intra-articular fragments, anterior fracture-dislocation (ORIF for olecranon), fracture dislocations with coronoid and radial head fractures (*Terrible triad*), persistent instability and late diagnosed (after 2 months) posterior dislocations in children.

Complications

- Injury to neurovascular structures may occur and must be detected early to prevent catastrophic sequelae.

- Associated fractures of radial head and neck (50–60%), coronoid (10%) and medial or lateral epicondyles (10%) are commonly seen with elbow dislocation.

- Myositis ossificans and ligamentous calcification occurs commonly following elbow dislocation.

- Stiffness is the commonest complication of elbow dislocation.

- Recurrent dislocation may occur due to persistent instability.

- Missed or late diagnosed dislocation is managed by open reduction or excision arthroplasty.

Elbow Injuries in Children

Elbow injuries account for 8–9% of all pediatric fractures. Elbow injuries in children are different from adults due to several peculiar anatomic features. The distal humeral bone is mainly cancellous and undergoing remodelling in children. This fact, along with the hyperextension possible in a pediatric elbow makes supracondylar fracture a very common fracture in this age group. In fact intercondylar fractures and elbow dislocations are much less common in children. Radial neck fractures (usually epiphyseal injuries) are much more common in children than radial head fractures. Medial epicondyle and lateral condyle fractures are other common fractures in children in this region.

Several ossification centers are present around elbow and they sometimes make diagnosis of a fracture difficult. It is always helpful to take radiographs of the opposite elbow for comparison. Average age of appearance of various secondary ossification centers around the elbow is (in order of appearance) capitellum 1 year (6m–2 years), radial head 3 years (2–4 years), medial (internal) epicondyle 5 years (4–6 years), trochlea 7 years (6–8 years), olecranon 9 years (8–10 years), and lateral (external) epicondyle 11 years (10–12 years); [CRITOE]. Around 10–12 years of age the epiphyses fuse to each other and to the metaphysis.

Common Pediatric Injuries Around Elbow

Supracondylar fracture of Humerus

Supracondylar fracture of the humerus is the commonest fracture around elbow in children constituting about 69% of elbow fractures in children. Supracondylar fracture is usually a transverse fracture running just proximal to trochlea and capitellum. The fracture is common during 5–10 years of age and is rare in adults.

Mechanism of injury

Supracondylar fracture usually results from a fall on the out stretched hand. It can also be caused by direct injury as a fall on the point of the elbow.

Classification

Supracondylar fractures are of two types according to the mechanism of injury.

Extension type is caused by the force, which displaces the distal fragment (i.e. the lower end of the humerus) posteriorly. It is the common type and constitutes almost 97.7% of the fractures. This is the type which results from the fall on the out stretched hand.

Flexion type is caused by a force which displaces the distal fragment anteriorly. This type of supracondylar fracture constitutes about 2.3% of fractures.

Extension type of supracondylar fracture of the humerus is further classified by *Gartland* according to the degree of displacement:

I)   Undisplaced

II) Displaced with intact posterior cortex.

III) Displaced without cortical contact

   Posteromedial displacement of distal fragment with varus angulation-more common.

   Posterlateral displacement of the distal fragment with valgus angulation.

The characteristic displacements in a supracondylar fracture in extension are posterior shift, medial/lateral shift, anterior angulation, posterior and medial tilt, internal rotation and overriding.

Evaluation of a child with supracondylar fracture of humerus

Patients present with a history of fall following which the elbow becomes painful and swollen. There may an obvious deformity and child is unable to move the elbow. Distal humerus is tender. The normal relationship between olecranon and medial and lateral epicondyles is preserved. Dimpling of the skin over the anterior aspect of the distal arm suggests button holing of the spike of the proximal fracture fragment through the brachialis muscle and tethering the skin. Movements at the elbow are not permitted due to pain. Distal neurovascular examination must be performed in all cases.

In cases presenting late with severe swelling around the elbow, with or without encircling bandages, careful examination to rule out Volkmann's ischemia must be performed. Tense forearm, severe pain in the forearm, impairment of two point discrimination sense and pain on passive extension of fingers all suggest Volkmann's ischemia. It is important to note that radial pulse may still be palpable in the presence of established Volkmann's ischemia.

Imaging Anteroposterior and lateral views of the elbow are usually sufficient to confirm the presence of fracture, type and degree of displacement and presence of comminution (Fig. 23.6a,b).

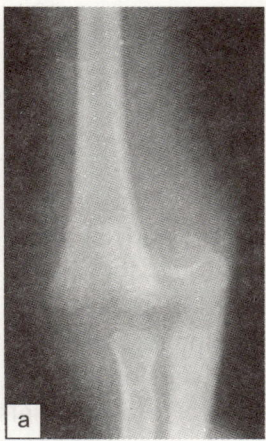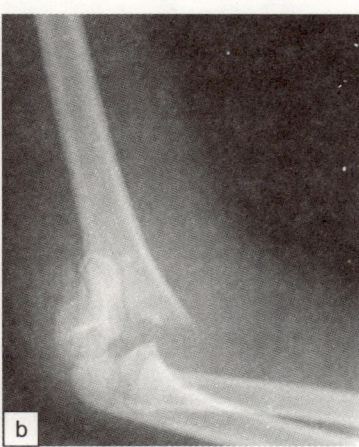

Fig. 23.6a,b. Displaced supracondylar fracture of humerus

After the reduction the lateral and anteroposterior "shoot through" x-rays (*Jones* view) are taken to confirm the adequacy of reduction. The following facts should be remembered.

- An undisplaced fracture is often betrayed by the "fat pad" sign suggesting hemarthrosis.

- A minimally displaced fracture is discerned by extending the anterior humeral line distally. Normally it divides distal humeral physis into anterior one third and posterior two thirds. Subtle posterior tilt of the distal fragment will diminish the fraction of distal physis anterior to the anterior humeral line.

- Sharp spike like appearance of proximal fragment suggests rotational deformity.

- Crescent shaped overlap between the distal humeral physis and olecranon on the lateral view suggests residual medial tilt, which may result in a cubitus varus deformity.

Treatment

Conservative treatment: Undisplaced fractures are treated in above elbow plaster slab in 120° flexion at the elbow for 3 weeks.

Displaced fractures needing manipulative reduction include:

- fracture with less than 50% bony contact

- posterior tilt of the distal fragment by more than 15°

- lateral or medial tilting of 10° or more

- presence of rotational deformity

- evidence of arterial obstruction in the presence of displacement and/or angulation of the fracture.

Technique of manipulative reduction of extension type fracture

The reduction is performed under general anesthesia. Radial pulse is palpated. Traction is applied to the forearm with the elbow in 20° of flexion while the assistant applies the countertraction at the arm. The fracture fragments are disimpacted. The medial and lateral displacements are corrected and the elbow gently flexed to 120° with a hand on the radial pulse. Disappearance of radial pulse at any stage warrants a reduction in the flexion at the elbow till the pulse just returns. At this stage, pronating the forearm tightens the medial periosteal hinge in cases with medial tilt/ lateral angulation (i.e. with varus deformity). Cases with lateral tilt/medial angulation (i.e. with valgus deformity) are managed with the forearm supinated.

Flexion of the elbow over 90° stretches the triceps over the fracture. Triceps than acts as an internal splint and stabilizes the fracture fragments.

Technique of manipulative reduction of flexion type fracture

Flexion type of supracondylar fractures are stable in extension. To reduce these fractures, traction is applied to the elbow in the flexed position to disimpact the fracture fragments. The elbow is then gradually extended and angulation reduced. An above elbow plaster slab is applied in 10° flexion for three weeks. At this time the slab is removed and elbow is gently flexed.

Alternatively, Sultanpur method of reduction may be used where in a plaster cuff is applied to the arm extending upto the distal end of the proximal fragment. Once this sets the distal fragment is pushed back against this cast with elbow in about 110 degrees flexion and the cast is quickly completed.

This method avoids immobilizing the elbow in the extension, thereby reducing the risk of stiffness in this position. Stiffness of the elbow in extension greatly compromises function.

After care The plaster immobilization is continued for 4 weeks (slightly more in older children). Lack of the tenderness at the fracture site and the x-rays suggest union. Active elbow exercises are started at this stage. A sling may be worn for a few days and discarded as early as the patient is comfortable.

Percutaneous Pinning If image intensifier is available and during reduction it is discovered that the reduction is achievable but unstable, percutaneous pinning may be performed. Two kirschner wires are used and both are introduced from the lateral side-either parallel to each other or in a crossed manner. The ends of the wires are bent to avoid migration. The wires are removed after 3 weeks. Percutaneous fixation is also useful for flexion type of supracondylar fractures where it obviates the need for immobilization of the elbow in near extension.

Open Reduction and Pinning is used for irreducible fractures, cases where closed reduction cannot be maintained due to inability to flex elbow above 90° (due to severe swelling and disappearance of radial pulse) and in cases with associated vascular injury. A medial, lateral or anterior approach is used and the fracture is openly reduced and stabilized by crossed K-wires inserted from medial and lateral epicondyles (Fig. 23.6c,d). K-wires are removed after 6 weeks.

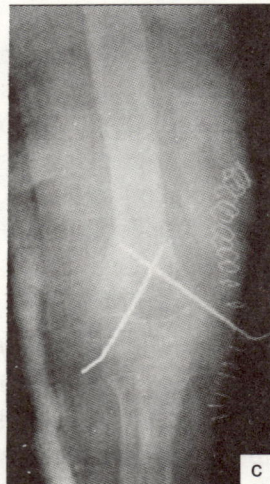 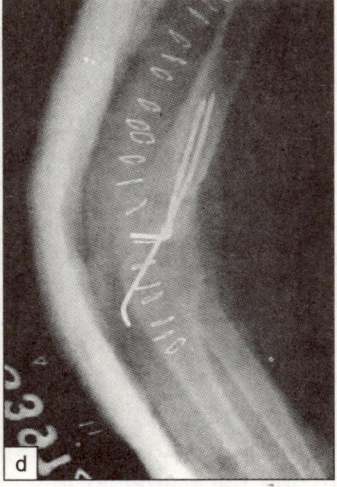

Fig. 23.6c,d. Displaced supracondylar fracture treated by open reduction and cross K-wire fixation

Traction Skin (*Dunlop*) or skeletal (olecranon pin) traction is often useful in cases where the reduction is difficult to achieve or maintain due to significant soft tissue swelling or comminution of the fracture fragments. Traction is also indicated in cases with minimal circulatory impairment, when brachial artery exploration is not indicated. Traction obviates the need for above 90° flexion at the elbow. Traction can be discontinued at 2–3 weeks and plaster slab can be applied till the fracture unites.

Complications

1. Vascular injury Vascular injury is associated with less than 1% cases of supra condylar fractures. The vascular injury can be due to kinking over the proximal fragment, spasm of the vessel, extrinsic pressure by fracture hematoma and swelling, internal thrombus, intimal tear, contusion of the vessel, or partial or complete tear of the brachial artery.

Tethering of the skin overlying a prominent spike of proximal fragment in the absence of a palpable radial pulse suggests entrapment of the neurovascular bundle and is an indication for urgent exploration. Excessive swelling and bruising around elbow may suggest vascular injury. Other signs of vascular compromise should be looked for in these cases. Often the patient may present with Volkmann's ischemia or rarely frank gangrene of the fingers.

When a patient with vascular compromise is seen, all the encircling bandages are removed. Fracture is reduced by gentle manipulation and the radial pulse checked. If the radial pulse does not return the brachial artery is explored. Peroperatively, the local pressure on the vessel is relieved. The spasm of brachial artery is relieved by local application of xylocaine or papaverine or by stripping the adventitia of the vessel, thus effecting sympathectomy. Spasm, which does not get relieved by these manoeuvres, is possibly an intimal tear and needs expert vascular intervention (Fig. 23.6e). Laceration of the artery needs repair. The fracture should be openly reduced and stabilized with k wires in all these cases.

Acute Volkamann's ischemia is managed by urgent fasciotomy extending right from elbow distally upto the carpal tunnel. The wound is closed secondarily after 3–5 days or skin grafted.

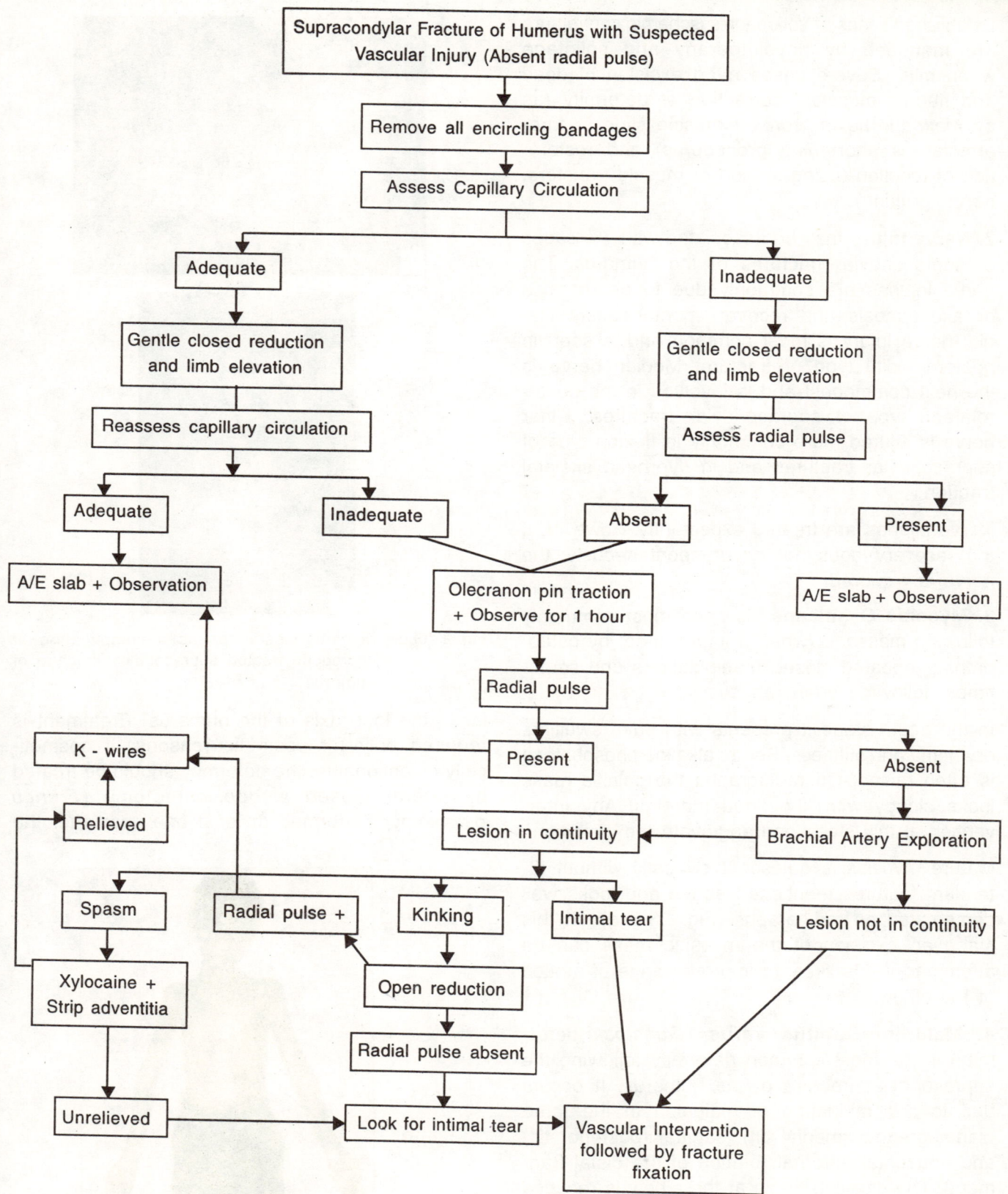

Fig. 23.6e. Algorithm for management of a patient with supracondylar fracture of the humerus with suspected vascular injury

Established cases of Volkmann's ischemic contracture are managed by physiotherapy and splintage when mild. Severe cases need excision of dead and fibrotic muscles, correction of deformity (as by *Maxpage* flexor-pronator muscle slide or forearm/carpus shortening procedures) and restoration of function (using tendon or muscle transfers, nerve grafting).

2. Nerve Injury may be associated with 7% cases of supracondylar fractures of the humerus. The nerve injuries are commonly due to neuropraxia or axonotmesis and recover spontaneously. Radial nerve injury is most common and is seen in posteromedial type of fracture. Median nerve is the next commonest and is involved in the posterolateral type of supracondylar fractures. Ulnar nerve is injured more commonly in flexion type of supracondylar fractures and in overhead skeletal traction.

Nerve injuries are treated expectantly. However, if the recovery does not occur spontaneously, the nerve is explored.

3. Myositis Ossificans is seen most commonly following massage (when fracture is set by osteopaths), repeated closed manipulations and sometimes, following open reduction.

In the acute stage it presents with pain, swelling, erythema and stiffness. Serum alkaline phosphatase is often raised. On radiographs the calcific mass looks cloudy with ill-defined margins. Any intervention at this stage can aggravate the condition.

Mature myositis is quiescent clinically without attendant features mentioned above and looks well demarcated on radiographs (Fig. 23.6f,g). At this stage an excision of the myositic mass can be attempted if it is likely to improve range of motion at the elbow.

4. Malunion-Cubitus varus (*Gunstock* deformity) is the most common deformity following the supracondylar fracture of the humerus. It occurs due to a combination of malunion in the three planes-coronal (medial tilt), sagittal (posterior tilt) and horizontal (internal rotation of the distal fragment). The carrying angle at the elbow is reduced and patient has unsightly deformity (Fig. 23.6h). Radiographs show crescent sign and reduced *Baumann's* angle (angle between the line along lateral condylar epiphysis and a line perpendicu-

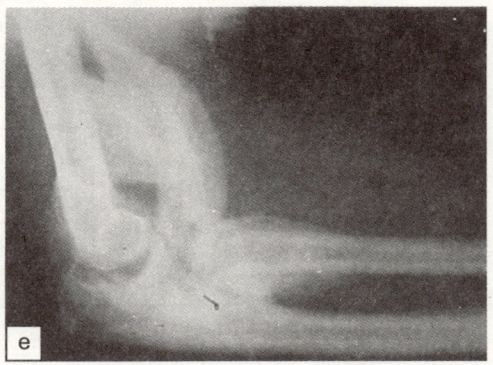

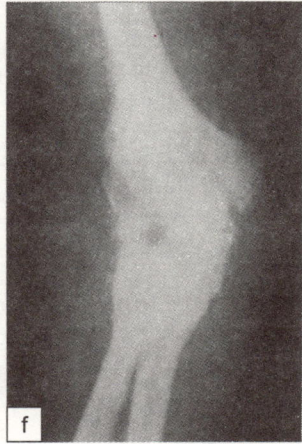

Fig. 23.6f,g. Myositis ossificans as a complication of improperly treated supracondylar fracture of humerus

lar to the long axis of the humerus). Treatment is required only for cosmetic reasons. If cosmetically objectionable, the deformity should be treated by lateral closed wedge osteotomy (*French osteotomy*) performed at least one year after the

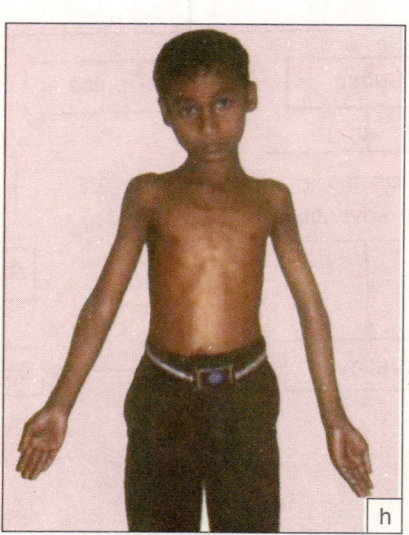

Fig. 23.6h. Cubitus varus (left elbow) following malunited supracondylar fracture of humerus

fracture. Cubitus valgus occurs *rarely*, following the posterolateral type of fracture. This deformity is not cosmetically as objectionable as cubitus varus. A longstanding deformity, however, may result in tardy ulnar nerve palsy, which requires anterior transposition of the ulnar nerve.

5. Stiffness of the elbow

Minimal loss of flexion is common even in the well-treated supracondylar fractures. Severe stiffness may result in cases with myositis ossificans or when late open reduction is attempted (more than 5 days after injury).

Trans condylar fractures

These are type I epiphyseal injuries which usually occur in children less than 3 years of age. Type II epiphyseal injury may occur in older children. The displacement is usually posteromedial. The radiographs confirm the injury and displacement. Treatment is by closed reduction and immobilization in flexion and pronation. Unstable reductions or irreducible fractures are managed by percutaneous or open pinning.

Fractures of the medial epicondyle

Fractures of the medial epicondyle are common between 8–14 years of age. Almost 50% of fractures of the medial epicondyle are associated with elbow dislocations.

Mechanism of injury

The medial epicondyle is fractured by a valgus pull with extension when it is avulsed by the flexor muscle mass and the ulnar collateral ligament. Due to this mechanism, ulnar nerve injury is commonly associated.

Classification

Fracture of the medial epicondyle can be undisplaced or displaced. Displacement can sometimes be intraarticular with the fragment trapped into the joint.

Evaluation of a child with fracture of medial epicondyle

Patient presents with the history of forcible abduction at the elbow followed by pain and tenderness, on the medial aspect of the elbow. Bruising may be present over the medial sides. Ulnar nerve should always be tested.

Imaging

Anteroposterior and lateral views of the elbow should be taken. Radiographs of the opposite elbow taken for comparison can be extremely useful. X-rays confirm the fracture and its displacement (Fig. 23.7). Intraarticular displacement of medial epicondylar fragment should be suspected when the medial epiphysis is not seen in A.P view in a child over 6 years age, when it is seen on the lateral film, and, when the medial epicondylar fragment is seen at the level of the joint line.

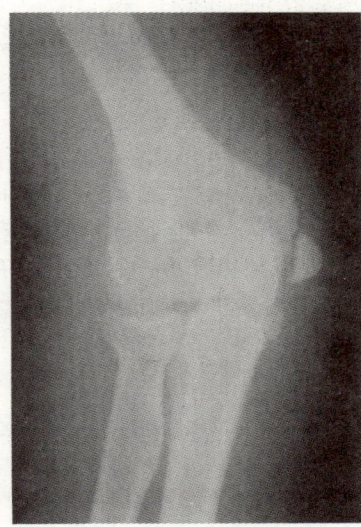

Fig. 23.7. Fracture medial epicondyle of humerus

Treatment

Conservative treatment is adequate when the fragment is displaced less than 2 mm. Above elbow plaster slab for 3 weeks followed by active exercises is adequate for all cases. Displaced fractures are treated by open reduction and K wire fixation.

Intraarticular displacement of the medial epicondylar fragment is managed by manipulation under anaesthesia. If this method fails, medial epicondyle is retrieved surgically and fixed to its bed using K wire or soft tissue suture. K wire is removed after 3 weeks.

The indications for surgery in fractures of medial epicondyle humerus are:

➤ Displaced fracture in individuals with athletic pursuits.

➤ Acute post traumatic ulnar nerve palsy and

➢ Acute incarceration of the medial epicondyle in the elbow joint with failed attempts at closed manipulation

The methods of closed removal of the incarcerated fragment are as follows:

• *Robert's* manipulative method: extension of elbow, supination of forearm, dorsiflexion of wrist and sudden hyperextension of the fingers causing tension on the common flexor origin may help in removal of the incarcerated fragment. This is effective when done before 24 hours.

• Faradic stimulation has been used by some.

• Distension of the joint by air/ fluid may help in extraction.

Complications

1. Ulnar nerve injury is common in these fractures. Most ulnar nerve palsies in these injuries are lesions in continuity, i.e. neuropraxia. Recovery usually begins within 3–6 weeks. Tardy ulnar nerve palsy may also occur long after these fractures.

2. Stiffness of the elbow may occur.

3. Weakness of forearm muscle (flexor-pronator group) may occur if a significantly displaced medial epicondylar fracture is left untreated.

Fracture of the medial condyle

This is a rare injury in children and is often missed. Injury is seen between 8–14 years of age. It is caused by an extension and valgus stress. The fracture is classified by Milch according to anatomical location as type I (fracture line passes through the apex of trochlea) and type II (fracture line passes through the capitello-trochlear groove). Milch I is caused by impaction by radial head while Milch II is caused by impaction by olecranon. The fragment displaces anteromedially by pull of flexors and medial collateral ligament. Impacted or undisplaced fractures are treated in an above elbow cast. Displaced fractures, especially with rotation, are treated with open reduction and internal fixation. Complications include non-union with cubitus varus, delayed union and tardy ulnar nerve palsy.

Fracture of the lateral epicondyle

It is a very rare injury and is often missed as it is confused with the normal physeal line. The epiphysis usually appears at the age of 11 years and fuses 2–3 years later. Avulsion of the lateral epicondyle occurs following adduction stress. Comparison with radiographs of the opposite side is extremely helpful. If the displacement is less than 2 mm, the injury is treated in above elbow slab for 3 weeks. Greater displacements need open reduction and fixation with K wire or soft tissue suture.

Fracture of the lateral condyle

The fracture of the lateral condyle occurs in 16.8% of elbow fractures and in 54.2% of physeal injuries around elbow. The injury is common between 4 to 8 years of age.

Mechanism of injury

Extension and varus forces lead to avulsion of the lateral condyle. Lateral condylar fractures can also be caused by valgus stress over the elbow in which case it is fractured by shearing force.

The fragment is displaced by forearm extensors or the lateral ligament.

Classification

Lateral condyle fractures are divided into two types according to Milch. In type I, the fracture line extends lateral to trochlea through the capitello-trochlear groove. It is a type IV epiphyseal injury. In type II, the fracture line extends into the apex of the trochlea. It is a type II injury.

The lateral condyle fractures can also be classified as undisplaced, displaced or rotated.

Evaluation of a child with lateral condyle fracture

Child presents with history of trauma followed by pain and swelling of the elbow. Tenderness is present over lateral aspect of the elbow. Crepitus may be present over the lateral aspect. Movements of the elbow are painfully restricted.

Imaging

Plain radiographs of the elbow confirm the diagnosis and degree of displacement of the fragment. Size of the fragment as visualized on the x-ray is much smaller than the real size of the fragment when encountered during the surgery due to the large cartilaginous component of the fragment.

Treatment

Undisplaced fractures are treated in above elbow cast for 4 weeks. However, radiographs should be taken at weekly intervals to ensure that no late displacement of the fracture occurs.

For displaced fractures, especially with rotation, conservative treatment is not effective. Open reduction and internal fixation with k wires is recommended (Fig. 23.8a,b). The blood supply to the fragment enters from the posterior aspect and this aspect of the fragment should not be stripped of the soft tissues. Following surgery above elbow cast is applied for four weeks. Active exercises are started at the end of this period.

Complications

- Delayed union or non-union is common in these cases. Non union leads to progressive cubitus valgus deformity (Fig. 23.8c) and tardy ulnar nerve palsy. The latter is treated by anterior transposition of ulnar nerve. Supracondylar osteotomy may be indicated sometimes to correct the deformity.

- Avascular necrosis of the fragment occurs in operated cases where excessive soft tissue stripping is done.

- Premature physeal growth arrest may occur. *Fishtail deformity* may occur (Fig. 23.8d).

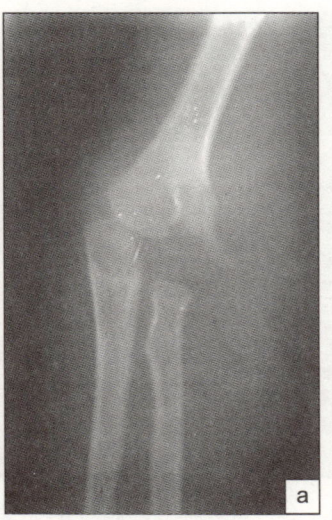
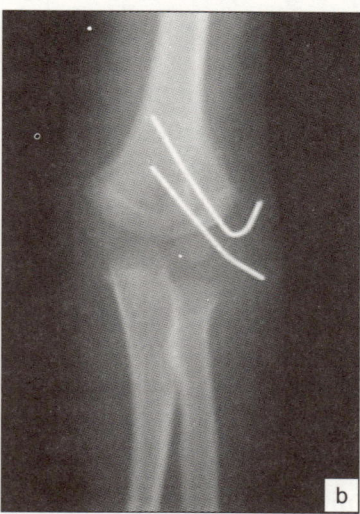

Fig. 23.8a,b. Pre and post-operative X-rays of a patient with fracture of lateral condyle humerus treated by open reduction and internal fixation with K-wires

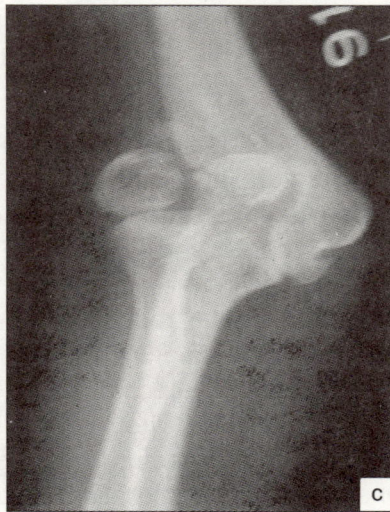

Fig. 23.8c. Non-union of fracture of lateral condyle with cubitus valgus

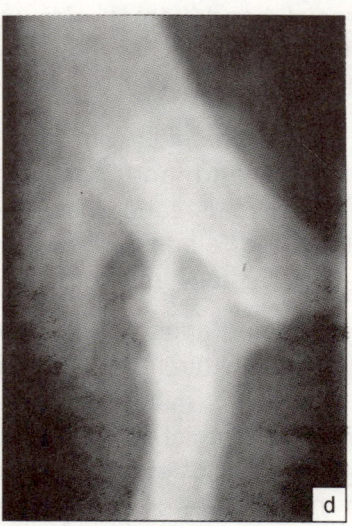

Fig. 23.8d. Fish tail deformity of elbow

- Lateral condylar overgrowth may be seen.
- Myositis ossificans may occur.
- Cubitus valgus occurs due to non union and/or epiphyseal growth arrest and can be progressive

Pulled elbow (Nursemaids elbow; *Guyrand's* elbow)

Pulled elbow occurs in young children (2–3 years old) due to ligamentous laxity. It is a hyperpronation injury, which leads to subluxation of radial head and partial displacement of the annular ligament. The parents give history of fall or pulling the child by holding his/her hands with forearm pronated. The child is often crying and refuses to use his upper limb, which hangs by the side of the body. Radiographs do not reveal any abnormalities and are not needed for diagnosis or treatment. Treatment consists of supination of the forearm with elbow flexed. The resumption of hand usage by the patient is immediate. No after care is required.

Fracture of Radial Neck

Fractures of radial neck occur in children. Metaphyseal compression is most common but often these injuries are type II epiphyseal injuries. These fractures may be associated with other injuries around elbow in almost half the cases.

Mechanism of injury This injury is caused by fall on the outstretched hand.

Classification Radial neck fractures can be undisplaced or displaced. Displaced fractures with the tilt of radial head from horizontal less than 30° are treated differently from those with more than 30° tilt.

Evaluation Patient presents with history of fall on the outstretched hand and pain in the elbow following that. There is tenderness over the lateral aspect of the elbow. Elbow and forearm movements are painfully restricted.

Imaging Plain radiographs confirm the diagnosis and displacement of the fragment (Fig. 23.9a,b). Diagnosis is extremely difficult in a child younger than 3 years when radial head is not visualized on x-rays. High index of suspicion is required for diagnosis in these cases.

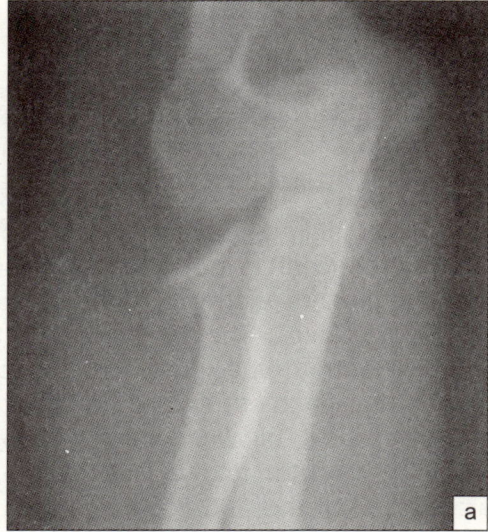

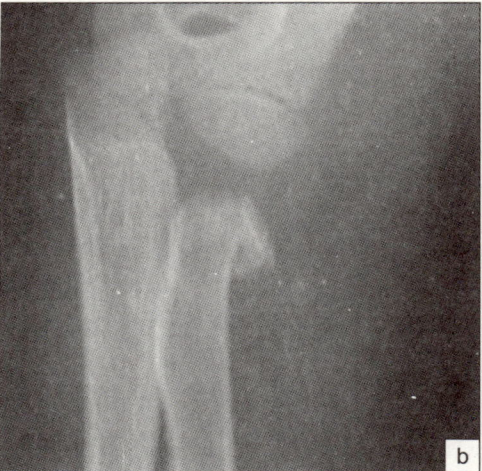

Fig. 23.9.   (a) Fracture of radial neck (angulation more than 45°) and (b) completely displaced fracture

Treatment   Undisplaced fractures and fractures with less than 30° tilt of the radial head are treated conservatively in a plaster slab for two weeks.

Greater displacement is treated by manipulation to reduce the fracture under anesthesia. With the elbow extended a varus stress is applied to the elbow that one hand and the radial head is pushed into place with the fingers of the other hand. Failing manipulative reduction, open reduction is performed. The fracture is usually stable after reduction and is treated in a POP slab for two weeks. Transcapitellar wire into the head and neck of radius to fix the fracture has high rate of complications (breakage, migration of wire) and should be avoided.

Injuries of the Forearm, Wrist and Hand

Forearm fractures

The radius and ulna are held together at the proximal and distal radio-ulnar joints, by annular ligament proximally, interosseous membrane along the length and the triangular fibrocartilage distally. These anatomical features do not allow only one forearm bone to fracture and shorten without disrupting either proximal or distal articulation between the two bones. The commonest fracture dislocation of this type is a fracture of ulna with dislocation of the radial head-the *Monteggia* fracture dislocation. A fracture of the shaft of radius associated with dislocation of inferior radio-ulnar joint is called *Galeazzi* fracture dislocation.

Fractures of the forearm bones are common in all age groups. In adults these fractures often result from high–energy trauma, often with associated musculo-skeletal and systemic injuries.

Mechanism of injury

Fractures of the radius and ulna can be caused by direct as well as indirect injury. Direct injury is commonly due to warding off blows, which commonly results in ulna fractures (Fig. 24.1). These fractures are transverse and may be compound. Indirect injury occurs due to fall on outstretched hand and produces oblique or spiral fractures. Monteggia fracture dislocation can be the result of hyperpronation (indirect) or night stick (direct) injuries.

Classification

Forearm fractures are classified according to the location or configuration of the fractures. They are also characterized by the presence of dislocation of radio-ulnar or radio-humeral joints.

Monteggia fractures are classified into four types by *Bado* (Table 24.1):

Table 24.1. Monteggia fracture dislocation: Bado's classification

Type	Ulnar angulation	Radial head dislocation	Mechanism of injury	Reduced in
I	Anterior	Anterior	Pronation hyperextension	Supination hyper flexion
II	Posterior	Posterior	Supination hyperflexion	Pronation hyperextension
III	Lateral	Lateral	Valgus force	Often needs ORIF
IV	Anterior	Anterior + fracture of upper 1/3rd Radius	Fall on outstretched hand, hyperpronation	Supination

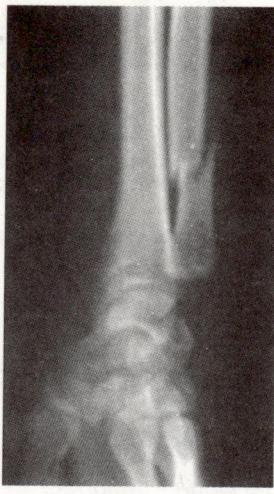

Fig. 24.1. X-Ray showing night stick fracture lower 1/3rd of ulna

1. *Anterior type* (Type I) has anterior dislocation of radial head with proximal third ulna fracture angulated anteriorly. This is the commonest type (60%) (Fig. 24.2a,b).

2. *Posterior type* (Type II) has posterior dislocation of radial head with proximal third ulna fracture angulated posteriorly (Fig. 24.2c).

3. *Lateral type* (Type III) has lateral radial head dislocation with lateral angulation of proximal ulnar fracture.

4. Type IV Proximal third both bone forearm fractures with anterior dislocation of the radial head.

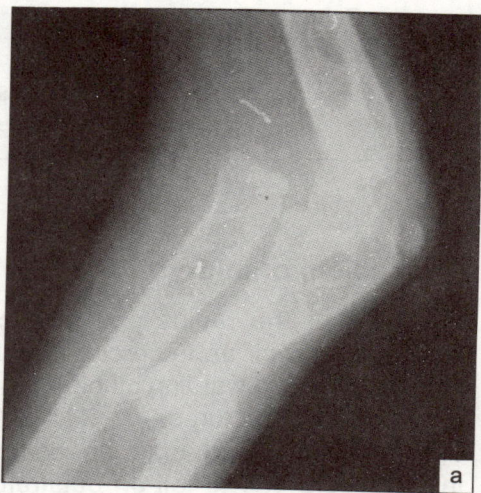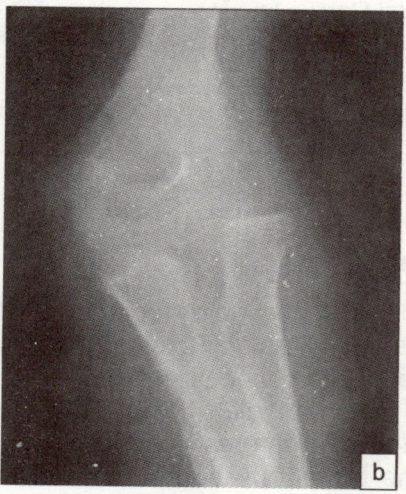

Fig. 24.2a,b. Type I Monteggia fracture dislocation. Note the anterior dislocation of radial head and fractured proximal one-third ulna with anterior angulation

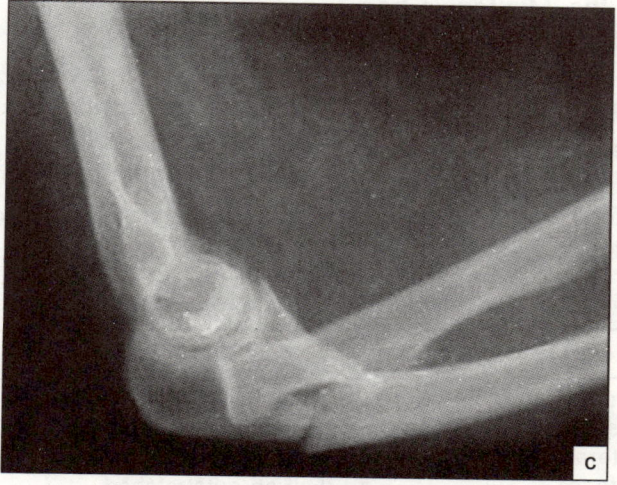

Fig. 24.2c. Type II Monteggia fracture dislocation. Note the posterior dislocation of radial head and fracture proximal 1/3rd ulna with posterior angulation

Monteggia Variants in children

Type I Plastic deformation of proximal one-third of ulna

Type II Greenstick fracture of proximal one-third of ulna

Type III Isolated radial head dislocation

Type IV Fracture of both bones forearm with radial fracture proximal to ulna.

Hume's fracture refers to the fracture of the proximal third of ulna with anterior dislocation of the radial head in children.

Evaluation

Patient presents with the history of injury to the forearm followed by pain, swelling and inability to move it. Deformity is obvious in most cases. Tenderness, crepitus and abnormal mobility are easily elicited. Skin should be carefully inspected for any breech. A detailed neurological and vascular examination must be done. In patients with high energy injuries, careful examination should be performed to rule out associated injuries.

Imaging Radiographs should include anteroposterior and lateral views of the forearm including the wrist and elbow to rule out disruption of distal or proximal joints.

It is extremely important to assess the rotational alignment of the forearm bones to prevent malunion with resultant loss of function. An AP view taken in full supination projects radial tuberosity medially (in full pronation, the tuberosity appears on the lateral side on AP view) and the radial styloid laterally. A lateral view in mid prone position depicts coronoid process anteriorly, radial tuberosity posteriorly (radial tuberosity disappears on AP view taken in mid prone position), the radial styloid anteriorly and the ulnar styloid posteriorly. These radiographic details help in ascertaining the rotational malalignment of the forearm bones following reduction. In addition, discrepancy between the diameter of fragments at the fracture site and difference in the width of the interosseous space between the proximal fragments and the distal fragments also suggest rotational malalignment.

It should be remembered that in the proximal third fractures of the forearm bones, the proximal fragment of radius is supinated by biceps while the distal fragment is pronated by pronator teres and pronator quadratus. In the mid or distal third fractures the proximal fragment is in neutral position as the biceps and pronator teres are both attached to it.

Greenstick fractures in children are seen on x-rays as breech of only one cortex. Torus fractures caused by compression force are seen as buckling of the cortex in metaphyseal region.

Treatment

The treatment of displaced fractures of both bones of the forearm in adults is open reduction and internal fixation (Fig. 24.3a-d). (Anatomical reduction and rigid fixation prevents any restriction of rotations and allows early mobilization). Fixation can be performed using 6 or 7 hole AO 3.5 mm DCPs. Primary bone grafting should be considered in cases where more than one-third cortical comminution is present. Sometimes fixation can also be achieved by intramedullary nails.

Conservative treatment is used in children, in undisplaced or minimally displaced fractures in adults, fractures in elderly and in patients in whom anaesthesia or surgery is contraindicated. Manipulation under anaesthesia is attempted in patients with displaced fracture, preferably under image intensifier and the forearm is immobilized

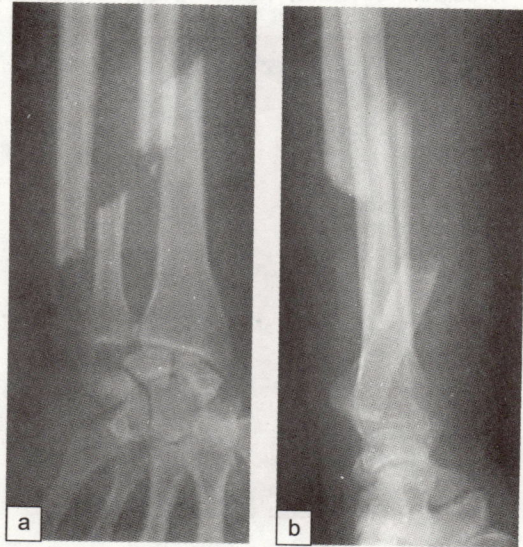

Fig. 24.3a,b. Preoperative X-rays showing fracture of both bones of the forearm

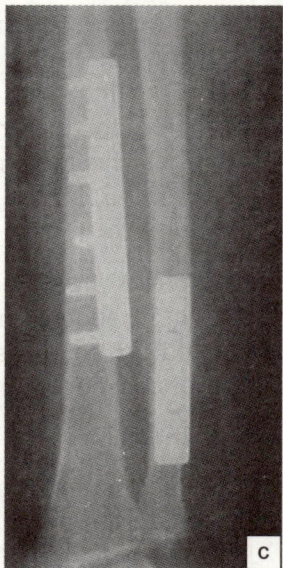
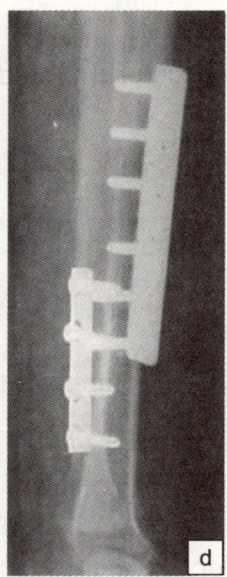

Fig. 24.3c,d.   Postoperative X-rays following open reduction and internal fixation

in above elbow cast with elbow in 90° flexion for 12–16 weeks. Close follow up must be done for these patients, as there is a very high incidence of redisplacement. Weekly x-rays should be taken during the first 3 weeks and plaster checked for loosening or breakage. Undisplaced fractures can be managed by replacing the long arm cast with a functional fracture brace with good interosseous moulding in the second week.

Monteggia fracture – dislocations are treated with open reduction and rigid internal fixation of ulna using AO 3.5 mm DCP. Radial head generally gets reduced spontaneously at this stage. (Fig. 24.4) Irreducible radial head is an indication for

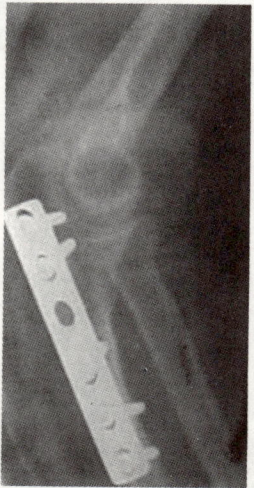

Fig. 24.4.   Post operative X-ray following open reduction and internal fixation of ulna following Monteggia Fracture Dislocation. Note the spontaneous reduction of radial head

open reduction to address infolding of the annular ligament, entrapment of posterior interosseous nerve or incarceration of the radial head behind the lateral epicondyle. After surgery the limb is immobilized in above elbow cast in 110° flexion (to keep the anteriorly unstable radial head reduced) except in type II Monteggia where posteriorly dislocated head is stable in less than 90° (usually 70°) flexion after the reduction. The immobilization is discontinued after 6 weeks.

Galeazzi fracture dislocation This consists of a fracture of the lower one-third of the radius with dislocation of the distal radioulnar joint (DRUJ) (Fig. 24.5a,b). It is often referred to as a fracture of necessity (cf lateral condylar physis injuries). This is because the fracture of distal radius is preferably immobilized in full pronation while the most common dislocation of the DRUJ is posterior which is stable only in full supination. The injury must therefore be treated with open reduction and internal fixation of radius (through an anterior approach using AO 3.5 mm DCP) and above elbow cast in supination for 6 weeks for the more common type with dorsal subluxation of ulna. Volar subluxation of ulna is treated with immobilization in pronation after internal fixation of the radius fracture.

Open fractures of the forearm bones are treated with debridement and irrigation. Primary fixation and delayed primary closure can be done in clean wounds without crushing and or contamination when presenting early. Type III compound

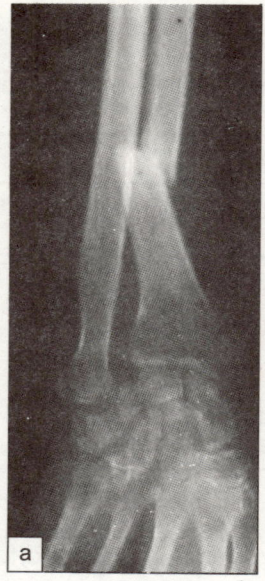 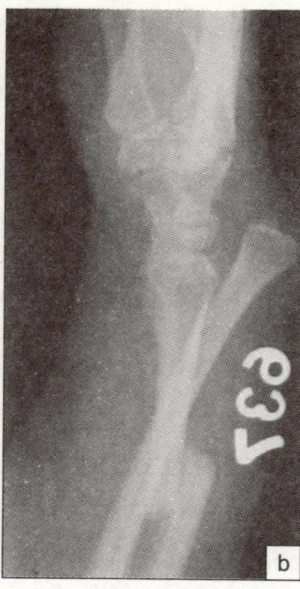

Fig. 24.5a,b.   Galeazzi Fracture Dislocation. Note the dorsal dislocation of the inferior radioulnar joint

fractures are treated by external fixation after debridement and irrigation.

Complications

1. Compartment syndrome may occur in patients with gunshot wounds, open fractures and fractures with vascular injury. High index of suspicion is needed for early diagnosis. Compartment pressures should be measured in doubtful cases. Early fasciotomy can preserve function.

2. Neurologic injury is otherwise uncommon in these fractures but posterior interosseous nerve palsy may complicate Monteggia fracture-dislocation.

3. Non union is seen after conservative treatment if immobilization is ineffective or discontinued too soon. Comminuted fractures and fractures which are not rigidly fixed at surgery are also prone to develop non-union. Treatment of non union is autogenous bone grafting and rigid internal fixation.

4. Malunion is common with conservative treatment. It leads to deformity and restricted rotations. Severe malunion may warrant recreating the fracture followed by anatomical reduction and rigid internal fixation. Malunited Monteggia fracture-dislocations present with persistent radial head dislocation. Treatment includes ulnar

osteotomy, plating after anatomic reduction and radial head excision in adults. In children, radial head should not be excised in order to avoid progressive instability at the elbow. Attempt should be made in these cases to openly reduce radial head and reconstruct the annular ligament using a fascial (*Bell-Tawse* procedure: fascial strip is taken from the tricipital fascia) or tendon graft.

5. Cross Union occurs in 3% cases and is common if the fractures are at the same level (most common in upper one-third fractures) or are fixed by single incision allowing the fracture hematomas to communicate, if the fractures are caused by high-energy injuries, cases with infection, associated closed head injuries, if bone grafts are placed on the interosseous membrane during surgery and also following radial head excision. Cross union (proximal radio-ulnar synostosis) occurs more commonly following Monteggia fracture-dislocation.

6. Hardware related complications such as loosening, infection, breakage etc.

7. Missed associated dislocation   Radial head dislocation is frequently missed when associated with proximal ulnar fractures. A useful clue is that normally in a lateral view of the elbow, throughout the range of flexion, a line along the longitudinal axis of the radius should always bisect capitellum.

Persistent radial head dislocation in adults is treated with radial head excision. Distal ulnar dislocation is often missed when associated with distal radius shaft fractures. Clues to dislocation of the distal radio-ulnar joint are styloid fracture, radial shortening more than 5 mm, dislocation of distal ulna on the lateral view and widening of the distal radio-ulnar joint on the anteroposterior view.

Persistent distal ulnar dislocation in adults becomes symptomatic and is treated with excision of the distal end of ulna (Darrach's procedure) leaving the ulnar styloid behind with the attachment of the ulnar collateral ligament.

Injuries of the Wrist

Fractures of the distal radius

General Considerations

Distal radius fractures constitute nearly three fourth

of all forearm fractures and one tenth of all bony injuries. Nearly one half of these fractures are intra-ollarticular, involving radiocarpal or distal radio-ulnar joint.

Mechanism of injury Distal radius fractures occur in older, osteoporotic patients due to low energy trauma such as fall on the outstretched hand. Younger patients sustain these fractures during sports or by high-energy injuries and therefore commonly have associated musculoskeletal and systemic injuries.

Mechanism of injury is very important determinant of the type of distal radius fracture. **Bending forces** cause Colles', Smith's fractures; **shearing forces** result in Barton's fracture, Reverse Barton's fractures, radial styloid fractures and simple articular fractures. **Compression forces** result in intra-articular fractures and complex articular fractures. In addition, there can be avulsion fractures and the combination of various types.

Classification Several classification systems are available. One of the most commonly used classifications is the one by Frykman. It classifies distal radius fractures into types I to VIII depending on extension into radio-carpal, distal radio-ulnar, or both joints, and presence or absence of ulnar styloid fractures (all even number classes have ulnar styloid fractures associated with distal radius fracture).

Type I is extra-articular fracture of distal radius with ulnar styloid intact;

Type II is Type I with styloid fracture

Type III is intraarticular fracture with extension into radiocarpal joint, with intact ulnar styloid

Type IV is same fracture with associated ulnar styloid fracture

Type V is distal radius fracture with extension into distal radio-ulnar joint – ulnar styloid intact

Type VI is same as type V with fracture of ulnar styloid

Type VII is distal radius fracture with extension into both radiocarpal as well as the distal radio-ulnar joints without ulnar styloid fracture

Type VIII is type VII with ulnar styloid fracture.

Universal classification by Sarmiento devised in

1990 is also quite popular and is shown in Table 24.2.

Table 24.2. Universal Classification of Distal Radius Fractures

Type	Description
Type I	Non articular undisplaced
Type II	Non articular displaced
Type III	Intra-articular undisplaced
Type IV	Intra-articular displaced
IV A:	Reducible, stable
IV B:	Reducible, unstable
IV C:	Irreducible, unstable

Evaluation

Patients are usually elderly (females more often than males) with history of trivial fall on the outstretched hand. Often there is past history of one or more osteoporotic fractures.

Wrist is deformed and may look like "*dinner fork*" after classical Colle's fracture or reverse of that following Smith's fracture. Tenderness can be localised to distal radius and styloid in addition to ulnar styloid and/or distal radio-ulnar joint. Skin should be carefully examined for any breech. Attempted movements at the wrist are painfully restricted. In younger patients with high-energy trauma, careful examination must be performed to rule out associated injuries.

Thorough neurovascular examination must be performed in all cases. Median nerve is most frequently injured in these fractures and must be examined for functional integrity.

Imaging Plain anteroposterior and lateral radiographs are generally adequate. Normal anteroposterior radiograph shows 23° inclination of the distal radial articular surface and the tip of the radial styloid is 11 mm distal to tip of the ulnar styloid. Normal lateral view shows a normal volar tilt of 11°.

When evaluating radiographs taken after reduction of the distal radius fracture it should be remembered that the following displacements are not acceptable :

a) More than 10° loss of volar tilt.

b) More than 1-2 mm articular step off.

c) Radius shortening more than 2 mm.

d) Persistent distal radio-ulnar joint dislocation.

e) Displacement of ulnar styloid fracture more than 4 mm.

Sophisticated imaging modalities are rarely required. Computerized Tomography helps in delineation of severe articular injuries and is the most effective method of imaging the damage to the distal radio-ulnar joint. Magnetic Resonance Imaging is useful in diagnosing associated soft tissue injuries such as triangular fibrocartilage injuries.

Principles of treatment of distal radius fractures include anatomic restoration of joint surface and radio-ulnar relationship, prevention of secondary displacement, achievement of union and regaining functional range of motion. Key factors determining the result after treatment are the quality and the stability of reduction (i.e. ability to maintain the reduced position in a cast) which is compromised by advanced age, significant osteoporosis, severe initial displacement (esp. dorsal tilt >20°, radial shortening > 5 mm),

metaphyseal comminution, intra-articular extension and associated ulnar fracture.

Distal radius fractures can be treated by a variety of methods such as conservative treatment (with plaster cast or Sarmiento's functional bracing), percutaneous pinning, external fixator or open reduction and internal fixation.

Conservative treatment is indicated for undisplaced and displaced stable fractures with weekly radiographs to detect any redisplacement of the fracture in the plaster.

Percutaneous pinning is suited for maintaining the volar tilt and is useful mainly for extraarticular fractures. It does not prevent shortening in comminuted fractures. Percutaneous pinning can be used as an adjunct to external fixator or ORIF also.

ORIF is ideally suited for marginal or partial articular fractures typically Volar Barton fractures (Fig. 24.6a-d). ORIF can also be used for complex intraarticular fractures.

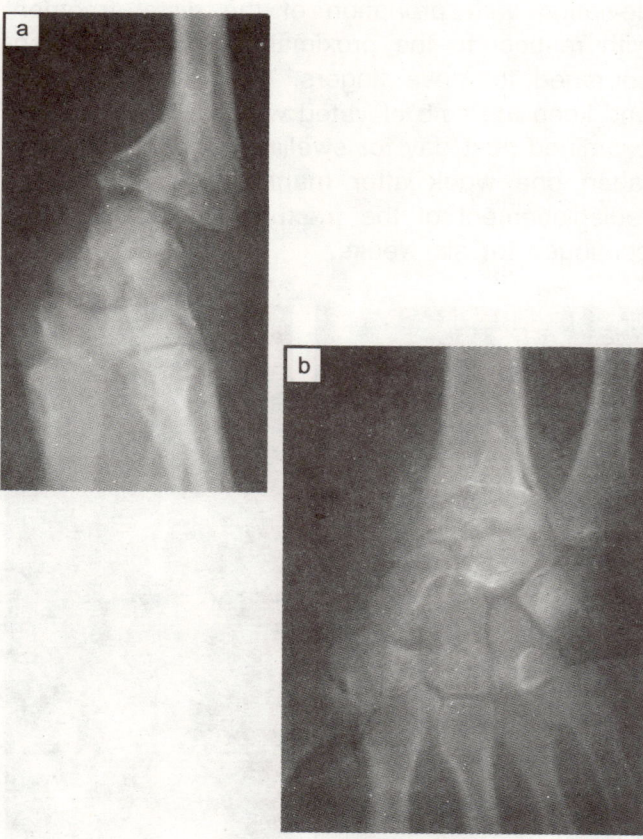
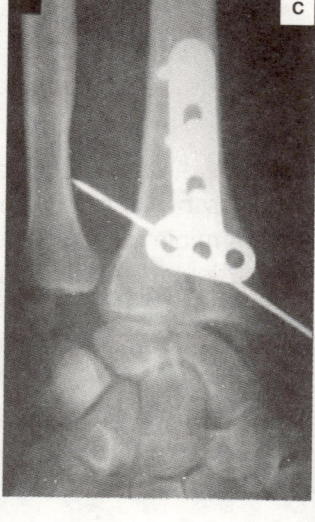
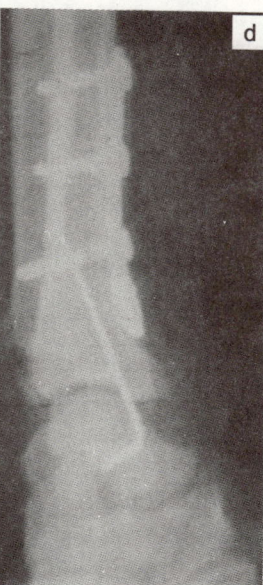

Fig. 24.6a,b. Volar Barton Fracture (Lower end radius). Note the volar subluxation of wrist in Fig. 24.6A

Fig. 24.6c,d.   Volar Barton fracture shown in fig. 24.6a,b treated by buttress plating. Note the K-wire used to stablise radial styloid fragment

External fixation is the treatment of choice for unstable extra-articular fractures with comminution and with unstable comminuted intra-articular fractures (Fig. 24.6e). External fixators have a high incidence of complications (15% to 60%) including pin tract infections, pin loosening and stiffness of wrist and hand.

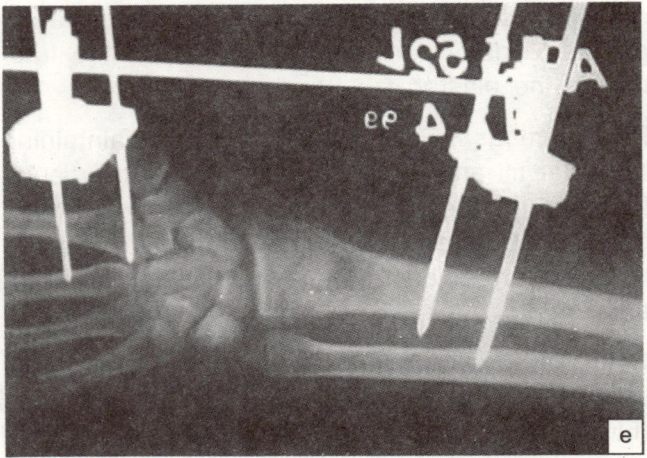

Fig. 24.6e. Unstable comminuted intraarticular distal radius fracture treated by external fixation

Complex distal radius fractures may require a combination using K-wire fixation, external fixation and ORIF.

Recently arthroscopy assisted fixation of the intra-articular distal radius fractures is being performed at some centers. Arthroscopy is minimally invasive, it allows visualization of the articular surface and helps in anatomical reduction of intra-articular fractures. It also allows diagnosis of soft tissue injuries such as ligament injuries and injuries to the triangular fibrocartilage.

Specific Distal Radius Injuries

Colles' Fracture

Colles' fracture is classically a fracture of the distal radius within 2.5 cm of the wrist at the meta-diaphyseal junction with a characteristic deformity. Most commonly it affects elderly osteoporotic women following a fall on the outstretched hand. The classic Colles' fracture has six displacements namely, dorsal displacement, dorsal tilt, lateral displacement, lateral tilt, impaction (or proximal migration) and, supination. These displacements give the deformity its typical "*dinner fork*" appear-

ance. The distal fragment while displacing often avulses the ulnar styloid to which it is attached by triangular fibrocartilage.

Plain radiographs show all the deformities (Fig. 24.7a,b) except the rotation. Ulnar styloid is commonly avulsed in displaced fractures while an intact ulnar styloid in these cases implies tear of the triangular fibrocartilage.

Treatment of Colles' fracture is conservative in the majority of cases. Undisplaced fractures are treated in a below elbow cast for six weeks. Displaced fractures are treated by manipulation and Colles' cast. Criteria for acceptable reduction are mentioned before and include restoration of length (less than 2 mm shortening of radius), ulnar tilt and volar tilt (less than 10° dorsal tilt on the lateral view). For manipulation the patient is anaesthetised and traction applied along the line of the forearm with the elbow flexed at 90° to disimpact the fracture while an assistant applies counter traction at the arm. Once the fracture is disimpacted the displacements are reduced and Colles' cast applied in palmar flexion and ulnar deviation with pronation of the distal fragment with respect to the proximal. The patient is encouraged to move fingers, elbow, and shoulder and keep the limb elevated with a sling. Patient is examined next day for swelling. Check x-rays are taken one week after manipulation to rule out redisplacement of the fracture. Immobilization is continued for six weeks.

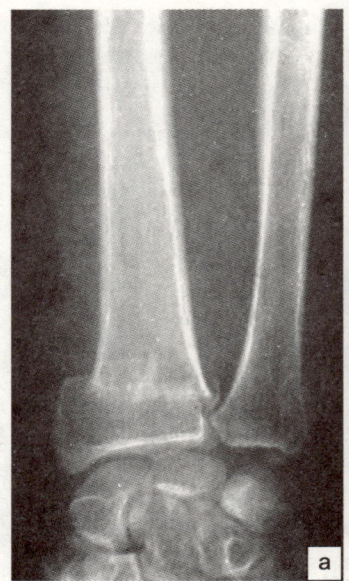
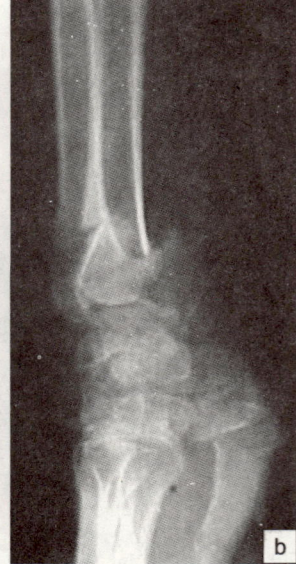

Fig. 24.7a,b. X-ray appearance of Colles' fracture

Comminuted fractures often make achieving and/ or maintaining the reduction difficult. These cases can be treated by percutaneous K-wire fixation or external fixator. External fixators can be non-bridging (i.e. stabilizing only the fracture fragments without spanning the wrist) or bridging (proximal pins in the radius shaft while distal pins are passed in the second metacarpal). Bridging fixators can consist of connecting rods between the pins without a joint or may include a ball and socket joint at the level of wrist to allow early movements and avoid stiffness.

In young patients with displaced fractures, open reduction and internal fixation using specially designed T plates and screws can be performed with good results.

Complications

Complications are quite common with Colles' fracture and diligent care and caution must be exercised to prevent these complications and treat them early upon their occurrence.

1. Malunion with manus valgus and prominence of the distal ulna is a common complication. It is commonly seen with comminuted fractures or with failed conservative treatment (inadequate reduction or inability to maintain the reduction). The other problems include malunion with residual impaction (leading to radial shortening), dorsal tilt (restricted palmar flexion). Manus valgus leads to restriction of ulnar deviation at the wrist. The patient develops ulnar impingement syndrome due to the relative lengthening of the ulna and consequent ulnocarpal impingement. Pain on the ulnar aspect of the wrist can also occur due to triangular fibrocartilage complex injuries. Most cases however are symptom free and do not need any treatment, especially the patients who are elderly with low demand function. Patients with pain and/or restriction of forearm rotations and young patients with severe deformity are treated with corrective osteotomy, ORIF and excision of distal 1 inch of ulna. In elderly patients with symptoms, only distal ulnar excision may suffice.

2. Stiffness of the fingers and shoulder is quite common after Colles' fracture despite adequate physiotherapy. Early physiotherapy of the joints should be encouraged.

3. Neurologic injury: Median nerve is most commonly involved. The injuries are closed and usually there is neuropraxia due to fracture displacement or hematoma. Expectant treatment is the method of choice to manage these injuries. Sometimes, extreme flexion at the wrist following manipulation and plaster application (*Cotton Loader's* position) can cause median nerve compression.

4. Sudeck's Osteodystrophy may occur in 0.1 – 10.3% cases following Colles' fracture. Patient has pain, swelling, discoloration and stiffness of the finger joints. Wrist x-rays show diffuse osteoporosis if the affliction is of more than a few weeks' duration. Early physiotherapy, along with drugs to relieve pain can relieve most patients. Stellate ganglion block may be needed for the resistant cases.

5. Rupture of Extensor Pollicis Longus (EPL) may follow Colles' fracture. Usually it occurs late, about *2* months after the fracture, and is attributed to the attrition rupture of EPL due to the roughness at the fracture site. However, it may sometimes occur early (7–14 days) and even in undisplaced fracture (1% cases). An ischemic theory is postulated for those cases.

   The treatment is transfer of extensor indicis to distal stump of EPL as the ruptured ends of EPL are not suitable for end to end repair.

6. Associated Injuries: Colles' fracture may sometimes be complicated by associated injuries such as the fracture of the scaphoid. Undisplaced scaphoid fractures are treated in plaster and take much longer to heal as compared to Colles' fracture. Displaced scaphoid fractures may be treated by open reduction and Herbert screw or K-wire fixation.

Smith's fracture

Smith's fracture is more like a reverse Colles' fracture. It is sustained by fall on the back of the hand and the distal fragment is displaced anteriorly, tilted anteriorly and impacted (proximally displaced). The fracture is treated by manipulation under anaesthesia and immobilization in an above elbow cast in supination and dorsiflexion. Weekly check x-rays are required during the first 3 weeks to look for redisplacement, which is treated by remanipulation. Immobilization is continued for 6 weeks. Unstable reduction as in cases with severe comminution can be managed by percutaneous K-wire fixation and plaster cast application or with an external fixator.

Barton's fractures

Barton's fractures are the radial rim fractures or the partial articular fractures. These fractures may involve the volar rim with volar displacement of part of the distal radial articular surface with the carpus: the so-called *Volar Barton fracture*. This is by far much more common of the two types. Dorsal rim fractures with dorsal displacement of the part of radial articular surface and the carpus are called the *Dorsal Barton fractures* (Fig. 24.8a).

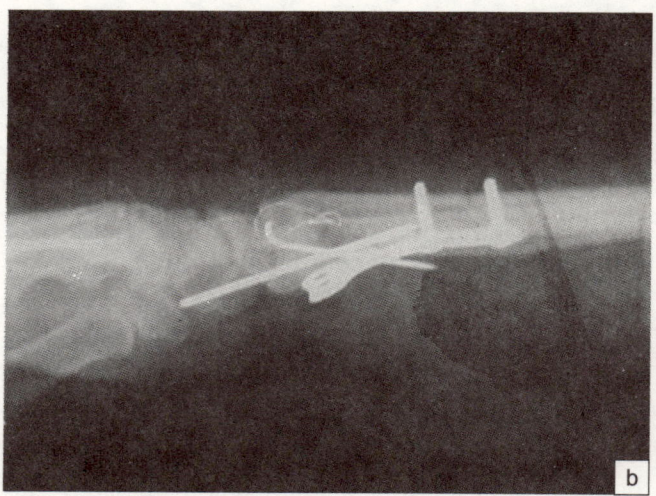

Fig. 24.8b. Volar Barton fracture treated with T-plate and K-wire fixation

Radial Styloid Fracture is also called *Chauffeur's fracture* (Fig. 24.8c) as it is sometimes caused by kickback from an engine-starting handle. Fracture is partially articular and has an oblique configuration. The fragment is usually only slightly displaced. A below elbow plaster cast applied for 6 weeks is adequate. Displaced fractures should be treated by open reduction and internal fixation using kirschner wires or lag screw. Persistent displacement is likely to lead to wrist osteoarthritis. Associated injuries must be diligently looked for in the patients with radial styloid fractures so as not to miss serious trans-styloid, perilunate dislocations.

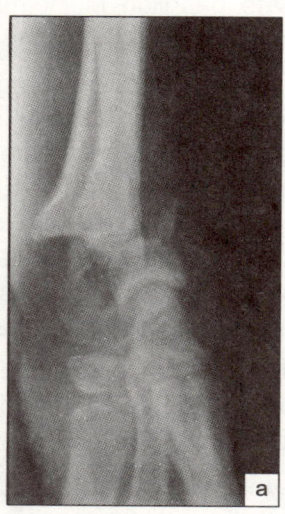

Fig. 24.8a. Dorsal Barton fracture. Note the dorsal subluxation of wrist

Treatment of Volar Barton's fracture: In most cases conservative treatment is attempted first by reduction of the fracture and immobilization of the limb in above elbow plaster cast in supination and dorsiflexion (slight palmarflexion according to some) for eight weeks. Inability to achieve or maintain reduction is an indication for open reduction and internal fixation using specially designed T- or Ellis plates (Fig. 24.8b). Fractures with marked comminution can be treated by external fixator for 6 weeks.

Complications of Volar Barton fracture include malunion (due to difficulty of achieving and maintaining the reduction) and osteoarthritis of the wrist joint.

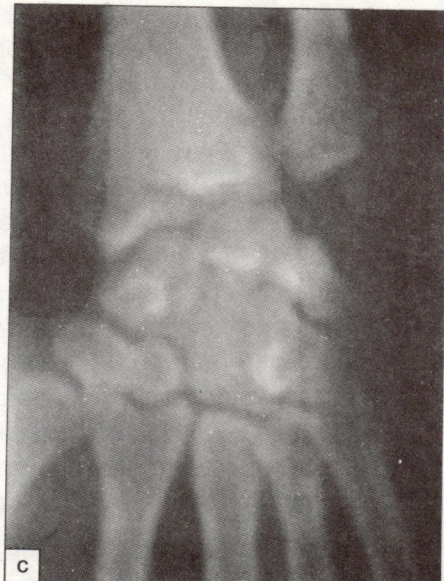

Fig. 24.8c. Fracture of the radial styloid. Note the fracture of ulnar styloid

Injuries of Distal Radio Ulnar Joint (DRUJ)

Dislocation of the DRUJ may occur with or without the distal radius fracture. Dorsal dislocation is by far most common and is caused by fall on the hand with pronated forearm. Injury is evident on lateral radiographs and is treated by reduction (by supinating the forearm) and immobilization in an above elbow plaster with forearm in supination and wrist neutral. Volar subluxation is uncommon, is caused by fall on supinated hand and is reduced by pronating the forearm.

Irreducible DRUJ dislocation may be due to the entrapment of extensor carpi ulnaris, TFC or fractured ulnar styloid in the joint and needs open reduction.

Instability of the DRUJ may occur late after distal radius fracture and is often disabling. It can be due to avulsion of radial attachment of Triangular Fibrocartilage (TFC), massive tears of TFC or avulsion of ulnar styloid process.

Clinically, patient has weak grip, limited forearm rotations and instability. Clinical and radiologic assessment of the reduction and stability of the DRUJ at the time of treatment of distal radius fracture is essential. Management is by distal ulnar excision (Darrach) or distal radioulnar joint arthrodesis and creation of proximal ulnar pseudarthrosis (*Sauve-Kapandji Procedure*).

Distal Radius Epiphyseal injury

Distal radius epiphyseal injuries are common in adolescents. These are usually Salter Harris type II injuries and occur following fall on the outstretched hand. Diagnosis is easily made on radiographs. Anatomic reduction is mandatory for satisfactory results. Reduction should be done early. Displaced fractures are treated by manipulative reduction and below elbow Colles' plaster cast for 3 – 4 weeks. Growth disturbance is rare.

Fracture of the Scaphoid

Scaphoid is the most commonly fractured carpal bone. The injury most commonly occurs in the young adults. Scaphoid has a unique blood supply, which enters the bone from dorsal and distal direction. The proximal pole of the scaphoid therefore is at risk of avascular necrosis following fractures.

Mechanism of injury

Scaphoid fracture occurs due to fall on the outstretched hand with forced dorsiflexion of the wrist. Scaphoid fracture may also occur due to "kickback" from the starting handle of the engines.

Classification

Scaphoid fractures are classified by level (distal pole or tuberosity (Fig. 24.9a), waist (Fig. 24.9b) or proximal pole fractures), direction (horizontal/oblique), stability (stable/unstable) or chronicity (acute, delayed union, non-union). Herbert defined stable fractures as fractures of the tubercle and hairline fractures of the waist. Unstable fractures

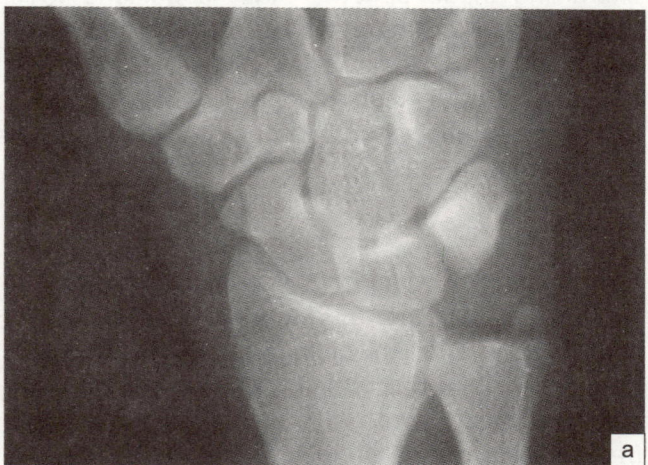

Fig. 24.9a.   Fracture of tuberosity of scaphoid

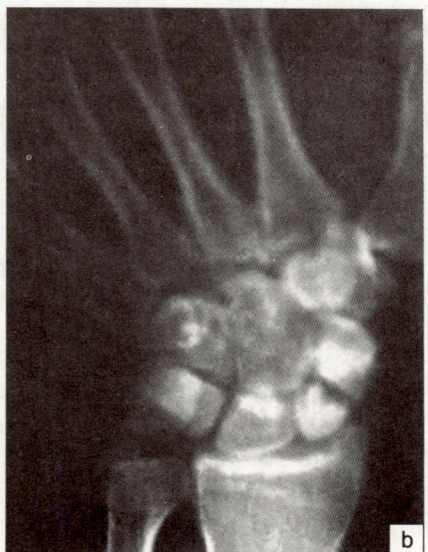

Fig. 24.9b.   Fracture of waist of Scaphoid

include oblique fractures of the distal third, displaced fractures of the waist, proximal pole fractures, fractures associated with carpal dislocations and, comminuted fractures.

Evaluation

Presentation in a case of scaphoid fracture is often subtle. A high index of suspicion is necessary to avoid missing the diagnosis. Patient presents with a history of fall followed by pain in the wrist. Attempted movements especially radial deviation at the wrist are painful but usually not restricted. Resisted pinch between thumb and the index finger on the affected side is painful. There is tenderness in the *anatomic snuffbox* and over the scaphoid tuberosity anteriorly. When clinically examining these patients other conditions which can give rise to tenderness in the anatomic snuffbox should be kept in mind. These include wrist sprain, injury to scapholunate ligament, fracture of the radial styloid and Bennett's fracture of the thumb metacarpal.

Imaging

Imaging for the scaphoid should include an AP view of the wrist (preferably in ulnar deviation), a lateral view and an oblique view of the wrist. These x-rays taken initially at the time of injury diagnose only two third of the cases. If the fracture scaphoid is suspected strongly but the x-rays are normal, patient is given a scaphoid cast for 2 weeks. The x-rays are repeated out of plaster after two weeks and if fracture scaphoid is present, it is usually discernible on the x-rays by this time.

For suspected fracture of scaphoid with normal radiographs, other imaging modalities are helpful. MRI is the most sensitive investigation to diagnose fracture scaphoid early. CT scan, tomography or bone scan can also detect fracture of the scaphoid when the radiographs are normal.

On plain x-rays, scaphoid fractures are usually not displaced. However, if displaced, associated carpal injuries such as trans-scaphoid perilunate dislocations must be looked for. A displaced scaphoid fracture is deemed unstable when it is displaced more than 1 mm, is angulated more than 15°, when on lateral x-ray of wrist scapholunate angle is more than 45° or the capitolunate angle is more than 15°.

Treatment

Most cases are undisplaced and do not need reduction. Fracture is immobilized in a below elbow plaster applied in "*Glass holding position*" (with wrist in slight extension and thumb abducted and pronated). The plaster includes the thumb upto base of the nail. The plaster is continued for 8–12 weeks.

Displaced fractures are treated by open reduction and internal fixation using specially designed Herbert screw or kirschner wires.

Complications

1. **Avascular necrosis** occurs when scaphoid with predominantly distal entry of blood vessels fractures through waist or proximal pole rendering the proximal fragment avascular (Fig. 24.9c). Almost one-third fractures of the proximal pole get avascular necrosis. Avascular necrosis sets in immediately after injury but may be visible on plain x-rays only after 1 to 2 months. Avascular scaphoid gradually collapses and leads to radiocarpal osteoarthritis. A painful stiff wrist often results. A symptomatic osteoarthritic wrist due to avascular necrosis of scaphoid is treated by excision of the avascular fragment of the scaphoid (if less than one fourth of scaphoid) or the radial styloid.

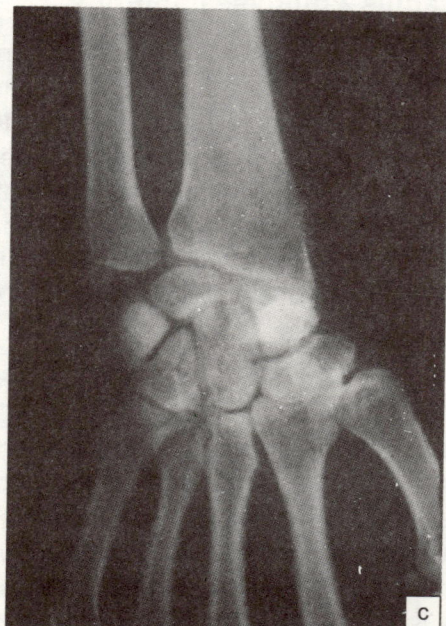

Fig. 24.9c. Avascular necrosis of proximal pole of scaphoid following fracture

2. Delayed union, and non union occur frequently and are managed by cortico-cancellous bone grafting (commonly from the iliac crest) with or without internal fixation with a Herbert screw and plaster cast application for 8–12 weeks.

3. Sudeck's Osteodystrophy

4. Osteoarthritis of the wrist occurs usually following avascular necrosis or non union. It can be treated conservatively with an orthotic device and NSAID's. Recalcitrant cases are treated by scaphoid excision with four corner fusion, proximal row carpectomy or wrist arthrodesis.

Other Carpal Bone Fractures

Triquetral fractures are common fractures and are caused by dorsiflexion and ulnar deviation force impinging ulnar styloid into triquetral and shearing off a flake. These fractures are mostly asymptomatic. Fracture is seen on lateral x-ray of the wrist. CT scan is extremely useful for diagnosing subtle fractures not apparent on plain x-rays.

Patient is treated in a below elbow cast for 3 weeks.

Hook of the hamate fractures are common among golfers and tennis players. These fractures can also result from a direct injury to the palm or following a fall on the outstretched hand. Patient presents with pain and tenderness over the hamate with or without ulnar nerve symptoms. Carpal tunnel view shows these fractures well but CT scan is the imaging modality of choice in these cases.

Injury is treated in a below elbow plaster cast for 6 weeks. If non union occurs and is symptomatic, excision of the fragment is treatment of choice.

Capitate Fracture

Capitate fractures are commonly associated with perilunate dislocations and scaphoid fractures. The hyperextension injury to the wrist results in fracture of the neck of capitate along with the fracture of wrist or the scaphoid. The proximal fragment of capitate often rotates by 180°.

High index of suspicion is required to diagnose these injuries. X-rays and CT scan confirm the diagnosis. Open reduction and internal fixation is the treatment of choice in these cases. Non union

and avascular necrosis are the common complications and are treated by scapho-lunato-capitate arthrodesis.

Carpal ligament injuries

Injury to the carpal ligaments leads to carpal instabilities wherein normal carpal alignment is lost. These instabilities can occur early or late after the injuries and can be static (present at rest and diagnosed on standard x-rays) or dynamic (routine radiographs are normal and instability occurs during the movements/use of hand).

Dorsal Intercalated Segmental Instability (DISI) occurs when scapholunate ligament is torn and lunate is tilted dorsally to an extended position. This is the commonest form of carpal instability.

Volar intercalated Segmental Instability (VISI) results from injury to the lunato-triquetral ligament. The lunate gets flexed in these cases.

Mechanism of Injury

Dorsiflexion, ulnar deviation and inter carpal supination lead to progressive carpal ligament injury. Progressive injury to scapholunate, capitolunate, and triquetrolunate ligaments can lead to progressive perilunate instability. In the perilunate dislocation, the lunate remains in place while the rest of carpus dislocates and comes to lie dorsally. However, in the final stage of perilunate dislocation the dorsal radiocarpal ligament is also torn and the lunate dislocates. The lunate may dislocate anteriorly or posteriorly.

Anterior dislocation is by far most common.

Imaging

Plain wrist radiographs can diagnose static carpal instabilities. It is important to note alignment of carpal bones and height of the carpus. Posteroanterior x-ray of the wrist can demonstrate scapholunate dissociation (injury to scapholunate ligament) as increased scapholunate interval (>2mm *Terry-Thomas sign*), foreshortened scaphoid and "*ring*" sign which is cortical outline of the scaphoid tuberosity.

Direction in, which distal articular surface of lunate is facing and its relationship with capitate help to decide the diagnosis and type of lunate dislocation or perilunate dislocation. Lunate dislocation shows volar tilt of distal articular surface ("*spilled tea cup sign*"). A dislocated lunate looks quadrilateral, which has prolonged distal projection instead of the normal crescent shape.

Lateral radiographs also divulge useful information about carpal instabilities. Note is made of scapholunate (normal 30°–60°; DISI >70°), capitolunate (normal up to 15°; increased in DISI) and radiolunate (normal up to 10°, increased in lunate dislocation) angles. Clenched fist postero-anterior x-rays can sometimes diagnose subtle carpal instabilities, which are not apparent on standard x-rays.

Evaluation of a Patient with Perilunate Dislocation

Patient presents with history of injury followed by pain and limitation of movements. High index of suspicion is required to diagnose these injuries. Associated musculo-skeletal and systemic injuries are common and must be looked for. Median nerve is frequently injured in cases with volar dislocation of lunate. Therefore, median nerve injury must be looked for.

Diagnosis of these injuries is based mainly on radiographs. Associated fractures of scaphoid, radial styloid and/or capitate must be looked for. Widely displaced scaphoid fragments following fracture must always raise suspicion of an associated perilunate dislocation.

Treatment of perilunate dislocations is closed reduction. Longitudinal traction is given to the wrist using finger trap traction.

The wrist is dorsiflexed. Direct pressure is exerted on to the dorsally dislocated capitate to reduce it onto the lunate. The wrist is then palmarflexed and immobilized in plaster cast for 6 weeks. In unstable cases, closed reduction can be supplemented by percutaneous pinning. Open reduction is required for irreducible dislocations – acute or chronic (Fig. 24.9d,e).

Complications

Incidence of complications is high with nearly half of the patients developing some complication.

Median nerve compression occurs due to compression by anteriorly dislocated lunate. Early reduction leads to spontaneous recovery of the nerve function.

Avascular necrosis of lunate can occur following lunate dislocation. Subsequent collapse of lunate over the years leads to osteoarthritis and stiffness of the intercarpal and wrist joints.

Stiffness of wrist and reduced function (pinch and grip strength) are common complications.

Osteoarthritis of the intercarpal and wrist joints is a frequent complication of carpal ligament injuries and perilunate dislocation.

Sudeck's osteodystrophy may commonly occur following the carpal ligament injuries.

Missed dislocations are difficult to treat. Closed reduction is not possible after one week. Open reduction is required in these cases. Avascular necrosis and median nerve injury may occur.

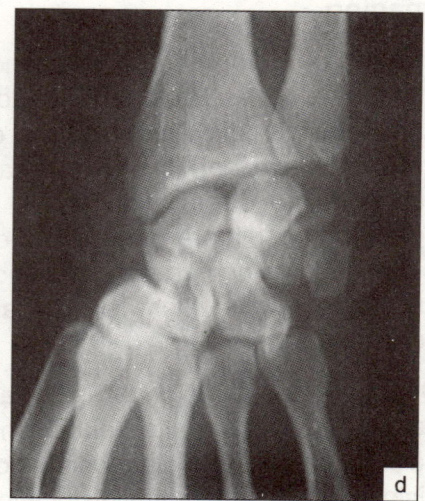 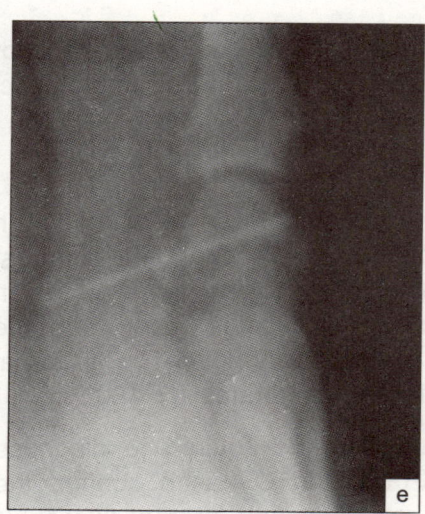

Fig. 24.9d,e. Post operative X-rays following ORIF of Trans scaphoid Perilunate dislocation with K-wire

Stiffness and poor function are common outcomes.

Fractures and Dislocations of Hand

General Considerations

Certain important principles must be followed while treating the injuries of the hand. First and foremost is the assessment of the injury to neurovascular structures, tendons and the soft tissue envelope (skin, subcutaneous tissues). Secondly, radiographic assessment must be made about the configuration of the fracture fragments, alignment of fractures and stability of the fracture. Acceptable alignment is up to 10° angulation in shaft or up to 45° angulation in neck of metacarpal, no rotational malalignment and at least 50% bony contact. Unstable fractures are comminuted fractures, spiral or oblique fractures, multiple fractures and displaced articular fractures.

Plain radiographs are adequate to assess the fractures. However, radiographic evidence of healing may occur very late and mobilization of hand joints should be done after 3 weeks for phalangeal fractures and after four weeks for metacarpal fractures.

Splinting of the hand should be in "position of function" as far as possible i.e. wrist extension (30°), metacarpophalangeal joint flexion (70°), extension at IP joints and abduction and apposition of thumb. Metacarpophalangeal joint, should never be immobilized in extension. Immobilization should be continued only for the minimum period required. Uninjured areas of hand should not be immobilized as far as possible. In open fractures irrigation, debridement to remove necrotic or foreign material and stabilization of fractures should be done.

Fractures of the Metacarpals

1. Thumb metacarpal fractures

a) Intraarticular fractures

i)   Bennett's fracture

Bennett's fracture is an intra-articular fracture-dislocation where the fracture line is vertical and extends into the first carpometacarpal joint (trapezometacarpal joint). The small volar ulnar fragment is displaced proximally and radially by the pull of the abductor pollicis longus (APL).

Mechanism of Injury   Injury occurs due to an axial force directed through the long axis of the thumb as in a fall or below on the clenched first (as in boxers). Forced abduction of the thumb metacarpal may also lead to these fractures.

Clinically patient has pain, tenderness and swelling over the radial aspect of the base of the first metacarpal. Attempted movements of the thumb are painful. The injury must be differentiated from the scaphoid fractures. In Bennett's the tenderness is not in the anatomical snuff box but distal to it.

Imaging of this fracture needs a true AP view and a true lateral view of the thumb metacarpal. Diagnosis is confirmed and size of proximal fragment and displacement of distal fragment are noted (Fig. 24.10a).

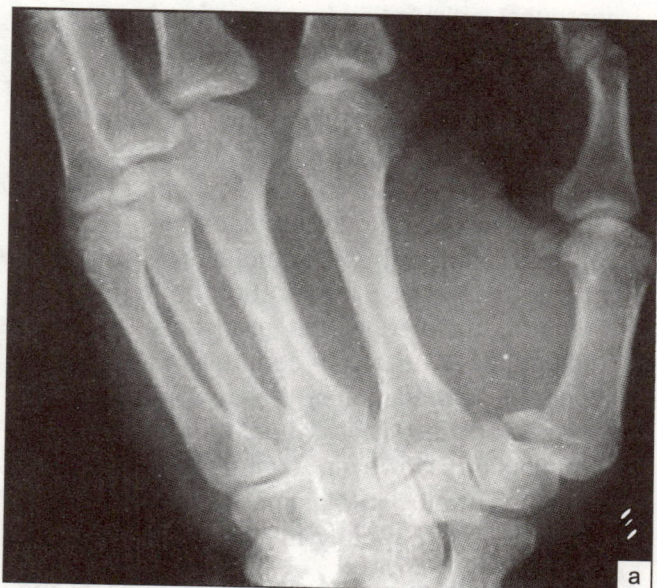

Fig. 24.10a. X-rays of a patient with Bennett's fracture

Treatment consists of closed reduction (Fig. 24.10b) and immobilization. Reduction is achieved by traction to the thumb followed by its abduction. Direct pressure is then applied to the lateral aspect of base of the thumb. A thumb spica is then applied for 4 to 6 weeks. Weekly check x-ray should be taken for 2 to 3 weeks to check for redisplacement. Percutaneous K-wires can be used to stabilize the fracture in cases with unstable reduction. Open reduction and

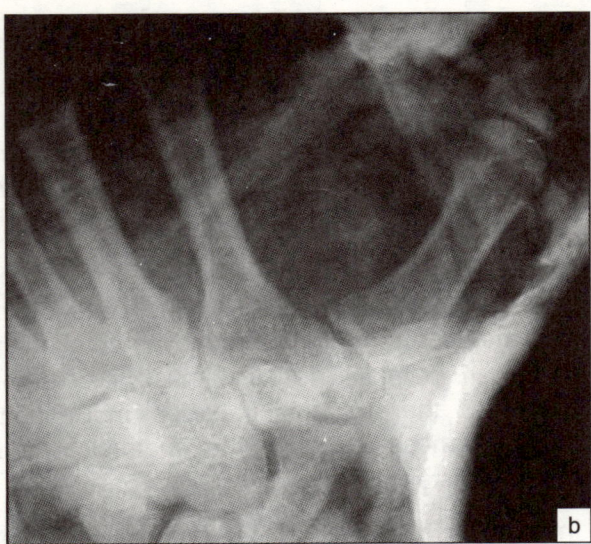

Fig. 24.10b. Same patient after closed reduction and thumb spica application

internal fixation are indicated for irreducible fractures, for unacceptable reductions (with non-congruent articular surface) or where reduction is unstable. An AO small fragment screw or two kirschner wires are used for fixation.

ii) Rolando's fracture

Rolando's fracture is a Y or T shaped fracture of the base of the thumb metacarpal extending vertically into the trapezio-metacarpal joint. The mechanism and presentation is similar to Bennett's fracture but the prognosis is worse. Restoration of articular congruity is the most important determinant of the outcome. ORIF is the method of choice when there is minimal comminution. However, comminuted fractures should be treated in plaster cast or in external fixator followed by early motion of the joint.

Complications of intraarticular fractures of the thumb metacarpal are stiffness and secondary osteoarthritis resulting from articular incongruity.

b) **Extra-articular fractures**

Extra-articular fractures of the base of thumb metacarpal in adults can be transverse or oblique and undisplaced or displaced. These fractures are treated by closed manipulation and plaster for 6 weeks.

In **children**, these fractures are usually greenstick and are treated by manipulation and plaster immobilization for 4 weeks.

Thumb metacarpal is extremely mobile and slight malunions are well tolerated and do not compromise function. Gross displacements are corrected and plaster applied.

2. Index, Long, Ring and Little finger metacarpal fractures

General Considerations

The index and long finger metacarpals are fixed and relatively stable. These metacarpals cannot compensate for more than 10° of angulation because of their relative immobility. The ring and little finger metacarpals are more mobile (with 20° and 30° movements at base respectively) and therefore angulation from 20 to 30 degrees is acceptable in these metacarpals. Greater displacements are acceptable at the metaphysis and neck as compared to the shaft.

Fracture configuration determines the displacement of metacarpal fractures. Spiral fractures lead to rotational malalignment while the oblique fractures lead to overriding (Fig. 24.11a,b). The transverse fractures tend to angulate dorsally due to the pull of the interossei (Fig. 24.11c).

Types of Metacarpal Fractures Metacarpal fractures are divided into the fractures of the head, neck, shaft and base.

Mechanism of injury Metacarpal fractures can occur due to axial force (as in boxing) or due to crush injuries. Crush injuries may lead to the fracture of multiple metacarpals with severe soft tissue injures. These fractures are often open.

Evaluation Patient with metacarpal fractures presents with pain, tenderness, swelling and deformity. Attempted movements are painful. Soft tissues and distal neurovascular status should be carefully assessed. Associated injuries must be looked for.

Metacarpal head fractures These intraarticular fractures are uncommon. Third metacarpal is most commonly involved. Crushing is the most common causative mechanism; open fractures therefore, are common. Treatment is open reduction and internal fixation to restore anatomy. Comminuted fractures are treated by external fixation and early movements of the joint. Stiffness of the MCP joint is the most common complication and significantly compromises hand function.

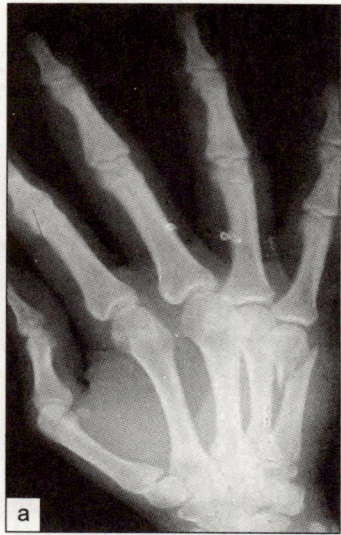 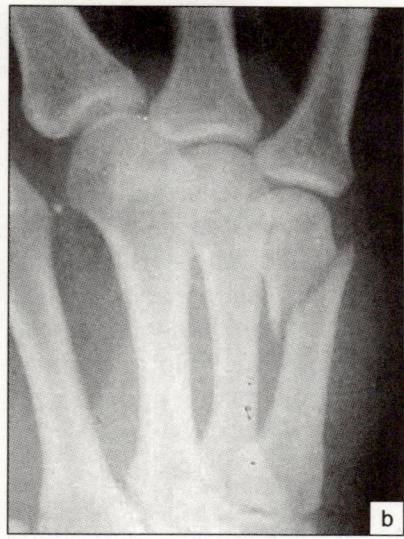

Fig. 24.11a,b. Radiographs showing oblique, unstable fracture of the shaft of 5th metacarpal

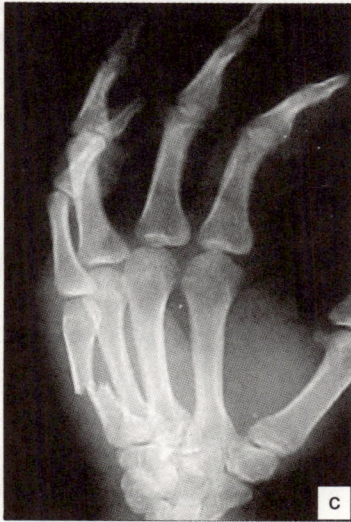

Fig. 24.11c. Dorsal angulation of fracture of 5th metacarpal

Metacarpal neck fractures

These fractures most commonly affect ring and the little finger. Impact of clenched fist against a surface is the most common mechanism. Fracture of neck of 5th metacarpal is termed *Boxer's* fracture. Angulation and impaction are common in this fracture.

These fractures are treated conservatively in most cases. Angulation up to 10° is acceptable in index and long fingers while angulation up to 30° may be acceptable in the ring and little fingers. No rotational malalignment should be accepted. Malrotation leads to overlapping of fingers in flexion. Excessive dorsal angulation leads to loss of the prominence of knuckle and pseudo-clawing.

Metacarpal neck fractures are treated with closed reduction and plaster slab for 3 weeks. Grossly displaced and open fractures need K-wire fixation. The latter can be passed transversely to fix the distal fragment to the adjacent metacarpal to prevent displacement.

Metacarpal shaft fractures

Commonest metacarpal shaft fracture is a spiral fracture. The transverse undisplaced fractures are treated in plaster cast for 3 weeks. Displaced transverse fractures are manipulated to correct angulation and dorsal displacement of the distal fragment and immobilized in plaster. Persistently displaced transverse fractures are treated with ORIF using box wiring, percutaneous or open pinning using K-wires or mini plates and screws. Oblique or spiral fractures (especially with more than 2 to 3 mm shortening) are difficult to treat conservatively and are treated with ORIF using inter-fragmentary screws, mini plates and screws or kirschner wires (open or percutaneous). Multiple metacarpal fractures are unstable and often need internal fixation using mini plates and screws or intramedullary kirschner wires.

Metacarpal base fractures

Fractures of the base of metacarpals are often due to crushing injuries and are often associated with fracture- dislocations of the carpometacarpal joints. Anatomic reduction is important in these cases to prevent posttraumatic osteoarthritis.

Fractures of the base of 5th metacarpal are also called *reverse Bennett's fractures*. These fractures are treated by closed reduction and plaster cast for 6 weeks. Unstable fractures are treated by closed reduction and percutaneous pinning. ORIF is done if articular congruity cannot be restored by closed means. Comminuted fractures are treated by external fixator and ligamentotaxis.

3. Fractures of the phalanges

(a) Fractures of the proximal and middle phalanges

General Considerations

Phalangeal fracture can occur due to direct injury (as in crush injury) or hyperextension injury.

Types Fractures of the proximal and middle phalanges can involve the base, shaft, neck, intercondylar region or the epiphysis. Proximal phalanx fractures angulate volarwards (due to pull of interossei). Middle phalanx fractures involving neck angulate volarwards dues to extensors pulling distal fragment dorsally while the base fractures (proximal to the insertion of FDS) angulate dorsally.

Evaluation Diagnosis is usually easy because of the pain, tenderness, swelling and deformity over the injured digit. Associated injuries should be looked for.

Imaging Plain radiographs are adequate for diagnosis. X-rays reveal the type of fracture, location, displacement and comminution (Fig. 24.12a).

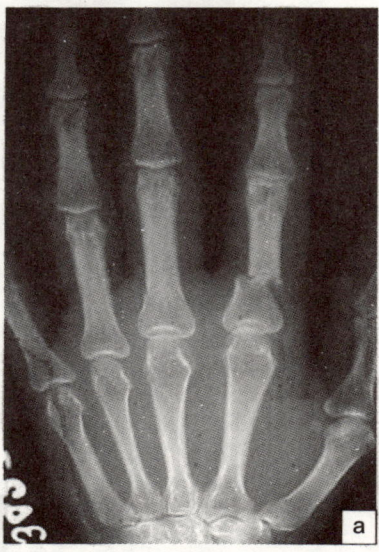

Fig. 24.12a. Transverse fracture of the proximal phalanx of index finger

Treatment is conservative in most cases and consists of splinting for 3 weeks (Fig. 24.12b,c). Irreducible, unstable or intra-articular fractures need pinning with K wires or ORIF.

Base fractures

Base of the phalanx fractures can be intra-articular or extra-articular. Extra-articular fractures do not angulate as much as shaft fractures but lead to greater functional impairment. Treatment is reduction followed by plaster slab or ball bandage. ORIF is done for irreducible or unstable fractures.

Intra-articular fracture of the base of the phalanx can be treated with splintage if undisplaced. If the intra-articular fracture is displaced, is unstable (vertical fracture line) and involves >10–15% of articular surface of base of proximal phalanx or if > 20% of articular surface is avulsed by collateral ligament attachment, ORIF is the treatment of choice. K-wire, mini screw or tension band wiring can be used for fixation.

Phalanx Shaft Fracture

Undisplaced shaft fractures are treated by *buddy splinting* or *Garter strapping*. Fractures angulated more than 10° are manipulated and immobilized

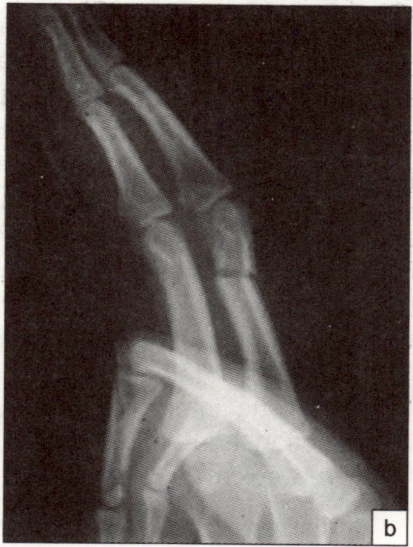
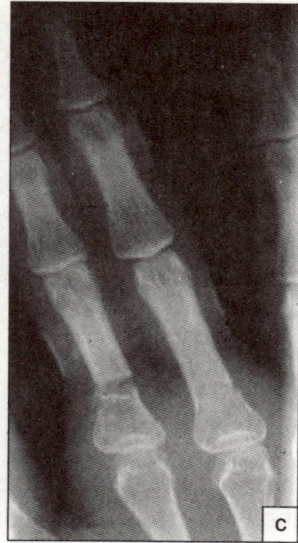

Fig. 24.12b,c. Check x-ray following strapping for proximal phalanx fracture

with the affected finger flexed (as with a "ball bandage") as extension tends to displace these fractures.

Progressive range of motion is encouraged.

Unstable or irreducible transverse fractures and oblique fractures need open reduction and internal fixation using k-wires, mini screws, intraosseous wiring or tension band wiring.

Neck fractures are uncommon in adults. They are easily reduced but often need percutaneous k-wire fixation to maintain reduction. Immobilization is continued for 6 weeks.

Fracture of intercondylar region

Fractures involving one or both condyles of the phalanges are caused by angulatory forces. Restoration of anatomy is the most important factor governing the outcome. Undisplaced fractures are treated with splint for 2 weeks followed by mobilization with strapping. Displaced fractures need open reduction, internal fixation and early movements of the joint.

b) Fractures of the Distal Phalanx

Distal phalanx fractures are the commonest fractures in hand and account for more than 50% cases. Direct trauma or crushing is the commonest mechanism. Middle finger and the thumb are the most commonly affected digits. Soft tissue injuries especially to the nail and skin are extremely common. Fractures are usually stable

and reduction is needed only for fractures involving articular surface. Dorsal splinting of distal interphalangeal joint provides comfort and can be discontinued after 3 weeks.

Avulsion fractures of the distal phalanx involving extensor surface are common injuries (*Mallet finger*) and occur following forced flexion of DIP joint. Treatment is in a mallet finger splint for 6 weeks. ORIF is indicated if joint fragment involves > 1/3rd of articular surface, if displacement is >2 mm, if there is incongruity of articular surface or if there is volar subluxation of the phalanx. Avulsion injuries involving the flexor surface need reattachment, which is done using a pull out technique to reattach FDP insertion.

Complications of the phalanx fractures include stiffness of fingers and malunion. Open injuries may sometimes lead to amputation of the digit(s).

Dislocations in the Hand

Dislocation of carpometacarpal joint (CMC)

Dislocations of CMC joints are high-energy injuries and are associated with severe injuries to the soft tissues. Dislocations of the carpometacarpal joint most commonly involve the articulation between the fourth and fifth metacarpals and the hamate. These dislocations are commonly associated with fractures and more commonly occur in a dorsal direction.

Dislocation of the thumb CMC joint results from

forcible abduction of the thumb. Clinically, the presentation is often similar to Bennett's fracture but true lateral x-ray of the first ray with maximal pronation of the hand and the thumb reveals the true injury.

Treatment of CMC dislocations is closed reduction and plaster cast for 4 weeks. Unstable reductions can be managed by percutaneous K-wire fixation. ORIF may be required for late cases.

Metacarpophalangeal joint (MCP) dislocations

First MCP joint dislocation Dorsal dislocation is much more common than volar. Dislocation of the thumb MCP joint results from forcible hyperextension of the thumb. The phalanx dislocates dorsally while the metacarpal head often buttonholes through the anterior capsule. Plain x-rays confirm the diagnosis (Fig. 24.13a,b). Treatment consists for closed reduction followed by a plaster splint for 3 weeks.

Buttonholing of the anterior capsule by the metacarpal head should be suspected if closed manipulation fails. Open reduction is indicated in such cases (Fig. 24.13c).

Injury to the ulnar collateral ligament (*Gamekeeper's thumb, skier's thumb*): This injury results from forcible abduction of the thumb. Pain and tenderness over the medial side of MCP joint following an injury should raise the suspicion of this injury. Plain x-rays are taken to rule out avulsion fractures from the proximal phalanx. Stress x-rays are needed to rule out instability. An opening medially of more than 30-45 degrees suggests complete tear of the ulnar collateral ligament and may be associated with interposition of the adductor hood between the ruptured ligament and its insertion (*Stener Lesion*) in 75% cases. This soft tissue interposition is an indication for open reduction and repair of the ligament followed by thumb spica for 6 weeks.

Partial tears of the ulnar collateral ligament (opening less than 30–45 degrees on stress x-rays) are treated with thumb spica for 4–6 weeks. A missed or inadequately treated injury leads to chronic instability with progressive subluxation of the MCP joint. These injuries can only be managed by reconstruction of capsulo-ligamentous complex using palmaris longus free graft or by fusion of the MCP joint.

Metacarpophalangeal joint dislocation of other fingers

These involve the little or the index finger. Dorsal dislocation is the commonest type and results

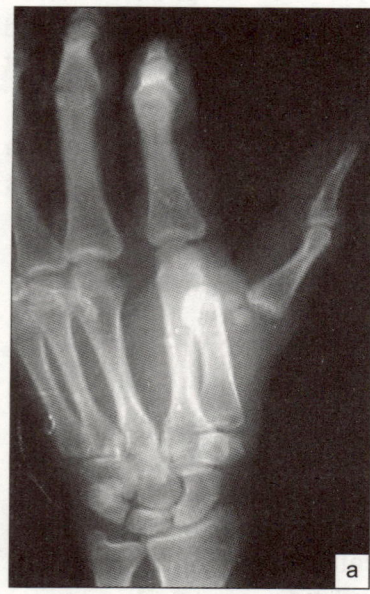 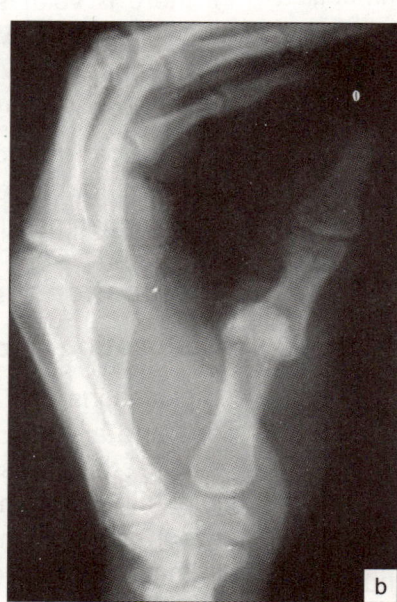 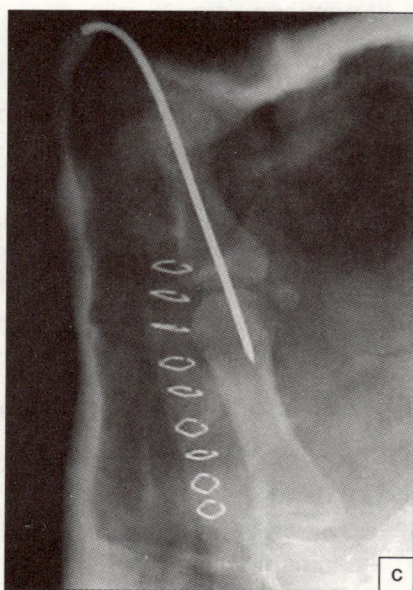

Fig. 24.13a,b. X-rays of a patient with complex MCP joint dislocation of thumb
Fig. 24.13c.   X-rays of the same patient following open reduction

from forcible hyperextension. Simple dislocations are suggested on plain radiographs by acute angulation between the axes of metacarpal and the proximal phalanx.

These dislocations are reduced by closed method, splinted in 50° flexion for 3 weeks and then strapped with progressive mobilization.

Complex MCP dislocations are irreducible MCP dislocations which are caused by interposition of the volar plate and buttonholing of the capsule. The metacarpal head is incarcerated between the lumbricals radially, flexor tendons ulnarly and deep transverse metacarpal ligament dorsally (*Kaplan's complex*) (Fig. 24.14). Complex dislocation is suspected clinically when the deformity is not severe and/or there is puckering of the volar skin. Radiologically, if the proximal phalanx and the metacarpal are *parallel* and/or there is a *sesamoid bone entrapped in the joint*, they point towards a complex MCP dislocation.

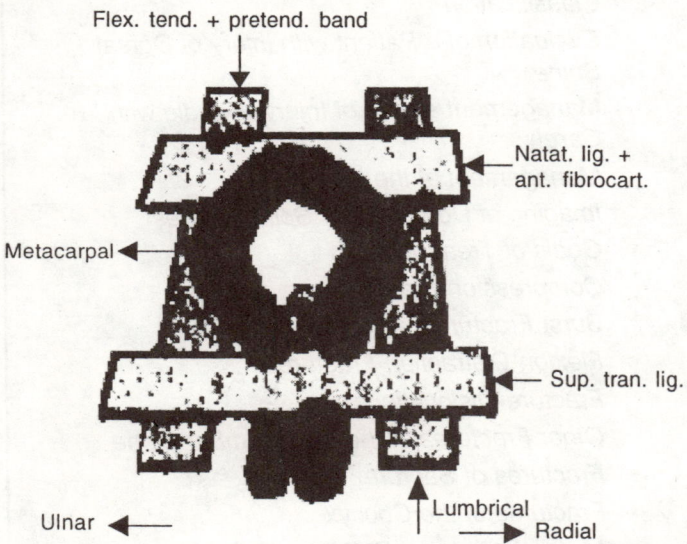

Fig. 24.14.   Anatomy of the dislocation of the metacarpophalangeal joint of the index finger and the mechanism of locking of the metacarpal head

Complex MCP dislocation needs open reduction which is possible only after dividing the interposed volar plate. Mobilization of the joint is started after 2 weeks with extension block splints.

Dislocation of the interphalangeal joints

Dislocations of the IP joints are most commonly dorsal (Fig. 24.15a,b) and occur following hyperextension injuries. The collateral ligaments are almost always (at least partially) disrupted and the volar plate is avulsed. Closed reduction and extension block splinting (to prevent hyperextension) for 3 weeks is adequate.

When associated with fractures of the articular surface, articular congruity must be restored and early range of motion exercises must be started. ORIF with intraosseous wiring, K-wires or mini screw is often indicated to restore articular congruity. Cases with interposition of volar plate or flexor tendon need open reduction.

Volar dislocation of the PIP joint is uncommon compared to dorsal dislocation but is a much more severe injury. The condyles of the proximal phalanx buttonhole through the extensor expansion. These injuries are often irreducible and need open reduction followed by early, protected motion.

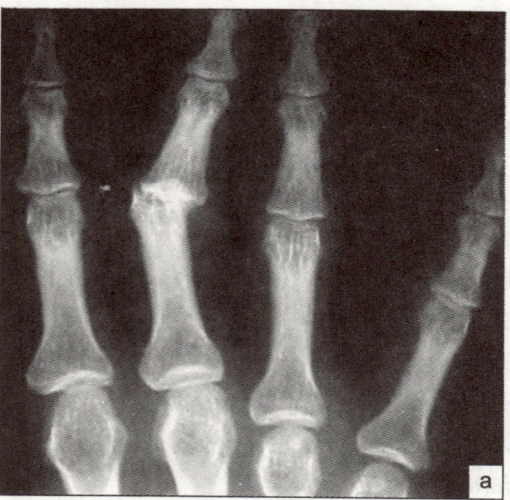

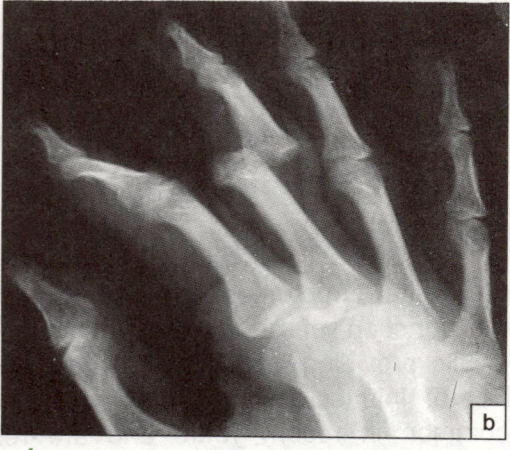

Fig. 24.15a,b. Proximal Interphalangeal joint dislocation of middle finger (Note the dorsal direction of dislocation)

CHAPTER 25

Fracture-Dislocation of the Spine

Overview of Spinal Injuries

Spine is a vital structure of the body, which has the twin function of supporting the head and torso (while providing mobility) and protecting the spinal cord. Injuries to the spine have become very common in recent years and are responsible for considerable morbidity and mortality. High-energy accidents such as resulting from motor vehicular accidents, diving accidents, falls, sports and gunshot wounds are the most common culprits. The most important factor, which determines the outcome and prognosis after spinal injury, is spinal stability or breach there of. Several structures act together to stabilise the normal spine and protect the cord (Table 25.1).

In addition muscles attached to and acting on the spine also move as well as protect it.

Table 25.1. Structures supporting the spine and protecting spinal cord

	Anterior	*Posterior*
Osseous elements	Vertebral body	Posterior elements (neural arch consisting of twin pedicles, laminae and transverse processes and a spinous process)
Joints	Intervertebral disc	Facet joints
Ligaments	Anterior longitudinal ligament (ALL) Posterior longitudinal ligament (PLL)	Ligamentum Flavum Interspinous ligament Supraspinous ligament

Stability of Spine

Injury to the stabilising structures mentioned above can compromise the stability of the spine. The spine is said to be unstable if it is liable to give rise to pain, deformity or displacement and/or neurological deficit on application of physiological loads. A severe injury disrupts the supporting structures and can displace the fractured segments enough so as to injure the spinal cord. Thorough knowledge of the anatomy of the spine and its stabilising structures, the mechanism of injury and detailed local neurological and radiological examination are mandatory to prevent displacement of the unstable spine further aggravating the spinal cord injury, so called "*second accident*".

Spinal Cord Injury (SCI)

Dislocation, fracture or a fracture - dislocation of the vertebra can result in direct crushing of the neural elements and compromise of the neural canal. Haemorrhage and oedema occurring in the spinal cord due to the injury further aggravate the neurological damage. The spectrum of the neurological deficit is determined by the type of neural tissue damaged and the extent of the injury and includes the following states:

Spinal Shock is a state of spinal cord "concussion" or dysfunction occurring immediately after a severe injury and occurs even without any permanent damage. It is therefore difficult to predict the recovery of spinal cord function during the spinal shock. It is characterised by complete motor, sensory and visceral paralysis and areflexia. Superficial reflexes such as anal wink and bulbocavernosus reflexes (anal sphincter con-

traction with squeezing of glans penis or clitoris) are absent. Spinal shock invariably starts regressing before 48 hours and the recovery is marked by the return of bulbocavernosus reflex. Return of the bulbocavernosus reflex is accompanied by spasticity, hyperreflexia and clonus. At this stage any preserved neurological function such as sacral sensations indicates partial/or incomplete SCI. Absence of any motor/sensory function at this stage indicates complete SCI.

1. Complete Spinal Cord Injury is usually caused by burst fractures, canal compromise leading to spinal cord compression or complete transection of cord due to fracture dislocations. The complete spinal cord injury is characterised initially by spinal shock. After the spinal shock abates, the total loss of sensations persists. Spasticity occurs and flexor spasms are common. Hyperreflexia and clonus are seen. Injuries to the upper cervical cord leading to complete transection are fatal due to injury to vital centres. Injuries above C_4 level lead to diaphragmatic palsy with resultant respiratory embarrassment. Injuries to the lower cervical cord leads to quadriplegia below the injured level. Neurological examination in these cases reveals an upper motor neuron type of paralysis. Injuries to the cord at the level of thoracic spine lead to paraplegia (UMN) below the level of injury. Complete transection of the neural tissues at the dorsolumbar junction may lead to division of cord as well as the roots (cauda equina). Features suggestive of a combination of the upper motor neuron and lower motor neuron lesions are seen in these cases. In injuries above the S_2 level an upper motor neuron type of urinary bladder paralysis (*automatic* or *cord bladder*) occurs. Sensations of vescical filling are absent.

Bladder empties reflexly in response to any stimulus in the perineum and there is minimal residual urine.

In cases of complete cord transection below S_2 level, a lower motor neuron type of bladder (*autonomous bladder*) occurs. The bladder function depends on the detrusor muscle. Manual pressure effects emptying in these cases, where, large residual volumes of urine commonly occur.

The prognosis for the recovery of complete SCI is poor and the patients have to live without function below the injury level.

2. Incomplete Syndromes

Partial neurologic function below the level of the injury has potential for some recovery and often has a well-described syndromal picture.

a) Central Cord Syndrome (Central Cord Involvement) is most common and usually occurs following hyperextension injury in the elderly (>50 years with pre existing spondylosis). Motor power and sensations of the upper extremities are affected more than that in the lower extremities. Perianal sensations are usually spared (sacral sparing).

b) Anterior Cord Syndrome (Anterior Cord Involvement) is less common and usually is seen following the flexion/compression injuries. Motor paralysis, more in lower extremities than upper and sensory anaesthesia occurs below the level of injury. However, proprioception, deep pressure and vibratory sensations are preserved as the posterior cord escapes injury. This type of syndrome has the worst prognosis.

c) Brown - Sequard Syndrome (Lateral Cord Involvement) occurs due to damage to one half of the cord, mostly due to penetrating injuries. The syndrome is characterised by ipsilateral motor loss and contralateral loss of pain and temperature sensations. It has the best prognosis.

d) Posterior cord syndrome (Posterior Cord Involvement) occurs rarely and is characterised by loss of deep pressure, pain and proprioception. Only crude touch sensation is spared below the level of injury. Motor function may be preserved.

Nerve Root Injury

Nerve root injury can occur due to compression fracture, burst fracture, facet joint dislocation or herniated disc. Injury to nerve root occurs either at the neural foramen or in the injuries below the level of L_1 vertebra (injuries to cauda equina). Clinically the nerve root injury has all the features of peripheral nerve injury (flaccid paralysis of LMN type). Injured nerve roots have good prognosis for recovery (like a peripheral nerve) if the injury is neuropraxia or axonotmesis. Complete nerve injuries (neurotmesis), however, do not recover.

Combined Spinal Cord and Nerve Root Injury

Injury to the spine at D_{12}–L_1 level can result in the damage to both the cord as well as the nerve roots. An injury to all the nerve roots is unusual so preservation (and regeneration of function in some injured roots) of function in some lumbar nerve roots may allow useful function to the patient.

Principles of Imaging in fractures and dislocations of the spine

Initial evaluation of spinal injury is always by conventional radiography. Plain X-rays localise the injured area and assist in decision making for more comprehensive imaging. X-rays of chest, pelvis and long bones below the level of injury should be obtained in all cases with head or spinal cord injury.

Conventional tomography has been replaced by CT and MRI but is still useful sometimes (e.g. for diagnosing Type II odontoid fracture, and *Chance* fractures where horizontal fracture lines may be extending into pedicles). Computed Tomography (CT) is extremely useful for axial plane imaging and shows fractures and the spinal canal dimensions. It is extremely effective in defining bony pathology in the spinal canal and articular pillars and is helpful in planning stabilisation or reconstruction.

Magnetic Resonance Imaging (MRI) is useful for visualising the soft tissues. Intramedullary contusions, hematomas, ligament tears, cord oedema and disc herniations are very well visualised with MRI. Rupture of ALL or PLL and haemorrhage in posterior ligaments seen on MRI can diagnose instability. MRI, however, has the disadvantages of availability and cost. It does not show bony details well and is inaccessible for patients on bulky life support systems.

Electromyography (EMG), nerve conduction studies and bone scan are not useful in acute cervical spine injuries.

Cervical Spine Injuries: An Overview

Cervical Spine Injuries range from minor strains and soft tissue injuries to life-threatening fracture- dislocations. It is extremely important to identify cervical injuries in any trauma situation and act accordingly. Cervical spine injury should be suspected in high speed motor vehicle collisions, fall from height, in patients with facial lacerations or fractures, and in patients with head injury. Any patient who complains of neck pain, stiffness, transient weakness or numbness at the time of injury or persistent neurological deficit should be presumed to have cervical spine injury.

Management at site of injury

A rapid and accurate evaluation should be done at the site of accident to protect spinal cord from further injury. The neck is immobilised using a spine board with a rigid cervical collar and sandbag. During the initial evaluation, headgear (such as helmet) should not be removed. Neck should not be manipulated in any way.

Management at hospital (in Casualty)

Rapid assessment and resuscitation or surgical care (if required) take preference over everything else. Once the patient is stable, a coherent history should be obtained and a more thorough examination can be done. Neck must be examined carefully. There may be localised tenderness, deformity and/or spasm of the neck. No attempt should be made to test the neck movements. Detailed neurological examination should be performed and patient sent for imaging. Neurologic examination should give a clue to the level of injury and guides subsequent management. It is especially important to note whether the neurologic injury is complete or incomplete.

Imaging studies

Conventional radiography remains the primary modality in the initial evaluation of patients with spinal injuries including the cervical spine. The best initial screening imaging technique is the cross table lateral view x-ray with the patient immobile on the spine board. It is reported to detect 85% of cervical spine injuries. The C_7–T_1 junction must be seen as 10% of cervical spine fractures occur at that level. An open mouth AP view for C_1 vertebra and odontoid is also required.

X-rays in flexion and extension are contraindicated in patients with neurological deficit in acute phase. Oblique views are sometimes required for suspected facet joint dislocations or fractures through the lateral masses.

Trauma Radiological Series for cervical spine injuries should include the following:

1. Lateral cervical radiograph
2. Open mouth anteroposterior view (AP)
3. Radiograph for cervico-thoracic junction (*swimmer's view* if required)

Retropharyngeal soft tissue swelling can provide a clue about the spinal injury when vertebrae look normal on x-rays. A value greater than 7 mm in the upper cervical spine opposite C_3 suggests injury. Instability is suggested by a combination of 3.5 mm horizontal translation, greater than 11° kyphosis, widening of the disc space and spinous process splaying. The presence of greater than 50% subluxation of one vertebral body over another is suggestive of bilateral facet joint dislocation, which is again a very unstable injury (Fig. 25.1).

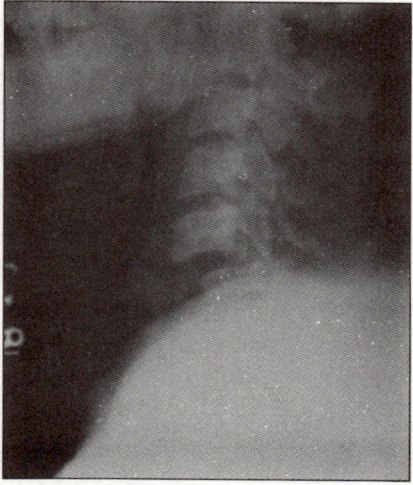

Fig. 25.1. Fracture dislocation C_5–C_6. Note that it is highly unstable injury with bilateral facet dislocation

Magnetic resonance imaging is indicated in patients with cervical spine injury with normal radiographs. MRI is very useful in detecting post-traumatic disc prolapse.

Injury Pattern

Injury pattern in cervical spine injury is related to the mechanism of injury as shown in Table 25.2.

Treatment

Treatment of any cervical spine injury is immobilisation. Stable injuries (without neurological deficit) are immobilised in a rigid cervical brace (such as SOMI brace or four poster collar) for 8–12 weeks.

Unstable injuries are treated with initial skeletal traction with 5–10 pounds with periodic check x-rays for follow up. Additional 5 pounds weight for each vertebra level is used for stabilisation and reduction up to a maximum of 40 pounds. Once the reduction of displacement is achieved, the traction weights are reduced by half. The traction is maintained for 3–6 weeks and then the patient is mobilised in a brace for another 6 weeks.

Unstable injuries with neurological deficit are treated with an aim to protect any uninjured (but at risk) neurological tissue and salvage the injured (but still viable) neural tissues of the spinal cord. Immediate immobilisation of the neck is done. Oxygen inhalation should be given in cases with respiratory embarrassment. Intubation, if required, should preferably be done using fiberoptic equipment. Tracheostomy should be performed if necessary. The impact of injury on the neural tissues is minimised by maintaining adequate perfusion pressures (since hypotension is known to aggravate neural injury) and the use of high dose steroids. Methyl prednisolone should be injected in an initial bolus of 30mg/kg within 6 hours of injury and then infused at 5.4 mg/kg/hour for the next 23 hours.

Attempt is made to indirectly decompress the spinal cord by realigning the spinal column by traction. *Sillar's manoeuvre* is sometimes attempted for the closed reduction of unilateral facet joint dislocations. It should however be attempted only under general anaesthesia by experienced surgeons as an improperly performed manoeuvre may lead to deterioration of neurologic status. In this manoeuvre the head is turned towards the side opposite the facet dislocation and traction is given with the neck slightly flexed. Severe cord injuries with residual compression by either bone or soft tissues are best treated by operative decompression (through an anterior, posterior or combined approach), reduction and stabilisation. The ultimate goal is to achieve bony fusion of the involved segment in proper alignment.

Upper Cervical Spine Injuries

1. Occiput-C_1 dislocation (Atlanto-Occipital dislocation)

Occiput-C_1 dislocation is a rare and usually fatal injury. It is caused by rotation, hyperextension,

Table 25.2. Cervical Spine Injuries-Injury Patterns

Mechanism of injury	Pattern of injury	Remarks
Flexion	Anterior vertebral body compression	Stable injury (If posterior ligament complex is intact)
Flexion-Rotation	Unilateral or bilateral facet dislocation ± fracture through lamina or vertebral body	Unstable injury
Axial loading	Burst fracture	Disruption of the whole vertebral body with bony elements pushed posteriorly in the canal.
	Atlas fracture	
Hyperextension	"Tear drop" fracture	Avulsion fracture (avulsed by ALL)
Lateral flexion	Fractures of lateral masses, pedicles or facet joints	Usually stable

translation and/or distraction. Lateral radiograph establishes the type of dislocation viz. anterior, posterior or longitudinal. This is always an unstable injury.

Management of the patients who survive is by immobilisation in halo-pelvic traction and early occipito-cervical fusion (extending up to C_2 vertebra). Halo stabilisation is continued post operatively till fusion is achieved.

2. Fracture of Atlas (C_1)

Fracture of the atlas is caused by axial load (e.g. fall on the head). Three types of injury patterns may occur depending on the position of the head at the time of impact.

Jefferson Fracture is caused by isolated axial load. The vertical compression force drives the occipital condyles into the lateral masses of the atlas and breaks the ring of atlas and/or lateral masses at one or more sites. The patient presents with neck pain without any neurological deficit.

Imaging Radiologically the fracture is diagnosed by the anteroposterior open mouth view.

Fracture Stability is determined by the lateral mass spreading. If the lateral masses spread more than 7 mm, it indicates tear of the transverse ligament and the fracture is deemed unstable.

Management of stable fractures is by/rigid cervicothoracic brace for 3 months. Unstable fractures are treated initially by halo pelvic or skull traction for 8 weeks followed by the cervico-thoracic brace for further 8 weeks.

Anterior arch fractures are caused by axial loading in flexion. These fractures are usually unstable and are treated by halo traction for 8 weeks followed by cervico-thoracic brace for further 8 weeks. Residual C_1–C_2 instability, if any, is treated by Occiput – C_2 fusion.

Posterior arch fractures result when axial load is applied on the extended head. These fractures are usually stable and are treated in a rigid cervicothoracic brace for 3 months.

Complications of atlas fracture include vertebral artery injury and injury to the cranial nerve VIII. Malunion is common. Concomitant injury to spinal cord, though rare, is fatal in these injuries.

3. C_1–C_2 Subluxation (Atlanto-axial instability)

Atlanto-axial subluxation occurs due to rupture of the transverse ligament and/or fracture of the odontoid process. The latter is responsible for the stability between the odontoid process and the anterior arch of the atlas. Severe flexion and compression force results in the rupture of transverse ligament and anterior subluxation of the atlas on the axis. A severe compromise of the spinal canal occurs in these cases, by the posteriorly displaced intact odontoid process and posterior margin of the atlas. Severe cord compression and death may occur. If, however, odontoid process also fractures as happens more commonly, it remains attached to anterior arch of the atlas and the spinal cord may escape injury. Severe hyperextension and compression forces can lead to odontoid fracture and posterior subluxation of the atlas and axis. These injuries suggest an intact transverse ligament and rupture of apical and alar ligaments. Posterior subluxation with or without fracture is rare.

Imaging A lateral view of the cervical spine can diagnose the atlanto-axial instability and its severity. Both the lateral and the anterior open mouth odontoid views can diagnose the odontoid fracture if present.

Fracture stability Atlanto-axial instability is always an unstable injury.

Management of atlanto-axial subluxation consists of reduction by skull traction followed by C_1–C_2 fusion.

Rotatory subluxation of C_1–C_2

Rotatory subluxations are caused by rotatory force applied to the head. Patient presents with torticollis and neck pain.

Radiological imaging consists of open mouth odontoid view which shows increased distance between the odontoid and lateral mass on one side with decrease in the distance on the opposite side (*winking eye* sign). Tomograms or computerised axial tomography can be helpful in confirming the diagnosis.

Management is with skull traction for reduction of subluxation followed by rigid cervicothoracic brace for 3 months. A residual atlanto-axial instability or recurrence requires posterior C_1–C_2 fusion.

4. Fractures of axis (C₂)

a) Odontoid fractures

Mechanism of injury causing odontoid fracture is not well understood though many authors believe that flexion is the most common mechanism (in almost 80% of the cases). Odontoid fractures are best visualised in AP (open mouth) and lateral radiographs. Tomograms and CT scan may sometimes be helpful.

Anderson and D' olonzo have described 3 types of odontoid fractures.

Type I Occurs as an oblique fracture at the tip of odontoid and is the most uncommon (2–3%) of all fracture types. It is believed to be stable if it is displaced less than 2 mm. It is important to differentiate it from Os odontoideum, which is a congenital ossicle at the site of tip of the odontoid. Type I fractures are treated in a rigid cervicothoracic orthosis for 6–8 weeks.

Type II Occurs at the junction of the odontoid and the body of C₂ vertebra. It is the commonest type of odontoid fracture (60%). Nearly 16% cases are associated with fracture of the atlas. The non union rate in this fracture is the highest (36%). These are unstable fractures and sudden or gradual anterior displacement of atlas on axis may occur

Minimally displaced (<5 mm) type II fractures are treated by skull traction for 6 weeks followed by rigid cervicothoracic brace for 8–10 weeks.

When the displacement is more than 5 mm or posterior displacement of the odontoid along with atlas on the axis, reduction and posterior C₁-C₂ fusion is done. Odontoid screws are used at some centres anteriorly to fix the type II odontoid fracture.

Type III fractures occur within the superior part of C₂ body. These fractures occur through the cancellous area and unite readily. Treatment with immobilisation using Minerva cast/halo cast or rigid cervico-thoracic brace for 8–12 weeks is usually sufficient.

b) C₂ Isthmus fracture (*Hangman's fracture*)

Hangman's fracture is traumatic spondylolisthesis of C₂ over C₃ resulting from fractures of the pars interarticularis. It is caused by hyperextension-distraction force. Neurological injuries are uncommon. However, the injuries may be associated with other injuries to the cervical spine, which may be missed.

Management is by skull traction to reduce the displacement followed by immobilisation for 12 weeks. Anterior C₂–C₃ fusion or C₁–C₃ posterior cervical fusion may be required for cases with unacceptable reductions (> 10 degrees angulation or > 4 mm translation) or cases with non union.

5. Lower Cervical Spine Injuries (C₃–C₇)

(a) Compression Fractures

i) Wedge Compression Fractures are most common at C₄–C₅ and C₅–C₆ levels. Flexion forces result in the anterior wedge compression fracture of the vertebral body. Posterior ligaments escape damage and these injuries are generally stable. Spinal canal compromise is rare and usually there is no neurological deficit.

Imaging Lateral view of the cervical spine shows reduction of the anterior height of the vertebral body in comparison to the posterior height.

Fracture Stability Severe compression injuries can damage posterior ligaments and compromise the fracture stability. Radiologically, a translation of vertebral body more than 3.5 mm or angulation more than 11° suggests instability.

Management of stable compression fracture is by immobilisation in a rigid cervico-thoracic orthosis for 8–12 weeks. Unstable fractures without neurological deficit are treated with posterior cervical spinal fusion. Fractures with neurological deficit are treated by decompression performed through anterior approach and anterior spinal fusion using iliac crest tricortical graft with or without internal fixation. The various techniques of anterior cervical spine fusion are Cloward technique, Bailey-Badgley technique and Robinson-Smith technique based on the shape of graft and biomechanical aspects of fusion.

ii) Burst Fractures Burst fractures most commonly involve the vertebral bodies C₅ or C₆ vertebrae. These fractures are most often caused by compression-flexion forces or axial loading of the spine. The vertebral body explodes (bursts) into multiple fragments. Posterior wall involvement leads to encroachment of the spinal canal and often, neurological deficit.

Imaging Plain radiographs (lateral and AP views of cervical spine) demonstrate comminuted fracture of vertebral body with fracture extending to end plates. Lateral view also shows retropulsion of bony fragments into the neural canal. In cases with neurological deficit CT scan shows encroachment of spinal canal by retropulsed bony fragments and also the presence of free bony fragments within the canal with the resultant compression of the cord. MRI is very effective in demonstrating the injury to the cord.

Fracture Stability The important factor to decide the stability in the burst fractures of the vertebral body is whether the posterior ligaments are injured or not. Fracture of posterior wall and /or posterior elements, canal encroachment by retropulsed bony fragments and the presence of neurological deficit suggest highly unstable injury.

Management of burst fractures without neurological deficit is immobilisation in a rigid cervico-thoracic brace for 8–12 weeks. Fractures with complete neurological deficit are treated in skull traction for 6 weeks followed by a cervico-thoracic brace for another 6 weeks. Fractures, which are associated with incomplete neurological or deteriorating neurological state, are treated by decompression and fusion with or without internal fixation. Anterior approach is used in cases where the posterior stability is present whereas combined anterior and posterior approach (anterior decompression and fusion plus posterior fusion) is used when posterior elements are unstable.

Complications of compression injuries are compromise of the spinal canal, neurological deficit and late deformity (posttraumatic cervical kyphosis). Kyphosis also occurs commonly when injury to posterior elements is not recognised and only anterior decompression and fusion is performed.

(b) Disruption of facet joints

Pure facetal dislocations (without associated fractures)

Facet joints are commonly injured in the cervical spine by flexion or distraction force combined with rotation. These forces result in disruption of posterior ligaments and facet joint capsule on one or both sides depending on the severity. Since the facet joints in cervical spine are inclined in horizontal plane the articular surfaces, in the presence of injury to stabilising soft tissue structures can subluxate without causing an associated fracture. Facetal dislocations occur most commonly at C_5–C_6 and C_6–C_7 levels.

i) **Unilateral facet dislocations** are diagnosed on x-rays following the injury to the cervical spine. Lateral X-ray of the cervical spine reveals a step off between adjacent vertebrae. The vertebra above slips forward by less than 25% of its diameter. The anteroposterior view shows the spinous process at the involved level to have fallen out of line with the rest of spinous processes.

ii) **Bilateral facet dislocations** occur following more severe injuries and are often associated with nerve root or spinal cord injuries (75% cases). The lateral x-rays of the cervical spine show 25–50% anterior translation of the vertebral body.

MRI may show the damage to cord by disruption of osseous anatomy or by a ruptured nucleus pulposus (which occur in about 7% cases).

Management of facet joint dislocations is by skull traction to reduce the dislocation. Skull traction is continued for 6 weeks after reduction. The cervical spine is then immobilised in a rigid cervico-thoracic brace for 6–8 weeks. In cases where traction fails to achieve reduction in the presence of neurological deficit, open reduction is indicated. Posterior spinal fusion should be combined with reduction in these cases. In cases where MRI shows ruptured disc with prolapse and compression of the spinal cord, anterior discectomy, decompression and fusion is indicated.

Complications of facet dislocations are spinal cord and/or nerve root injury and disc herniation.

(c) Fracture Dislocation of Cervical Spine

Fracture dislocation of the cervical spine is the most unstable injury and occurs following violent trauma to the neck. Flexion, axial compression and rotation forces in combination disrupt the bony and soft tissue integrity of the cervical spine. Compression fracture of vertebral bodies with or without neural arch fracture and dislocation of facet joints occur. Variable degree of canal compromise with resultant complete or incomplete neurological deficit is seen.

Imaging Plain X-rays demonstrate dislocation/ subluxation of vertebra on the one below with compromise of the spinal canal. A teardrop (triangular bony fragment from antero inferior part of the vertebral body) may be seen. CT scan delineates vertebral fracture fragments and spinal canal compromise. MRI demonstrates the extent of cord compression and damage.

Fracture Stability Translation more than 3.5 mm or angulation more than 11 degrees between adjacent cervical vertebrae suggests instability.

Management Suspected fracture dislocations of the cervical spine need utmost care while handling the patient as a little carelessness can damage an intact cord or aggravate an incomplete spinal cord injury. Neck should be immobilised at the site of injury itself and should be supported by sandbags on either side.

Once the patient reaches hospital, resuscitation and detailed neurological examination are carried out.

Heavy skull traction with neck in extension is applied with an attempt to reduce the dislocation. After the dislocation is reduced, the traction is reduced and maintained for the next 8–12 weeks.

Patients with incomplete neurological deficit or deteriorating neurological status need decompression, reduction and posterior spinal fusion with or without internal fixation.

(d) Hyperextension/ Acceleration-Deceleration/Whiplash Injuries

Hyperextension injuries commonly occur following sudden acceleration injuries as in cases of passengers in a stationary car, which is hit from behind by another car; or, sudden deceleration where following sudden braking of the car the head hits the windscreen. The hyperextension force thus exerted can cause an avulsion fracture from anterior body or rupture of anterior longitudinal ligament anteriorly and fractures of the lamina posteriorly. During the hyperextension, the vertebral bodies may displace enough so as to injure the spinal cord. Spinal cord injury in hyperextension injury occurs more frequently in patients with degenerative changes in the spine and a central cord syndrome is the commonest presentation. Sudden hyperextension may also lead to injury to trachea (leading to hoarseness of voice), oesophagus (leading to dysphagia), vertebral artery or neck muscles.

The patient may have abrasions on the forehead or facial laceration, which may suggest a hyperextension injury.

Imaging The spine may spring back and no abnormality may be seen on the lateral x-rays of spine. However, a small avulsed bony fragment anteriorly, an increased soft tissue prevertebral shadow, and/or fracture of lamina can all point to the whiplash (Fig. 25.2).

MRI can demonstrate injury to ligaments and spinal cord.

Fracture Instability The posterior ligament complex remains intact and therefore, these injuries are stable in flexion.

Management in patients with intact spinal cord consists of immobilisation of the neck in slight flexion in rigid cervico-thoracic brace. In patients with spinal cord injury, treatment consists of skeletal traction in slight flexion for 8–12 weeks. If

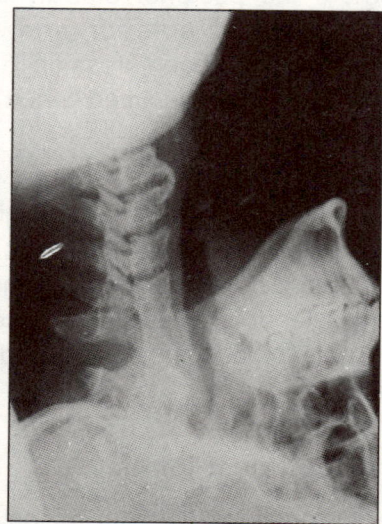

Fig. 25.2. Whiplash injury C_5–C_6. Note that the injury occurs in stiff cervical spine (Anterior osteophytes at C_5–C_6 are seen)

the patient does not show signs of recovery, care of the quadriplegic is instituted.

e) Other Fractures of Lower Cervical Spine

i) Spinous process avulsion fractures occur following sudden, forceful flexion of the neck.

Clay Shoveler's Fracture is avulsion fracture of the spinous process of the C_7 vertebra.

The treatment of spinous process avulsions is symptomatic with analgesics and cervical orthosis (if pain is severe).

ii) Lateral mass, lamina, pedicle, articular process fractures are mostly stable and are treated with a rigid cervico-thoracic orthosis for 8 to 12 weeks. Unstable injury patterns are treated with spinal fusion (anterior or posterior depending on injury) with or without fixation.

Dorsolumbar Spine Injuries

An Overview

Most dorsal and lumbar spine fractures (60%) occur at the junction (D_{10}–L_2) of the kyphotic dorsal spine and lordotic lumbar spine. The fractures of the upper dorsal spine (D_1–D_9) are usually stable. Only very severe injuries leading to fractures of multiple ribs, fracture of sternum or flexion rotation injuries leading to disruption of spinal integrity are unstable.

The mechanism of injury determines the severity and the pattern of the fracture. Low energy compression fractures seen in elderly often result from minor falls whereas fall from height and motor vehicle accidents lead to high energy fracture-dislocations. Seat belt injuries are often associated with abdominal injuries.

Classification of the dorsolumbar spine injuries is based on the involvement of the three columns described by Denis (Table 25.3).

One or more of these columns can fail due to the injury and produce various specific fracture patterns. The fracture patterns are given in Table 25.4.

In addition to the injuries outlined above, dorsolumbar spine may sustain minor fractures such as fracture of the transverse processes, pars interarticularis, spinous processes or articular process fractures. These fractures are of no serious consequence and do not compromise structural or neurologic function.

Evaluation of a patient with injury of dorsal spine

High index of suspicion is important to avoid missing the dorso-lumbar spine injury in an injured patient. Any complaints of pain/soreness in the back, paraesthesiae or anaesthesia in lower limbs or inability to move the lower limbs should alert the physician about the possibility of dorsolumbar spinal injury. All injured patients especially those who have fallen from height or involved in high-energy motor vehicle accident should be presumed to have spinal injury unless it has been ruled out after thorough clinical examination and radiologic imaging. Till such time the patient should be turned and transferred as a log using 3–4 persons.

Clinical examination of the spine in these patients may reveal tenderness at the spinous processes. A step or abnormal gap may be palpable between the spinous processes. Local swelling, ecchymoses, spasm of paraspinal muscles, bruises, or alteration of normal sagittal contours of spine may also point to spinal injury. Detailed neurological examination helps in establishing a baseline for monitoring neurological deficit and any deterioration thereof in addition to treating injury. Careful examination should be performed to look for associated injuries.

Table 25.3. Columns of Spine - after Denis

Anterior	Middle	Posterior
Anterior Longitudinal Ligament	Posterior Longitudinal Ligament	Pedicles, Facet Joints Bony neural arch
Anterior 1/2 of vertebral body	Posterior 1/2 of vertebral body	Ligamentum flavum
Anterior aspect of annulus fibrosus	Posterior part of annulus fibrosus	Interspinous ligaments Supraspinous ligament

Table 25.4. Injury patterns of dorsal and lumbar spine

Type of fracture	Column injured			Stability	Remarks
	Ant	Middle	Post		
Compression	F.C	I	I	S (mostly) *Loss of ant. *height < 50% *kyphosis < 30%	Commonest # type, Pathologic in osteoporotic patients, Progressive late kyphosis may occur
Burst	F (F.C)	F (F.C)	I	S (if) *loss of height < 50% *kyphosis < 20-25% *<50% canal compromise *Posterior column intact	"Blow out" #, May be confused with compression #, 3 column injuries may have dural tears and CSF leak
Flexion-distraction	F (F.C) or I	F (F.D)	F (F.D)	U	Seat belt injuries Chance fractures Associated abdominal injuries
Fracture-dislocation	F (Compression rotation shear)	F (Distraction rotation shear)	F (Distraction rotation shear)	U	Severe neurologic injury

F : Fails   I : Intact   S : Stable   U : Unstable
F.C. Fails in compression   F.D. Fails in distraction

Management at site of injury (*Handle with Care!*)

The patient should be assessed for vital functions and chest, abdominal and head injuries are looked for. Airway must be established immediately in cases with respiratory embarrassment. All patients with spinal injuries are treated as if they have neurologic deficit and are transferred in one piece using 3–4 persons. The number of transfers should be kept to a minimum. Patient should be transferred on a wooden board or stretcher and should not be dumped on the back seat of car and rushed to hospital.

Management at the hospital

Resuscitation should be the topmost priority once the patient reaches hospital. Steroids should be given as early as possible to patients with neurologic injury. Patient is taken for imaging after detailed neurologic examination and should always be accompanied by a resident while proceeding for x-rays. The x-rays should be taken on the trolley itself as far as possible to avoid further transfers.

Imaging of Dorsolumbar Spine Injuries

Radiologic evaluation must include the *entire* spine to avoid missing other spine fractures (in addition to the most prominent one).

Plain radiographs (Anteroposterior and Lateral) adequately visualise vertebral bodies, transverse processes, pedicles, laminae and spinous processes. Fracture dislocations with compromise of neural canal are readily appreciated. However, one must remember that serious neurological deficit may be present with normal radiographic picture in cases where severe ligamentous disruption causes significant displacement of vertebrae and spinal cord injury. Spontaneous reduction may occur in these cases and clinical examination and MRI remain the mainstay of diagnosis.

In children spinal cord injury may occur without any radiological changes, this well accepted condition called *Spinal Cord Injury without Radiologic Abnormality (SCIWORA)*.

Imaging of other areas may be indicated to rule out associated osseous injuries as in cases of fall from height where calcaneus may be fractured bilaterally.

CT scan is useful for delineating bony injury especially the retropulsed fragment of a burst fracture compressing the cord anteriorly.

MRI is especially useful in evaluating spinal cord and ligamentous injuries (as in flexion-distraction injuries). MRI is especially helpful in cases where a mismatch is found between the injury seen and the neurological deficit present.

Goals of treatment in dorsolumbar injuries are to prevent further neurologic injury and restore spinal stability and alignment while preserving neurologic function. Internal fixation may be necessary to mobilise the patient early and reduce overall morbidity.

A secondary goal of treatment in patients with dorsolumbar injuries is prevention of late pain and deformity.

Compression Fractures

Compression fractures are the most common fracture pattern and occur in 60–80% of all dorsolumbar spine fractures. A flexion force leading to disruption of anterior column (while middle column remains intact) causes compression fractures. Neurologic function usually remains intact. Multiple compression fractures leading to kyphosis are often seen in osteoporotic elderly patients following trivial injuries.

Imaging   Plain radiographs are adequate for evaluation. Lateral radiographs reveal a loss of anterior height of the vertebral body, which becomes wedge shaped. No compromise of the canal is seen.

CT and MRI are useful to assess the damage and compression of the cord in cases associated with neurological deficit.

Fracture Stability

If loss of anterior height of the vertebra is >50% or more than 30° of kyphosis is present, the spine is deemed unstable.

Treatment

Stable fractures are treated with immobilisation in a hyperextension (Anterior Spinal Hyperextension Brace) brace for 3 months. However, elderly osteoporotic patients with pathologic fractures are immobilised in brace only till their symptoms are relieved to avoid further osteoporosis due to immobilisation. Salmon calcitonin is the drug of choice in the treatment of pain due to osteoporotic wedge compression fractures.

Unstable fractures   The treatment of these fractures is controversial. They are often treated in brace and followed up closely for occurrence of pain, neurologic deficit or progression of deformity. In case these complications occur, posterior instrumentation and fusion is performed. Many people recommend posterior instrumentation and fusion primarily for these patients.

Vertebroplasty has been recently described for compression fractures where height of vertebral body is restored and Polymethylmethacrylate (PMMA) is injected percutaneously in the vertebral body to provide stability and pain relief.

Burst Fractures   Burst fractures are reported to represent 17% of major spine fractures.

Burst fractures of the vertebral body are caused by the axial loading (with or without flexion rotation and lateral bending) of spine similar to wedge compression fractures. Anterior and middle columns always fail while the posterior column may fail in tension or compression in very severe injuries. Laminar or pedicular fractures and ligamentous injuries may be associated with posterior column disruption. Posterosuperior end plate may retropulse and compress the spinal cord. Neurological deficit occurs in 50% of patients with posterior column injury and dural tears and cerebrospinal fluid leaks should be looked for in these cases.

Imaging   Plain radiographs in burst fractures show an anterior, central or lateral compression with comminuted fracture of the body seen as multiple fracture lines in the vertebral body (Fig. 25.3a,b).

CT scan shows the retropulsion of the bony fragments posteriorly and compromise of the neural canal. It also shows the degree of disruption and comminution of involved vertebra and predicts its future load bearing capacity.

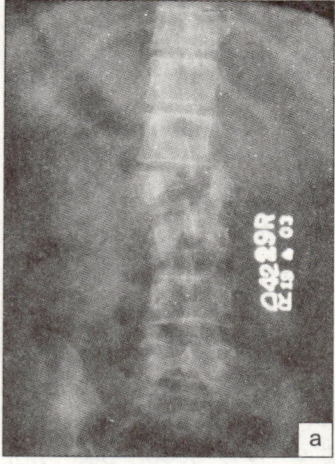

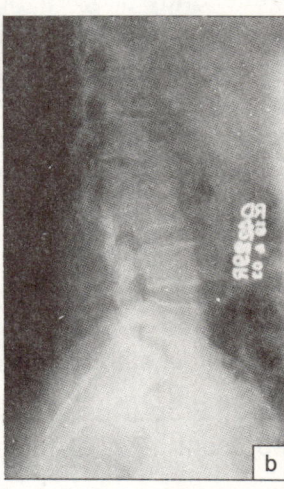

Fig. 25.3a,b. Plain radiograph AP and lateral of unstable burst fracture of L₂ vertebra. Note the comminution of vertebral body

MRI shows the extent of injury to the spinal cord and the posterior ligaments (Fig. 25.4a,b).

Fracture Stability Burst fractures are considered unstable if there is greater than 50% vertebral body compression, greater than 50% canal compromise and more than 20° kyphosis with posterior column disruption.

Treatment

Stable burst fractures without neurologic deficit are treated nonoperatively in a hyperextension brace for 3–4 months.

Unstable fractures with involvement of 3 columns and more than 50% compromise of the neural canal are associated with high incidence of neurologic deficit, increasing kyphosis and pain. These patients should be considered for stabilisation and fusion.

Patients with incomplete or progressive neuro-

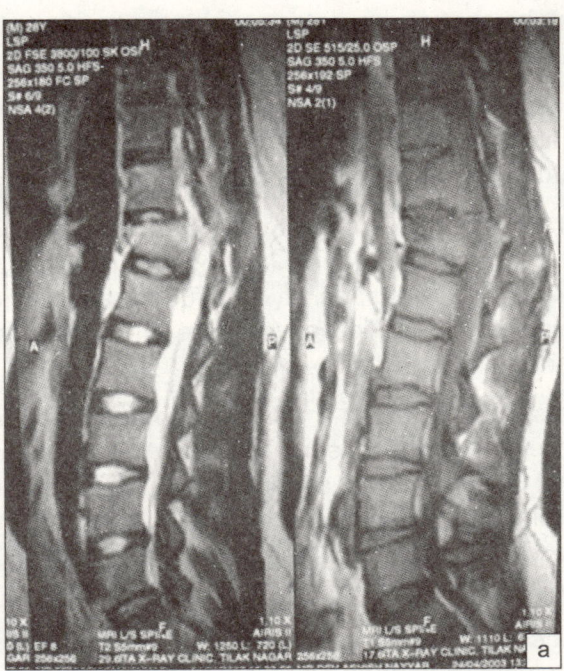

Fig. 25.4a. MRI appearance of D₁₂ fracture with compression of spinal cord

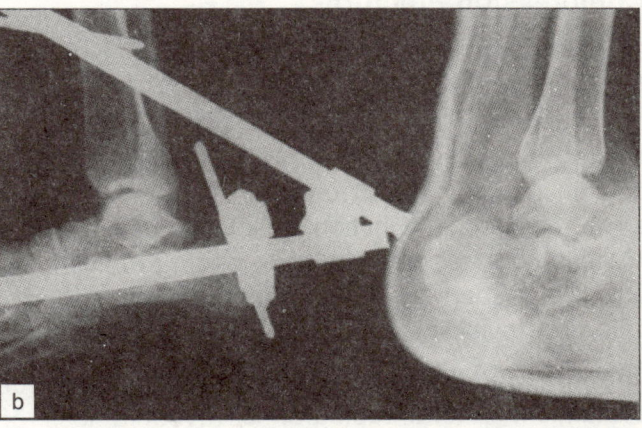

Fig. 25.4b. Bilateral calcaneal fracture in the same patient

logic deficit need early decompression and stabilisation of the spine.

Patients with complete neurologic deficit are treated with indirect reduction and stabilisation of the spine using instrumentation to improve mobilisation and reduce the complication rate.

Anterior versus Posterior Approach for Decompression of Spinal Canal after Burst Fractures

Anterior versus posterior approach for decompression and fusion in these injuries is controversial. Anterior approach provides visualisation of the canal and is also more effective in direct removal of all offending fracture fragments from the spinal canal. Anterior column can be supported, bone grafted and reconstructed using instrumentation better by the anterior approach. Anterior approach is indicated for severe initial canal compromise (>60%), residual canal compromise after posterior approach and posterior skin wounds. Newer anterior spine systems have good stability and enhanced safety compared to older systems. Disadvantages of the anterior approach are that in the presence of significant posterior column disruption it has to be combined with posterior approach. Consequently the morbidity is considerably increased. Also, significant subluxations cannot be reduced by the anterior approach.

Posterior approach involves indirect reduction using distraction or transpedicular decompression. Advantage of posterior approach is reduced morbidity but the disadvantage is that it is less efficient than anterior approach in decompression of canal and reconstitution of the anterior column. Posterior skin wounds or sores also preclude posterior approach.

Flexion-Distraction Fractures

Flexion-distraction injuries are also called *"seat - belt fractures"* since they are sustained by passengers wearing only lap seat belt in automobile accidents. During sudden deceleration, acute forward flexion of the spine across the seat belt pushes it forward on the lower part of spine, which is fixed. These injuries have anterior column compression and distraction of the posterior column. These injuries can be of three types osseous, osseoligamentous or ligamentous. The classic *Chance fracture* occurs when the distraction occurs through the bone and a horizontal splitting of vertebra (from spinous process or lamina posteriorly, through pedicles and extending into vertebral body anteriorly) results.

The anterior longitudinal ligament is intact in flexion distraction injuries (cf. fracture dislocations where ALL is torn) while disruption of interspinous, and supraspinous ligaments and ligamentum flavum creates posterior column instability. These injuries usually do not have neurological deficit but may be associated with herniation of the intervertebral disc giving rise to neurologic deficit.

These injuries may at times be associated with intra-abdominal injuries.

Imaging   Plain x-rays can demonstrate the osseous injuries quite well. When the axis of rotation in the flexion distraction injury is in the posterior part of vertebral body, compression fracture of the body may be seen.

CT scan can show bony injury on sagittal reconstruction.

MRI helps in delineation of ligamentous damage or a prolapsed intervertebral disc causing cord compression.

Fracture Stability

The flexion distraction injuries are quite unstable injuries by virtue of widespread ligamentous and/or osseous damage to the spine.

Management

Purely osseous injuries (especially with angulation less than 30 degrees) are treated non-operatively in a brace for 3 months. Osseous injuries which are severely displaced with angulation more than 30° are treated with reduction and spinal fusion.

Osseoligamentous injuries are treated conservatively if ligament damage is not extensive and adequate bony apposition can be obtained non operatively. Otherwise they are treated with short segment compression instrumentation and posterior spinal fusion.

Ligamentous injuries are treated with reduction and posterior spinal fusion.

For reduction of flexion distraction injuries, distraction techniques should never be used, as they are likely to aggravate the displacement. Compression instrumentation applied posteriorly combined with spinal fusion is treatment method of choice. Incomplete neurologic injuries should be decompressed before instrumentation and spinal fusion.

If severe anterior compression (loss of >50% anterior height of body) exists along with posterior ligamentous instability, combined anterior and posterior surgery is indicated.

Fracture-Dislocations of dorsolumbar spine

These are extremely unstable 3 column injuries

caused by flexion, rotation and shear injuries. These injuries are usually associated with severe neurologic complications (75% cases). One half of these have transection of the cord.

These injuries are more common in lumbar spine and relatively uncommon in thoracic spine due to the stabilising influence of sternum and the rib cage. If fracture - dislocation occurs in the dorsal spine, fractures are often seen at multiple levels.

Imaging Plain radiographs show translation of one spinal segment over the segment below at the site of injury on AP and lateral radiographs. The vertebral bodies may be intact (in posteroanterior shear injuries) or may show anterior wedging (in flexion - rotation injuries). The dislocated vertebral segment may sustain fractures of the posterior elements including laminae, articular facets and spinous processes and these may be fractured at several levels. The flexion distraction type of fracture dislocation may lead to bilateral facet joint dislocation (akin to cervical spine facet joint dislocation).

Fracture dislocation of the flexion-distraction type resembles seat belt injuries involving the failure of the middle and posterior column but is differentiated by intact ALL in the latter.

CT scan is particularly useful to fully evaluate bony injuries, especially in the dorsal spine.

MRI is useful to reveal the injury to spinal cord, ligamentous injuries and soft intervertebral disc herniations.

Fracture Stability

Fracture dislocations of spine are (always) the most unstable injuries.

Management

In the absence of neurological deficit, postural reduction (in prone position) followed by plaster jacket for 3 months followed by Thoraco Lumbo Sacral (TLSO) brace for 6 months has been practiced in the past.

Where the postural reduction is not possible (mostly due to locked facets), open reduction, instrumentation and spinal fusion by posterior approach are indicated.

In cases with incomplete neurologic deficit, early decompression should be done. Many surgeons recommend a posterior alignment procedure with instrumentation first, followed by the anterior decompression if necessary.

Early stabilisation prevents further injury in these cases.

In cases with complete neurologic deficit, most people recommend early stabilisation of spine across multiple segments proximal and distal to the area of injury. Anterior column decompression with either anterior or posterior (or both) fusion is done if canal compromise is severe (>60%) or there is significant translation at the level of the injury. This is followed by early rehabilitation to reduce the overall morbidity and mortality.

Other fractures of the dorsolumbar spine

Many other types of major and minor fractures of various parts of vertebral body may occur. These are usually stable fractures and are not associated with neurologic deficit.

1. Fractures of pars interarticularis (Traumatic Spondylolysis)

Severe hyperextension injury to the spine can result in fracture of the lamina. Anterior part of vertebral body may also sustain fracture in these injuries due to avulsion of A.L.L. A break in pars interarticularis (spondylolysis) may be seen on lateral x-rays but may sometimes need special oblique views for diagnosis.

These injuries are uncommon but carry with them the risk of spondylolisthesis (slip of vertebral body on vertebra below) later in life due to break in pars. Therefore, these fractures are treated with immobilisation in a brace (TLSO) for 3–4 months with the hope of achieving union. The non-union of pars interarticularis leading to spondylolisthesis is treated by posterolateral spinal fusion with or without reduction and posterior spinal instrumentation.

2. Fracture of lumbar transverse processes

Fractures of transverse processes occur in the lumbar spine. Patient gives history of violent injury or fall. Tenderness is elicited on both sides of midline and there is severe spasm of the back. The injury occurs following an indirect injury when psoas major and quadratus lumborum (both attached to transverse processes) contract violently. Multiple transverse processes are usually avulsed on both sides of midline. Injury to posterior abdominal wall and occasionally to kidney may be associated with this injury. Retroperitoneal hematoma is always associated with the lumbar transverse process fractures and when large, can cause hypotension and/or paralytic ileus.

Imaging Anteroposterior plain radiographs adequately demonstrate avulsion of the transverse processes.

Ultrasound may define the size of retroperitoneal hematoma and evaluate kidneys for injury.

Management is bed rest with pillow under the knees to keep the hips and knees flexed and relax psoas to relieve pain. Patient is gradually mobilised out of bed as the pain abates.

Paralytic ileus is treated expectantly with stoppage of oral feeds, nasogastric suction, and intravenous fluids and electrolyte administration.

Fractures of Sacrum

Fractures of the sacrum are commonly related to the pelvis fractures. They occur mostly due to high-energy trauma except the insufficiency fractures in osteoporotic patients, which occur following trivial injuries. Fractures of sacrum associated with pelvis fractures have high incidence of associated injuries such as the bladder and urethral injuries. Neurologic injury may occur in up to 50% of patients due to injury to roots traversing sacral foramina and/or injury to cauda equina terminations in the central canal.

Evaluation of patients with sacral fractures must include assessment of vitals (esp. hemodynamic status) and detailed neurologic examination including perianal sensations and anal sphincter tone. Posterior skin overlying sacrum may show bruising and/or ecchymosis. Bladder function may be impaired especially in transverse fractures occurring at S_1 to S_3.

Imaging Radiographic evaluation of sacrum fracture should include AP view of pelvis, inlet and outlet views. An AP film showing asymmetry or break in arcuate lines strongly suggests sacrum fracture. Fracture in the sacrum can be vertical (medial, through or lateral to foramina), horizontal or H-shaped Table 25.5.

Table 25.5. Danis classification of Sacral Fractures

Vertical fracture	
Type I	Lateral to foramina
Type II	Through the foramina
Type III	Medial to foramina
Horizontal fractures	
H shaped fractures	

CT Scan can help diagnose the sacral fractures definitely and define the extent of damage.

Bone Scan is useful to diagnose occult or insufficiency fractures.

Fracture Stability

In sacral fractures it is important to determine the stability of the associated pelvis fracture. Fracture of transverse process of L_5, avulsion fracture of ischial spine, asymmetry of sacral foramina and proximal migration of the injured hemipelvis suggest instability.

Management Initial treatment of sacral fractures is resuscitation and hemodynamic stabilisation when severe pelvic fractures are associated. Definitive treatment of the sacral fractures is governed by the pattern of associated pelvis injury and neurologic deficit. Sacral fractures can be ignored in the presence of other severe visceral, soft tissue or open injuries.

Sacral fractures associated with stable pelvic ring and intact neurologic function are treated with bed rest for 4–6 weeks followed by corset and protected weight bearing.

Vertical fractures associated with unstable pelvis fracture are treated according to the pelvic injury pattern.

Transverse fractures, often associated with neurologic deficit, should be treated by posterior decompression and stabilisation.

Fractures of the Coccyx

Coccygeal injuries occur due to fall in sitting

position. Either a fracture of the coccyx or disruption of the sacrococcygeal joint may result from the fall. Patients complain of pain and discomfort while sitting.

Plain radiographs demonstrate the fracture or dislocation and its displacement.

Management of displaced fractures or dislocations is by manipulation of the coccyx under anaesthesia by a gloved finger in the rectum. After reduction the injury is treated like undisplaced fracture with NSAIDs and sitz bath. Patient is advised to avoid sitting for long intervals or on the hard surface. Microwave diathermy helps in the relief of pain. If pain persists, trial of local anaesthetic infiltration may be given. Recalcitrant cases can be treated with excision of the coccyx.

Management of a Patient with Residual Neurologic Deficit

The principles of management of quadriplegic and paraplegic patients are:

1. *Assess the disability*

Rehabilitative measures for patients with neurological deficit depend on the level of injury/lesion, and the corresponding disabilities. Realistic goals then must be set for rehabilitation depending on the visceral (bladder/bowel) function, likely dependence on others for activities of daily living and expected status of ambulation.

2. *Bladder Care*

Bladder care must be started immediately after injury. Intermittent catheterization under aseptic precautions is used to manage the retention. When intermittent catheterization is not available, bladder training can be undertaken by introducing an indwelling catheter and clamping it. The urine is allowed to drain every 4 hours by releasing the clamp. The process is continued till the bladder develops the reflex pattern of emptying. Autonomous bladders (LMN) are emptied by manual pressure while automatic bladder (UMN-Lesion above L_1) empty reflexly.

3. *Chest Care*

Hypostatic pneumonia should be prevented by aggressive chest physiotherapy.

4. *Decubitus sore prevention*

This is the most important aspect of management and should begin by education of the patients and relatives. The most effective method is meticulous nursing care. Two-hourly turning round the clock is imperative to prevent development of pressure necrosis of the skin. Waterbed, air mattresses and electrically operated beds (alpha beds) are useful but not obligatory. Good skin care and avoiding wrinkles in the bed linen can also help in sore prevention. Once bedsores develop, secondary suturing, local transposition/rotation skin flap or myocutaneous flap after shaving the underlying bony prominence can be used to provide skin cover.

5. *Exercises to prevent joint contractions*

The physiotherapy should be started early to prevent contractures in the joints. The joints should be moved through the range of motion and kept in neutral/functional position.

6. *Family Education*

The family should be involved with the care of a paraplegic/quadriplegic. They should be taught skin care, bladder and bowel care, physiotherapy for chest and limbs, and above all, should be told to provide moral support to the patients.

7. *Generate Confidence (Psychological support)*

Patient should be involved in vocational training and rehabilitation and attempt should be made to generate self-esteem in the patient.

8. *Habit Reflex (Bowel Care)*

Bowel training should be undertaken in the form of stimulation of bowel reflex every 2–3 days with suppositories till habit reflex to evacuate bowels is established. Stool softeners are often required.

9. Initiate sexual, vocational and social rehabilitation.

Fractures of the Pelvis and Acetabulum

Pelvis Fractures

The pelvic ring is made of 3 bones, two innominate bones and sacrum and 3 joints – two sacroiliac joints posteriorly and symphysis pubis anteriorly.

Anterior, interosseous and posterior sacroiliac ligaments stabilise the sacroiliac joint. Interosseous and posterior sacroiliac ligaments, especially former, are very strong and resist the vertical shear injuries. Anterior sacroiliac ligaments are weak and resist anteroposterior compression as in "open book" injury. Symphyseal and sacrospinous ligaments are the other restraints, which resist anteroposterior compression (Fig. 26.1a,b).

Mechanism of Pelvis Fractures

Pelvis fractures are caused by high-energy blunt trauma. These patients often have associated serious, life threatening visceral and/or vascular injuries. Young patients often sustain pelvis frac-

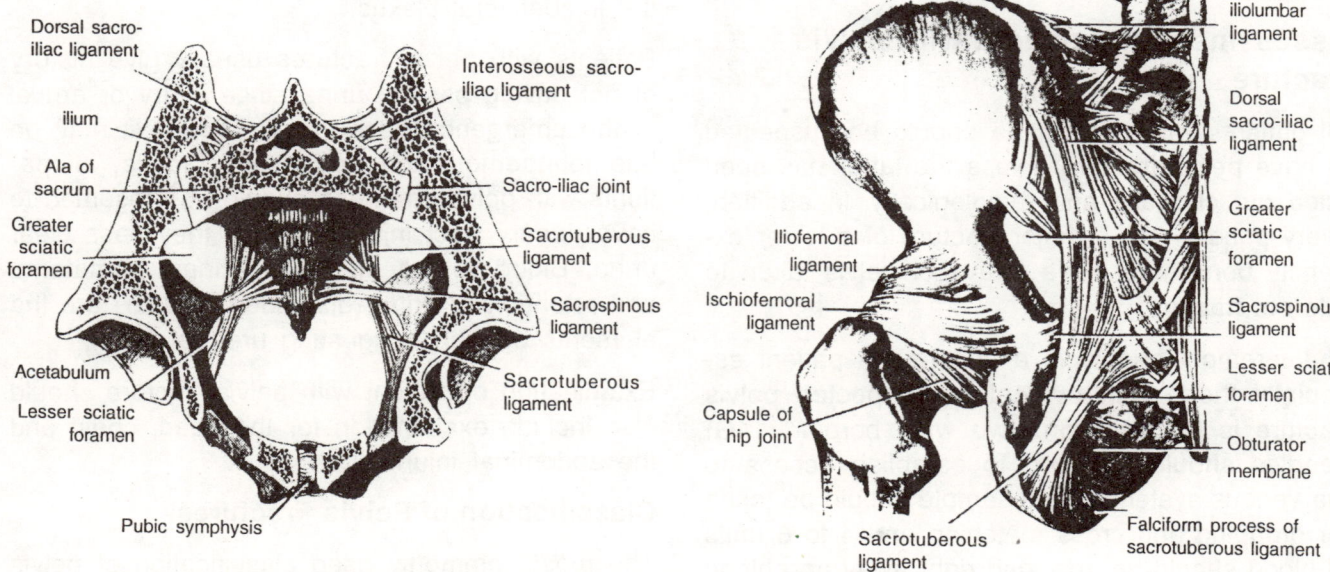

Fig. 26.1a,b Ligamentous support contributing to stability of pelvis—(a) anterior and (b) posterior views

tures due to high-speed vehicular crash or fall from height and also often have head and abdominal injuries. Most patients also have other extremity fractures. Elderly patients may however sustain pelvis fractures following fall from standing height.

The mechanical force causing pelvis fracture can be anteroposterior compression ("*Straddle*" fractures), lateral compression (motor vehicle crash or a pedestrian struck by motor vehicle) or vertical shear (*Malgaigne's* fracture). In addition, minor avulsion fractures can be caused by sudden violent contraction of the muscle attached to that site. Certain fractures such as iliac wing fractures can be caused by direct trauma.

The ligaments disrupted in pelvic fractures have been shown in Table 26.1.

Table 26.1. Ligaments disrupted in pelvic fractures

Ligaments disrupted	Resultant injury
1. a) Symphyseal ligaments ↓	Anteroposterior compression
b) Sacro-spinous ligament ↓	
c) Anterior sacroiliac ↓	(Open book injury)
d) Interosseous sacroiliac ligaments	
2. Posterior sacroiliac ligaments, Iliolumbar ligament	Vertically unstable fracture

Assessment of a patient with pelvis fracture

All patients with polytrauma should be suspected to have pelvis fracture unless the latter has been ruled out clinically and radiologically. In addition, every patient with a major fracture of a lower extremity bone must have x-rays of pelvis taken to rule out fracture.

The foremost priority in a polytrauma patient especially those with evident or suspected pelvis fracture is resuscitation. Two wide bore (# 14G) needles should be used to establish access to the venous system. Blood sample should be taken for grouping and cross matching and 4 to 6 units of blood should be arranged right away and blood bank instructed about the possible need for an-

other 4–6 units. Pelvis should be trussed (with a belt or drawer sheet) where open book injury is suspected. Patient should not be shifted frequently for the fear of disturbing the retroperitoneal hematoma and precipitating hypotension.

Diagnostic phase can then continue simultaneously with resuscitation. Flanks are inspected for abrasions, contusions or hematoma. Large hematoma may be seen above the inguinal ligament. Severe anterior injury with disruption of genitourinary floor is often associated with scrotal hematoma in males and labial swelling in females.

Pelvic ring stability is assessed by pelvic compression test to detect pain and abnormal movement. Internal and external rotation forces are applied to the iliac crests to determine any abnormal opening or closing of the pelvic ring suggesting rotational instability.

Palpation of the pubic symphysis may elicit tenderness or reveal abnormal gap.

All male patients should have rectal examination to assess the prostate and feel for bony fragments and/or large hematoma. Vaginal lacerations suggest the possibility of open fracture. All female patients should undergo a pelvic speculum examination.

Lower limbs should be examined for associated fractures, rotational deformities and shortening (in vertical shear injuries). Neurologic examination of the extremities is important to diagnose injuries to the lumbosacral plexus.

Patients with pelvis fractures usually give history of not having passed urine since injury or arrival in the emergency department. Though it may be due to haemorrhage and hypovolaemia, all patients with pelvis fractures should be presumed to have urinary tract injuries unless they pass clear urine. Blood at the meatus, perineal hematoma and retention of urine (distended bladder) are the elements of triad suggesting urethral injury.

Examination of patient with pelvis fracture should also include examination for the head, chest and the abdominal injuries.

Classification of Pelvis Fractures

The most commonly used classification of pelvis fractures is the one according to Marvan Tile Classification

TYPE A fractures are **stable** fractures. They do not involve the posterior weight-bearing arch of the pelvis. There is no compromise of the posterior pelvic complex and the pelvic floor. Examples are avulsion fractures, iliac wing fractures and transverse fractures of the sacrum.

TYPE B fractures are **rotationally unstable** and **vertically stable**. These fractures have incomplete disruptions of the posterior pelvic complex. These injuries can be external rotation injuries (open book or anterior compression) or internal rotation injuries (lateral compression).

TYPE C fractures are **vertically** and **rotationally unstable.** These injuries are caused by vertical shear forces.

These fractures are associated with complete bony or ligamentous disruption of the posterior pelvic complex and the pelvic floor.

Imaging of Pelvic Injuries

An AP radiograph of pelvis should be taken in all patients with suspected pelvic fracture initially for screening. Anterior ring fractures are appreciated on this view though subtle sacral fractures and sacroiliac disruptions can be missed.

Pelvic inlet and outlet views are done when a pelvic fracture is detected on AP film.

An inlet view of the pelvis is taken with the x-ray beam directed 60° caudally and the patient supine (Fig. 26.2a-c). This view demonstrates displacement of the pelvis in AP plane, rotational deformities of the hemipelvis as well as sacral crush fractures.

The outlet view of the pelvis is taken with the x-ray beam directed 45° cranially and the patient supine (Fig. 26.3a-c). This view demonstrates superior displacement of the pelvis, rotational deformities of the hemipelvis as well as fractures through the sacral foramina.

Signs suggestive of instability of the pelvis on plain radiographs are fracture of the L_5 transverse process, avulsion fracture of the sacrospinous ligament from the sacrum or the ischial spine, bilateral pelvic injuries, displacement of posterior sacroiliac complex more than 1 cm, posterior fracture with gap (rather than impaction) and vertical pubic rami fractures.

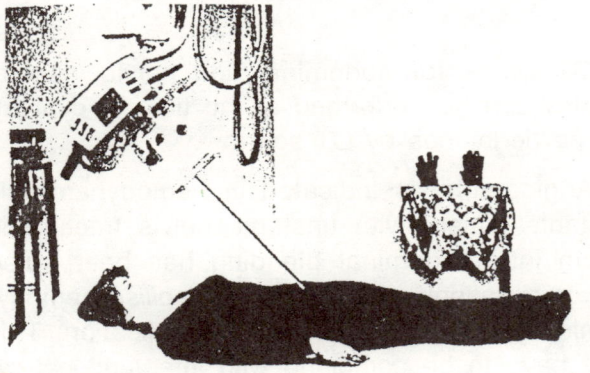
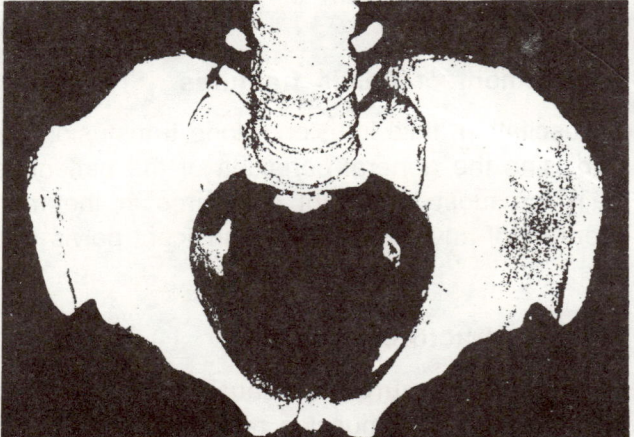
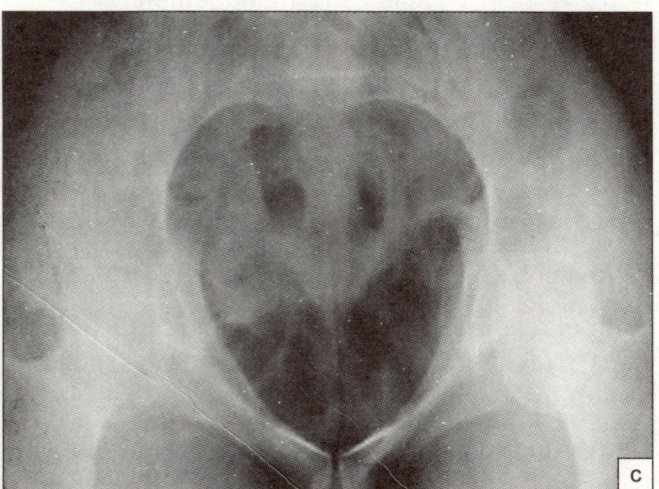

Fig. 26.2a-c. Inlet view of Pelvis (a) Bony Inlet (b) Positioning of patient for radiograph (c) Inlet view X-ray

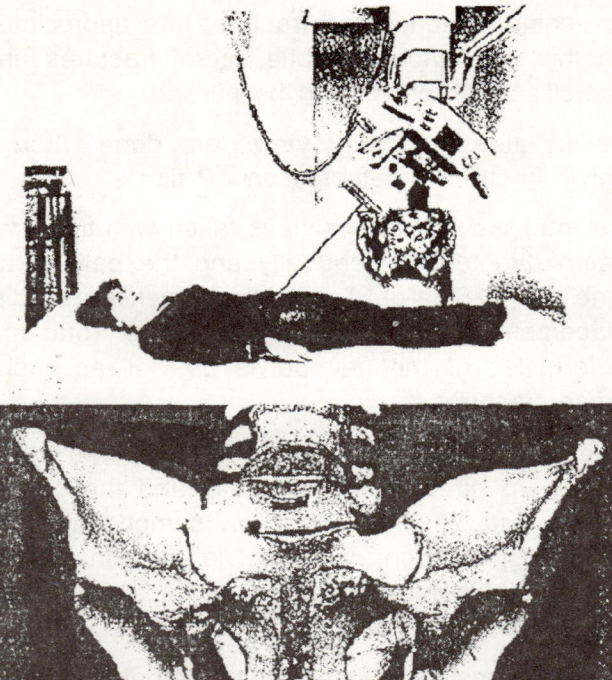

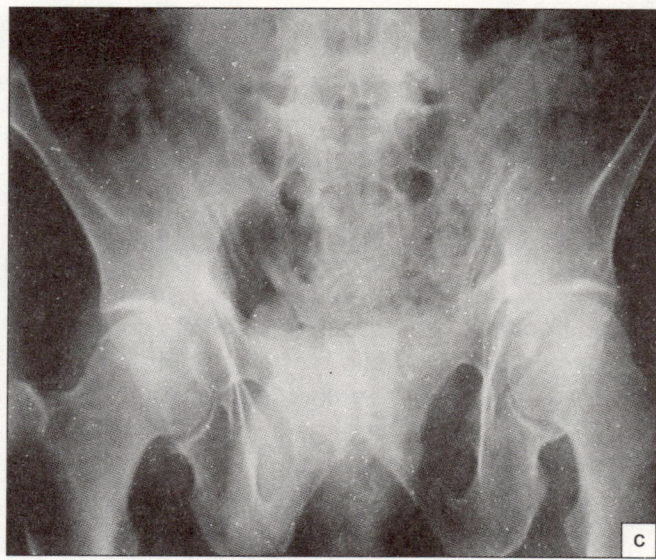

Fig. 26.3-c. Outlet view of Pelvis (a) Bony outlet (b) Positioning of patient for radiograph (c) Outlet view X-ray

CT Scan has considerably enhanced the assessment and the diagnosis of the posterior pelvic ring injuries (especially sacral fractures and sacroiliac joint disruptions). Up to one third of pelvis fractures detected on CT scan are missed on plain x-rays.

Two- and three- dimensional reconstructions provide excellent images, help to determine stability and assist in deciding the management.

CT done to assess pelvis fractures should be done from iliac crest to ischial tuberosities to avoid overlooking fractures (CT for abdomen and pelvis usually end at the level of symphysis pubis).

Special Investigations

1. Imaging of the lower urinary tract

Retrograde urethrogram, cystogram and intravenous pyelogram (IVP) are used to evaluate injuries to the urinary tract.

Ultrasound (u/s) examination is indicated in cases with visceral injuries especially the bladder injuries.

2. CT scans for abdominal and pelvic visceral injuries can be performed at the time of evaluating pelvic injuries by CT scan.

3. Angiography is indicated in hemodynamically unstable patient with unstable pelvis fracture in whom intra-abdominal bleeding has been ruled out or a patient *who does not stabilise* hemodynamically after external fixator application. This may have to be combined with interventional radiology where gelfoam or coil may be used to stop bleeding.

Management of Pelvis fractures

Resuscitation, fluid infusion, blood transfusion and stabilising the general condition of the patient remain the most important measures in the management of any patient with significant pelvis fracture.

1. Stable fractures

a) **Avulsion fractures** are caused by sudden violent contraction of muscles resulting in a piece of bone breaking off from its attachment to pelvis

(Table 26.2). Avulsion fractures are sustained most commonly by young adults during contact sports. Pain and localised tenderness point to the area of injury and the diagnosis. Plain radiographs demonstrate the size and displacement of the fragment besides confirming the diagnosis. Avulsion fractures are treated with rest, NSAIDs, fomentation and gradual mobilisation as tolerated by the patient.

Table 26.2. Avulsion fractures of pelvis

Avulsion type Fracture	Muscle responsible
1. Anterior Superior Iliac Spine (ASIS)	Sartorius
2. Anterior Inferior Iliac Spine (AIIS)	Rectus femoris
3. Ischial Tuberosity	Hamstrings
4. Iliac crest	Quadratus lumborum

b) **Iliac Wing fractures** (*Duverney*) are caused by direct trauma or fall from height. These fractures may be associated with severe troublesome local hemorrhage. Resuscitation must be initiated early. Fractures unite readily and rapidly. Bed rest, NSAIDs and gradual physiotherapy as tolerated allow the patient to be back on his feet quickly. Open iliac wing fractures are treated with internal fixation after irrigation and debridement.

c) **Fractures of pubis** occur following direct injury and are treated expectantly with rest, NSAIDs and early mobilisation.

d) **Single break in the pelvic ring** includes fractures of both superior and inferior pubic rami on one side (commonest), disruption (or opening) of symphysis pubis, fracture of iliac wing extending to ilioischial line or fractures and /or dislocation of one sacroiliac joint. Single break in pelvic ring is a stable injury and displacement of fragments is minimal. These patients mainly complain of pain, which gets worse on ambulation. Plain radiographs confirm the diagnosis. Special care should be taken to avoid overlooking a subtle posterior complex injury such as fracture of sacrum or sacroiliac joint disruption. A prominence or fracture of the ischial spine with fracture of the contralateral superior and inferior pubic ramus suggests a bucket handle injury and it is *not* a stable injury.

These injuries respond to NSAIDs and bed rest for a couple of weeks and the patient is gradually mobilised. Pubic symphysis disruptions of up to 2.5 cm are treated conservatively while larger displacements need anterior stabilisation.

2. Unstable fractures

After stabilising the general condition of the patient, the treatment of unstable pelvis fractures aims to restore stability of the pelvis to allow healing and mobilisation. Table 26.3 shows the indications for stabilisation of the injured pelvis.

Acute stabilisation of pelvis in casualty

Rapid stabilisation of the pelvis in an acute setting in casualty can be done using a Ganz C-clamp, which is a pelvic resuscitative clamp. The C-clamp is an invasive device, which is applied to the posterior pelvis to reduce it.

An anterior AO tubular type of external fixator can also control the unstable hemipelvis in the hemodynamically unstable patient. This type of fixator serves as the definite stabilisation for open book injuries (where posterior and interosseous sacroiliac ligaments are intact and function as tension band) and as provisional stabilisation for the other

Table 26.3. Pelvis Fractures: Indications for stabilisation

EARLY
Absolute	Acute hemorrhagic blood loss associated with unstable pelvis fracture
	Open pelvis fractures with perineal injuries
Relative	Multiply injured patient with associated fractures

DELAYED
Absolute	Displacement of symphysis more than 2.5 cm
	Displaced sarcoiliac joint disruptions (Dislocations/Fracture- Dislocations)
	Severe rotational deformity when limb cannot be brought to neutral
	Vertical shear injuries with limb length discrepancy >2 cm
Relative	Locked symphysis pubis
	Tilt fracture (displaced superior ramus fracture projecting posteriorly into perineum). Tilt fractures lead to dyspareunia in females
	Sacral fracture with compression of sacral nerves
	Sacral fractures with gap more than 5 mm

posterior complex injuries in unstable pelvis fractures.

Other measures which can be used for stabilizing the pelvis in acute setting are tying a broad belt, broad sheet, or any other truss (hammock sling) around the pelvis, vacuum bean bag and pneumatic anti shock garment.

Once the patient is stabilised, decision is made regarding the definitive management.

If facilities and expertise for open reduction and stabilisation are not available, the unstable pelvis fracture should be treated by skeletal traction for 6 weeks. Canvas slings can be used to achieve and maintain reduction of open book type of injuries.

Another method of treating open book injuries aims to achieve manual reduction by lateral compression followed by well padded double spica cast for maintaining the reduction.

Internal fixation of unstable pelvis fractures can be done anteriorly as well as posteriorly.

Anteriorly, the separation of symphysis pubis can be treated by reduction and internal fixation with plate and screws through a *Pfannensteil* incision. The plate and screws fixation acts as tension band in open book injuries. In cases where posterior instability is also present but only anterior stabilisation is being done, two plates can be applied at 90° to each other.

Posteriorly, the unstable posterior pelvic complex can be fixed anteriorly, posteriorly or percutaneously. Anterior approach involves fixing a fracture close to S I joint or an S I joint disruption using a 2- or 3- hole plate and screws anteriorly through a retroperitoneal approach. Special care, however, should be taken to avoid injury to L_5 nerve root.

Posterior approach is used to fix the posterior pelvic disruptions using contoured reconstruction plate with screws or transiliac bars. Posterior approach needs image control to avoid injury to anterior neurovascular structures and has high incidence of skin breakdown and infection.

Percutaneous fixation for sacroiliac dislocations and sacral fractures using ilio sacral screw (from outer table of the iliac wing, across the sacroiliac joint into the S1 body) is an excellent option which avoids the potential soft tissue complications of the posterior approach.

Complications of the Pelvic Fractures

Pelvis fractures are associated with many troublesome and potentially fatal complications. The mortality in various pelvis fractures is reported in 6-25% cases.

1. Hemorrhage

Retroperitoneal hematoma and intraabdominal bleeding (due to concomitant abdominal injury) are the main causes of hypovolaemia, shock and death in patients with pelvis fractures. Fluid resuscitation should be started immediately on receiving the patient with pelvis fracture in casualty. Continuing hemodynamic instability in a patient with unstable pelvic fracture is indication for determining the presence of the intra-abdominal bleed (Fig. 26.4 algorithm). Laparotomy and pelvic stabilisation are performed if there is evidence of intra-abdominal bleeding. If there is no intra-abdominal bleeding, immediate stabilisation of pelvis should be performed. If patient still remains hemodynamically unstable, arteriography/angiography to determine the source of bleeding and coil or embolize the bleeders is performed. Where facilitates for angiography and interventional radiology are not available, ligation of internal iliac arteries can control troublesome bleeding.

2. Injuries to urinary tract

Straddle fractures (bilateral superior and inferior pubic rami fracture) are most commonly associated with rupture of the urethra. Rupture of the urethra is common in males and commonly membranous urethra is injured. Extraperitoneal rupture of the bladder can occur with extravasation of urine occurring in the perivesical space. Patients with pelvis fractures are examined carefully for injury to urinary tract and special imaging techniques are performed if deemed necessary. Urologist should be consulted for the management of injuries to the urinary tract.

3. Visceral Injuries

Injuries to viscera (bowel, rectum) can occur in severe pelvic injuries and need laparotomy to deal with them.

4. Other associated injuries

Injuries to perineum, vaginal lacerations, testicular injuries and rupture of the diaphragm can occur

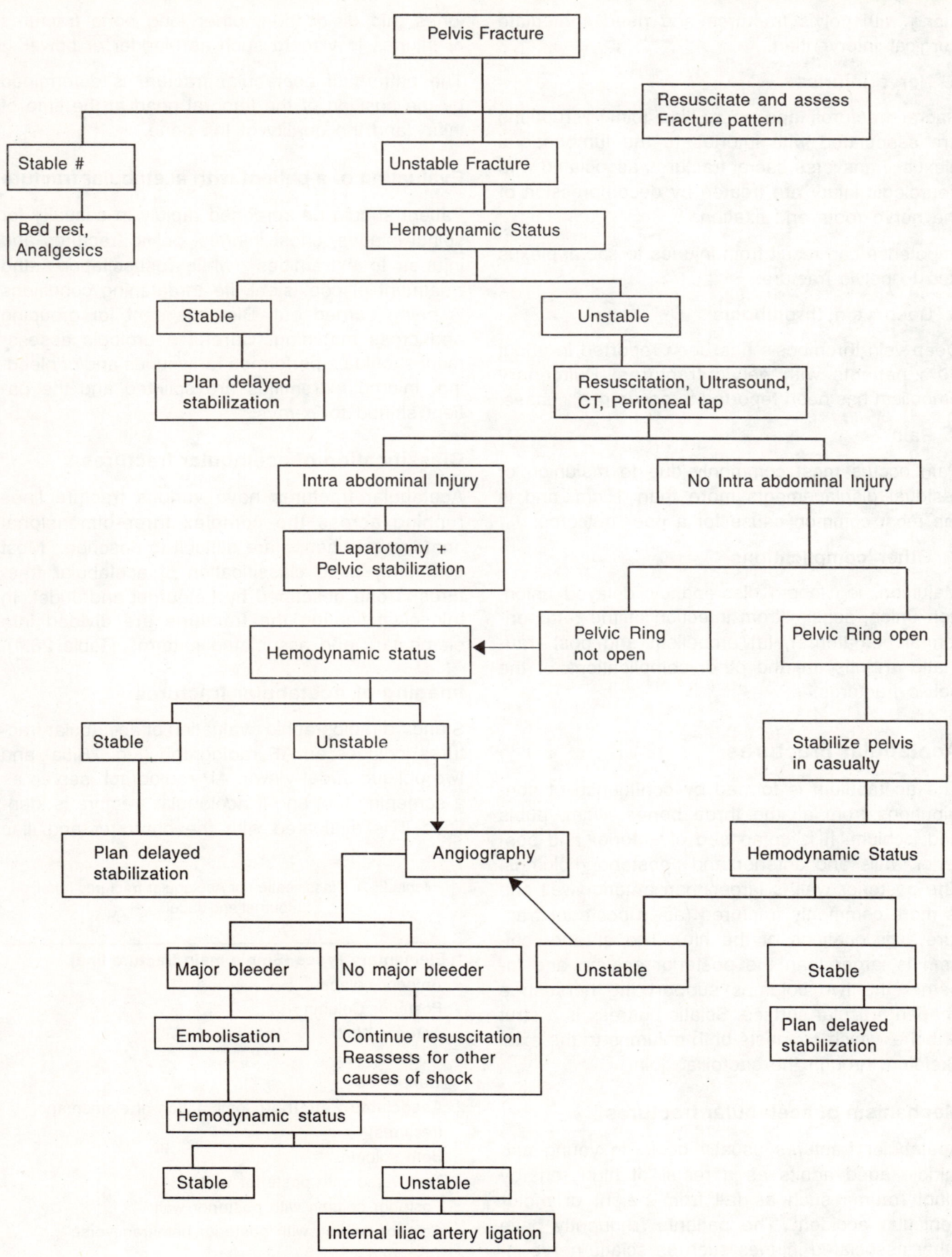

Fig. 26.4. Algorithm for management of Pelvic Fractures

along with pelvis fractures and need immediate surgical intervention.

5. Nerve injuries

Sacral fractures and sacro-iliac joint disruptions are associated with injuries to the lumbosacral plexus. Transverse sacral fractures associated with neurologic injury are treated by decompression of the nerve roots and fixation.

Impotence can result from injuries to sacral plexus due to pelvic fracture.

6. Deep vein thrombosis

Deep vein thrombosis has been reported in about 60% patients with pelvic fractures. Pulmonary embolism has been reported to occur in 2% cases.

7. Pain

Pain occurs most commonly due to malunion or residual displacements more than 1 cm. and is the most common cause for a poor outcome.

8. Other complications

Malunion, leg length discrepancy, delayed union, non union, sepsis (from infection of the retroperitoneal hematoma), fat embolism and post traumatic arthritis are the other complications of the pelvic fractures.

Acetabular Fractures

The acetabulum is formed by confluence of contributions from all the three bones: ilium, pubis and ischium. It is comprised of anterior and posterior walls and anterior and posterior columns. The posterior wall is larger than anterior wall and is more commonly fractured (as in posterior fracture - dislocations of the hip). The anterior column is larger than the posterior column and together the two columns support the horseshoe shaped articular surface. Sciatic buttress is a strut of bone, which connects both columns to the axial skeleton through the sacroiliac joint.

Mechanism of acetabular fractures

Acetabular fractures usually occur in young and middle aged adults as a result of high -energy blunt trauma such as fall from height or motor vehicular accident. The patients frequently have other associated injuries such as sciatic nerve in-

juries, hip dislocation, other long bone fractures or injuries to viscera such as bladder or bowel.

The pattern of acetabular fracture is determined by the position of the femoral head at the time of injury and the quality of the bone.

Evaluation of a patient with acetabular fracture

Patient should be screened rapidly in casualty for spinal injuries, chest injuries, pelvic fractures and injuries to extremities while resuscitation and treatment of coexistent life threatening conditions is being carried out. Blood is sent for grouping and cross matching. Careful neurologic assessment should be performed for wounds and/or bleeding. Injured extremities are splinted and the patient shifted for x-rays.

Classification of acetabular fractures

Acetabular fractures have various fracture lines running across the complex three-dimensional anatomy and hence are difficult to describe. Most commonly used classification of acetabular fractures is one described by Letournel and Judet. In this classification the fractures are divided into elementary and associated patterns (Table 26.4).

Imaging of Acetabular fractures

Standard radiographic evaluation of acetabular fractures includes an AP radiograph (Fig. 26.5a) and two oblique Judet views. AP radiograph serves as a screening tool and if acetabular fracture is identified it is evaluated with the obturator and iliac

Table 26.4. Classification of Acetabular fractures (after Letournel and Judet)

---

1. **Elementary Types (Single main fracture line)**
   Anterior column
   Posterior Column
   Anterior Wall
   Posterior wall
   Transverse
2. **Associated Patterns** (Combination of elementary fractures)
   Both column
   Transverse with posterior wall
   Posterior column with posterior wall
   Anterior column with posterior hemitransverse
   T-Shaped.

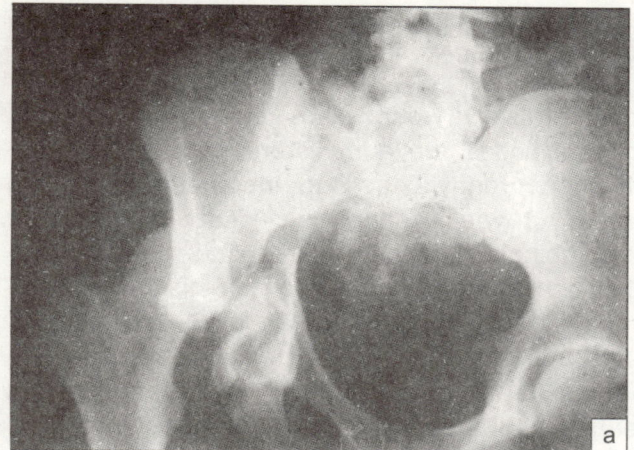

Fig. 26.5a. AP view of a patient with acetabular fracture. Note the posterior column with posterior wall fracture and associated posterior dislocation of hip

oblique Judet views. The **obturator oblique view** is taken with the patient turned 45° to the contralateral (unaffected) side. The obturator view shows obturator foramen in its entirety and is best for the imaging of the anterior column and the posterior wall

The **Iliac oblique view** is taken with the patient turned 45° to ipsilateral (affected) side. The Iliac view shows the ilium in its entirety and is best for the imaging of the posterior column and the anterior wall.

Computerised Tomography (CT) is extremely useful in the acetabular fractures. It shows intraarticular

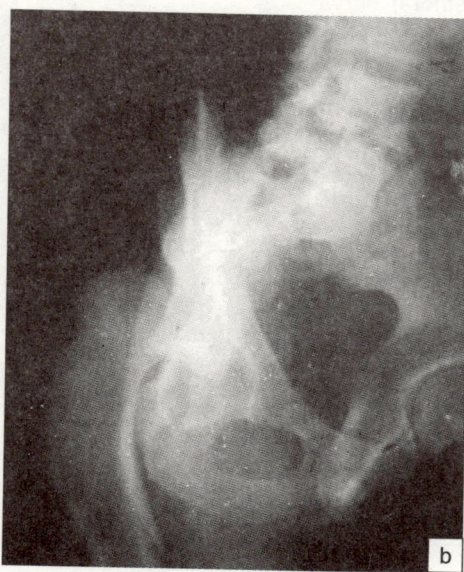

Fig. 26.5b. Obturator view of the same patient

fragments and femoral head fractures which are frequently missed on plain x-rays.

It is useful for showing articular discontinuity, rotation of fragments and marginal impaction injuries. CT evaluation of posterior wall fragment can determine the hip stability. Fragments less than or equal to 20% of posterior wall are associated with a stable hip (Treat conservatively) while fragments larger than 40% of posterior wall are unstable (Treat surgically). 3-D reconstruction can improve fracture visualisation and may help in surgical planning.

Treatment

If acetabular fractures are associated with unstable pelvis fractures or other life threatening injuries, the treatment of associated injuries takes preference over acetabular fracture. However, a hip dislocation with acetabular fracture must be reduced early pending definitive treatment of the acetabular fracture.

Conservative treatment of acetabular fractures is indicated for

1. Undisplaced or minimally displaced fractures

2. Those that involve only small areas of weight bearing articular surface

3. Severe osteoporosis, sepsis, and serious systemic illness precluding operative treatment are also indications for non operative treatment

4. Certain displaced **both column** fractures may reveal so-called "secondary congruence" and can be treated conservatively.

Conservative treatment involves longitudinal (upper tibial pin) traction in bed for 10–12 weeks. Trochanteric (lateral) traction is seldom useful or indicated.

Surgical Treatment

The aims of surgical treatment of acetabular fractures are to provide stability and pain relief initially to allow early mobilisation (Fig. 26.5c). The ultimate aims are the prevention of posttraumatic arthritis and loss of function. Indications for surgical treatment of acetabular fractures are irreducible fracture / dislocations, greater than 3mm step in articular surface, loss of acetabular

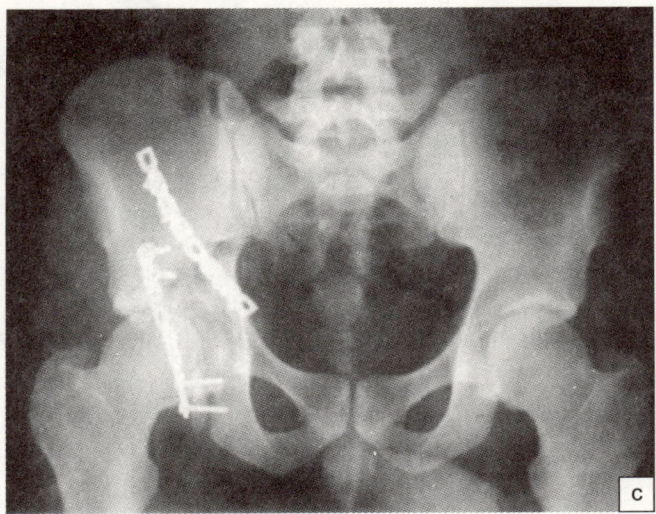

Fig. 26.5c. Both columns fracture of acetabulum fixed by combined anterior and posterior approach

congruency, posterior wall fractures greater than 40% in size and intraarticular fractures. The various surgical approaches and the region that can be accessed through them are shown in Table 26.5. Each approach has certain complications associated with its use.

Fixation of acetabular fractures is achieved by using special reconstruction plates, 3.5 mm dynamic compression plates and cancellous screws inserted percutaneously.

Postoperatively, wounds are drained for 48 hours and antibiotics are administered. Heterotopic ossification prophylaxis (Cap Indomethacin 75 mg daily for 2 weeks) should be used when posterior or combined approaches are used. Low molecular weight heparin should be administered subcutaneously for DVT prophylaxis for 3–6 weeks. Patients are mobilised out of bed as early as comfortable and are encouraged to walk non-weight bearing. Full weight bearing is allowed after 8 to 10 weeks.

Complications

Serious complications occur commonly after acetabular fractures and also after their surgical treatment. Hemorrhage, sepsis, injury to neurovascular structures, deep vein thrombosis, heterotopic ossification and posttraumatic arthritis are some of the common complications. Intra-articular penetration of hardware is likely during surgery and can be avoided by intraoperative use of fluoroscopy. Total hip replacement done following acetabular fracture has a worse outcome compared with THA for osteoarthritis.

Table 26.5. Surgical approaches for acetabular fractures

Approach	Regions exposed	Complications
Ilioinguinal (anterior)	*Anterior wall *Anterior column(including quadrilateral plate, superior pubic ramus, and symphysis pubis)	Injury to *femoral nerve *femoral vessels *lateral cutaneous nerve of thigh *bleeding from corona mortis
Kocher-Langenbeck (posterior)	*Posterior wall *Posterior column *Sciatic notch	*Injury to sciatic nerve *Damage to blood supply of femoral head
Extensile approaches i) Combined anterior and posterior	Both columns	Incomplete simultaneous both column visualisation
ii) Extended iliofemoral (lateral)	Lateral aspect of innominate bone and both columns (if superior gluteal artery is not patent)	*Heterotopic ossification *Gluteal muscle necrosis
iii) Triradiate	Both columns	*Skin necrosis *Inadequate visualisation

Injuries of the Hip and Thigh

- *Dislocation of Hip Joint*
- *Femoral Neck Fractures*
- *Intertrochanteric Fractures of Femur*
- *Subtrochanteric Fractures of the Femur*
- *Fractures of the Femoral Shaft*
- *Supracondylar Femur Fractures*
- *Distal Femoral Epiphyseal Injury*

Dislocation of Hip Joint

The hip joint is inherently quite stable. *Bony* stability is provided by ball and socket configuration which ensures that nearly 70% of the femoral head is covered by the acetabulum and labrum at all times. *Soft tissue* stability is provided by the iliofemoral ligament (anterior) and Wischiofemoral ligament (posterior) in addition to the hip joint capsule. Understandably, therefore, the hip joint dislocations are caused by high-energy trauma.

Mechanism of Injury

Hip joint dislocations are mostly caused by road traffic accidents. A direct axial blow to the femur pushes the head out of acetabulum. The position of the thigh at the time of the impact determines the direction of the hip dislocation. Direct axial blow to hip, which is adducted, flexed and inter-nally rotated (as in dashboard injuries) leads to posterior dislocation of the hip. These injuries are often associated with fractures of the posterior actabular wall. If the limb is abducted and flexed at the time of injury, it leads to anterior dislocation. A direct impact over the trochanter may drive the femoral head through the floor of the acetabulum and result in central fracture dislocation of the hip. Central fracture dislocation may occur commonly in epileptic patients.

Classification

Hip dislocations can be divided according to the direction of the dislocation namely anterior, posterior (Fig. 27.1a) and central. The anterior dislocations may be further divided into superior (head is dislocated above the superior pubic ramus) and inferior (or thyroid type-head in this case is dislocated within the obturator foramen) (Fig. 27.1b).

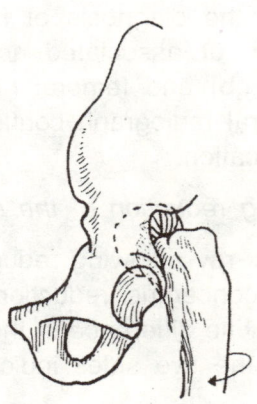

Fig. 27.1a. Posterior dislocation of hip-line diagram

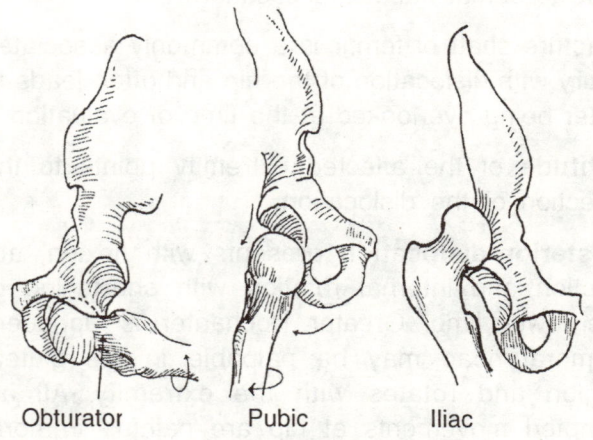

Obturator   Pubic   Iliac

Fig. 27.1b.Types of anterior dislocation of hip-line diagram

Posterior dislocation of the hip has been classified by Thompson-Epstein (Table 27.1).

Table 27.1. Thompson-Epstein classification of Posterior Dislocation of Hip

I: Posterior dislocation with or without small posterior acetabular wall fragment. Stable on closed reduction.

II: Posterior dislocation with large posterior wall fragment. Unstable after reduction

III: Posterior dislocation with large comminuted posterior acetabular wall fragment

IV: Posterior dislocation with acetabular roof fracture

V: Posterior dislocation with **femoral head fracture** (Classified by Pipkin)
    Va   below fovea
    Vb   above fovea
    Vc   with fracture neck of femur
    Vd   with acetabular fracture

Evaluation of a Patient with Suspected Hip Dislocation

Hip dislocation should be suspected in any young adult who sustains high velocity trauma and presents to the casualty with shortening and abnormal attitude of the lower extremity. The injury is rare in children (as *all* dislocations are rare since the remodelling bone fails before strong ligaments) and elderly (as fracture of osteoporotic bone occurs more readily than dislocation).

Vital functions must be assessed before musculoskeletal system in these patients due to the high incidence of associated head, chest, abdominal and/ or pelvic injuries. A dislocated hip may be the cause of shock due to pain or intrapelvic haemorrhage (due to cental fracture dislocation).

Fracture shaft of femur is a commonly associated injury with dislocation of the hip and often leads to latter being overlooked at the time of evaluation.

Attitude of the affected extremity points to the direction of the dislocation.

Posterior dislocation presents with flexion, adduction and internal rotation with shortening of the lower limb. Greater trochanter is upridden. Femoral head may be palpable in the gluteal region and rotates with the extremity. All attempted movements at hip are painful. Femoral artery is not readily palpable as the bony support is lacking posteriorly (*Narath sign*).

Anterior dislocation presents with flexion, abduction and external rotation (Fig. 27.2). The limb appears longer. Attempted movements at the hip are painful.

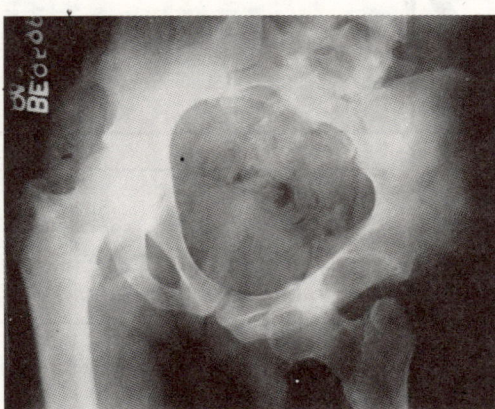

Fig. 27.2.   Anterior dislocation of left hip. Note the abduction and external rotation of the hip

Central fracture dislocation is difficult to diagnose clinically. The limb is usually in neutral position. The attempted movements at the hip are extremely painful. The distance of trochanter from the midline is reduced on the affected side. The bitrochanteric manual compression test is painful.

Neurovascular assessment must be done in every case of suspected dislocation of the hip. The sciatic nerve lies close to the posterior capsule and is at risk for injury in the cases with posterior dislocation of the hip.

Imaging for Hip Dislocations

Plain radiographs: An anteroposterior x-ray of pelvis with both hips is an excellent screening modality for hip dislocation in a patient with polytrauma. AP view allows the diagnosis of hip dislocation and identification of associated acetabular fractures (Fig. 27.3a,b) and femoral head fractures. Cross table lateral radiograph confirms the direction of the dislocation.

Imaging following reduction of the dislocation

Anteroposterior x-ray following reduction is useful to confirm the concentric reduction. Asymmetric joint space or subtle difference in the medial clear space between the two sides indicates incarcerated fragments.

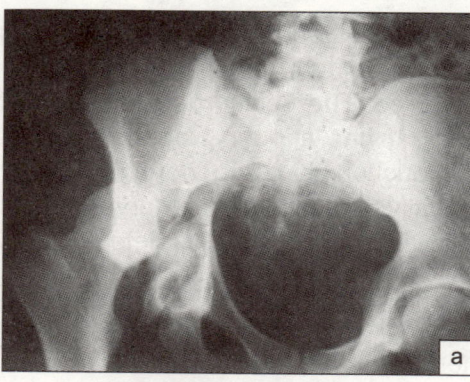

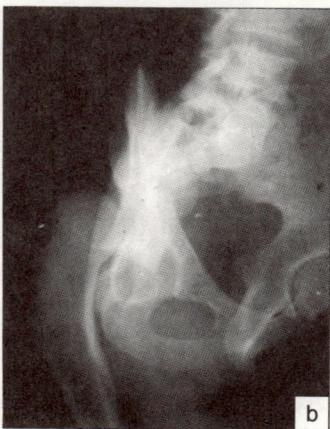

Fig. 27.3a,b. X-rays showing posterior dislocation of hip. Note the associated acetabular fracture

CT Scan is not indicated for adequately reduced simple dislocations but is done preferably following the reduction of all fracture dislocations to confirm concentricity of reduction and diagnose incarcerated bony fragments. CT scan is extremely useful when surgical treatment is contemplated for fracture dislocations to assess comminution of the fragments, for irreducible dislocations and / or for unstable reductions.

MRI allows evaluation of the viability of the head when avascular necrosis is suspected. MRI also is a useful tool for the evaluation of the labrum.

Treatment

Dislocation of hip is an emergency and its management takes precedence even over the head injury. Femoral head should be reduced promptly into the acetabulum under general anaesthesia with full muscle relaxation. Reduction must be achieved within 6 hours of injury. Delayed reduction is associated with problems in closed reduction. The incidence of avascular necrosis also increases with the time to reduction.

Manoeuvres for reduction of posterior dislocation

Bigelow's Manoeuvre

Patient should be preferably put on the floor and pelvis is stabilised by one person. Another person should apply traction along the axis of the thigh with hip and knee flexed to right angle. Femoral head is felt to reduce in the acetabulum with a jerk.

Stimson's gravity method

Patient is put prone on a table with hip flexed to a right angle beyond the edge of the table. With the knee also flexed to 90°, longitudinal traction along the axis of the thigh assisted with gravity is used to reduce the dislocation.

Following reduction, skeletal traction is applied through the upper tibial pin with hip abducted to about 20° and fully extended. Traction is continued for six weeks followed by gradual hip mobilisation and protected, graduated weight bearing for the next 6 weeks.

Reduction of anterior dislocation (Allis Manoeuvre)

Traction is applied along the axis of the thigh and the hip is gently adducted and internally rotated to achieve reduction. Treatment after reduction is same as for posterior dislocation.

Reduction of central fracture dislocation is achieved by applying upper tibial pin skeletal traction. Periodic x-rays reveal the gradual reduction of the medially displaced head. Rarely, lateral traction through trochanter via a schanz pin inserted in the neck of femur may be required to pull the femoral head laterally out of the fractured floor of the acetabulum.

Operative Treatment

Operative treatment is indicated for

1. Irreducible dislocation
2. Unstable hip following closed reduction
3. Incarcerated bony fragment leading to incongruent reduction
4. Concomitant fracture fixation of:
   a) large posterior wall fragment

b) femoral head and /or neck fracture in a young patient

5. Fracture of head, neck and/or acetabulum in elderly patients where arthroplasty is indicated.

6. Sciatic nerve palsy appearing after the closed reduction of hip dislocation.

Complications

1. Irreducible dislocation

Failure of closed reduction of a hip dislocation can occur due to entrapment of a bony fragment, interposition of soft tissue (labrum, capsule) or due to buttonholing of the femoral head out of the hip joint capsule.

An irreducible dislocation is an indication for open reduction.

2. Associated fractures

Fractures of the acetabular margin are the most common fractures associated with hip dislocation. The acetabular fragment usually falls in place once the dislocation is reduced. Persistently displaced large fragment is treated by open reduction and internal fixation using cancellous screws or buttress plating using reconstruction plates.

Femoral head, femoral neck and femoral shaft fractures are the other fractures associated with hip dislocation.

Femoral head and/or femoral neck fractures associated with hip dislocation are best treated by internal fixation in young adults and arthroplasty in the elderly patients.

Fracture shaft of femur can often lead to missed diagnosis of ipsilateral dislocation of the hip. If, in a fracture shaft of femur, the proximal fragment is adducted rather than abducted, ipsilateral posterior dislocation of hip should be suspected. Securing pelvis x-rays for all patients with major lower limb trauma can avoid the complication of missed hip dislocation.

Fracture shaft of femur associated with hip dislocation is an indication for internal fixation of the shaft fracture.

3. Neurovascular injury

Sciatic nerve injury has been reported in up to 20% cases of posterior dislocation of the hip joint. The lateral popliteal component is more commonly involved. The sciatic nerve injury is treated expectantly. It has a poor prognosis for recovery. If open reduction is being done for hip dislocation, clinically injured sciatic nerve must be explored and inspected for complete transection.

A sciatic nerve palsy, which presents for the first time after reduction is an indication for exploration of the nerve.

Femoral artery or nerve can be damaged during anterior dislocation of the hip. The femoral nerve injury is treated expectantly while femoral arterial injury needs urgent angiography and repair.

Superior gluteal artery injury may occur in patients with central fracture dislocation.

4. Avascular necrosis of femoral head

Avascular necrosis of femoral head occurs in about 15% cases of hip dislocation. Prompt reduction can reduce the incidence. Sartorius or quadratus femoris based muscle pedicle bone grafts can be used in an attempt to improve vascularisation of the femoral head in young adults. Avascular necrosis resulting in secondary osteoarthritis in young patients can be treated by arthrodesis of the hip while in elderly patient, replacement arthroplasty is the treatment of choice.

5. Myositis Ossificans

Myositis ossificans can occur following hip dislocation (2% cases). It is more likely to occur in patients treated surgically, patients mobilised early and those with head injury. The functional compromise is not always proportionate to the amount of bone seen on radiographs but stiffness of hip occurs commonly in these cases.

6. Secondary Osteoarthritis

Secondary osteoarthritis occurs as a sequel to avascular necrosis with deformation of femoral head due to collapse or in cases of acetabular incongruity arising from central fracture dislocation of hip or malunited acetabular wall fracture. It takes many years to develop. Patient develops painful restriction of movements, limp and shortening. In a young adult with unilateral affliction, arthrodesis of hip is the treatment of choice though it is not suitable for the Indian society and habits. Elderly patients with secondary osteoarthritis are best treated with replacement arthroplasty.

7. Recurrent dislocation

Recurrent dislocation is an unusual complication of hip dislocation. It needs CT (for evaluation of bony structures-most commonly large posterior acetabular fragment) and MRI (for evaluation of labrum) to elicit the cause of instability so that remedial operative intervention can be undertaken.

8. Neglected hip dislocation

It is a clinical entity peculiar to our country where the hip has remained dislocated for weeks to months without treatment. In such neglected dislocations the patients must be put on heavy skeletal traction through the upper tibial pins, and heavy sedation and muscle relaxation. Gupta and Saravat described a method of closed reduction of these neglected fractures by heavy skeletal traction (up to 18 Kgs) followed by gradual reduction of weights with the limb in increasing degrees of abduction.

In some cases it may be possible to achieve gradual reduction using this method. In others it brings the femoral head closer to the acetabulum so that open reduction is rendered easier. Open reduction in the late cases is fraught with the dangers of sciatic nerve injury and avascular necrosis but restores anatomy, making subsequent reconstructive surgery easier.

A pain-free persistent dislocation in a young adult can be treated with intertrochanteric osteotomy to correct disabling adduction and internal rotation deformity.

Femoral Neck Fractures

Fractures of the femoral neck occur most commonly in elderly individuals who sustain low energy fractures from falls while walking or standing. The indirect injury leads to rotational strain on the osteoporotic neck of femur, which fails. Rarely (5% or less), the femoral neck fractures occur in high-energy trauma (as in the vehicular trauma or fall from height) in patients younger than 50 years of age. Femoral neck fractures occur more frequently in patients with medical comorbidities including disturbances of vision, balance and neurologic diseases.

Relevant anatomy

The adult femoral neck shaft angle is approximately 130° while the femoral neck anteversion is approximately 10 degrees. Vascularity of femoral head must be understood in detail (Fig. 27.4a,b) for a rational approach to surgical management of the femoral neck fractures (Table 27.2).

Compromise of vascularity of femoral head following fracture of femoral neck.

A femoral neck fracture leads to:

1. Interruption of vascular supply from nutrient artery due to fractures of the femoral neck;

2. Disruption or kinking of the lateral epiphyseal arterial system due to direct pressure from fracture fragments; and,

3. Intra-articular hematoma which leads to pressure elevation in the joint resulting in compromise of blood flow through the retinacular vessels.

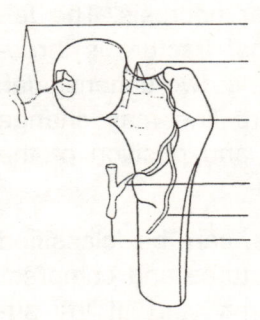

Obturator artery and the foveal artery

Ascending cervical branches of the arterial ring

Arterial ring of the femoral neck

Medial femoral circumflex artery

First perforator artery

Profunda femoris artery

Posterior

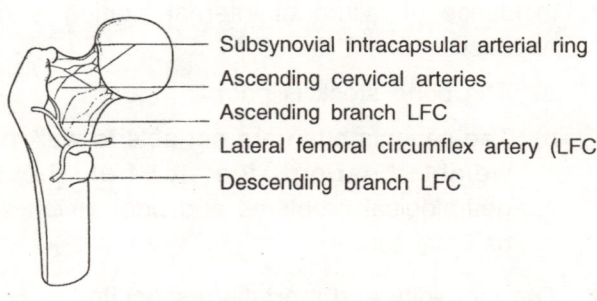

Subsynovial intracapsular arterial ring

Ascending cervical arteries

Ascending branch LFC

Lateral femoral circumflex artery (LFC)

Descending branch LFC

Anterior

Fig. 27.4a,b. Posterior (a) and anterior (b) views of the hip, showing the extraosseous blood supply to the femoral head.

Table 27.2. Blood supply of femoral head

Vessel	Branch of	Location supplied	Area of femoral head
1. Lateral epiphyseal artery	Medial femoral circumflex (Profunda femoris system)	Retinacular reflection at the posterior superior capsule femoral neck (Ascending cervical arteries)	Most of the femoral head (90%)
2. Inferior metaphyseal artery	Ascending portion of lateral femoral circumflex	Midportion of anterior hip capsule	Anterior and inferior metaphyseal bone
3. Medial epiphyseal artery	Artery of ligamentum teres (obturator arterial system)	through ligamentum teres	(Variable) Medial part of the head

The "problem" fracture

The femoral neck fracture is called *the problem fracture* because of its peculiar characteristics:

1. It is difficult to achieve union because
   a) The periosteum in femoral neck region is deficient in cambium layer.
   b) The synovial fluid washes away the fracture hematoma since the fracture is intra-capsular.
   c) Vascularity of the femoral head is compromised following fracture.
   d) It is difficult to get secure purchase on the proximal fragment, which is small and osteoporotic; inadequate fixation contributes to non-union.
   e) There is significant comminution of the posterior cortex at the fracture site, which predisposes to collapse into retroversion and implant failure.

2. Incidence of failure of internal fixation is high because
   a) The bone stock is poor
   b) The patients often are not able to walk non-weight bearing due to frail health, neurological problems and poor vision and/or balance.

3. The morbidity and mortality associated with the fracture is high due to the high incidence of comorbidities in the elderly patients who are most prone to this fracture.

Classification

1. Traumatic fractures
2. Insufficiency/fatigue fractures

The traumatic fractures are classified by Garden's classification and Pauwel's classification.

Garden's classification of femoral neck fractures includes incomplete (Type I), complete undisplaced (Type II), incomplete displaced (Type III) and complete displaced (Type IV). The trabecular alignment of the acetabulum and proximal femur is variably disturbed based on the fracture type (Fig. 27.4c).

Pauwel's classification (Fig. 27.4d) is based on orientation of the fracture with respect to a horizontal line through the superior margin of acetabulum with Type I having 30°, Type II having 50° and Type III having 70° inclination of the fracture line. Fracture line is more vertical with progression from type I to III and hence increasing shear forces are placed across the fracture site. Type III has the worst prognosis and the highest incidence of avascular necrosis. The fallacy of this classification is that fracture is three-dimensional while the x-ray is two-dimensional. The orientation of the fracture line may change with direction of x-ray beam and position of the patient.

The insufficiency fractures can be classified into tension or transverse fractures and compression fractures. Tension fractures start at the superior lateral neck and they invariably displace. They must be fixed operatively before they displace. The compression fractures occur in the

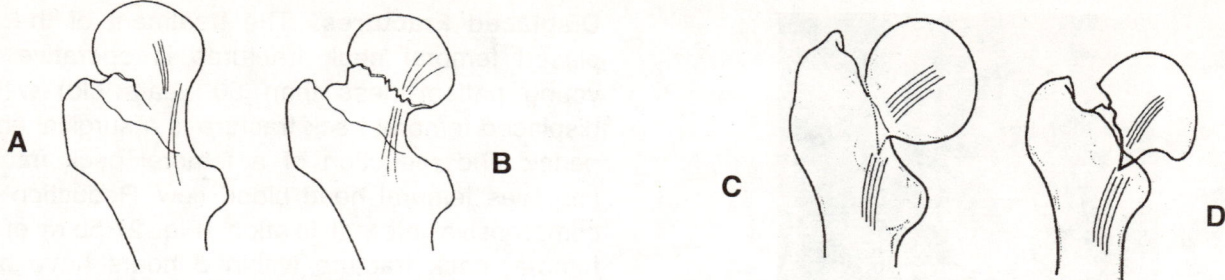

Fig. 27.4c.   Garden classification of femoral neck fractures. A: Stage I: Incomplete fracture that is abducted and impacted. B: Stage II: Complete fracture without displacement. Note that the compression trabeculae are aligned. C: Stage III: Complete facture with partial displacement. The neck is still in apposition posteroinferiorly; therefore, the fragments have rotated in opposite directions like two cogwheels. Note that the compression trabeculae are angulated. D: Stage IV: Complete fracture with full displacement. Contact between the fracture surfaces is lost. The distal fragment is in full external rotation and lies anterior to the proximal fragment. The proximal fragment is free to resume its natural position in the acetabulum; therefore, the compression trabeculae lie in their normal alignment.

inferior neck, seldom displace and can be treated with observation.

The **impacted** or abducted fracture is a type of undisplaced femoral neck fracture where the distal fragment impacts into the proximal in valgus position. These patients are often able to get up and walk even after having sustained a femoral neck fracture. The patient can actively internally rotate the leg, perform active straight leg raising and has no shortening.

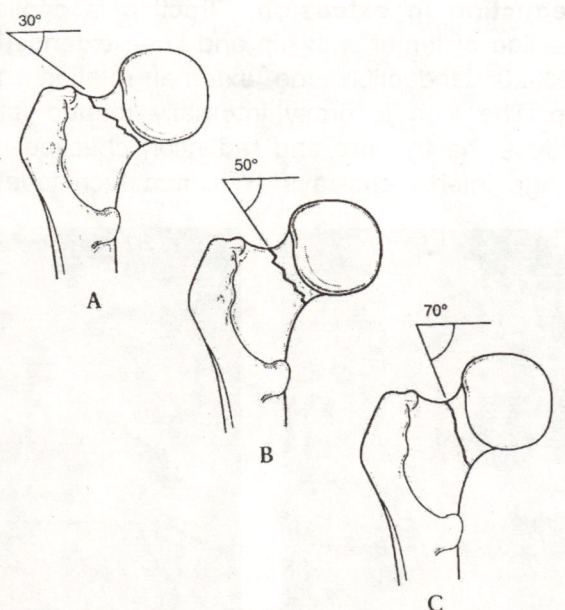

Fig. 27.4d.   Pauwels's classification of intracapsular hip fractures. A: Type I: Fracture is 30° to 49° from the horizontal. B: Type II: Fracture is 50° to 69° from the horizontal. C: Type III: Fracture is 70° or more from the horizontal.

Evaluation of a patient with suspected femoral neck fracture

Patient with femoral neck fracture usually complains of pain in the hip and inability to walk following injury.

The limb is shortened and lying in an attitude of external rotation. There is tenderness in Scarpa's triangle. Attempted movements at the hip are painful. Telescoping should not be attempted in a fresh fracture.

A patient with impacted fracture may present without shortening or deformity and may walk to the casualty.

Imaging of femoral neck fractures

Plain radiographs An AP view of pelvis provides the screening tool for the fracture of femoral neck. Fracture line can be appreciated in most cases. Shenton's line is broken in cases with displaced femoral neck fracture and lesser trochanter is prominent suggesting external rotation of the extremity (Fig. 27.5a). A lateral (cross table or frog leg) radiograph is also taken to confirm the fracture and the displacement of fragments.

Occult fractures or cases with high clinical suspicion of fracture (severe hip pain and inability to bear weight following injury) with normal radiographs are best detected by MRI (most sensitive) or bone scan.

MRI shows occult fractures earlier than bone

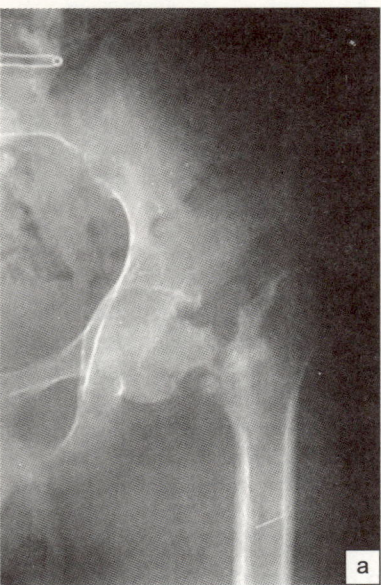

Fig. 27.5a. Displaced fracture neck of femur. Note the fracture line and the broken Shenton's line

scan, provides better anatomic information and is useful in assessing femoral head viability. MRI can show other abnormalities, which can mimic fracture neck femur and/or hip pain such as muscle tears and pelvic insufficiency fractures.

CT scan is useful for assessing the comminution of the posterior cortex.

Treatment

Treatment of femoral neck fracture depends on the displacement of fragments and physiologic age of the patient.

Undisplaced fractures

All undisplaced fractures, which are not impacted and tension type of insufficiency fractures, are best treated by internal fixation before displacement occurs in both young and elderly patients. Displacement rate of up to 30% has been reported in the undisplaced fractures without fixation.

Valgus impaction fractures can be treated conservatively in traction for 6 weeks. Patients are then mobilised non-weight bearing with crutches for a further period of 6 weeks. The patients on conservative treatment should have periodic radiographic examination to rule out displacement. Compression type of insufficiency fractures can also be treated conservatively and patient administered calcium, vitamin D and diphosphonates to improve bone mass.

Displaced Fractures The treatment of the displaced femoral neck fractures is operative. A young patient (less than 50 years old) with a displaced femoral neck fracture is a surgical emergency. The reduction of a femoral neck fracture improves femoral head blood flow. Reduction and compressive internal fixation (Fig. 27.5b,c) of the femoral neck fracture within 8 hours have been shown to reduce the incidence of avascular necrosis of the femoral head.

The treatment plan for fracture neck of femur is shown in Table 27.3.

Fractures of femoral neck in children are treated with closed reduction and internal fixation using multiple Moore's or Knowle's pins. Surgery is done on the fracture table with the image intensifier. The fracture can be reduced in flexion or extension.

Reduction in flexion Traction is applied in the line of femur with the hip and the knee in 90° flexion and internal rotation at the hip. With the traction and internal rotation at the hip maintained, the hip is gradually extended and abducted. Reduction is checked under image intensifier/x-rays (Leadbetter technique).

Reduction in extension Traction is applied in the line of femur with hip and knee extended and 15°–20° abduction and external rotation at the hip. The limb is firmly internally rotated fully to reduce the fracture and reduction checked under image intensifier/x-rays (Whitman technique).

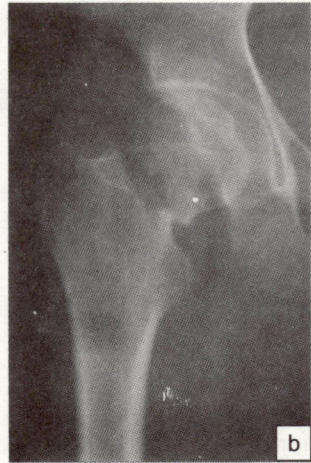 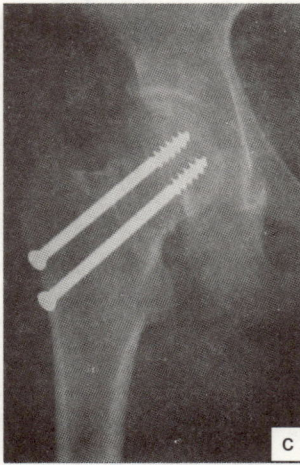

Fig. 27.5b,c. Pre and post operative X-rays showing fracture neck of femur treated by closed reduction and cancellous screw fixation

Table 27.3. Surgical Treament of Displaced Femoral Neck Fracture

Age group	Activity level	Functional demands	Bone quality	Operative procedure	Timing of surgery
Children	+++ (high)	High	Good	Reduction + internal fixation (Moore's pins or Knowle's pins)	As soon as possible (ASAP)
Young Adult <50 years	+++ (high)	High	Good	Reduction + internal fixation (3 AO screws or DHS with side plate ± derotation cancellous screw superiorly)	ASAP
Elderly patients	++ (high)	High	Good	Reduction + internal fixation (3 AO screws or DHS with side plate)	ASAP
Elderly patients with medical problems	+ (low)	Low	Poor	Hemireplacement arthroplasty	After managing correctable medical conditions

Following reduction, the pins are inserted from the greater trochanter into the head of the femur. Pins should not cross the physis. The patients should be immobilised in a one and a half hip spica for 8–12 weeks following fixation.

Fractures of the femoral neck in young adults are treated with compressive internal fixation using three **parallel** 6.5 mm partially threaded cancellous screws with washers (or 7.0 mm cannulated screws with washers) in the configuration of an inverted triangle. The lowermost screw should not be distal to the lesser trochanter to avoid the formation of stress riser, which can give rise to subtrochantric fracture. At least one screw should be placed within 3 to 5 mm of subchondral bone. All the threads should be in the femoral head fragment only in order to achieve compression at the fracture site.

When a stable anatomic configuration cannot be achieved, a compression hip screw/Dynamic hip screw with side plate and a superior derotation cancellous screw should be used to transfer loads to the lateral shaft.

If the closed reduction cannot be achieved, open reduction by anterior Smith Peterson's approach must be done. Angulation greater than 20 degrees on lateral x-ray is associated with high incidence of failure. Anterior approach has the advantage of not subjecting the vascular supply of femoral head to risk. Also, anterior capsulotomy has been shown to decompress capsular hematoma and relieve tamponade.

After treatment After the surgery the patient starts walking non weight bearing with crutches for 3 months. Check x-rays are taken at this stage and if radiologic evidence of union is appreciated, gradual weight bearing is started.

Replacement arthroplasty In elderly patient with low activity level and functional demands and poor bone quality, hemiarthroplasty is the treatment of choice (Fig. 27.6a,b). Posterior or posterolateral approach is used though, some people

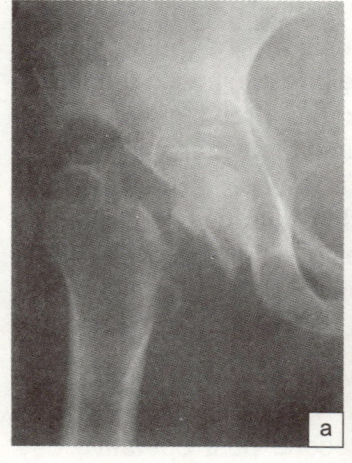
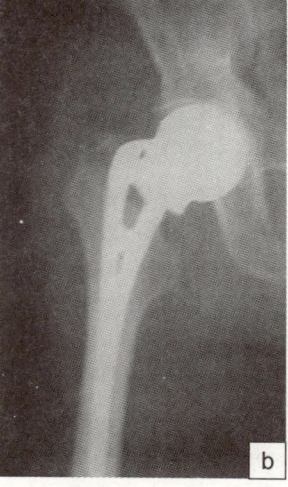

Fig. 27.6a,b. Fracture neck of femur treated by hemi-replacement arthroplasty using Austin Moore prosthesis

prefer direct lateral approach of Hardinge. The femoral head and neck are replaced by a metallic implant inserted in the femoral medullary canal. The prosthesis can be fixed to femur by cement or just by press fit (cementless).

Austin Moore prosthesis is inserted without cement and relies for fixation to femur on bony in growth through the fenestration provided in the stem. Presence of 1cm calcar is mandatory for the use of this prosthesis. The presence of a fin provides greater rotational stability. However, these prostheses often subside (or sink) in femoral medullary canal; also, once bone grows through fenestration, these implants are very difficult to extract.

Thompson's prosthesis is used in cases where calcar is deficient and/or the bone stock is too poor for cementless prosthesis. Thompson prosthesis is used with cement and obviates the problem of prosthesis sinking in the shaft. However, these prostheses often migrate superiorly and/or medially into the acetabulum resulting in erosion and /or protrusio acetabuli.

Bipolar prosthesis was designed to prevent acetabular erosion by a cemented hemiarthroplasty. The dual bearing in a bipolar prosthesis results in movements occurring predominantly at the low friction inner bearing (Metallic head-Polyethylene liner) while the movements at the outer bearing (Acetabulum – Metal shell) is minimised leading to reduced wear. However the problems of bipolar prosthesis is that it may start behaving like a unipolar after a while due to loss of movement at inner bearing due to fibrin deposition. Also, if dislocated, a bipolar prosthesis is more difficult to reduce. Rarely disassembly of bipolar prosthesis has been reported.

After treatment Following hemireplacement, the patient is encouraged to walk full weight bearing with support from the second post operative day. Hip abductor muscle strengthening exercises are started. After 6 weeks patient is encouraged to walk with a cane on the contralateral side.

Complications of hemireplacement include sciatic nerve injury, haemorrhage, periprosthetic femoral shaft fractures, dislocation, limb length discrepancy, infection and myositis ossificans.

Non-operative treatment of femoral neck fractures

If, due to medical co-morbidities or any other reason, the surgery is not possible in an elderly patient, the patient should be mobilized as early as the pain permits. Nonunion with shortening can be accepted in these cases to avoid the complications of prolonged recumbency. If, subsequently the symptoms warrant and the medical conditions improve, the non-union can be treated at a later date.

Non operative treatment should also be chosen in non-ambulatory patients who sustain femoral neck fracture.

Neglected/Missed Fractures of Femoral Neck

If a femoral neck fracture is not treated, the femoral neck starts getting resorbed by the end of four weeks and marked up riding of greater trochanter occurs. Accurate anatomical reduction becomes impossible in these cases. The following methods of treatment are available for those cases which are neglected / detected after three weeks

In **children** with neglected femoral neck fracture, an intertrochanteric valgus or abduction osteotomy with internal fixation and/or spica is the method of choice. Free fibular graft can be used across the fractures in these cases to provide fixation and enhance bone stock.

In **young adults,** muscle pedicle bone graft (MPBG) based on sartorius or quadratus femoris muscle(Meyer's Procedure) can be used to augment vascularity and bone stock in the neck region. Screws are used for fixation of the fracture from greater trochanter into the femoral head. Cancellous grafts from iliac crest are used to fill the defect in the femoral neck. A young adult with non-union of femoral neck fracture and a viable head can be treated by intertrochanteric valgus osteotomy with fixation of fracture. Osteotomy changes the orientation of the fracture line thus converting shearing forces into compressive forces.

Other methods which have been used to treat the neglected femoral neck fractures are the Pauwel's (reposition) osteotomy and McMurray's (inter-trochanteric displacement) osteotomy. These are not preferred these days because they distort the proximal femoral anatomy and make subsequent total hip arthroplasty difficult.

In **elderly individuals,** replacement arthroplasty is the treatment of choice for neglected femoral neck fractures.

Total hip arthroplasty (THA) in femoral neck fractures

THA in femoral neck fractures is indicated for fractures occurring in arthritic hip (e.g. rheumatoid arthritis, OA), fractures with associated injuries to acetabular articular cartilage, fracture associated with hip dislocation or acetabular fractures and cases with failed osteosynthesis for femoral neck fractures.

In **elderly individuals**, replacement arthroplasty is the treatment of choice for neglected femoral neck fractures.

Ipsilateral femoral neck and shaft fractures are reported in 3% cases of femoral shaft fractures. Almost 30% of the femoral neck fractures occurring in association with the shaft fractures are missed initially. This can be easily avoided by securing AP X-rays of pelvis with both hips in **ALL** cases with polytrauma and/or major lower limb trauma. The anatomic reduction and fixation of femoral neck fracture is the priority is these cases. The various treatment modalities available for treatment of this combination of injuries are:

1. Second generation cephalomedullary nails: These nails allow fixation of femoral neck and shaft fracture with a single implant. Some of the newer nails such as RECON Nail (Zimmer), Miss-a-nail (AO) are now available for use.

2. Dynamic hip screw with long side plate (to fix shaft fracture). A derotation cancellous screw can be inserted from trochanter to the head just proximal to the lag screw.

3. AO screw fixation of the femoral neck fracture with retrograde femoral nailing for shaft fracture (especially for the lower one third or lower half femoral fractures).

4. AO screws fixation of femoral neck fracture with plating for the femoral shaft fracture.

Newer techniques

New high-strength cement (such as Norion SRS – an osteoconductive carbonated apatite) can be injected in the fracture site to fill defects in the bone, enhance fixation of fracture and improve the bone strength.

Complications of femoral neck fractures

1. Complications of recumbency such as pneumonia, decubitus sores, deep vein thrombosis, pulmonary thrombo-embolism, and urinary tract infection are common in the elderly patients with femoral neck fractures.

2. Avascular necrosis is reported in 10% of undisplaced fractures and 40% of displaced femoral neck fractures. Displacement of fracture, delay in internal fixation, valgus reduction and associated dislocation of hip predispose to avascular necrosis. MRI is the earliest investigation to confirm osteonecrosis. Bone scan is also useful but less sensitive and becomes positive later than MRI. Plain x-rays show changes of osteonecrosis only after a few months. Changes of osteonecrosis may make their appearance for the first time on plain x-ray up to two years after injury. Plain X-rays of patients with osteonecrosis show increased sclerosis followed by collapse of weight bearing surface. Non-union and failure of fixation may also occur. Avascular necrosis can lead to non union and secondary osteoarthritis of the hip. Avascular necrosis may not be sufficiently symptomatic in elderly patients to warrant any treatment. In symptomatic elderly patients with avascular necrosis with or without union, replacement arthroplasty is the treatment of choice.

In young adult with avascular necrosis, muscle pedicle bone grafting, based on sartorius or quadratus femoris muscle, remains the treatment of choice. Young adult with avascular necrosis involving less than 50% of femoral head can be treated by valgus intertrochanteric osteotomy (to bring viable portion of femoral head in the weight bearing area) and internal fixation.

3. Non Union is defined as no healing 3 months post injury (Fig. 27.6c,d). Non Union has been reported in 10–30% cases with avascular necrosis and the incidence is higher in displaced frac-

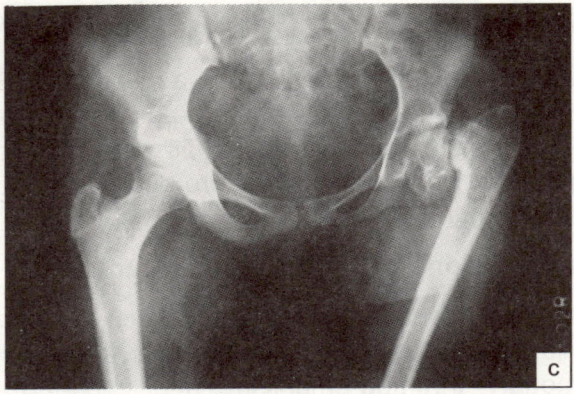

Fig. 27.6c. Non union of fracture neck of femur. Note the upriding of the greater trochanter

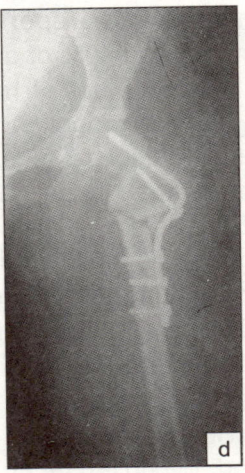

Fig. 27.6d. Non union of fracture neck of femur in a child treated with valgus osteotomy and internal fixation

tures and in patients with poor bone quality. Treatment of non union is carried out based on principles elucidated above.

4. Secondary Osteoarthritis results from collapse of femoral head secondary to osteonecrosis. Unilateral secondary osteoarthritis in a young patient is best treated by arthrodesis of the hip while replacement arthroplasty (THA) is the treatment of choice in elderly.

Intertrochanteric Fractures of Femur

Intertrochanteric fractures occur in a region extending from the base of the neck to the distal extent of the lesser trochanter. These fractures account for half of all hip fractures.

Intertrochanteric fractures occur most commonly in elderly patients due to a fall resulting in a direct impact on the greater trochanter as well as tor-sional force applied to the femur. Osteoporosis, unstable gait and impaired vision are recognised as risk factors for the trochanteric fractures. In younger people, the fracture occurs due to high-speed trauma due to road traffic accident or fall from height.

Relevant Anatomy

Intertrochanteric region provides attachement to abductor musculature on the greater trochanter and iliopsoas on the lesser trochanter. Presence and size of the bony fragments avulsed by these muscles also contribute to the fracture pattern.

Bony anatomy of intertrochanteric region is extremely important since it is an indicator of quality of bone and dictates the optimal position of fixation devices for secure purchase in the femoral head. An estimate of the degree of osteoporosis can be made by the study of trabecular pattern of the proximal femur. Secondary trabeculae are lost early in osteoporosis. Loss of the primary tensile trabeculae suggests moderate osteoporosis while loss of primary compressive trabeculae suggests severe osteoporosis. The site of crossing of primary compressive and primary tensile trabeculae in the centre of the femoral head has the maximum density of trabecular bone and provides good purchase needed for implant stability.

Classification

Boyd and Griffin have classified the intertrochanteric fractures into type I (undisplaced), II (displaced), III (reverse obliquity) and IV (Subtrochanteric extension).

Jensen and Evans classified these fractures into stable and unstable depending on the ability to achieve anatomical reduction and stability following fixation. Fractures with posteromedial comminution (3- and 4- part fractures) and reverse obliquity fractures are classified as unstable fractures.

Evaluation of a patient with suspected intertrochanteric fracture

Patients with intertrochanteric fractures are usually older than patients with femoral neck fractures. There is a history of fall with inability to get up and walk after the fall. Pain and swelling are mainly over the trochanteric area (cf pain over Scarpa's triangle in femoral neck fracture).

Ecchymosis may appear over the trochanter in an injury a few days old. Shortening and external rotation are much more marked in the patients with trochanteric fractures vis-a-vis femoral neck fractures. Attempted hip movements are extremely painful. Since these elderly patients frequently have medical comorbidities, an evaluation of their status must be done initially with an attempt to stabilise them within the next 12 to 24 hours.

Imaging An anteroposterior view of the affected hip in internal rotation and a lateral view are sufficient to diagnose the fracture, displacement of fragments and the degree of comminution (Fig. 27.7). Size of posteromedial fragement must be noted as larger the size of the fragment, more unstable is the fracture pattern.

If a fracture is suspected strongly on clinical grounds, MRI can help in detection of or ruling out the fracture.

Treatment

Intertrochanteric region is the region of cancellous bone with abundant blood supply. The fractures in this region unite readily. The reason for choosing surgical treatment is to reduce the period of recumbency with its attendant complications and reduce the hospital stay and cost. Also, anatomic reduction and internal fixation decreases the chances of malunion, which is common after conservative treatment.

Conservative treatment can be chosen in young patients if there is local (e.g. poor skin condition) or systemic disorder precluding surgery. These patients are treated with skin or skeletal traction for 10–12 weeks followed by mobilisation and gradual weight bearing.

Conservative or non-operative treatment can be chosen in elderly patients with comorbidities who are high-risk candidates for anaesthesia and/or surgery. These patients are mobilised quickly out of bed and encouraged to walk with support. It is explained that some shortening and deformity will persist once the fracture unites. Non surgical treatment should also be chosen for non-ambulatory and terminally sick patients.

Surgical treatment is chosen to reduce the period of recumbency, hospital stay and the cost. Patient becomes comfortable, can be mobilised out of bed early and the nursing care becomes easy.

The successful outcome after surgical treatment depends on the bone quality, fracture pattern, quality of reduction and stability of fracture fixation.

The most suitable implant for fixation of intertrochanteric fracture is the dynamic hip screw with angle side plate (Fig. 27.8a). It allows secure fixation of the fracture. At the same time it permits controlled impaction which reduces the risk of failure of fixation.

The DHS fixation is done on a fracture table under the control of image intensifier. The frac-

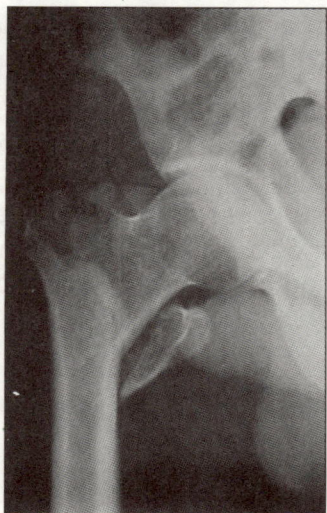

Fig. 27.7. AP X-ray showing 4-part intertrochanteric fracture

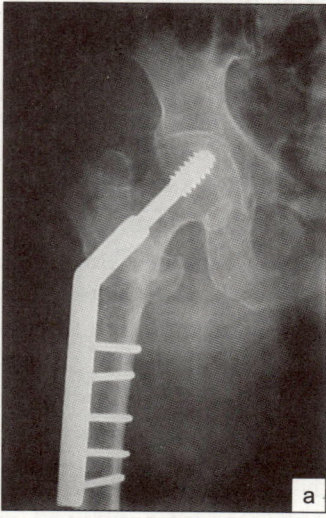

Fig. 27.8a. Radiograph showing intertrochanteric fracture treated by Dynamic Hip Screw

ture is reduced by traction in line of thigh with hip extended and in 15°–20° abduction followed by firmly internally rotating the limb.

The reduction is checked under the image intensifier. The principles of fixation are

- The ideal location of the implant is in the centre of the femoral head in both AP as well as the lateral views.

- The tip of the compression screw should be within 10 mm of the subchondral bone on both AP and lateral views for best results.

- TAD (Tip Apex Distance-sum of distance between the tip of the screw and outline of the femoral head on AP and lateral views) should not be more than 25 mm.

- A short barrel plate should be used in cases with severe comminution and in cases where a short lag screw is used to allow more collapse.

- Compression screw should be passed **after** releasing the traction completely.

- Compression screw should not be used in severely osteoportic bone to avoid pulling out the lag screw.

Postoperative care

The patient is allowed to sit up as soon as the pain permits. The patients with stable fracture pattern and secure fixation are allowed to partially weight bear as tolerated. Patients with severely comminuted fractures are only allowed toe-touch weight bearing till callus is seen on x-rays.

Internal fixation of intertrochanteric fractures with other devices

Reverse obliquity trochanteric fractures are **not** treated by dynamic hip screw and need either 95-degree blade plate (Fig. 27.8b) or 95° dynamic compression screw with side plate. Cephalomedullary devices (e.g. gamma nail) offering intramedullary fixation with screw fixation across the fracture site into the femoral head have been used with success for the treatment of trochanteric fractures.

Ender's condylocephalic nails are also used for fixation of trochanteric fractures. Usually 3 nails are inserted from the medial femoral condyle.

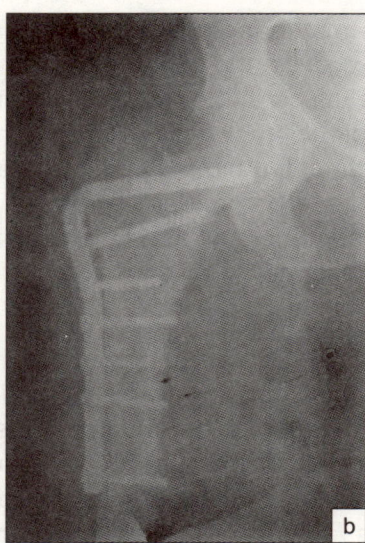

Fig. 27.8b. 95° condylar blade plate fixation for inter-trochanteric fracture

These nails traverse the medullary canal and fan out in the femoral head and provide secure fixation.

Prosthetic replacement may rarely be indicated for pathological fractures or severely comminuted fractures in extremely osteoporotic bone. It is imperative to repair the greater trochanter in these cases to preserve the abductor mechanism.

Complications

1. Intertrochanteric fractures are associated with greater morbidity and mortality than femoral neck fractures. These fractures are often associated with systemic complications of fractures in the old age such as deep vein thrombosis, pulmonary thrombo-embolism, hypostatic pneumonia, decubitus sores etc.

2. *Malunion with coxa vara* is the most common local complication of intertrochanteric fractures. It can follow both conservative as well as the surgical treatment. Coxa vara results in shortening and limping and may warrant valgus osteotomy of the proximal femur with internal fixation (Fig. 27.8c,d).

3. Complications related to fixation devices such as implant failure, screw cut out and infection.

4. Non union occurs in less than 1% cases and is treated by revision internal fixation and bone grafting.

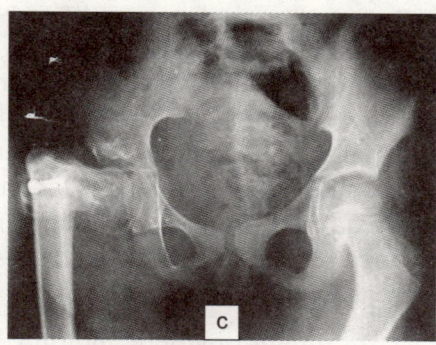

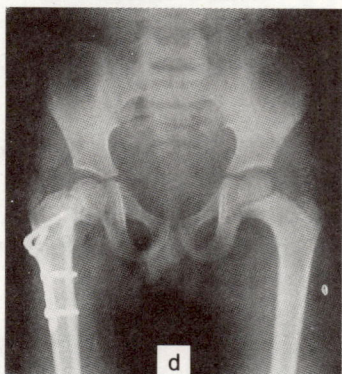

Fig. 27.8c,d. Malunited intertrochanteric fracture with coxa vara, treated by valgus osteotomy and internal fixation with blade plate

5. Avascular necrosis occurs in less than 1% cases and is treated by replacement arthroplasty.

Subtrochanteric Fractures of the Femur

Subtrochanteric region of the femur extends from the upper level of the lesser trochanter and extends 5 cm distally. Unlike the intertrochanteric region, this area is composed of thick cortical bone. Though the bone is enveloped by well vascularised musculature it heals more slowly than the metaphyseal area and is more prone to develop delayed or non union. Strong muscular pull from the hip abductors, iliopsoas and short external rotators on the proximal fragment sub-

ject the fractures in this area to large bending moments. These fractures therefore are prone to malunion or implant failure leading to non-union of the fractures.

Mechanism of injury

Elderly patients with osteopenic bone sustain subtrochanteric fractures following a trivial fall. This age group is also prone to pathological fractures secondary to metastatic or primary tumours.

Young patients sustain these fractures following high-energy trauma. The fractures in these cases are typically more comminuted despite the better bone quality.

Classification

Russell-Taylor classification (Table 27.4) is most commonly used to describe subtrochanteric fractures and choose suitable internal fixation device.

Evaluation of a patient with suspected subtrochanteric fracture

Subtrochanteric fractures are associated with history of trivial trauma in elderly or high-energy trauma in younger patients. A history of low-energy trauma resulting in a subtrochanteric fracture in a young patient should lead to search for a pathologic process.

Subtrochanteric fractures occurring due to high velocity trauma are often associated with other injuries. A thorough examination must be performed in casualty to look for these injuries. Vitals must be assessed and venous line must be accessed. Blood should be sent for grouping and cross matching.

Patients present with severe pain and inability to

Table 27.4. Russell-Taylor Classification of subtrochanteric fractures

Type	Extension into piriformis fossa		Lesser Trochanter Fractures		Choice of internal fixation device
	Yes	No	Yes	No	
IA		+		+	Intramedullary fixation
IB		+	+		Intramedullary fixation
IIA	+			+	Extramedullary fixation
IIB	+		+		Extramedullary fixation

walk after the injury. Marked swelling of the thigh is seen. The limb is short and lies externally rotated. Distal neurovascular status must be assessed.

Imaging

Anteroposterior and lateral radiograph of the affected thigh with hip are adequate to confirm the fracture and ascertain the degree of comminution (especially postero-medially). The presence of any pathologic lesion in the region is looked for. X-rays of the whole femur including the knee joint and x-rays of pelvis with both hips must be examined to rule out associated skeletal injuries in the ipsilateral extremity.

Oblique radiographs, tomograms and bone scan help in the diagnosis of non-union with implants in situ.

Treatment

The aim of treatment of these fractures is to achieve sound healing of the fracture in acceptable alignment. This can be done more readily by operative means, which allow adequate reduction, stable fixation, early mobilisation and healing in good alignment.

Conservative treatment

All subtrochanteric fractures are placed in traction initially to immobilise the limb and relieve pain, restore limb length, reduce thigh swelling and improve alignment. X-rays taken in traction allow better assessment of the fracture pattern and comminution.

Traction as definitive treatment, however, is demanding. The proximal fragment in these cases is in flexion, abduction and external rotation and 90–90 (90° flexion at hip and 90° flexion at the knee) traction is required to align distal fragment with the proximal fragment. The hip and knee flexion is gradually reduced after 3 weeks and patient is put in a cast brace after 4–6 weeks. Partial weight bearing is allowed with crutches and cast brace is removed after 16–20 weeks of injury.

Traction treatment requires diligence, excellent care and prolonged immobilisation. Malunion may occur. This treatment is mainly reserved for children and those adults who are medically unfit for surgery.

Surgical treatment

In cases where piriformis fossa is intact, intramedullary devices such as second generation interlocking nails with fixation into femoral head and neck are the ideal implants. Reconstruction nail and gamma nail are the usual implants used in these cases. All comminuted fractures should be treated with static locking.

In cases where fracture extends into the piriformis fossa, an extramedullary device such as dynamic condylar screw, dynamic hip screw or 95° angle blade plate is used.

Enders flexible condylocephalic nails have been advocated for subtrochanteric fractures but high incidence of complications such as migration of nail, loss of fixation and malunion has been reported.

Fractures with medial comminution (especially with involvement of lesser trochanter) must be bone grafted.

Complications

Complications of conservative treatment include the complications of prolonged recumbency, malunion and non union.

Complications of surgical treatment include the complications related to implants such as implant failure, cut out and infection. Loss of fixation results in nonunion or malunion.

Malunion resulting in rotational differences and shortening is a common complication. Severe unacceptable malunion is treated with corrective osteotomy and intra-or extramedullary fixation.

Non union occurs due to extensive comminution, failure of fixation or failure of implant. Treatment of non-union is revision internal fixation with reamed statically locked intramedullary nailing. Those fractures, which anyway require opening of the fracture site to remove the failed implants, must be supplemented with iliac crest cancellous bone grafting.

Fractures of the femoral shaft

Fractures of the femoral shaft result from severe injuries and are commonly associated with other serious injuries. The bone is enveloped by well vascularised musculature, which sustains considerable trauma in association with the shaft fracture. The compound femoral fractures are uncommon due to thick overlying soft tissue envelope. Considerable bleeding occurs from femur fracture and up to 1500 ml blood may be lost without any evidence of external bleeding.

Mechanism of Injury

Severe trauma, as in motor vehicular accidents, fall from height or natural calamities (as in earthquakes) leads to femoral shaft fracture. Bomb blast and gunshot wounds can lead to femoral shaft fractures along with severe injury to the soft tissues.

Pathological fractures of the femoral shaft occur commonly in association with various benign and malignant lesions located in the shaft.

Classification

Femoral shaft fractures may be transverse, oblique, spiral (Fig. 27.9a), comminuted (with or without a triangular "butterfly" fragment) or segmental (Fig. 27.9b).

Winquist and Hansen classified femoral shaft fractures depending on the degree of comminution. They divided femoral shaft fractures into types 0 to IV (0: no comminution; I: Transverse with <25% comminution of fracture surface area; II: 25–50% comminution; III: >50% comminution; and IV: Extensive comminution with no cortical contact between the fragments).

Evaluation of a patient with suspected femoral shaft fracture

Any patient with suspected femoral shaft fracture must undergo a quick assessment of vital parameters and resuscitation should be instituted immediately. Two wide bore no. 14 venflons must be used to access venous system and samples sent for blood group and cross matching, and, hematocrit. Intravenous ringer lactate infusion should be started. Patient should be evaluated to rule out cranial, abdominal, thoracic and pelvic injuries.

Local examination reveals marked shortening, swelling and deformity of the thigh. The attempted movements are painful and the patient is unable to lift the leg. Any breech in the skin should be presumed to be an open fracture. Severely tense

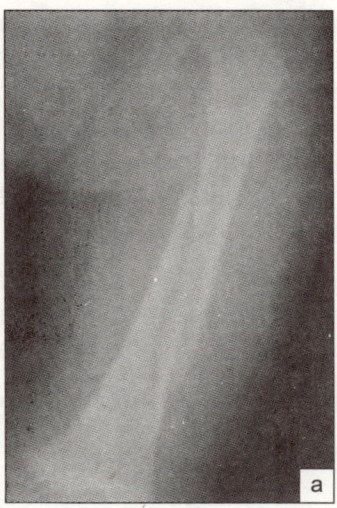

Fig. 27.9a. Spiral fracture of shaft of femur

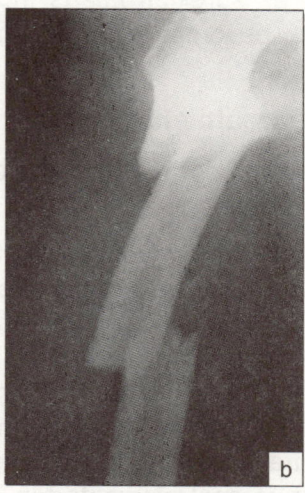

Fig. 27.9b. Segmental fracture shaft femur

thigh should raise the suspicion of a compartment syndrome and warrants pressure measurement of the thigh compartments. A careful and detailed neurovascular examination of the extremity should be performed. Other skeletal injuries commonly associated with femoral shaft fracture should be looked for and include acetabular fractures, pelvic ring fracture, ipsilateral hip dislocation, patella fracture and ligamentous disruptions of the knee.

Imaging

Imaging for suspected femoral shaft fracture should include anteroposterior and lateral radiographs of the entire femur. Ipsilateral hip and knee x-rays must be taken to look for associated fractures. An anteroposterior view of pelvis must be taken in all patients with femoral shaft fractures as a screening tool for pelvic ring injury or acetabular fractures. An internal rotation view of the hip to visualise femoral neck is mandatory to rule out associated femoral neck fracture. Adduction of the proximal fracture fragment indicates associated posterior dislocation of the ipsilateral hip.

An angiography should be performed to investigate any patient, presenting with femoral shaft fracture and a compromise in vascularity.

Treatment of femoral shaft fractures

All patients with femoral shaft fracture are treated initially with resuscitation, intravenous fluid infusion, blood transfusion and splintage. The femoral shaft fracture can be treated by both conservative as well as surgical means though, surgical treatment has become the mainstay in recent times.

Conservative treatment

Conservative treatment is the method of choice in infants and children.

Infants younger than 2 years are treated in the Gallow's or Bryant's traction. Adhesive tape is applied on bilateral legs and traction rope through the tape is attached to an overhead point so that buttocks of the infant are just off the bed. Body weight acts to align the fragments and 3 weeks in this traction are sufficient to achieve union. This type of traction is contraindicated in older children as it can lead to compromise of the vascularity to the lower limbs.

Older children can be treated in fixed skin traction on Thomas splint or by sliding traction through an upper tibial (tensioned) kirschner wire with the thigh supported on a pillow. The fracture usually takes about 6 weeks to heal.

Adults Conservative treatment of fracture shaft of femur in adults is out of vogue and is limited to the patients who cannot be taken up for any type of anaesthesia due to medical conditions. Conservative treatment, however, was practised widely in the past. Conservative treatment involves skeletal traction through an upper tibial steinmann pin using balanced traction. Patient is encouraged to perform ankle and quadriceps exercises and patella is moved side to side everyday to prevent

adhesions. Periodic check x-rays are mandatory and any displacements are corrected by applying padding on the thigh. Distraction at the fracture site by applying excessive weights on the traction should be avoided. After 4–6 weeks when the fracture site becomes non-tender, knee mobilisation is begun using the Pearson's knee flexion attachment. The fracture unites usually in 12–16 weeks. Functional cast bracing is a method of treating femoral shaft fractures wherein at the end of 4–6 weeks of traction (when the fracture becomes sticky), a snugly fitting cast brace is applied with hinges extending from thigh component of the cast brace to the leg component at the level of the knee. Cast brace prevents displacement of fragments while allowing knee mobilisation. Use of the limb results in compression at the fracture site and early union.

Surgical Treatment Surgical treatment allows appropriate reduction, stable internal fixation and early return to function. The cost of treatment, patient morbidity and period of hospitalisation are considerably reduced.

1. **Intramedullary nailing** is the treatment of choice for fixation of diaphyseal fractures of femur. Closed, antegrade, locked intramedullary nailing has been reported to result in 99% union rates (Fig. 27.9c-e).

Technique The intramedullary nailing is usually performed on a fracture table with the patient supine or in the lateral position. The fracture is reduced by traction through a supracondylar pin. Excessive traction should be avoided as it can lead to distraction, recurvatum (due to pull of gastrocnemius) and valgus (due to pull of iliotibial band). Femoral canal is opened from the piriformis fossa in line with the former and a ball tipped guide wire is passed. Femoral canal is reamed sequentially with flexible reamers to a size determined on preoperative x-rays to fit the femoral medullary canal snugly. The ball tipped guide wire is exchanged with an ordinary guide wire and the nail is inserted in an antegrade manner. The guide wire is removed and the proximal holes locked using a jig. The distal holes in the nail are locked free hand.

Postoperatively the knee is kept flexed to 60° on pillows and the patient is encouraged to perform

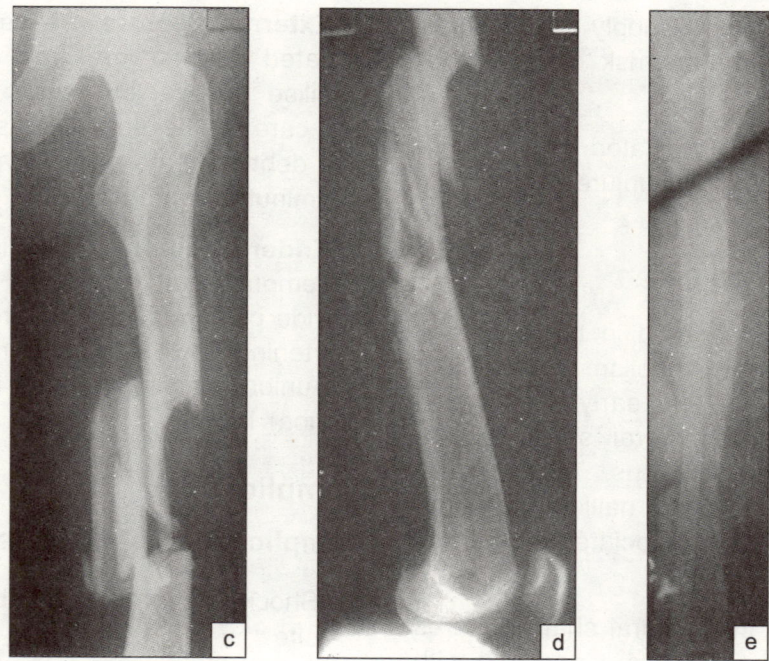

Fig. 27.9c-e. Pre and post operative X-rays of a patient with comminuted, segmental fracture shaft femur treated with interlocking nail

quadriceps exercises. The patient is mobilised out of the bed the next day and ambulates non weight bearing with crutches. Knee bending is encouraged. The fracture unites in 12–16 weeks and full weight bearing is allowed after union.

Kuntscher's Nail Versus Interlocking Nail

The principle of use of IM nail is to achieve 3–point fixation by insertion of a straight nail into a curved medullary canal. Kuntscher's (Cloverleaf) intramedullary nails were used in the past to treat femoral shaft fractures. The cloverleaf cross section of the Kuntscher's nail provides limited rotational stability. Interlocking nails have the advantages of preventing shortening and rotation and can be used in comminuted fractures. Kuntscher's nail, however, is still a useful device in cases where the facilities (such as fluoroscopy) or expertise is not available or when the patient cannot afford the expensive interlocking nail.

Antegrade Versus Retrograde Nailing

Interlocking nails were initially devised only for antegrade nailing but Kuntscher's nails have been used both in an antegrade (introduced from piriformis fossa) as well as retrograde manner (into the proximal fragment from the fracture site, out into the gluteal region and then pushed back in distal fragment). Retrograde insertion is easier especially when fracture has to be opened for irreducibility. Retrograde interlocking nails, which are introduced through the knee, are now available but are associated with inferior union rates and there are concerns over their effect on the knee function.

Open Versus Closed Nailing

Closed intramedullary nailing is preferred to the open nailing as the fracture hematoma is lost in the latter and fracture healing takes longer. Closed nailing can be done through a small incision with reduced morbidity to the patient. However, incidence of sciatic nerve injury (due to traction to the limb with hip flexed and knee extended) and compartment syndrome of the thigh is higher with the closed method.

Reamed Versus Unreamed Nail

Reaming enlarges the medullary canal thus allowing the use of a larger sized (stiffer) nail, improved contact of nail with medullary canal and generates osteogenic reamings which act as bone grafts. However, reaming generates heat and causes thermal damage to the bone. Also, it destroys the endosteal blood supply of the bone. There are concerns about the risk of fat embolism due to reaming.

Unreamed nail is presently indicated only in compound fractures or in multiply injured patient to reduce the operating time.

Early Versus Delayed Nailing

Delayed nailing was propagated in the past due to the fear of causing fat embolism by reaming. However, it is now known that early stabilisation (within 24 hours) of the femoral shaft fracture reduces pulmonary complications. The concern for the complications of early nailing, however, still exists in a patient with associated pulmonary contusion.

2. **Plating** is useful for the femoral shaft fractures in cases of fracture shaft femur associated with femoral neck fractures or in cases where facilities or expertise for interlocking nailing are not available. Plating is also useful if nailing has to be abandoned due to some complication (Fig. 27.9f). Minimally invasive plate osteosynthesis (often done percutaneously) or biologic plating are currently popular. Plating is done with an attempt to maintain soft tissue attachments to the bone and sometimes even without exposing the fracture site(using indirect reduction techniques).

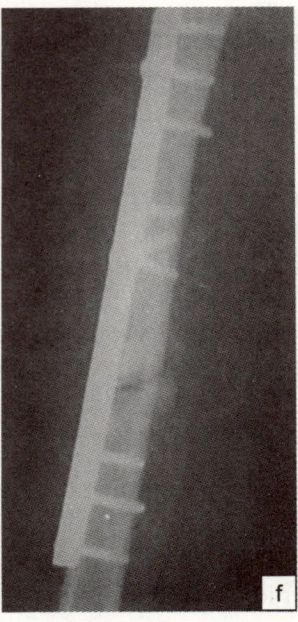

Fig. 27.9f. X-ray showing fracture shaft femur treated by dynamic compression plating

3. **External fixators** are useful for fractures associated with severe soft tissue injuries. They stabilise the fracture while permitting inspection and care of the soft tissues. Fixators allow multiple debridements and are also useful in severely comminuted fractures.

4. **Enders nailing** is practised at some centres for femoral shaft fractures. However, Enders nails provide poor rotational control and do not prevent shortening. Incidence of complications (malunion, non-union, backing out of implants with loss of fixation) is high.

Complications

Complications of fracture

1. Shock due to excessive bleeding at the fracture site

2. Fat embolism may occur as a complication of femoral shaft fracture and needs urgent care.

3. Injury to neurovascular structures may occur. Femoral artery and profunda femoris artery both are at risk of injury from sharp bony fragment. Urgent angiography, vascular repair and stabilisation of the fracture (external or internal) should be undertaken early.

    The injury to sciatic or femoral nerve by femoral shaft fracture is rare.

4. Knee stiffness is an important complication of femoral shaft fracture and may occur with conservative as well as surgical treatment. Knee stiffness can be due to both intraarticular (adhesions) as well as extraarticular (tethering of vastus intermedius at the fracture site) reasons. External fixation and infection following internal fixation can also lead to knee stiffness. Knee stiffness is treated by physiotherapy. Resistant cases may benefit by release of tethered quadriceps by **Quadricepsplasty.**

Complications of conservative treatment include complications of prolonged recumbency, malunion and non union.

Complications of surgical treatment include:

•   Injury to sciatic or pudendal nerves may occur due to traction

- Complications related to implants such as implant failure (Fig. 27.9g,h) (most commonly through the interlocking site close to the fracture site) and infection.

- Heterotopic ossification can occur following intramedullary nailing.

- Malunion resulting in rotational malalignment, shortening and angulation may occur in cases with implant failure. Severe unacceptable malunion (rotational malunion >15°, angulation >15°, shortening > 2 cm) is treated by corrective osteotomy and internal fixation with a nail or a plate.

- **Non Union** is not uncommon after femoral shaft fractures and is most commonly due to inadequate vascularity (soft tissue stripping by injury or surgery), inadequate immobilisation, and infection. Non union without infection is treated with exchange nailing with reaming to allow insertion of a bigger nail and promote osteogenesis. Plating and bone grafting can also be done if a marked deformity and / or obliteration of medullary canal are present.

- Infected non-union is treated by removal of the previous implant, debridement and insertion of gentamicin impregneated PMMA beads followed by reaming and nailing at a second stage after removal of beads. Alternatively, external fixator can be applied to stabilise the fracture after debridement followed by bone grafting once the infection is controlled.

Supracondylar femur fractures

The supracondylar region of the femur is variously defined as the region within 9 cm of the articular surface or from 5 cm above the metaphyseal flare to the articular surface. Supracondylar fractures account for almost 4% of all of the femur fractures and 31% of all femur fractures if hip fractures are excluded. The fractures in this region often extend into the knee joint as T- or Y-shaped fractures. Two distinct anatomical factors determine the course of this fracture; the first is the attachment of gastrocnemius to the distal fragment which flexes it. The second feature is the proximity of popliteal artery to the distal fragment. The combination of these two factors results in popliteal artery being at risk of laceration by a sharp edge of bone.

Mechanism of Injury

The young adults sustain supracondylar fracture due to high-energy trauma such as motor vehicular accident. The elderly patients with osteopenic bones sustain supracondylar fractures due to low energy trauma such as trivial falls. Another population of elderly people who sustain supracondylar femur fractures consists of patients who have undergone total knee replacement.

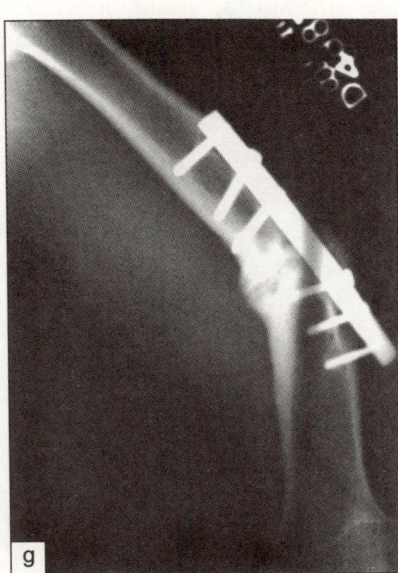

Fig. 27.9g. Malunion with implant failure following plating of femur

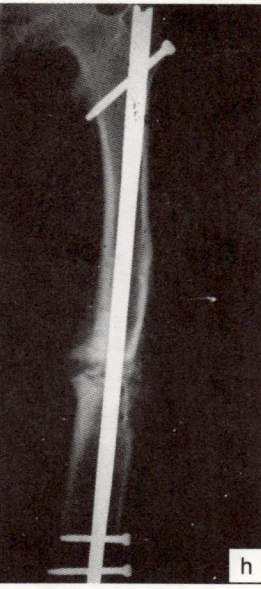

Fig. 27.9h. Non union of fracture following ILN femur

Classification

Supracondylar fractures have been classified by the AO group into extraarticular (Type A), unicondylar (Type B) and bicondylar (Type C).

Evaluation of a patient with supracondylar fracture

History of trauma and its severity is important to elicit in a patient with supracondylar fracture. A young patient who sustains high-energy trauma may have associated skeletal and extra skeletal injuries.

Local examination reveals swelling, deformity and shortening of the thigh. Patient has severe pain and does not allow movements of the knee. Hemarthrosis suggests intraarticular extension of the fracture or concomitant injury to knee ligaments. Skin must be examined for any breech. Distal neurovascular status must be checked to rule out injury to popliteal artery and/or lateral popliteal /tibial nerves.

Imaging   Plain radiographs (AP and lateral) of the knee provide sufficient information about the type and extent of the supracondylar fracture and displacement of fragments (Fig. 27.10a,b). Oblique views may be required sometimes to diagnose vertical or coronal splits (Hoffa fracture) of the femoral condyle. Radiographs of the femoral and tibial shafts are important to rule out associated fractures. Angiography is indicated in patients with suspected vascular injury.

Management of supracondylar fractures Aim of treatment of supracondylar fractures is to achieve union in correct alignment and restore function. This is extremely challenging in young patients due to severe comminution and in old patients due to comminution as well as osteopenia. In fractures with intraarticular extension the aim of treatment is to restore articular congruity and allow early motion of the knee.

Conservative Treatment

Conservative treatment of supracondylar fractures is limited to undisplaced fractures, impacted fractures with minimal displacement in osteoporotic patients, non-ambulatory patients and patients in whom medical conditions preclude surgery. These patients are treated in a cast splint or cast brace and allowed to walk non weight bearing. Early knee motion is encouraged (at 3 to 4 weeks) but weight bearing is permitted only after the fracture heals. Some people prefer to give skeletal traction (2 pin traction one through proximal tibia to allow traction in the direction of femur with knee flexed 30°–40° and other through the supracondylar area to pull the distal fragment vertically up) for 3–4 weeks to restore alignment and length followed by application of cast brace.

Surgical treatment

Surgical treatment is indicated for all displaced intra-articular fractures, malaligned and/or comminuted extra-articular fractures, polytrauma pa-

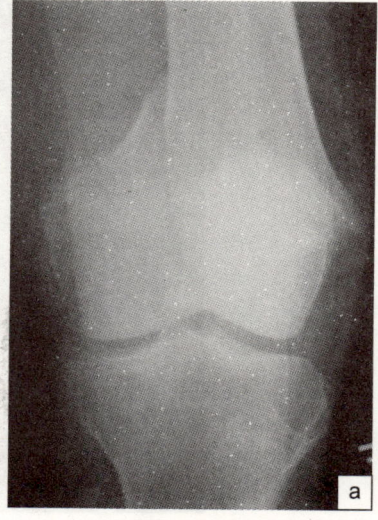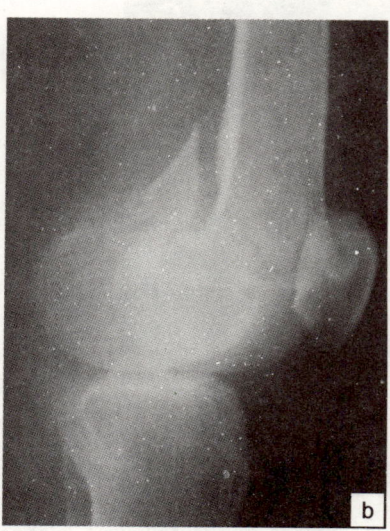

Fig. 27.10a,b.   Radiographs of a patient showing supra-condylar fracture

tients, coexistent vascular injury, coexistent supracondylar and upper tibial fractures (floating knee) and pathologic fractures.

Displaced extra-articular fractures   are treated by fixed angle devices such as condylar blade plate or dynamic condylar screw. Recently intramedullary devices (supracondylar nails) have become available which can be inserted retrogradely through the knee and can be locked using screws through the nail. Supracondylar nails are especially useful in patients with ipsilateral total knee arthroplasty in patients with floating knee and the patients who have femoral shaft fracture in addition to the supracondylar fracture.

Displaced unicondylar fractures are treated by open anatomic reduction and fixation with cancellous screws using washers.

Displaced intercondylar fractures are treated by open anatomic reduction of the articular fragments and their fixation using cancellous screws thus converting the intercondylar into a supracondylar fracture. The metaphyseal fragment can then be fixed to the diaphyseal fragment using a fixed angle device or an intramedullary device. If however, there is a coronal fracture line then none of these devices can be used. In these cases a special implant known as condylar buttress plate can be used on the lateral side to fix the intercondylar fracture (Fig. 27.10c,d).

Complications

Complications of the fracture include neurovascular injury (esp. popliteal artery injury), knee stiffness, malunion, nonunion and posttraumatic arthritis. In cases with popliteal artery injury, urgent angiography should be performed and vascular repair along with fixation of the fracture should be undertaken.

Complications of the conservative treatment include knee stiffness, malunion, nonunion and post traumatic arthritis.

Complications of surgical treatment include complications related to implants such as implant

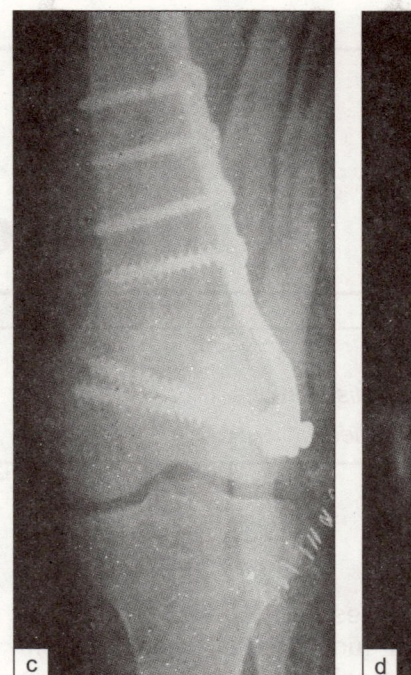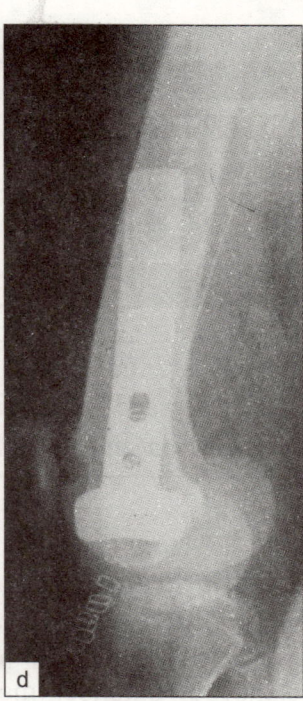

Fig. 27.10c,d. Buttress plating used to fix the supracondylar fracture

failure (or breakage), cutout and infection. Malunion with angular deformity, rotational malalignment and shortening may occur. Non union may occur due to implant failure. Poor bone quality may lead to implant cut out and malunion or nonunion.

Distal Femoral Epiphyseal Injury

Separation of the distal femoral epiphysis (Type 3 Salter and Harris type) is a rare injury, which occurs in adolescents. Classically, the injury is sustained by a severe hyperextension force when the person is trying to ride on a cart while running after it. The epiphysis is displaced anteriorly and laterally and sharp spike of the proximal fragment can injure the popliteal artery. The diagnosis is evident on x-rays. The treatment is urgent closed reduction under anaesthesia. The reduction may be stabilised by fixing the fragments using smooth kirschner wires. A long leg last is applied with knee flexed 60° for 6 weeks. The knee is mobilised at the end of this period and weight bearing started. The growth disturbance following the injury in uncommon.

Injuries of Knee and Leg

- Patellar fractures
- Traumatic Patellar dislocations
- Dislocation of the knee

- Tibial Spine Fractures
- Fractures of the Tibial Plateau
- Fractures of Tibia and fibula

Patellar fractures

Patella is the largest sesamoid bone in the body. It has the important functions of improving efficiency of extensor mechanism (by providing increased lever arm) and protecting the anterior knee joint from injury. A displaced fracture of the patella results in the disruption of extensor mechanism of the knee with serious functional consequences.

Mechanism of injury

The **indirect injury** occurs due to sudden violent contraction of the quadriceps muscle with the knee flexed (as happens while trying to break a fall). This injury results in transverse fracture of the patella with tear of the quadriceps expansion and lateral patellar retinaculae (Fig. 28.1a). Severe disruption of extensor mechanism may occur.

The **direct injury** to the front of the knee results in a comminuted or vertical fracture of the patella (Fig. 28.1b). These fractures are associated with minimal injury to the soft tissues and extensor mechanism is often intact.

Dislocation of the patella can lead to osteochondral fractures of the articular surface. These fractures are often missed.

Stress fractures of the patella are relatively rare and may present with anterior knee pain. Patellar stress fractures may occur due to complex combination of tension and bending forces leading to break in the patella. Stress fractures may occur

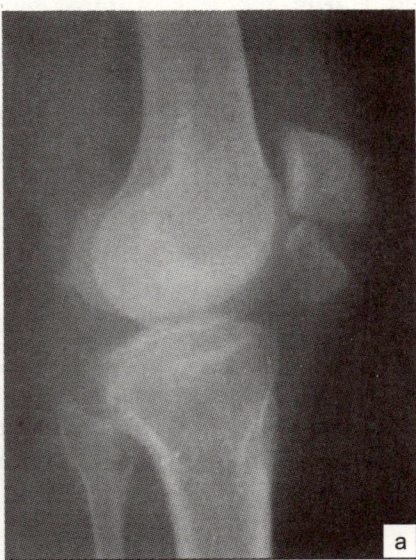

Fig. 28.1a. Transverse fracture of patella. Note the displacement of the fragments indicating disruption of extensor mechanism. This fracture has to be treated by open reduction and tension band wiring

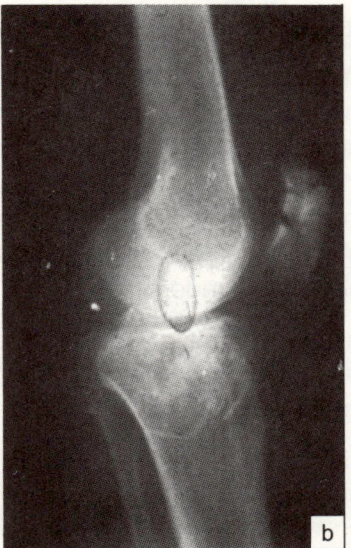

Fig. 28.1b. Undisplaced, stellate fracture of patella suggesting direct injury. Note: The extensor retinaculum is expected to be intact. Patient can be treated conservatively in cylinder POP cast

as periprosthetic fractures following total knee replacement or following anterior cruciate ligament (ACL) graft harvest for ACL reconstruction surgery.

Classification

Patellar fractures can be divided into various types as follows.

1. Depending on displacement of fragments
   - Undisplaced (<3 mm cortical separation or <2 mm of articular step off)
   - Displaced (>3 mm cortical separation or >2 mm of articular step off)
2. Depending on fracture configuration
   - Vertical (direct injury)
   - Stellate (direct injury)
   - Transverse (indirect injury)
     - Polar fractures (upper pole or lower pole fractures are variants of the transverse fracture).
     - Stress fractures are usually transverse.
3. Depending on involvement of articular surface
   - Intra-articular (most fractures belong to this type).
   - Extra-articular–fractures such as inferior pole fractures do not involve the articular surface.

Evaluation of a patient with patella fracture

Patient with patella fracture presents with a history of direct injury to the knee or a fall. Patient may give a history of inability to stand and walk (suggesting disruption of extensor mechanism) and a rapid swelling of the knee along with pain.

After thorough examination to rule out associated injuries, skin is meticulously examined to rule out an open fracture. Direct trauma producing patellar fracture may lacerate the prepatellar skin. Hemarthrosis is present. Patients with extensor disruption are unable to perform straight leg raising and there is a palpable gap between the fracture fragments. In patients with undisplaced, vertical or stellate fractures without extensor mechanism disruption, no such gap is felt and the patient is able to perform straight leg raising.

Imaging Patella must be visualised in all cases of polytrauma with lower limb injury and/or hemarthrosis of the knee. A routine of securing anteroposterior, lateral and skyline (sunrise) views of the knee should be followed. Lateral view is ideal for demonstrating separation of fragments and articular congruity.

Transverse fractures are best visualised in lateral view while the vertical fractures are appreciated on anteroposterior or, better still, on skyline views. Skyline view is also extremely useful in diagnosing the osteo-chondral fractures/fragments associated with patellar dislocation. Presence of fat globules in the joint on x-rays without any evident fracture line strongly suggests the presence of an intra-articular fracture.

Distinction should be made between patellar fractures and bipartite patella. Latter usually is seen on superolateral quadrant, has smooth cortical outline and is often bilateral.

Bone scan is a useful modality to diagnose occult stress fractures of the patella.

Magnetic Resonance Imaging (MRI) can diagnose osteochondral fragments, chondral flaps and ligament injuries.

Treatment of Patellar fractures

Conservative treatment

Undisplaced or minimally displaced (<3 mm displacement or less than 2 mm articular incongruity) fractures are treated with an above knee cylinder cast in full extension for six weeks. Patient is allowed weight bearing as tolerated. Range of motion exercises are started after 6 weeks. Conservative treatment is also advocated in displaced fractures in non-ambulatory patients or patients with medical comorbidities which preclude surgery.

Surgical treatment

Surgical treatment allows anatomic reduction of the displaced patellar fragments, repair of quadriceps expansion and lateral patellar retinaculae, early mobilisation and aggressive rehabilitation.

Open reduction and internal fixation is most commonly indicated for transverse displaced fractures. Osteosynthesis is achieved using tension band wiring (two parallel transosseous kirschner wires or cannulated compression screws with tension-band wiring in figure of 8 configuration). Large fragments can also be fixed using cancellous screws or circumferential wiring. Post operatively the patients are allowed to bear weight as tolerated in a hinged knee brace locked in full extension. The brace can be removed daily for gentle passive range of motion exercises. Straight leg raising is started after 2 weeks and active range of motion exercises are started after 6 weeks.

Comminuted (stellate) fractures are sometimes amenable to fixation using a combination of interfragmentary screws and circumferential (Fig. 28.1c) or the tension-band wiring. Tension band wiring is also extremely useful for fixation of periprosthetic fractures in patients with total knee arthroplasty.

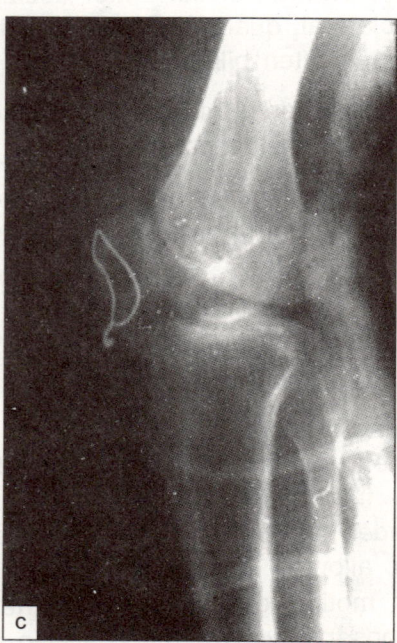

Fig. 28.1c. Fracture patella treated by circumferential/ encirclage wiring

Partial Patellectomy

Polar fractures with very small or extensively comminuted fragments are treated by excision of the fragment and reattachment of the quadriceps tendon or patellar tendon to **anterior** aspect of remaining patella using sutures through the bone. Knee is immobilised in the cylinder cast in full extension for 6 weeks following the surgery. Partial patellectomy can restore satisfactory function but more than 40% patellar resection leads to patellofemoral degeneration and unsatisfactory outcome.

Total Patellectomy

Patellectomy is reserved for extensively comminuted fractures in which anatomical reduction and fixation of fragments is not possible and excision of comminuted fragments would leave less than 60% of the host patella. Patellar fragments are meticulously excised (*"no soft tissue with bone, no bone with soft tissues"*) and quadriceps expansion and lateral retinaculae are repaired. Knee is immobilised in an above knee cylinder cast for 6 weeks. Lack of full flexion and/ or extension may occur after total patellectomy. Total patellectomy also compromises the results of subsequent total knee arthroplasty.

Osteochondral fractures

Large osteochondral fractures are treated with anatomic reduction and stabilisation using Herbert screws or biodegradable pins. Small osteochondral fragments are excised.

Arthroscopic treatment of patellar fractures

Vertical fractures, minimally displaced fractures and fractures without disruption of extensor mechanism can be treated by minimally invasive method using arthroscopy. Latter allows evacuation of intra-articular hematoma, lavage of the joint space, arthroscopic confirmation of anatomic reduction, diagnosis of occult osteochondral fractures, removal of loose bodies in the joint and percutaneous screw insertion. All these goals can be achieved without any disruption of the retinaculae.

Complications of patellar fractures are failure of fixation, infection, delayed union, non union, malunion, delayed patellofemoral degenerative arthritis and loss of knee movements.

Traumatic Patellar dislocations

Traumatic dislocation of the patella occurs in children and adolescents. The patella always dislocates laterally.

Mechanism of injury

Dislocation of the patella occurs following a direct injury with knee slightly flexed and quadriceps relaxed.

Evaluation

Patient presents with history of direct blow to the side of the knee and pain and inability to extend the knee following the injury. Swelling of the knee (due to hemarthrosis or effusion) may be seen. Patella is found to be lying lateral to knee joint on palpation and tenderness is often elicited medial to patella suggesting injury to medial soft tissues.

Imaging

Anteroposterior, lateral and skyline views should be taken. Skyline views are especially useful to demonstrate lateral dislocation (and subsequent reduction), congruity of reduction, osteochondral fractures and loose bodies in the patello-femoral joint.

MRI is useful to diagnose osteochondral fragments, chondral flaps and ligament injuries.

Treatment of the acute traumatic dislocation of patella is reduction with knee in full extension and immobilisation in an above knee cylinder cast for 4 weeks. After the cast removal, progressive range of motion and vastus medialis obliquus strengthening exercises are started.

Complications

Traumatic dislocations of patella may be complicated by recurrence. Recurrent dislocations are managed by repair of medial attenuated retinaculae, lateral retinacular release and proximal or distal realignment of extensor apparatus.

The other factors responsible for recurrent patellar dislocation apart from trauma are given in Table 28.1.

Table 28.1. Factors responsible for recurrent patellar dislocation

- Patella alta
- Hypoplastic patella
- Hypoplastic lateral femoral condyle
- Attenuation of VMO* complex
- Contracture of iliotibial band
- Genu valgum
- Abnormal Q# angle
- Excessive femoral anteversion
- Excessive extorsion of tibia
- Laterally placed tibial tuberosity

* Vastus Medialis Obliquus
# Quadriceps

Proximal realignment procedures aim to correct the imbalance between the medial and lateral patellar retinacula and involve a lateral retinacular release and medial plication/ strengthening procedures. Distal realignment is most often needed in patients with abnormally large Q (Quadriceps angle > 20°). The commonly used procedure is the Hauser procedure, which consists of osteotomy followed by distal and medial transfer of the tibial tuberosity. It is reserved for skeletally mature patients only.

Dislocation of the knee

Dislocation of the knee is a rare injury. It is caused by a high-energy trauma and the associated injuries are common. Dislocation of the knee results in disruption of joint capsule and most of the ligaments. The main stabilising structures of the knee joint include the medial and lateral collateral ligaments and the anterior and posterior cruciate ligaments. At least three of these four ligaments must be ruptured for a knee dislocation to occur.

Classification

Knee dislocations are classified depending on the direction of the displacement. Five major types of knee dislocations are anterior, posterior, medial, lateral and rotational (Fig. 28.2). Anteroposterior dislocation is most commonly associated with vascular injury.

Evaluation of a patient with knee dislocation

A patient with knee dislocation gives history of high-energy trauma such as motor vehicular accident or fall from height. Associated injuries must be looked for in these cases. The knee is deformed and painful and patient does not allow movements. Femoral and tibial condyles are prominent. Tense hemarthrosis does not occur due to disruption of the capsule and extravasation of blood out of the joint. Careful neurovascular examination must be performed to rule out injury to popliteal artery and/or lateral popliteal nerve. Diminished capillary refill or pulse, expanding hematoma, thrill or bruit and cold extremity suggest associated vascular injury.

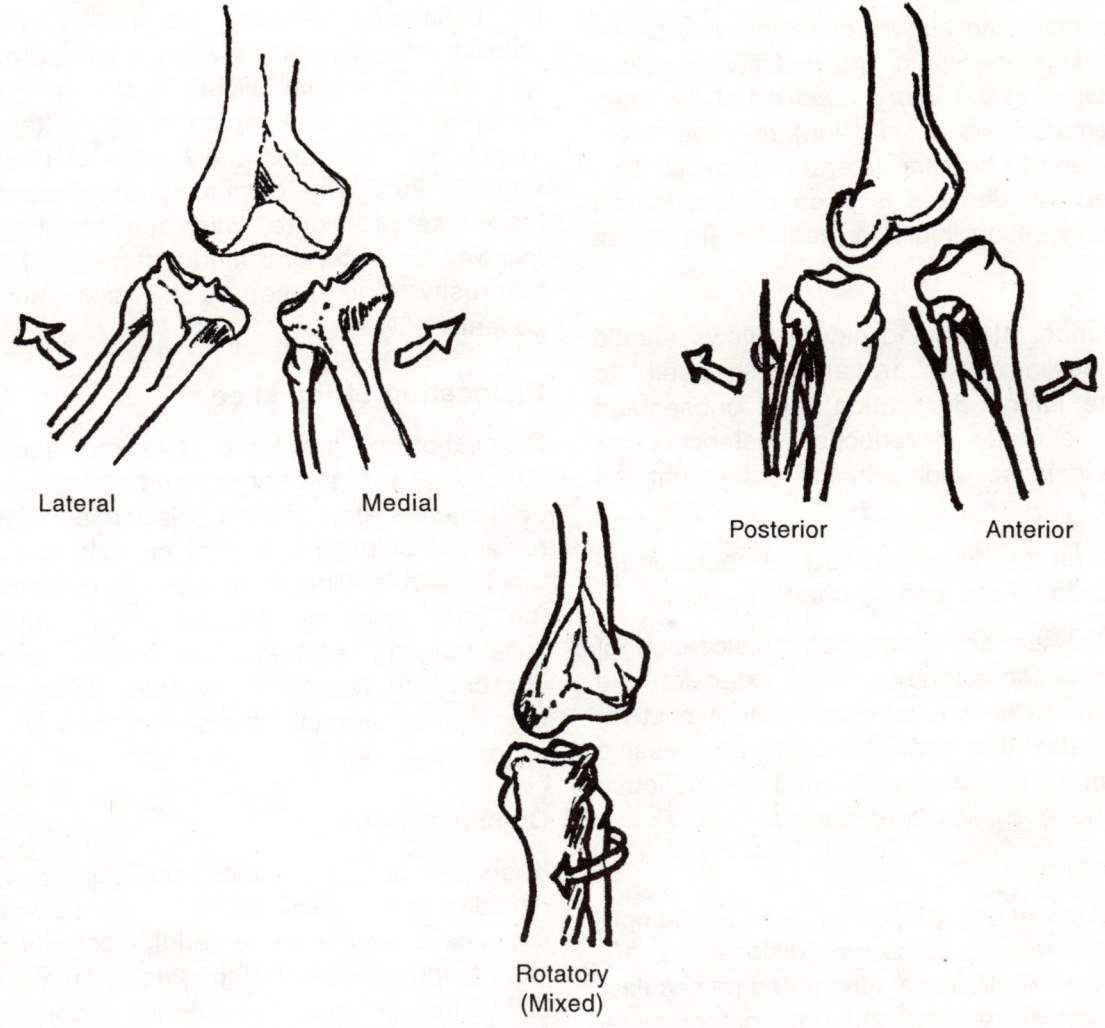

Lateral   Medial

Posterior   Anterior

Rotatory
(Mixed)

Fig. 28.2.   Classification of Knee Dislocations

Imaging

Anteroposterior and lateral views of the knee are usually sufficient to confirm the presence and direction of the dislocation. Oblique views are sometimes required to evaluate associated fractures. Fractures of the tibial spine and head of the fibula are commonly associated with knee dislocation.

Urgent angiography is indicated in cases of knee dislocation with associated popliteal artery injuries.

MRI is useful to evaluate associated soft tissue injuries.

Treatment

Knee dislocation should be treated as an emer-gency. Reduction is performed under anaesthesia followed by immobilisation in an above knee plaster cast for 3 months. Conservative treatment, however, is associated with knee stiffness. If closed manipulation fails to achieve reduction due to the interposition of soft tissues, open reduction is indicated. Open reduction with repair of ligaments can be undertaken early (within 3 weeks) or on a delayed basis. The aim of treatment is to attempt to achieve a painless and stable knee with near normal range of motion and strength. Vascular injuries are treated with urgent angiography and vascular repair using reverse saphenous vein graft.

Complications of the knee dislocation include neurovascular injuries, compartment syndrome, and stiffness of the knee.

Tibial Spine Fractures

Tibial spine fractures are avulsion fractures of the tibial attachment of the anterior cruciate ligament. This injury is quite commonly missed and high index of suspicion is required for diagnosis.

Mechanism of Injury Tibial spine fractures are caused by the hyperextension injury.

Classification

The fracture is classified according to degree of displacement of fragment as undisplaced, incompletely displaced (lifted off on one side while still attached to tibia on the other side), and completely displaced types.

Evaluation of a patient with tibial spine fracture

Patient presents with a history of injury to the knee followed by pain, swelling and inability to move the knee. Knee is held in an attitude of flexion and a tense hemarthrosis is present. Attempted movements of the knee are extremely painful.

Other knee injuries causing acute hemarthrosis are:

- Osteo-chondral fractures of patella
- Osteo-chondral fractures of distal femur and proximal tibia
- Peripheral meniscal tears (red-red zone)
- Injury to cruciate ligaments

Imaging

Anteroposterior and lateral x-rays confirm the presence of the fracture, size of the fragment and degree of its displacement.

Treatment

Conservative treatment consists of plaster immobilisation of undisplaced fracture and reduction of displaced fracture. Closed reduction of the fracture is done under anaesthesia by extending the knee fully and if adequacy of reduction is confirmed, immobilising it in a long leg cast for 6 weeks.

Irreducible fractures are treated by anatomic reduction of the fracture (arthroscopic or open) followed by fixation with a screw (if the fragment is large) or transosseous pull out wire sutures.

Complications of tibial spine fracture include stiffness and non union with ACL incompetence.

Fractures of the tibial plateau

Tibial plateau fractures are the fractures of the articular surface of the proximal tibia. These fractures disrupt the articular surface of a major weight bearing joint and often lead to articular incongruity, secondary osteoarthritis and stiffness of the knee. These fractures occur in young males with good bone stock and elderly females with osteopenia. Since proximal articular surface of tibia gives attachment to several important soft tissues, its fracture commonly injures menisci and cruciates. Also, the load bearing in lateral compartment is entirely through the lateral meniscus while the medial meniscus and the articular cartilage share the load bearing equally on the medial side. Therefore, patients with lateral plateau fractures fare well functionally despite imperfect reduction while the results in medial condylar fractures are worse.

Mechanism of Injury

Tibial plateau fractures are caused by axial loading with lateral (varus/valgus) bending stress. Valgus stress causes lateral condylar fractures and may injure medial collateral ligament. Varus stress causes medial condylar fractures and may injure lateral collateral ligament, popliteal artery and lateral popliteal nerve. Bicondylar fractures are caused by pure axial load on the extended knee.

Classification

The most commonly used classification of tibial plateau fractures is one described by Schatzker (Table 28.2). Fracture types are described from type I to VI and this classification allows planning appropriate treatment and dictates prognosis.

Evaluation of a patient with tibial plateau fracture

Patients with tibial plateau fractures are evaluated after assessment of vital parameters, search for associated injuries and resuscitation. Skin around the knee should be inspected for any breach.

Table 28.2. Tibial plateau fractures (after Schatzker)

Type	Mechanism	Age Group	Involved condyle	Bone stock	Associated injuries	Treatment	Prognosis
I (split/ wedge #) (Fig. 28.3a)	Valgus with Axial load	Young	Lateral	Good	Lateral meniscus - Tear - entrapment in # MCL* Disruption	*Undisplaced* Conservative *Displaced* ORIF (cancellous screws & buttress plate)	Excellent
II (split/de pression #) (Fig. 28.3b)	Valgus with Axial load	Elderly	Lateral	Poor	ACL tear + Lateral meniscus - Tear - entrapment in # MCL* Disruption	*Minimally displaced/stable* Conservative *Displaced* - Reduction - ORIF + BG - Arthroscopic repair of #	Good
III (Pure depression #) lateral plateau (central depression) (Fig. 28.3c)	Valgus with Axial load	Elderly	Lateral	Poor	ACL tear + Lateral meniscus - Tear - entrapment in # MCL* Disruption	*< 3 mm step/ stable* Conservative *> 3 mm step/ unstable* - ORIF + BG - Arthroscopic elevation of fragment	Good
IV (split/ depression #) Medial plateau split (Fig. 28.3d)	Varus	Young	Medial	Good	Avulsion of - intercondylar eminence of tibia (both cruciate disruption) - Fibular collateral ligament - Lat. Popliteal N. - Popliteal A injury	Surgical - ORIF (Screws & buttress plate) - Limited Internal+ Ext. Fixator	Fair
V (Bicondylar split #) Both plateaus split off, Metaphysis/ diaphysis remain in continuity (Fig. 28.3e)	Pure axial load on extended knee	Elderly	Both : Metaphysis intact	Poor	Meniscal injuries Articular cartilage injuries	Surgical - ORIF & buttress plate on the more comminuted side (Screws+ plate on other condyle) - Limited Internal+ Ext. Fixator	Guarded
VI Associated Plateau & Proximal Shaft # Metaphyseo diaphyseal separation (Fig. 28.3f)	Axial load	Elderly	Both : Metphyseal separation	Poor	ACL tear	Surgical - ORIF (Screws & buttress plate) - Limited Internal + Ext. Fixator	Guarded

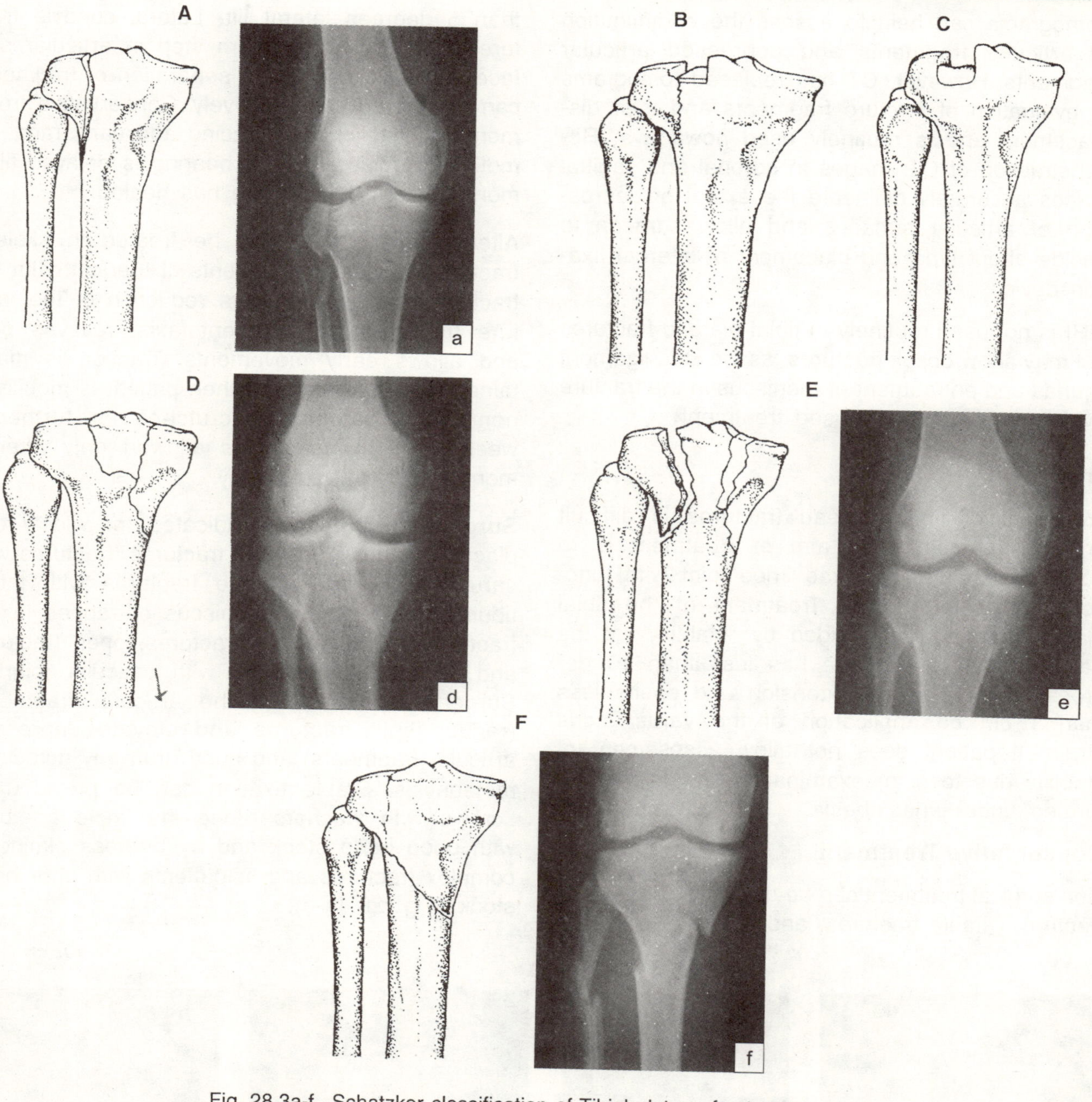

A

B

C

D

E

F

Fig. 28.3a-f. Schatzker classification of Tibial plateau fractures

Hemarthrosis is the rule and the knee appears deformed. Movements at the knee are not possible and any attempts at moving the knee are extremely painful. Limb should be examined above and below the knee for associated skeletal injuries in the limb.

Careful neurovascular examination must be performed in all patients with tibial plateau fractures to rule out injury to the lateral popliteal nerve and/or popliteal artery. Compartment syndrome may occur with tibial plateau fractures and must be diagnosed early.

Imaging

Imaging begins with the standard anteroposterior and lateral views of the knee. Additional anteroposterior view with beam tilted 10–15 degrees inferiorly (in the direction of normal posterior articular slope of the proximal tibia) allows better visualisation (*Moore view*). Oblique 45-degree views are taken to evaluate articular depression of tibial plateau. Internal rotation view shows lateral plateau while the external rotation view helps in assessing the medial plateau.

Tomograms can help to assess the comminution of articular fragments and depressed articular fragments. However, CT has replaced tomograms in evaluation of fracture fragments and their displacement and is routinely used nowadays. Reconstruction of CT images in coronal and sagittal planes accurately delineate the extent of depression of articular surfaces and allow surgeon to decide about type and placement of internal fixation devices.

MRI is not used routinely in tibial plateau fractures but may show occult fractures, associated ligament injuries and entrapment of meniscus in the fracture (which may preclude closed treatment).

Treatment

Treatment of tibial plateau fractures is difficult and controversial. The aim of treatment is to achieve a stable, pain-free knee joint with functional range of motion. Treatment of the tibial plateau fractures is decided by "stability" of the fracture—a stable fracture has less than 10 degrees of laxity in full extension and opens less than 1 cm on application of the varus/valgus strain. If patient does not allow assessment of stability due to pain, examination should be performed under anaesthesia.

Conservative Treatment

Non surgical treatment can be done for undisplaced fractures, stable fractures, and fractures with less than 5 degrees lateral tilt. Lateral condyle fractures with less than 3-mm step in articular surface and less than 5-mm separation of fragments can be treated conservatively. Conservative treatment consists of cast bracing and early range of motion exercises. Weight bearing is delayed till 3 months when the fracture has healed.

Alternatively, patient can be treated in skeletal traction with early movements of the joint with the traction on. Traction allows reduction of the fracture fragments by ligamentotaxis, relieves pain and allows early movements. Traction is maintained for six weeks and then patient is mobilised non-weight bearing on crutches for further 6 weeks. Weight bearing is allowed only after 3 months following the injury.

Surgical treatment is indicated for widely displaced fractures, unstable fractures, fractures with varus tilt (medial condyle fractures with intact fibula), fractures with meniscus entrapped in the fracture line, bicondylar fractures, open fractures and fractures associated with vascular injuries. Surgery aims to align the articular fragments (reduce split fractures and elevate depressed articular fragments) and bone graft any defects in metaphysis. Stable fixation can be provided by screws with washers alone in simple fractures with good bone stock and by buttress plating in complex fractures and in patients with poor bone stock (Fig. 28.4a-d).

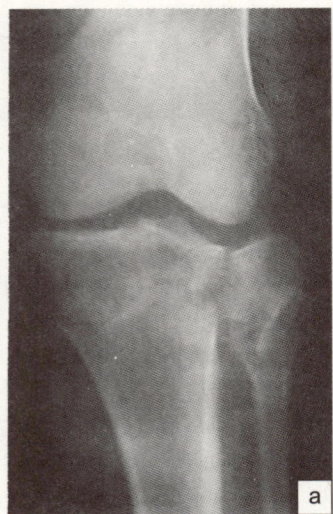 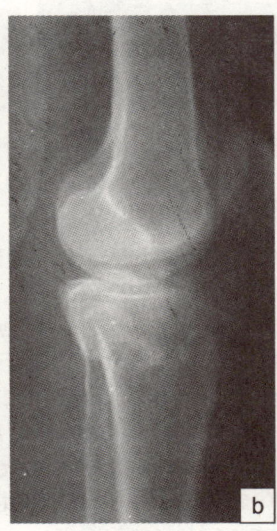 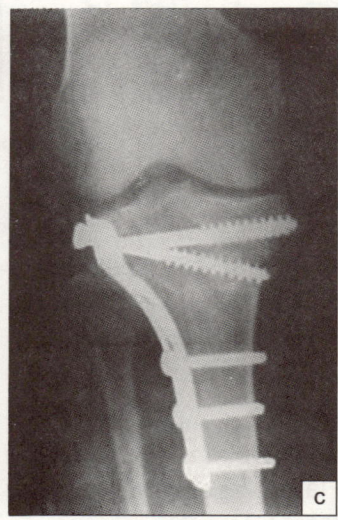 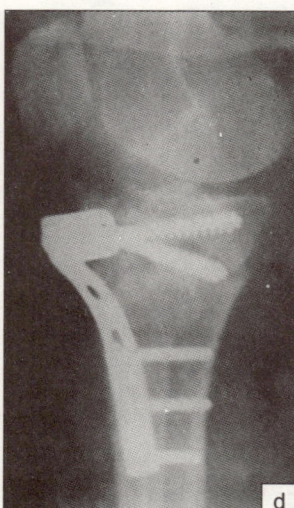

Fig. 28.4a-d. Pre and Post operative X-rays of a patient with bicondylar fracture of the tibial plateau treated by open reduction and buttress plating.

Limited internal fixation of the fracture with protection of the fragments against displacement by a fixator spanning the knee or a hybrid external fixator is a good method to treat complex fractures. The method is especially useful in cases where the condition of the soft tissues is poor. Further soft tissue injury due to surgery, avascularity of fragments due to soft tissue stripping and hardware related problems are minimised by this method.

Arthroscopy is being used increasingly to repair tibial plateau fractures under direct visualisation. Arthroscopic assisted fixation is suitable only for simple low energy fractures (Type I-III). Arthroscopy reduces iatrogenic soft tissue damage and has been shown to be safe. Arthroscopy is not suitable for repair of fractures with poor bone stock or comminution. Collateral ligaments, if torn, have to be repaired by an open method.

Complications of tibial plateau fractures include neurovascular injuries, compartment syndrome, avascular necrosis of fragments, malunion, nonunion, stiffness, post traumatic arthritis, deep vein thrombosis and hardware related problems.

Fractures of Tibia and fibula

Fractures of tibia and fibula are the commonest long bone fractures. The spectrum of injuries causing these fractures ranges from repetitive cyclic stress loading leading to fatigue fractures to extreme high-energy injuries leading to severe disruption and loss of soft tissue structures and bone. Close to one fourth of all the patients may present as open injuries and soft tissue management is the key factor in the management of these fractures.

Mechanism of injury

Road traffic accidents, fall from height and other high energy injuries can cause fractures of both bones of the leg by bending (angulatory) forces, torsion (rotatory) forces or a combination of the two. The type of injury determines the configuration of the fracture - torsion forces produce spiral fractures while direct injury (bending force)) produces a transverse fracture. High-energy torsion (as in skiing injuries) and combinations of bending with torsion or compression lead to comminuted fractures.

Classification

Tibial and fibular fractures can be classified as closed or open. Open fractures are classified by Gustilo's classification. No standardised classification for fracture pattern is available but a simple way is to classify these fractures into three types: simple [spiral, oblique or transverse (Fig. 28.5a,b)], fractures with a butterfly fragment and comminuted (including segmental and crush) fractures (Fig. 28.5c).

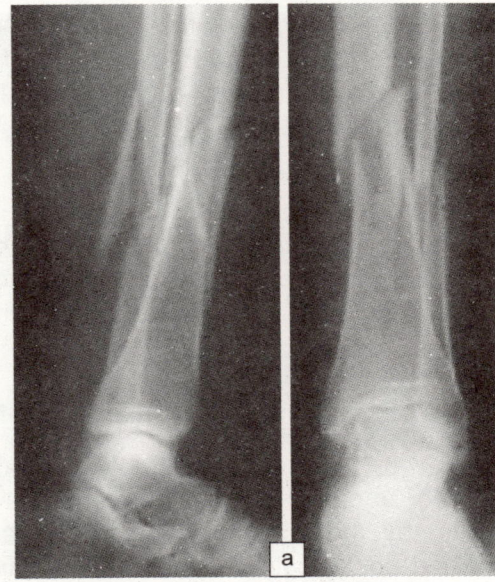

Fig. 28.5a. Oblique fracture of tibia with comminuted fracture of fibula

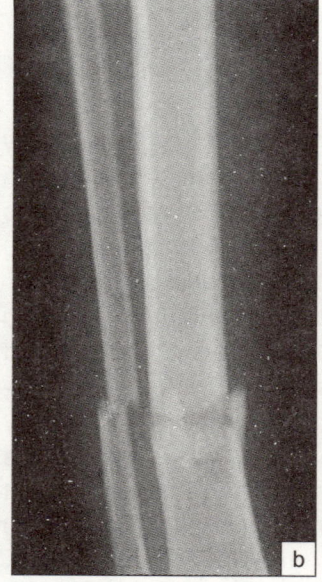

Fig. 28.5b. Transverse fracture of both bones leg

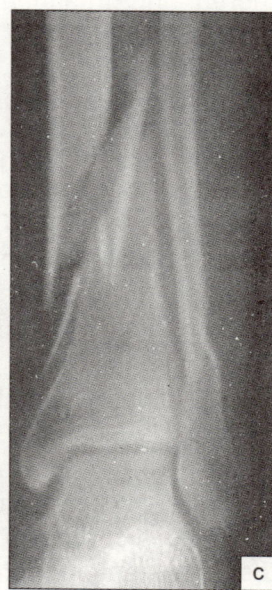

Fig. 28.5c. Comminuted fracture of the tibia

Evaluation of a patient with fracture of both bones of leg

Initial assessment includes vital function evaluation, examination for associated injuries and resuscitation. Other skeletal injuries in the affected extremity should be looked for. Local examination reveals deformity which is readily apparent since tibia is mostly subcutaneous. The limb is shortened in cases with displaced fractures. Pain, tenderness and abnormal mobility is present at the fracture site. Soft tissues are inspected circumferentially for skin wounds, ecchymosis and any evidence of compartment syndrome. Neurovascular examination of the limb is extremely important and should be recorded.

Imaging

Anteroposterior and lateral radiographs are adequate for diagnosis and assessment of the fracture. It is imperative to include ipsilateral knee and ankle in the radiographs.

Treatment of fractures of both bones of the leg

Treatment of fractures of both bones of the leg is determined by the condition of soft tissues and location and configuration of the fracture and the nature of associated injuries. In treatment of fractures of both bones of the leg, fibula is ignored and treatment is planned mainly for the tibia fracture.

Conservative Treatment

Conservative treatment is the most commonly used method of treating fractures of the both bones of the leg. This method is applicable to closed fractures and grade I compound (skin opening <1 cm, most likely from inside out) fractures. Fracture is reduced under anaesthesia and immobilised in an above knee plaster cast (Fig. 28.6a,b). Fractures where acceptable reduction is achieved are monitored with weekly check x-rays to detect redisplacement of the fracture. Accepted guidelines for reduction are at least 50% cortical contact, varus/valgus up to 10 degrees, anteroposterior angulation up to 10°, less than 10° rotational malalignment and less than 1 cm shortening. Early weight bearing and functional bracing expedite union and reduce the incidence of joint stiffness in these cases. Static quadriceps exercises are started from the beginning. The immobilisation is discarded after 12 to 16 weeks, once the radiological evidence of union appears.

Conservative treatment has the advantage of avoiding the risks of surgery and infection, reduced cost and universal availability. However, it has the disadvantages of ankle stiffness (25–40% cases), delayed union and higher incidence of malunion.

Contraindications to closed treatment are fractures with excessive initial shortening, fractures showing increasing angular deformity in cast, patients with neurovascular damage, patients with segmental bone loss and fractures with severe attendant soft tissue injuries.

Surgical Treatment

Surgical treatment is indicated for failure to achieve or maintain reduction, open fractures, fractures associated with vascular injury or compartment syndrome, polytrauma patient and patient with ipsilateral femur fracture (*floating knee injuries*).

Reamed intramedullary interlocking nailing is the most suitable operative treatment for tibial diaphyseal fractures. Tibial medullary canal is not suitable for ordinary unlocked medullary nailing due to its triangular cross section and lack of curvature. Interlocking screws prevent axial and

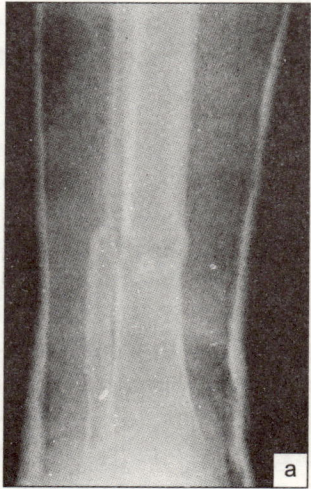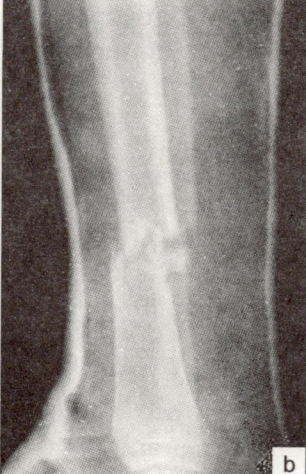

Fig. 28.6a,b.   AP and lateral radiographs showing conservative treatment of fracture of both bones of leg in an above knee plaster cast.

rotational deformities and maintain reduction. Reamed intramedullary nailing has lower time to union and non-union rates compared to conservative treatment (Fig. 28.7a,b).

Interlocking nailing is not suitable for proximal and distal metaphyseal fractures and malunions are common subsequent to its application in these situations.

Anterior knee pain is the most common complication of intramedullary nailing of tibia.

Open reduction and plate osteosynthesis is used only in unstable metaphyseal fractures and polytrauma patients where other techniques cannot be used. High complication rates have been reported with plating of tibial shaft fractures. Recently biological plating has been advocated where indirect reduction and minimally invasive techniques of plating have been described which retain soft tissue attachment of fracture fragments (Minimally Invasive Plate Osteosynthesis-MIPO).

External fixators are used mainly in compound fractures but are also advocated in closed fractures particularly in patients with polytrauma. External fixators are also useful in patients with burns, head injury or compartment syndromes. External fixators allow movements at the neighbouring joints and care of the soft tissues without disturbing the alignment of the fracture fragments. When intact diaphysis is present proximal and distal to the fracture, unilateral tubular fixator with schanz pins is applied to the medial surface of the tibia (Fig. 28.8a). In metaphyseal regions, tensioned kirschner wires connected to the ring frame provide stability. Ring frame is connected to the tubular frame fixed to the diaphysis by bicortical schanz screws (Hybrid fixator). External fixators are associated with higher incidence of delayed union and non-union.

Management of open tibial fractures

Open tibial fractures present the orthopaedist with a great challenge. The aim in the manage-

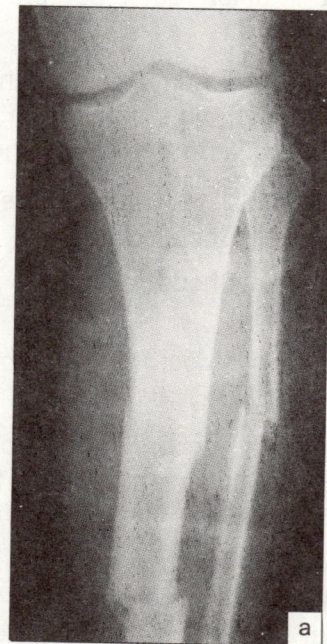

Fig. 28.7a.   Segmental fracture of both bones of the leg

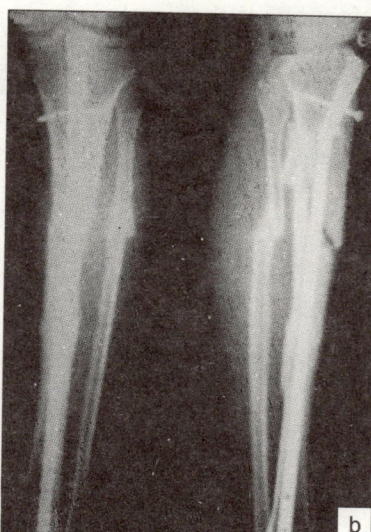

Fig. 28.7b.   Same fracture after treatment with interlocking nailing

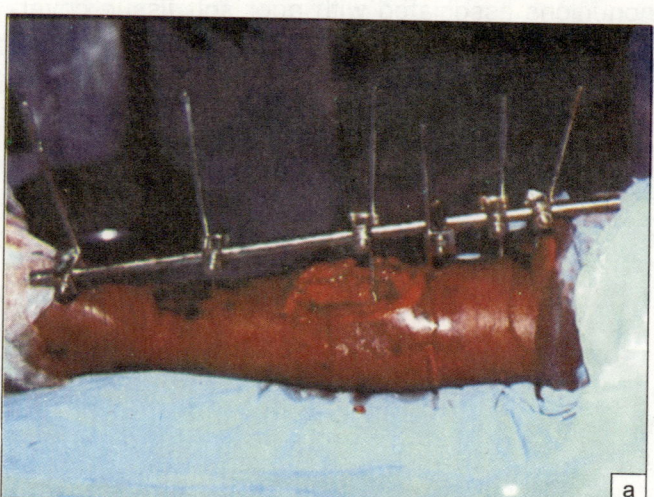

Fig. 28.8a. Open fracture of tibia stabilized by external fixator

ment of an open fracture is to convert it to a closed fracture. The management of compound fracture begins with radical debridement and thorough irrigation. Tap water can be used in abundance if sterile saline is not available. The fracture is then stabilised by external fixation or, rarely, by unreamed interlocking nail at some centres. The incidence of infection is significantly reduced if the micromotion at the fracture site is eliminated. Suitable parenteral antibiotic therapy is started. Repeated debridements are done every 24–48 hours as required. Once the underlying bed becomes healthy, soft tissue coverage is achieved. Bone grafting or bone transport techniques are often required to overcome the osseous defects in open fractures of the tibia.

Complications

Non-union, delayed union, malunion, compartment syndrome and hardware related complications are common after tibial fractures.

Non union is treated by compression plating and bone grafting or reamed intramedullary interlocked nailing. Phemister grafting, where osteoperiostal flaps are raised and cancellous "match-stick" grafts are placed under them is. an extremely useful technique to achieve union in cases where fibrous union is present, alignment of fragments is acceptable, neighbouring joints are not stiff and use of metallic implants is not desirable.

Ring fixator (Ilizarov) is a useful technique in nonunions associated with poor soft tissue coverage and / or bone loss. A corticotomy done at the time of surgery improves vascularity and also allows bone transport to manage the defect in the bone.

Compartment syndrome should be diagnosed early and compartment pressure monitoring is recommended in suspected cases. Fibulectomy effectively decompresses all compartments in cases with compartment syndrome. The wound should be left open and skin grafted/secondarily closed after 3–5 days.

Malunion, if not acceptable, is treated by corrective osteotomy, internal fixation and bone grafting.

Delayed union is treated by continued expectant treatment but if union does not progress, bone grafting is indicated.

The role of electrical stimulation in the treatment of delayed/nonunion tibia has been extensively researched. The different methods include:

1. Invasive methods (the cathode is surgically implanted into the fracture site)

2. Semi-invasive methods (electrodes are inserted through the skin)

3. Non-invasive methods: Pulsed Electro-magnetic field Therpy (PEMF)

Infection commonly occurs in the pin tracts of external fixator. Infection may occur following internal fixation or due to compound fracture.

Infection with implant in situ is treated by debridement and retention of implants if the latter is providing stability. Local antibiotic delivery systems (Gentamicin-PMMA beads (Septopal) or garamycin implant) and systemic antibiotics are used to suppress the infection. If the implant is not providing stability, it is removed, debridement and irrigation is performed and extremity is stabilised with external fixator. Bone grafting or bone transport may be required in these cases to treat nonunion and/or osseous defect subsequent to debridement.

Fractures of the Ankle and Foot

Fractures of the ankle Injuries around the ankle are very common. A steady increase in their incidence has been reported in the recent years. Ankle fractures must be evaluated carefully to assess the probable mechanism of injury and plan appropriate treatment. Failure to restore normal anatomy leads to painful restriction of ankle movements and degenerative arthritis.

Mechanism of injury Ankle fractures usually result from rotational forces. Most ankle injuries occur as a result of road traffic accidents (direct injury), fall from height or falls due to loss of balance (indirect injury). During the indirect injury due to fall, the foot is usually planted firmly on ground while the body of person twists and applies rotational force on ankle leading to sequential failure of soft tissues and bony structures.

Classification of ankle fractures An understanding of the terms supination and pronation of the foot is necessary to understand the classification of ankle fractures. Supination is a complex movement consisting of plantar flexion at the ankle, inversion at the subtalar joint and adduction of the forefoot while pronation consists of a combination of dorsiflexion at the ankle, eversion at the subtalar joint and abduction of the forefoot. The biomechanics of the ankle and foot is complex and interrelated with various movements occurring at the ankle, subtalar and midtarsal joints (talonavicular & calcaneocuboid joints). Classically bimalleolar fractures (fractures of medial and lateral malleolus)

are referred to as *Pott's* fractures. Trimalleolar fractures are referred to as *Cotton's* fractures.

Several classifications are available for the ankle fractures. *Lauge-Hansen* classification describes fracture patterns based on the position of the foot and the direction of the injuring force (Fig. 29.1a-e). This classification provides an understanding

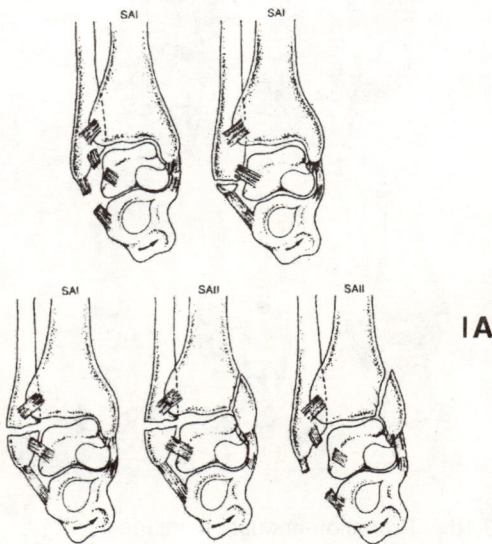

Fig. 29.1.   Lauge-Hansen classification of ankle fractures
Fig. 29.1a.   Stages of Supination-adduction (SA) injuries
SAI   Rupture of the lateral ligament, avulsion fracture of tip of lateral malleolus or transverse avulsion fracture of the lateral malleolus
SAII   SAI plus compression fracture of medial malleolus

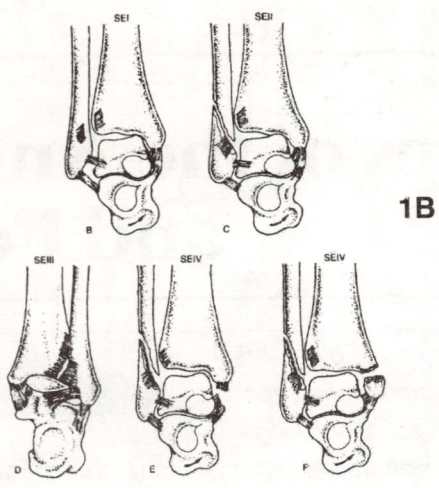

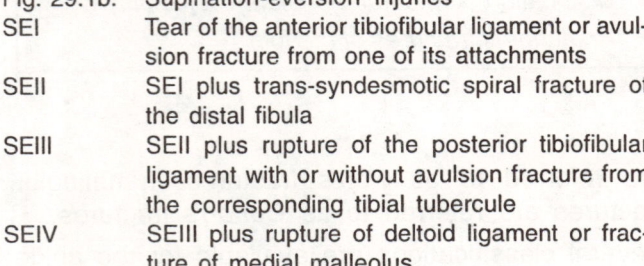

1B

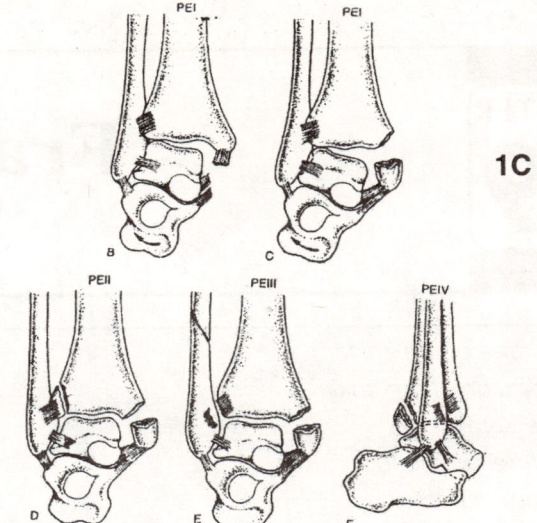

1C

Fig. 29.1b. Supination-eversion injuries

SEI	Tear of the anterior tibiofibular ligament or avulsion fracture from one of its attachments
SEII	SEI plus trans-syndesmotic spiral fracture of the distal fibula
SEIII	SEII plus rupture of the posterior tibiofibular ligament with or without avulsion fracture from the corresponding tibial tubercle
SEIV	SEIII plus rupture of deltoid ligament or fracture of medial malleolus

Fig. 29.1c. Pronation-eversion injuries

PEI	Disruption of the deltoid ligament or fracture of the medial malleolus
PEII	PEI plus tear of the anterior tibiofibular ligament or avulsion fracture of its attachment to tibia or fibula
PEIII	PEII plus supra-syndesmotic spiral fibular fracture
PEIV	PEIII plus rupture of posterior tibiofibular ligament or avulsion fracture from its tibial attachment

1D

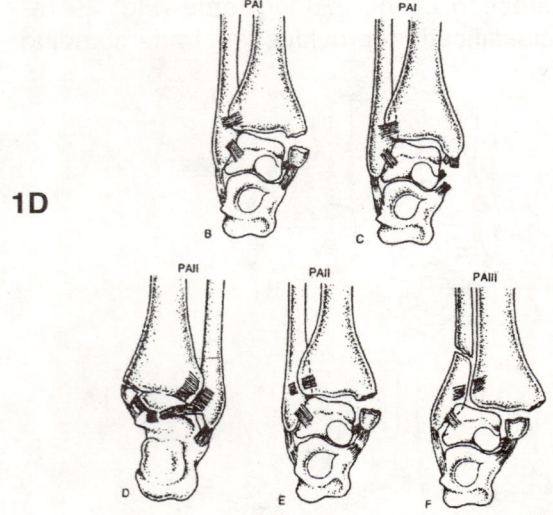

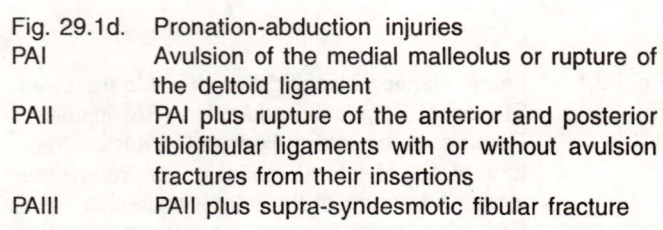

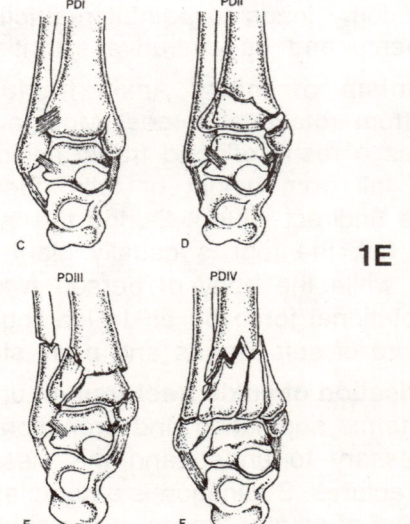

1E

Fig. 29.1d. Pronation-abduction injuries

PAI	Avulsion of the medial malleolus or rupture of the deltoid ligament
PAII	PAI plus rupture of the anterior and posterior tibiofibular ligaments with or without avulsion fractures from their insertions
PAIII	PAII plus supra-syndesmotic fibular fracture

Fig. 29.1e. Pronation-dorsiflexion injuries

PDI	Fracture of the medial malleolus
PDII	Avulsion of anterior lip fragment of tibia
PDIII	Transverse fracture in fibula level with tibial fracture
PDIV	Comminuted intra-articular tibial fracture

of mechanism of injuries and is especially useful for closed treatment where manoeuvres to reverse the injury pattern are used to achieve reduction. This classification divides fractures into supination-adduction, pronation-abduction, supination-external rotation (supination-eversion), pronation-external rotation (pronation-eversion) and vertical compression (pronation-dorsiflexion). For example supination external rotation injury refers to external rotation force applied to a foot, which is in supination. It is interesting to note that the radiographic appearance of the fracture patterns gives a clue to the underlying mechanism of injury (Table 29.1).

Table 29.1. Types and Management of ankle fractures

Fracture	Mechanism	Associated injuries	Radiographs	Treatment
Lateral malleolus	Abduction injury	Avulsion # of medial malleolus (bimalleolar) or Tear of deltoid ligament (bimalleolar equivalent)	Comm. fracture of lat. Malleolus at the level of syndesmosis, horizontal avulsion # of the medial malleolus	*Isolated Lat. Malleolus fracture–conservative treatment *Tension band wiring or screw fixation for medial malleolus & plaster
	Adduction injury	Fracture of medial malleolus (bimalleolar)	Horizontal avulsion # of lateral malleolus distal to syndesmosis, vertical fracture of medial malleolus	*Tension band wiring or oblique screw or intramedullary screw for lateral malleolus, *Screw fixation for displaced medial malleolus fracture.
Medial Malleolus	Adduction	Avulsion of lateral malleolus (bimalleolar)	Vertical fracture line of medial malleolus, Avulsion(horizontal) # of lateral malleolus	*Isolated, undisplaced # -conservative treatment *Displaced bimalleolar #: ORIF
	Abduction	Fracture of lateral malleolus at level of syndesmosis with comminution of lateral cortex (bimalleolar)	Horizontal avulsion # of medial malleolus, # of lat. Malleolus	*Displaced med. malleolus # - ORIF with screws, TBW or buttress plating
Trimalleolar fractures	Supination-External rotation	Rupture of anterior syndesmosis (Avulsion from anterolateral tibia: *Tillaux Chaput* fracture or from anterior aspect of lateral malleolus: *Leforte-Wagstaffe* lesion) (Interosseous tibio fibular lig. usually intact)	Avulsion # from syndesmosis (stage I) Spiral fractures of fibula at or just above syndesmosis (stage II) (# line directed down-ward, forward, medially) # of post. malleolus (stage III). Transverse # of med. malleolus or rupture of deltoid ligament (stage IV).	*Undisplaced fractures conservative treatment in plaster (6 weeks) *Displaced bimalleolar # ORIF *# Posterior Malleolus: operate if > 1/3rd articular surface > 2mm articular step
	Pronation External rotation	Rupture of anterior syndesmosis and interosseous ligament	Avulsion fracture of medial malleolus or rupture of deltoid lig. (stage I) Rupture of syndesmosis, (Gross diastasis-*Dupuytren fracture-dislocation* of ankle) (stage II) Spiral fracture of fibula anywhere above the fibular syndesmosis(# line directed upward, forward)- # of fibular neck-*Maissoneuve's* # (stage III) Posterior malleolus fracture-(stage IV)	*Closed reduction and plaster (6 weeks) *Irreducible # ORIF+ syndesmotic screw

Danis-Weber classification divides ankle fractures into three types depending on the position of the fibular fracture (i.e. distal, at or proximal to syndesmosis). The classification is given in Table 29.2.

Table 29.2. Danis Weber classification

Group	Fibular Fracture
A	Infrasyndesmotic (below the tibio fibular syndesmosis)
B	Transsyndesmotic (at the level of the tibio fibular syndesmosis)
C	Suprasyndesmotic (above the level of the tibio fibular syndesmosis)

Note   Group A through C represents progressively more unstable injuries

Evaluation of a patient with ankle fracture

Evaluation of ankle injury begins with a thorough history to elicit the mechanism of injury, any associated injuries and history of any preexisting local or systemic disorder, (e.g. peripheral vascular disease). Examination should assess the integrity of skin and extent of soft tissue injury. Ankle is deformed, painful and swollen and patient is unable to bear weight on it. Egg shaped swelling over the lateral malleolus suggests complete tear of the lateral ligament or fractures of lateral mealleolus (*Mckenzie's sign*). Attempt should be made to ascertain the location and extent of injury. Tenderness should be elicited over malleoli, entire fibula and over the medial and lateral ligaments. A careful neurovascular examination must be done in all cases. Fractures that are commonly associated with ankle fractures are:

1. Fractures of the foot: Talus, Calcaneum
2. Spinal fractures: (most commonly) Dorsolumbar junction.

Imaging for ankle fractures includes antero posterior, lateral and mortise views (AP view with ankle in 15° internal rotation). Entire fibula must be visualized so as not to miss proximal fractures (*Maisonneuve fracture*). Comparison views of the opposite unaffected ankle may help in exact evaluation of the injury. Radiographic evidence of disruption of the distal tibio-fibular syndesmosis should be looked for. Tibio-fibular overlap of less than 10mm on AP view or less than 1 mm on mortise view and posterior displacement of fibula on the lateral view all suggest the disruption of the syndesmosis. Stress abduction and stress external rotation views should be taken to assess the integrity of syndesmosis in suspect cases. Articular cartilage injury of the talar dome has been reported in nearly half the patients with ankle fractures and such injuries need CT or MRI for evaluation.

Treatment The aim of treatment of ankle fractures is to achieve anatomic reduction, restore stability and regain function. Closed treatment of ankle fractures is possible in a large number of cases and consists of long leg cast following reduction. Reduction manoeuvres strive to reverse the injury pattern evident on the x-rays. Widely displaced fractures, failed closed reduction or suspected bony osteochondral fragments or soft tissue interposition in the fracture (as periosteum, extensor retinaculum or tibialis posterior tendon in medial malleolus fractures) and open fractures are indications for surgical treatment.

Surgical treatment attempts anatomic reduction and stable internal fixation. Fibular fracture should always be fixed first to restore the length (except in supination adduction and laterally comminuted fractures).

Medial malleolus can be fixed by a variety of methods such as screws, tension band wiring or buttress plate. Posterior malleolus is fixed only if it constitutes more than 1/3rd articular surface and has an articular step more than 2 mm. Disruption of syndesmosis can be fixed either by a screw through the fibular plate or a separate trans-syndesmosis screw. A 3.5 mm cortical screw is passed 2 cm above joint line from posterolateral to anteromedial direction with the foot in full dorsiflexion. It should ideally have tricortical purchase. The syndesmotic screw is passed with the ankle in full dorsiflexion so as to enable the wider part of the talar dome to engage into the ankle mortise. This is to ensure that tightening the syndesmotic screw does not decrease the total capacity of the ankle mortise. The screw is used as a positional screw and not as a lag screw. Post operatively ankle movements should be started early. Weight bearing however is delayed till 8–12 weeks. Whenever a syndesmotic screw is used it should be removed before permitting weight bearing in order to prevent breakage of the screw. Compression fractures are treated by calcaneal pin traction or hinged external fixator and early active exercises. Compression fractures are commonly referred to as *Pilon* fractures and show varying degrees of articular comminution. The principle of limited internal fixation followed by external fixation is best employed in these cases. During the treatment of ankle fractures one must adhere to the basic principles in the management of intraarticular fractures, which include:

a) Early anatomic reduction

b) Stable internal fixation

c) Atraumatic surgical technique and

d) Early pain-free mobilization

A strict adherence to these AO principles can go a long way towards ensuring a good functional out come in these patients.

Open fractures are treated by irrigation and debridement and internal fixation using K wires or screws. Repeated debridements may be needed. Soft tissue management can be done either primarily or later as a secondary procedure depending on the condition of the soft tissues.

Complications of ankle fractures include stiffness of ankle, Sudeck's osteodystrophy, instability, malunion, degenerative arthritis, non union and hardware related complications (infection, breakage of implant)

Non union is most commonly seen in medial malleolus and may be due to soft tissue interposition. ORIF and bone grafting are used to treat non-union.

Malunion and secondary osteoarthritis may need arthrodesis of the ankle joint to alleviate pain in later years.

Hardware related problems are managed by removal of the implant (if fracture has healed) or with refixation and bone grafting if the fracture has not healed.

Dislocation of the ankle

Usually occurs along with fractures but may occur in isolation also in which case rupture of both medial and lateral ligaments occurs. Closed reduction and plaster application should be performed as soon as possible to decrease the risk of skin necrosis and vascular insult to the talus. For isolated dislocations immobilization is continued for 6 weeks. Fracture dislocations are reduced and then malleoli are fixed. Stability should be reassessed after skeletal stabilization. If the joint is still unstable, a smooth steinmann pin is passed from the heel, through the talus into the tibia (*Childress pin*) or an external fixator is applied for 6 weeks.

Open ankle dislocations are treated by meticulous debridement and irrigation. Joint should be stabilized by a fixator or Childress pin and ligamento-capsular repair is attempted. Repeated debridements may be needed. A delayed closure after 5–7 days is performed.

Ankle sprain

"Ankle sprain" belongs to the spectrum of injuries to the lateral ligament of the ankle and is the injury of the anterior talo-fibular ligament. It is the commonest ligament injury. Lateral ligament of the ankle has three distinct parts-anterior talofibular ligament resists talar inversion when the foot is plantarflexed and resists anterior subluxation of the talus with the foot in neutral position, calcaneofibular ligament resists talar inversion when the ankle is dorsiflexed. Consequently, inversion of the talus with ankle in plantar flexion injures the anterior talofibular ligament while inversion with foot in neutral position injures calcaneofibular ligament as well. The third part of the lateral ligament complex includes the posterior talo fibular ligament, which is injured least often.

Evaluation of a patient with ankle sprain reveals soft tissue swelling over the lateral malleolus. Partial ligament injuries are more painful than complete ligament tears, which are often painless. Stress tests performed by inverting the foot lead to increased opening on the lateral side as compared to the normal side. If pain is too severe to allow examination, it should be performed after injecting local anaesthetic agent or under general anaesthesia.

Imaging includes plain radiographs of the ankle, which are normal except soft tissue swelling over the lateral malleolus. Stress inversion AP radiographs may show abnormal talar tilt in ankle mortise (5°–10° tilt: partial tear, >10° tilt-complete

mortise (5°–10° tilt: partial tear, >10° tilt-complete tear). Lateral ankle radiograph with foot pulled forward (*Anterior drawer's test*) shows abnormal anterior shift of talus (4mm or more) with relation to distal tibial articular surface.

Treatment of ankle sprain is immobilization in a below knee cast for 3 weeks. Elevation on pillows is advised for the first few days for cases with severe swelling.

Complete tears of the lateral ligament are treated either by surgical repair or conservatively by plaster application for 6 weeks.

Chronic lateral ligament insufficiency (due to previously inadequately treated injuries) is a disabling condition with feeling of instability and giving way of the ankle. Attempts are made to strengthen muscles by wobble board exercises and 1/8 or 3/16 inch lateral wedge in the heel is given to avoid inversion. Recalcitrant cases are treated by reconstruction of the lateral ligaments using the tendon of peroneus brevis (Jones procedure).

Fractures of the foot

Fractures of the foot present with a challenge to the treating orthopedist. Increased incidence and recognition of these fractures have made it mandatory for the surgeons to accurately diagnose and efficiently treat these fractures. Foot fractures often occur in polytraumatized patients and may often be missed. These patients often end up with poor functional outcomes.

Calcaneal fractures

Calcaneus is the most commonly injured bone in the foot. Calcaneal fractures are bilateral in 5–10% cases. Almost 3/4th of calcaneal fractures are intra-articular while 1/4th are extraarticular.

Mechanism of injury

Axial loading (with force transmitted through the talus into the calcaneus) is the usual cause of calcaneal fractures. The injury is sustained most commonly due to fall from a height onto the heels. The fall can also cause fracture of the opposite calcaneus or fracture of the dorsolumbar spine.

Classification

Calcaneus fractures are classified into extra-articular and intra-articular (those involving subtalar joint and/or the calcaneocuboid joint).

Extra-articular fractures include fractures of the tuberosity, anterior process, medial process, body and sustentaculum tali.

Intra-articular

Fractures involving subtalar joint are divided by *Essex-Lopresti* into tongue (fracture extending backwards up to the tuberosity with the posterior facet of subtalar joint remaining intact) and joint depression type (fracture extends superiorly behind the posterior facet of subtalar joint resulting in its comminution).

Newer classifications (*Sanders*) are based on the involvement of the posterior facet seen on the CT scan (Fig. 29.2a).

Type I   undisplaced posterior facet

Type II   single fracture line involving posterior facet

Type III   two fracture lines involving the posterior facet

Type IV   three fracture lines involving the posterior facet

Type I to IV are further subdivided depending on where the fracture lines enter the subtalar joint (lateral, central, medial or sustentacular).

Evaluation of a patient with calcaneus fracture

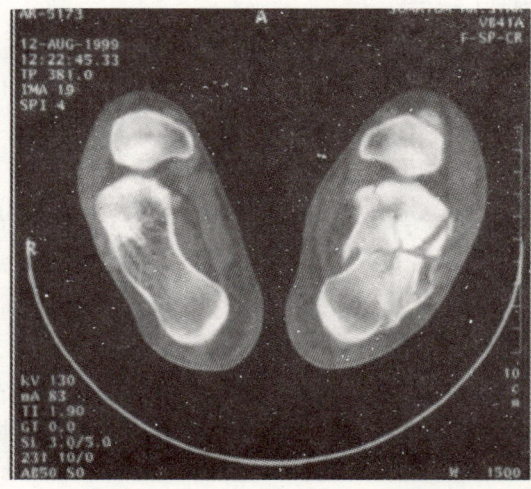

Fig. 29.2a. CT scan appearance of fracture calcaneum

should be elicited. Dorsolumbar junction injuries are reported in 10% cases while up to two third patients with calcaneal fractures may have other associated lower extremity injuries.

Local examination reveals a wider and shorter heel when viewed from behind. There is often tense swelling and ecchymosis around the heel. Marked local tenderness is present. Patient is often unable to bear weight on the affected heel. The opposite side must always be examined.

Imaging

The most helpful x-ray for evaluation of the calcaneal fracture is the lateral view. Lateral view shows calcaneal integrity, *Bohler's angle* (normal 25°–40°; < 20° indicates fracture) and the *crucial angle of Gissane* (normal–135°).

An axial view is taken with the x-ray beam directed 40° cephalad to the vertical and centered on the subtalar joint (Fig. 29.2b). Axial view

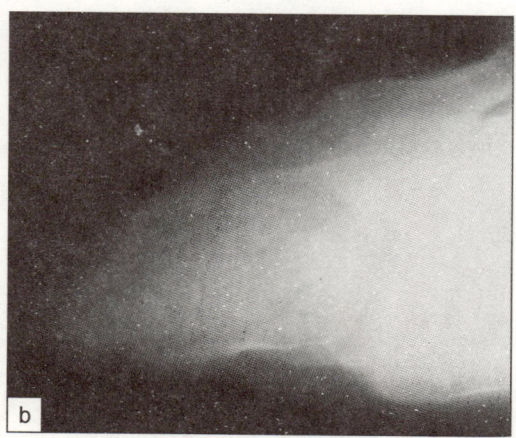

Fig. 29.2b.   Axial view of calcaneum

shows the sustentaculum tali, anterior and posterior talocalcaneal joints and the fracture lines.

Broden's oblique projection reveals the posterior facet of the subtalar joint and its involvement by the fracture (Fig. 29.3). CT scan is extremely valuable for assessing the severity of calcaneal fractures and involvement of the subtalar joint and also for planning surgery.

Treatment

Undisplaced or extra-articular fractures are treated conservatively in a below knee plaster cast with early aggressive range of motion exercises. Weight

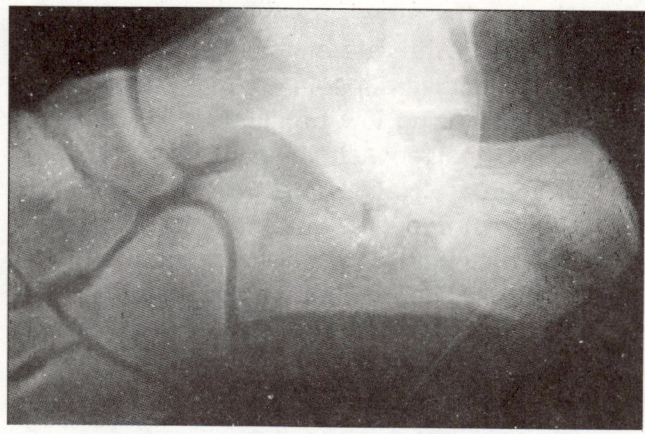

Fig. 29.3. Broden's view showing fracture of the calcaneum

bearing is avoided till the fracture heals (10–12 weeks). Conservative treatment is also recommended in elderly patients, patients with peripheral vascular insufficiency and the patients who are poor surgical risks.

Operative treatment is indicated for avulsion fractures of tendo achilles insertion (***to restore the function of tendo achilles***) and displaced intra-articular fractures of the calcaneus (to restore the height and congruency of the subtalar joint to decrease the risk of osteoarthritis) (Fig. 29.4a,b). Displaced

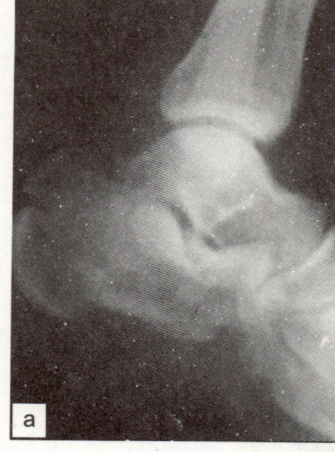

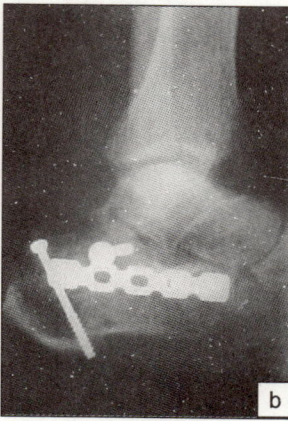

Fig. 29.4.   (a) Pre and (b) post operative X-rays showing fracture of calcaneum treated by ORIF. Note the fixation of tuberosity fragment and restoration of joint congruity

intraarticular fractures are treated by internal fixation through the lateral approach (sometimes medial or a combined medial and lateral approach may be used) using low profile implants such as 2.7 mm calcaneal reconstruction plates and screws. Limited internal fixation, or *Gissane spike* (or steinmann pin) reduction of major fragment are alternative methods of treatment for the calcaneus fractures. Non weight bearing is continued till fracture consolidates (10–12 weeks). Severely comminuted calcaneal fractures are treated by primary subtalar arthrodesis by many surgeons.

Complications Calcaneal fractures are associated with high incidence of complications. Malunion is the commonest complication. Persistent displacement of the main fragment leads to local heel pain, broadening of the heel and inability to wear normal shoes. In addition, impingement symptoms may arise from the lateral malleolus or the peroneal tendons. Reduced power of push off is seen consequent to reduced Bohler's angle (and efficiency of tendo achilles). Other complications include posttraumatic osteoarthritis of the subtalar joint, sural nerve injury, tarsal tunnel syndrome, persistent oedema around the heel and foot and skin problems.

Fractures of the Talus

Talus is a key bone in ankle, subtalar and talonavicular articulations. It is covered by the articular cartilage over most of its surfaces (60%). It does not give attachment to any muscles, hence its vascularity is limited. Blood supply to the talus is provided by blood vessels entering the dorsal neck, medial side of the body and the sinus tarsi area (Fig. 29.5a,b). Due to these unique anatomical factors, talus fractures present a great challenge with regard to management quite like the calcaneus fractures.

Mechanism of injury

Talus fractures are caused by high-energy inju-

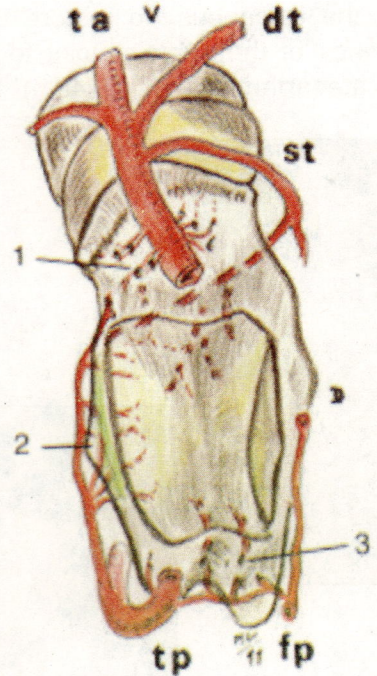

Fig. 29.5a. Superior aspect of the right talus-arterial supply
ta: anterior tibial artery
dt: lateral tarsal artery
st: artery of the sinus tarsi
tp: posterior tibial artery
fp: (posterior) peroneal artery
1- branch to neck of talus
2- medial osteoligamentous branches
3- posterior periosteal branches

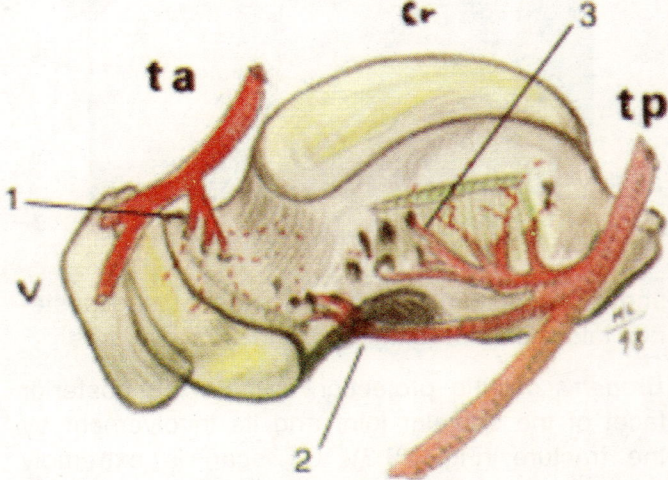

Fig. 29.5b. Medial aspect of right talus - arterial supply
t.a.: anterior tibial artery
t.p.: posterior tibial artery
1- branch to neck of talus
2- branch to roof of sinus tarsi
3- branches to deep fibres of medial ligament

ries (motor vehicular accidents) and fall from height. Forced dorsiflexion at the ankle as in car accidents and aircraft crash causes the talar neck fractures (*Aviator's astragalus*). Fractures of the posterior talar processes are caused by hyperplantarflexion.

Classification

Talar fractures are classified according to the location of the fracture viz. head, neck, body and process.

Fractures of the talar head are uncommon.

Fractures of the talar neck are the commonest and are classified into four types by *Hawkins and Canale* depending on the displacement of fracture. Type I are undisplaced fractures, type II are talar neck fractures with subtalar joint subluxation, type III are talar neck fractures with talar body dislocation (Fig. 29.6a) (subluxation of both the subtalar and tibiotalar joints), and rare type IV fractures include a talonavicular dislocation also.

Evaluation of a patient with talus fracture

Patient with talus fracture gives a history of high-energy vehicular injury or fall from height. Evaluation must be done for associated injuries and patient resuscitated if required. The foot is deformed, swollen and painful. Extruded body of talus may cause compression of the neurovascular structures and stretching of skin with impending sloughing of overlying skin. The incidence of injury to posterior tibial neurovascular bundle is not as high as may be expected in injuries with ankle joint subluxation. This is because the body of the talus subluxates posteromedially and is buttonholed between the posterior ankle capsule and the tendon of flexor hallucis longus which separates the talus from the neurovascular bundle, thus preventing injury. Diagnosis is made on x-rays.

Imaging

Anteroposterior and lateral radiographs of the ankle establish the diagnosis of talus fracture. *Canale view* (x-ray in maximum plantar flexion, 15° internal rotation and 15° cephalad tilt) helps in evaluating the talar neck alignment.

CT scan evaluates fracture morphology and intra-articular involvement.

Management

Talar neck fracture when undisplaced (Type I) can be treated with a below knee plaster cast for 8–12 weeks (Fig. 29.6b). Fracture is then assessed with x-ray for union and any evidence of avascular necrosis. Uncomplicated cases are initiated on gradual weight bearing and exercises for ankle, calf and the subtalar joint. Type II, III and IV are treated by ORIF using lag screws using anteromedial and/or anterolateral approaches. These patients should be treated as emergency to prevent necrosis

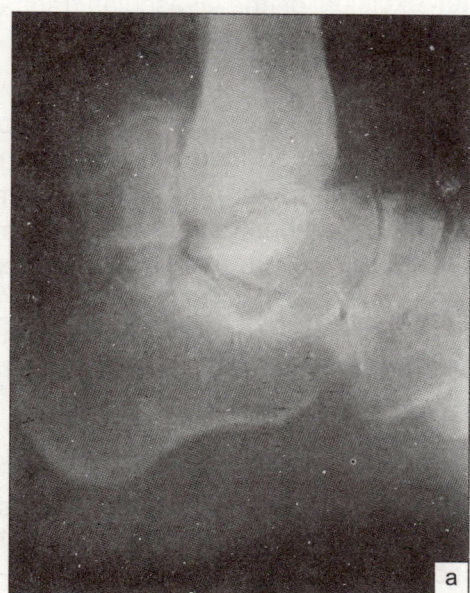

Fig. 29.6a. Type III Hawkin's talar neck fracture. Note the dislocation of talar body from the ankle joint

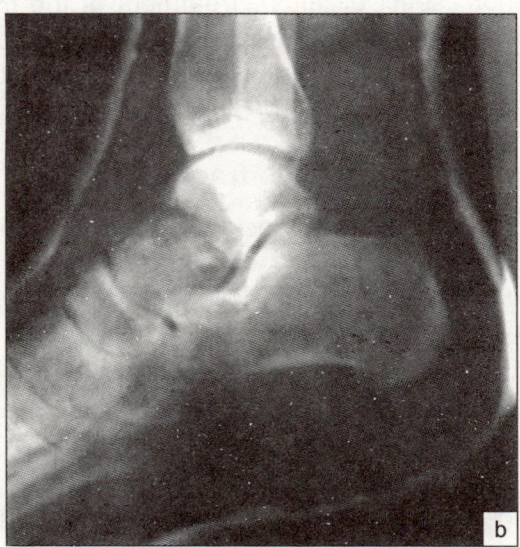

Fig. 29.6b. Minimally displaced talar neck fracture. Conservative treatment

of the overlying skin. If surgery is likely to be delayed, a closed reduction should be attempted with the help of calcaneal pin traction. The foot is plantar flexed and everted and position checked under x-ray. A satisfactory reduction is immobilized in below knee plaster cast. Even moderate degree of displacement (as less as 2 mm displacement) should not be accepted as it might lead to malunion in varus with alteration of subtalar joint contact characteristics. Patients are kept non-weight bearing for 12 weeks after surgery.

Fractures of the body of the talus are treated by open reduction and internal fixation of the fracture. These fractures have high incidence of avascular necrosis, delayed union, non-union and secondary osteoarthritis.

Fractures of talus head are treated with open reduction and internal fixation of the fragments. Patients are kept partial weight bearing for 6 weeks after fixation. Small fragments not suitable for fixation can be excised.

Fractures of the lateral talar process are common and frequently missed. Treatment is decided by the size of the fragment and displacement. Undisplaced fractures are treated in a below knee cast for 6 weeks. Small and extra articular fragments are excised while large fragments contributing to the posterior subtalar joint facet should be reduced and fixed with screws.

Fractures of the posterior process are often confused with os trigonum (sesamoid in relation to posterior aspect of talus). Treatment of the medial or the lateral tubercle fractures is by immobilization in a below knee cast for 6 weeks. Large displaced fragment needs ORIF with screw.

Complications of talus fractures

Complications of talar neck fractures include skin necrosis and circulatory embarrassment, avascular necrosis, delayed union, non-union and secondary osteoarthritis.

Avascular necrosis is common after talar neck and body fractures. Incidence of avascular necrosis varies according to the grade of talar neck fracture (type I–10%; type II–40%; type III–90% and type IV–100%). The diagnosis is evident on radiographs as increased density by 12 weeks post injury. Vascular talus shows radiolucent zone in the subchondral area of the talar dome (*Hawkin's sign*). Lack of appearance of this sign indicates avascular necrosis. MRI may be used to make early diagnosis of AVN of talus in conservatively treated patients but the limitation is the high incidence of false positive results. Established avascular necrosis should be treated by avoiding weight bearing for one year to avoid collapse and deformity of the avascular bone. Periodic (monthly) x-rays should be taken to check the progress of revascularisation. The basic principles of treatment of an avascular talus is to retain joint congruity by:

1. Relief of weight bearing stress, and

2. Maintain mobility of ankle and foot.

Conservative treatment includes complete non-weight bearing for a period ranging from 18–24 months (impractical option), and use of patellar tendon bearing cast to relieve weight.

Operative treatment is indicated in cases with established collapse of the talus leading to joint incongruity and severe pain. The options include

1. *Blair fusion*: excision of the avascular body and fusion of the tibia to head and neck of the talus

2. Complete talectomy with tibio-calcaneal fusion

3. Revascularisation procedures for the talus

Avascular necrosis in the presence of open fractures may lead to recalcitrant infection, which may heal only after excision of the avascular fragments.

Dislocation of the talus

Dislocations of the talus are the result of high-energy injuries. Forced inversion of plantar-flexed foot leads to the rupture of lateral ligament of ankle and talocalcaneal ligament. The talus remains in mortise while the talocalcaneal and talonavicular joints dislocate (Fig. 29.7a). Medial dislocations are more common (85%) than lateral (15%). Associated fractures are seen in half the cases.

Diagnosis is usually possible by x-rays.

Treatment is by closed reduction under anesthesia. For medial dislocation, the foot is plantarflexed, the traction is applied to the heel and the foot is everted. Position is checked under x-rays and below knee plaster cast is applied for 6 weeks.

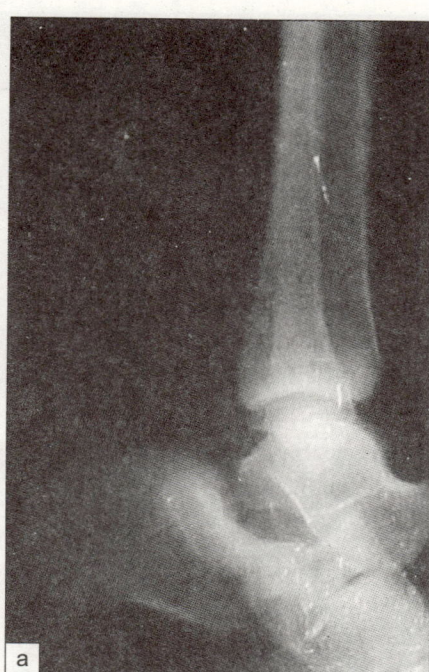

Fig. 29.7a. Dislocation of the talus. Note the dislocation of talocalcaneal and talonavicular joints; ankle mortise is normal

Irreducible dislocations are treated by open reduction. Talonavicular joint should be exposed first in the medial dislocation as irreducibility is due to buttonholing through the capsule or interposition of extensor digitorum brevis in the talonavicular joint. Irreducible lateral dislocation is due to interposition of the tibialis posterior tendon.

Complications

Complications of subtalar joint dislocation include necrosis of overlying skin, irreducibility and late subtalar osteoarthritis.

Total dislocation of talus

occurs with greater violence which leads to rupture of all the ligaments attached to talus. Talus dislocates out of the mortise and comes to lie in front of the ankle and laterally (in most cases; rarely, medially). This is an emergency since delay leads to sloughing of the skin stretched over the talus. Closed reduction is performed under anesthesia. A steinmann pin may be used through the calcaneus for traction if required. Irreducible dislocations warrant open reduction. Avascular necrosis occurs in 100% cases. About 50% of these injuries are open at the initial presentation.

Fractures of other tarsal bones

Fractures of navicular occur due to fall from height or road traffic accidents (Fig. 29.8a,b). They occur commonly in association with other injuries in the foot. Fractures of the navicular include the fractures of the tuberosity (avulsion of the tibialis posterior attachment), cortical avulsion fractures and body fractures. Avulsion fractures and other undisplaced fractures are treated in a below knee plaster cast for 6 weeks. Displaced fractures are treated with ORIF to restore anatomic joint surface using small fragment screws or kirschner wires.

Fractures of the cuboid can occur due to avulsion (adduction injury) or compression ("nut cracker" injury due to abduction injury). Undisplaced or minimally displaced fractures are treated in a non weight bearing cast for 6 weeks. Large displaced fragments are reduced and stabilized with

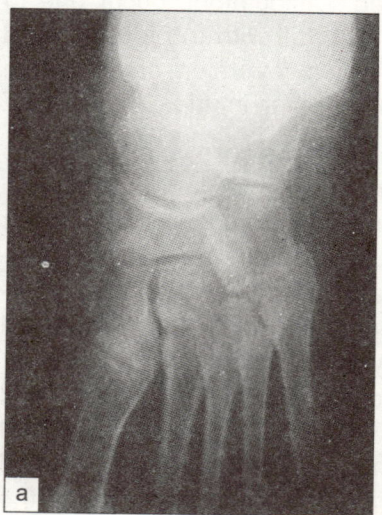

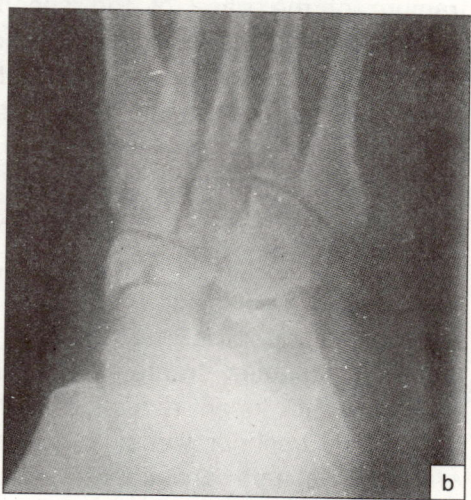

Fig. 29.8a,b. Fracture of the navicular

internal fixation and kept non weight bearing for 6 weeks.

Midtarsal dislocations

usually accompany subtalar dislocations. Both abduction and adduction types of dislocations may occur disrupting the articulation between talus and calcaneus posteriorly and navicular and cuboid anteriorly. Ligaments rupture and small avulsion fractures, most commonly of navicular, may be associated with dislocations. Treatment is by closed reduction under anesthesia. Unstable reductions are stabilized by percutaneous kirschner wires. Below knee plaster is applied for 6 weeks. Complications include stiffness of foot joints and secondary osteoarthritis.

Tarsometatarsal Dislocations (*Lisfranc Fracture Dislocations*)

Tarsometatarsal dislocations are uncommon and are often unrecognized. Dislocations occur due to fall on plantar flexed foot, fall with the foot trapped leading to forced inversion, eversion or abduction of the forefoot and in run-over injuries.

Tarsometatarsal dislocations are classified as homolateral (all metatarsals dislocated in one direction), isolated (medial dislocation of first or lateral dislocation of 2nd to fifth rays) and divergent (1st ray dislocated medially and rest laterally). Diagnosis is suggested by history and local swelling, pain, ecchymosis and inability to walk. The diagnosis is confirmed by AP, lateral and oblique views X-rays (Fig. 29.9a,b). Second metatarsal is the key to tarsometatarsal stability and lateral displacement of 2nd ray is not possible without the fracture of the base of the second metatarsal. Injuries may be subtle at times and need stress views. On oblique views medial border of the second metatarsal should align with medial border of middle cuneiform and medial border of the fourth metatarsal should align with medial border of cuboid. Alteration of this relationship suggests injury to Lisfranc joints.

Treatment of undisplaced fractures of the base of second metatarsal is in a below knee cast for 6 weeks. Displaced fractures and deformity are indications for open reduction and internal fixation using kirschner wires or lag screws. Postoperatively patients are kept in plaster for 8–10 weeks.

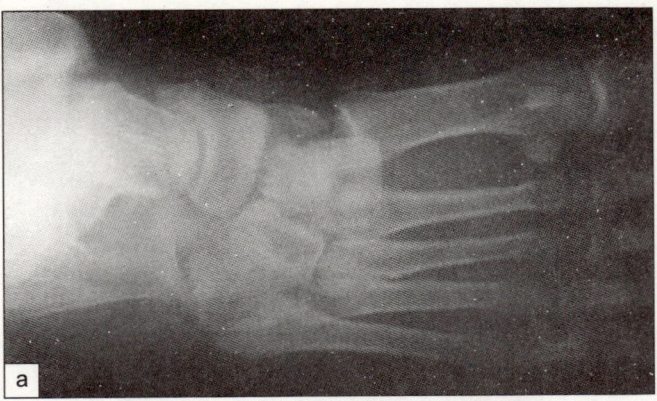

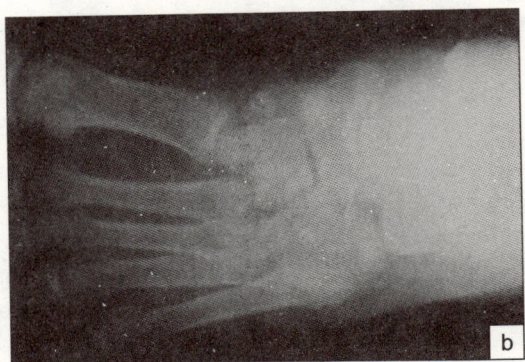

Fig. 29.9a,b. Radiographs of a patient with isolated lateral dislocation of 2nd-5th rays

Metatarsal fractures

Metatarsal fractures can occur as a result of direct (crush) or indirect (road traffic accidents) injuries or as stress fractures. Isolated metatarsal neck and shaft fractures usually are not malaligned and can be treated nonoperatively in a below knee plaster for 3 weeks. Displaced fractures or multiple metatarsal fractures (especially in polytrauma patients) should be treated by k-wire fixation either percutaneously or through limited dorsal incisions. Fractures with involvement of the joints are fixed rigidly using plates and screws. Post operatively, patients are kept non-weight bearing in plaster for 4–6 weeks.

"Jones Fracture" is a metadiaphyseal fracture at the base of 5th metatarsal, which is common in athletes during training (Fig. 29.10a). It does not occur due to inversion injury as commonly thought but may occur as stress fracture. Non union is common in these fractures. Treatment is below knee plaster cast for 8 weeks without weight bearing. Chronic non unions are treated by ORIF and bone grafting. Avulsion fracture of the base of the fifth metatarsal is the commonest fracture

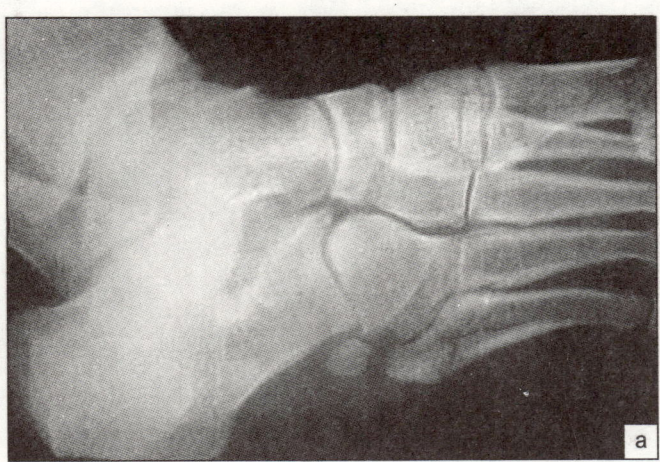

Fig. 29.10a. Avulsion fracture of the base of 5th metatarsal

of the lower limb. It is caused by sudden inversion strain leading to violent contraction of peroneus brevis and avulsion of its bony attachment. The fracture is mostly undisplaced and treated in a below knee walking cast for 3 weeks.

March fractures are fatigue fractures of the second metatarsal neck and shaft. X-rays are often normal and callus may be the first evidence of the fracture on X-rays (Fig. 29.10b). Below knee walking cast for 2–3 weeks and reducing the activity ameliorate the symptoms.

Dislocation of metatarsophalangeal joints

Dislocation of metatarsophalangeal joints is caused

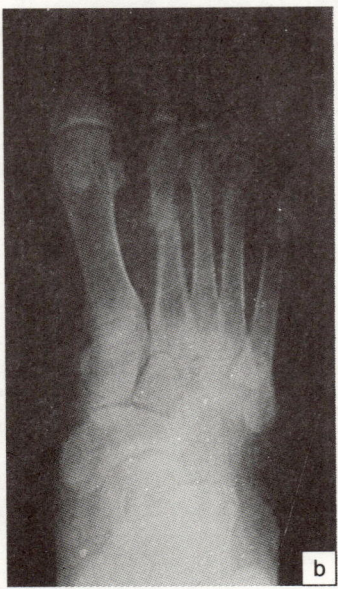

Fig. 29.10b. Stress fracture of the 2nd metatarsal shaft. Note the callus formation

by hyperextension injury (Fig. 29.11). One or more toes may be involved. Fracture of base of proximal phalanx may accompany dislocation. These injuries should be reduced by traction and the toes should be strapped together. Multiple dislocations are immobilized in a walking cast for 4 weeks. If the joints are unstable after reduction, kirschner wire fixation should be done.

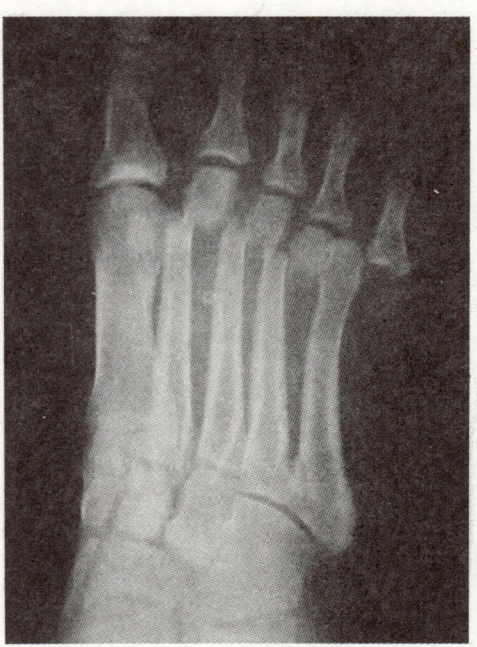

Fig. 29.11. Dislocation of 5th MTP joint. Note the multiple metatarsal neck fractures (2, 3, 4)

Phalangeal fractures of the foot

Fractures of the phalanges commonly occur due to crushing by fall of heavy objects. Distal phalanx of the hallux (big toe) is most commonly fractured and the injury is often compound. These fractures are treated with generous irrigation and debridement. Wound edges are loosely approximated. Nail should be retained as far as possible. Fractures of the tuft or even those running into DIP are ignored.

Proximal and middle phalangeal fractures can be treated by reduction and buddy splinting. Intraarticular fractures of the proximal phalanx are treated with ORIF. Displaced intra-articular fractures especially the fractures of the proximal phalanx may be treated with k-wires or low profile screws. Limited weight bearing is allowed after surgery in a protective shoe.

Miscellaneous

CHAPTER 30

Sports Injuries

- Rupture of the muscle belly
- Hematoma in a muscle belly
- Musculotendinous ruptures
- Injuries to muscle insertions
  - Tennis elbow
  - Golfer's elbow
  - Jumper's Knee
- Paratenonitis
- Tendon injuries
- Over use syndromes
  - Stress fractures
  - Chronic Compartment Syndrome
  - Shin Splints
  - Disruption of acromio-clavicular joint
- Sports injuries to the knee joint
  - Breast stroke knee

- Pellegrini-Stieda Disease
- Jogger's knee
- Iliotibial Band Friction syndrome
- Semimembranosus tendinitis
- Meniscal Tears
- Knee ligament injuries
  - Anterior cruciate ligament injury
  - Posterior cruciate ligament tear
  - Collateral Ligament Injuries
    - Medial Collateral Ligament (MCL)
    - Lateral Collateral Ligament (LCL injury)
  - Posterolateral Corner Injuries
  - Multiple Ligament Injury
- Anterior knee pain
- Miscellaneous conditions seen in sports persons

Sports medicine is a type of occupational health medicine, which deals with problems of the fittest persons in the society. It also identifies lesions, which are more likely to occur in sporting activities rather than everyday life. Some of the conditions commonly seen in athletes but not unique to them are described below.

Rupture of the muscle belly

Rupture of the muscle is seen most commonly in rectus femoris and hamstring. Patient feels sudden severe pain. A defect is sometimes palpable in the muscle. Muscle belly becomes prominent as the muscle contracts. Swelling and tenderness occur at the site of rupture immediately. Bruising may occur about 24 hours later.

Treatment is expectant with application of ice, elevation, analgesics and mobilization within the limits of comfort. Active contraction of muscle should be avoided for 6 weeks to avoid rerupture. Functional deficit is negligible though the defect in the muscle remains.

Hematoma in a muscle belly

Hematoma in a muscle belly usually occurs following a direct trauma or sometimes due to tear of central fibers. Quadriceps muscle is most commonly affected. Hematoma in the muscle is also called "Charley Horse". Hematoma gets organized and sometimes even ossified and restricts muscle movements. Ossification is more common if the muscle is mobilized too rapidly after injury.

Treatment is expectant. Ossified hematoma usually resolves within 2 years of injury. If it persists and interferes with function, it can be excised.

469

Musculotendinous rupture

Most commonly occurs in the medial belly of gastrocnemius ("Tennis leg"). It often occurs while playing tennis or squash. Common age group affected is 30–50 years. Presentation is similar to the muscle rupture and localized tenderness and defect can be palpated in the muscle belly.

Treatment is same as for muscle tear. Ultrasonic therapy can be given to reduce swelling. Complete recovery always occurs in about 8 weeks.

Injuries to muscle insertions

Tennis elbow is the commonest lesion of insertion of muscle or tendon into bone. Degeneration or a tear occurs in the insertion of the common extensor origin (esp. extensor carpi radialis brevis) on the lateral epicondyle. Injury occurs due to sharp flexion of the wrist while the extensors are contracted as while executing a back hand stroke in tennis.

Golfer's elbow is similar to tennis elbow in which common flexor attachment (esp. pronator teres-flexor carpi radialis interface) on the medial epicondyle of the humerus is torn. Symptoms are typically aggravated, when the golfer hits the ground instead of the ball.

Jumper's Knee (Patellar tendinitis) occurs at the insertion of patellar ligament onto the lower pole of patella. The condition is seen commonly in the basket ball and volley ball players. The patient cannot jump vigorously.

The treatment for these conditions is conservative initially with rest, ultrasonics and NSAIDS. Resistant cases can be treated with local hydrocortisone injections. The injections can be repeated after 4–6 weeks. If three injections do not relieve the symptoms, the area of tendon insertion is explored and tissues are drilled or scarified and necrotic areas are excised.

Paratenonitis

The paratenon of the tendon may become inflamed by repeated friction. Condition commonly affects achilles tendon and extensor tendons of the wrist. Paratenonitis at the heel is made worse by running on hard surfaces and wearing shoes with a worn heel. Proper footwear or a soft heel pad may resolve the problem. Injection of steroid in the paratenon and not tendon (caution steroid injection into the tendon can lead to rupture of the tendon) can relieve symptoms. In resistant cases paratenon must be explored and its adhesions with the tendon divided.

Tendon injuries

1. Peroneal tendon injuries can occur following violent dorsiflexion of the inverted foot. Diagnosis is confirmed by eliciting instability of the tendons with eversion and dorsiflexion of the foot. Acute injuries are treated with repair of fibro-osseous tunnel while chronic injuries need deepening of the peroneal groove or bone block operations.

2. Tibialis posterior tendon injury can occur in athletes. Rupture can be partial or complete. Partial ruptures are treated by debridement while the chronic ruptures are treated by flexor digitorum longus transfer.

3. Achilles tendon injuries: Tendinitis of the achilles tendon occurs due to over use and may lead to partial rupture. Complete rupture occurs due to forceful contraction of the tendo achilles with the foot fixed to ground. A gap may be felt in the tendo achilles. Thompson test is positive. (The patient is in prone position lying over the edge of the bed, normally compression of the calf leads to plantar flexion which is absent in cases of tendo achilles rupture). Both conservative and surgical treatments are possible but the incidence of re-rupture is lesser with the primary repair.

Over use syndromes

Stress fractures

Stress fractures arise due to repeated, unaccustomed, physical activity. Overuse is followed by insidious onset of pain. Common sites are tibial shaft, femoral neck, metatarsal shaft ("March fracture"), tarsal navicular and base of metatarsal (Jones fracture). Spondylolisthesis, due to stress fracture of the pars interarticularis occurs in athletes who hyperextend their spine such as fast bowlers in cricket and in javelin throwers. Condition is sometimes bilateral. Initial x-rays are normal and bone scan is diagnostic at this stage. Later on radiographs may show cortical thickening, fracture line or callus formation. Treatment includes protected weight bearing, rest, low impact exercise for conditioning and analgesics.

Following stress fractures need special care

Femoral neck stress fractures are also called insufficiency fractures. These can be tension or transverse type or compression type. Tension type stress fractures often displace and are more serious. They should be operated and internally fixed early.

Compression fractures do not displace and can be treated expectantly.

Tibial shaft stress fractures can sometimes be resistant to conservative treatment especially when associated with anterior bowing of shaft. If the stress fracture is visible for more than 6 months and bone scan is positive, bone grafting should be undertaken.

Fifth metatarsal base stress fracture at the junction of metaphysis and diaphysis (Jones fracture) in athletes should be treated aggressively. Early internal fixation (and bone grafting if required) should be done.

Chronic compartment syndrome Chronic or exertional compartment syndrome may be seen in runners and cyclists. The anterior and deep posterior compartments of leg are most commonly affected. Exercise results in increased pressure within enclosed fascial compartment leading to reduced local blood flow. Patients complain of gradual onset pain during exercise. Numbness and paraesthesiae may occur. Diagnosis is confirmed by documenting elevation of compartmental pressure by more than 15 cm of water above resting level fifteen minutes after exercise. The compartmental pressures also take much longer to return to resting levels (≤ 15 minutes) in exertional compartment syndrome as compared to normal state where they take only 3 to 4 minutes.

Treatment is mainly surgical, as most cases are refractory to conservative treatment. Fasciotomy of the affected compartments is done.

"Shin Splints"

Shin splints or tibial periostitis is characterized by pain and tenderness in the distal third of tibia posteromedially. Pain and tenderness are diffuse and are not localized as in stress fractures. Plain radiographs are normal. The bone scan may show linear streaking. Treatment is expectant and most cases resolve. Rarely fasciotomy and periosteal cauterization is required.

Disruption of acromio-clavicular joints can occur in javelin throwers (due to violent forward movement of the shoulder) and archers. Javelin throwers in addition can also suffer from spondylolysis and rupture of the rectus abdominis.

Sports injuries to the knee joint

Knee joint is especially prone to the athletic injuries. Knee ligament injuries and meniscal injuries are most commonly sustained injuries by the sports persons.

Breast stroke knee Pain and tenderness over distal insertion of medial ligament due to forceful adduction of legs against resistance of the water during breast stroke. Modifying training is the only treatment available.

Pellegrini-Stieda Disease

Calcification over the femoral attachment of the medial collateral ligament following injury and partial avulsion (as in valgus strain). Pain and tenderness are present locally. Rest, NSAIDs and ultrasonic therapy provide relief.

Jogger's knee is pain in the knee and patello femoral joint in joggers in 30–40 years age group due to loss of articular resilience. Treatment involves running on soft ground, proper footwear and analgesics.

Persistent symptoms warrant stopping the running.

Iliotibial Band Friction syndrome occurs commonly in runners and cyclists. The condition arises from the friction between the lateral femoral condyle and iliotibial band. Localized tenderness in the region of lateral epicondyle of femur is common. Treatment is rest and NSAIDs. Resistant cases warrant excision of a portion of iliotibial band.

Semimembranosus tendinitis occurs in male athletes. Tenderness is present over the semimembranosus tendon. Condition responds to stretching and strengthening.

Meniscal Tears

Meniscal tears are more common in medial meniscus. It is because the lateral meniscus is more circular, narrower and moves with movements of the knee due to its attachment to the popliteus while medial meniscus is less mobile due to its fixity to the deep portion of the medial collateral ligament. Up to 30% peripheral portion of the meniscus is vascular (red zone) and is amenable to repair. Rest of the meniscus is avascular and does not heal. Meniscal tears are defined according to their position (anterior 1/3rd, middle third or posterior third), the appearance (Parrot beak, flap, bucket handle), and orientation (longitudinal, horizontal, radial).

Traumatic tears of the meniscus in sports persons occur due to twisting injury in semi flexed and weight bearing knee and present with mechanical symptoms such as "catching" and locking.

On examination, joint line tenderness and pain with circumduction maneuvers (as in special tests such as McMurray's test, Apley's grinding test and Steinmann's test) can be elicited. MRI has revolutionized the imaging for meniscal tears and arthroscopy has revolutionized their treatment. Aim of treatment is to preserve as much meniscus as normal while removing unrepairable portions which are giving rise to symptoms. Meniscal tears that do not need treatment include partial thickness tears, tears less than 5 mm size and tears that cannot be displaced.

Partial menisectomy should be done for tears in avascular zone.

Tears in the vascular zone should be repaired. Meniscal transplantation (allografts) is still experimental technique under investigation.

Knee ligament injuries

Anterior cruciate ligament injury

Anterior cruciate ligament injuries are most often the result of non contact pivoting injuries. Sudden deceleration and change of direction are important clues in history of these patients. Football and skiing are the sports commonly associated with ACL injuries. O'Donohgue's triad seen in American footballers is a combination of ACL tear, medial meniscus tear and medial collateral ligament tear. These patients with ACL tear often report an audible 'POP' at the time of injury which is associated with immediate swelling due to hemarthrosis. The injury to the ACL can be a mid substance tear (80%) or avulsion from the femoral (18%) or tibial

(2%) attachments. Lachman's test is the most sensitive test for diagnosis in the acute stage. It is performed in 20-degree flexion at knee and a posterior to anterior force is applied to the tibia. Abnormal anterior translation of tibia suggests ACL tear. Pivot shift test performed under anesthesia is also a sensitive test. Anterior Drawer's test may be negative in acute stage due to pain and spasm. Plain x-ray may reveal the presence of associated avulsion fractures. MRI is a sensitive imaging modality to diagnose the ACL tears. Arthroscopy is the most accurate method of diagnosing partial or complete tears of ACL.

Treatment options for ACL tear include quadriceps exercises and functional bracing. However a higher incidence of complex meniscal tears and chondral injury has been reported over time in ACL deficient knees.

Operative treatment of ACL tear consists of arthroscopy assisted ACL reconstruction using autologous patellar tendon or hamstring tendon graft. Allografts or synthetic ACL substitutes (such as Gore-Tex) have also been used with variable success.

Incomplete ACL tears are treated according to the findings of clinical examination and functional stability. Immobilization in POP cast for 6 weeks is sufficient if they are chosen to be treated conservatively.

Avulsion fractures are treated with early surgery to internally fix the avulsed bony fragment.

Posterior cruciate ligament tear

Posterior cruciate ligament (PCL) is the primary restraint to posterior tibial translation. It also restrains external tibial rotation. The most common mechanisms leading to tear of PCL are: blow to the anterior tibia with the knee flexed as in dashboard injury, by hyperflexion of the knee with a plantar flexed foot without a blow, and hyper extension injury. Posterior Drawer's test, performed in 90° knee flexion is the most sensitive examination. Other sign of PCL tear is a posterior sag or gravity test (when the knee is viewed from the lateral side the tibia appears to sag posteriorly on the femur). Radiographs of the knee may sometimes reveal bony avulsion of the PCL insertion on tibia. MRI can diagnose PCL tear accurately.

Arthroscopy can reliably diagnose PCL tear and other associated injuries.

Treatment for PCL tears is mainly conservative. Majority of patients with isolated PCL tear does well with quadriceps rehabilitation. However, chronic PCL deficiency can lead to degenerative changes in the patello femoral and medial compartments. Indications for surgery include bony avulsion fractures where ligament is intact and good results can be achieved by primary repair. Other indications are associated injury to posterolateral corner, collateral ligaments or ACL.

Most often performed reconstruction for PCL tear is arthroscopic reconstruction of PCL using central third of patellar tendon (bone-tendon-bone).

3. Collateral ligament injuries

a) *Medial collateral Ligament (MCL) injury* is more common. Injury to medial collateral ligament occurs due to valgus (abduction) injury. Injuries at the femoral attachment of the ligament are most common. The diagnosis is based on history of abduction strain to the knee, localized pain and tenderness over the site of MCL. Valgus stress opening of the medial side of the knee joint tested at 30 degrees of flexion is diagnostic. The laxity of the joint is graded depending on the opening of the medial joint in millimeters. Opening of the medial joint between 1mm to 5 mm is grade 1, 6 mm to 10 mm opening is grade 2, 11 mm to 15 mm is grade 3 while more than 16 mm opening is grade 4. Laxity of the medial collateral ligament in full extension suggests injury to cruciates in addition to MCL. Plain x-rays reveal any associated fractures while arthroscopy/ MRI can diagnose associated injury to intra-articular structures.

Treatment of isolated MCL injuries is mainly non operative.

These injuries are immobilized in a POP or, better still, a hinged knee brace for 6 weeks. Quadriceps exercises are encouraged during this period. Chronic injuries, which do not respond to conservative treatment, can be treated by advancement and reinforcement of the ligament. If MCL injury is associated with intra-articular injury, only intra-articular injury is stabilized.

b) *Lateral collateral ligament (LCL) injury* Iso-lated injury to LCL is rare and is usually associated with cruciate ligament injury. The injury is caused by a varus (or adduction) stress. Injuries to lateral popliteal nerve are commonly associated due to the varus force causing LCL tear. The diagnostic clinical sign is lateral joint opening on varus stress applied in 30 degrees of flexion. The severity of injury is graded according to the grading of joint opening on stress in mm. Tests for cruciate injury should be performed. Lateral popliteal nerve should be carefully examined. Isolated lateral collateral ligament injuries are treated in a hinged brace for 6 weeks. Surgical repair of LCL complex is recommended if associated with injuries to other capsuloligamentous structures.

c) *Posterolateral Corner Injuries* Posterolateral corner includes the structures in the posterolateral corner namely LCL, arcuate ligament, popliteus tendon, lateral head of gastrocnemius, popliteofibular ligament, short lateral ligament, fabellofibular ligament and posterolateral capsule. Injuries to the posterolateral corner alone are rare injuries. These injuries are usually associated with other ligamentous injuries, especially PCL. These injuries are frequently missed.

Injuries are caused by excessive external rotation force. Examination reveals exaggerated external rotation as compared to opposite side. Other less reliable tests include external rotation recurvatum test, posterolateral drawer test and reverse pivot shift test.

Treatment of posterolateral corner injuries is early repair, which offers most consistent results. However these injuries often present late due to missed diagnosis. Reconstructive procedures recommended for chronic injuries include posterolateral corner advancement, biceps tenodesis or "split grafts" to reconstruct both the LCL and the popliteus/posterolateral corner.

d) *Multiple ligament injuries* represent severe injuries with severe soft tissue and often articular surface injury. These injuries are often associated with knee dislocation. A careful neurovascular examination must be performed in these cases. A high incidence (40%) of intraluminal tear or arterial thrombus has been reported which can compromise circulation immediately or even days after injury. An arteriogram should be performed in all cases where joint dislocation has been documented or both cruciates and a collateral ligament have been injured. Radiographs confirm the presence of dislocation and its direction. Treatment includes reduction of the dislocation and delayed reconstruction (or repair of bony avulsion) of the torn ligaments at 5–7 days after injury. Indications for emergency surgery include popliteal artery injury, open dislocations and irreducible dislocations. Risk of joint stiffness is quite high in these cases. Post operative rehabilitation is difficult and prolonged and needs a lot of devotion on the part of the patient.

Anterior knee pain

Anterior knee pain is diffuse, aching knee pain which is aggravated by running, climbing up or down the stairs, kneeling, squatting, yoga or other activities involving flexion of the knee. The etiology can be patellofemoral disease due to trauma (fracture or dislocation), malalignment syndrome, patella alta, weak vastus medialis, tight vastus lateralis or tight retinaculum. Other causes can be disorders of extensor expansion insertion, anterior fat pad disease (Hoffa's syndrome), chondromalacia, patellofemoral dysplasia or patellar instability. The treatment depends on specific diagnosis.

Miscellaneous conditions seen in sports persons

- Fast bowlers can get tear in the abdominal muscles.
- Footballers get degenerative changes in the pubic symphysis.
- Joggers can get *jogger's foot* where medial plantar nerve gets entrapped at the point where FHL & FDL cross due to external compression by orthotics.
- *Skier's hip* is proximal femoral fracture sustained by cross-country skiers.
- Distal clavicle osteolysis occurs in weight lifters.
- *"Burners"* or *"Stingers"* are brachial plexus injuries usually caused by minor traction or compression sustained by football players.
- *Little leaguer's shoulder* is a type I Salter-Harris epiphyseal injury of the proximal humerus.
- *Little Leaguer's elbow* is stress fracture of the medial epicondyle in adolescents sustained due to repetitive valgus force in throwing.
- *Jersey finger* is avulsion injury of Flexor digitorum profundus tendon.

Plaster and Traction

Plaster

The use of plaster of Paris (POP) as an external splint dates back to the 19th century. Plaster of Paris is a hemihydrate of calcium sulfate ($CaSO_4.1/2\ H_2O$) with unique characteristics. It is now available as commercial preparations like Gypsona. Plaster of Paris bandages are fabricated by impregnation of the ($CaSO_4.1/2\ H_2O$) powder into wide mesh starched cotton bandages. Recently other materials made of fiberglass have been introduced and have different setting characteristics and strength.

Indications The uses of plaster of Paris in orthopaedic practice are multiple. These include :

1. **Immobilization of fractures** POP is most commonly employed for the purpose of immobilization of fractures. Casts made of plaster of Paris are widely used for achieving and maintaining reduction, immobilization and definitive conservative management of several fractures (e.g. Colles' fracture, most fractures of shaft of humerus, fractures of the both bones of leg and fractures of the hand and foot).

2. **Deformity correction** can be achieved either by the application of serial corrective plasters after manipulation or by use of wedging casts. Serial casting technique has been employed for the correction of congenital talipes equino varus deformity very successfully. Also, the use of serial casts pre-operatively can help in stretching the skin and makes the soft tissue supple, thus helping at the time of surgical intervention. Serial casting can also be used in the correction of other congenital anomalies like congenital dislocation of knee where serial casts in increasing degrees of knee flexion are employed. Previously scoliotic curves were treated in localizer casts (Risser) prior to surgery.

Wedging of plasters is usually done to correct minor degrees of angulation at fracture site. The technique is most often used in correction of residual angulatory deformity after manipulation of fractures of both bones of the leg. It can be open wedge or closed wedge. Open wedging of the plasters is generally preferred. The method involves cutting the plaster cast on the concave side covering two thirds of the circumference, and opening of the linear cut, which provides deformity correction. The gap is held open by the use of cork or wood and reapplication of plaster bandage is done to repair the gap. The advantage of this method is that deformity at the fracture site can be corrected without changing the plaster cast. Care should be taken to avoid the formation of plaster sore (wedging should be done only after the plaster is dry). The following facts must be kept in mind while using wedging of plaster casts for correcting malalignment of fracture fragments:

a) The level of wedging must be carefully and accurately determined.

b) Wedging should be done preferably after 2 weeks (during the third week) when the fracture fragments have become "sticky" and will not redisplace.

c) Wedging is useful only for single bone fractures (such as humerus) or fracture of both bones of the leg where alignment of the second bone (fibula in this case) is not important. Wedging is **not** useful for correcting malalignment of fractures of both bones of the forearm and should not be used in these cases.

d) Wedging corrects only angulatory deformity. It does **not** correct the rotational malalignment.

e) Wedging of plaster can also be used in the treatment of deformities like flexion deformity of the knee, equinus at the ankle etc.

3. **Prevention of Deformity** Plaster splints can be used to prevent the occurrence of fixed deformities in conditions such as tuberculosis, rheumatoid arthritis and other inflammatory conditions. This is achieved by use of removable splints which hold the limb in desired functional position till the infection or inflammation subsides. These splints being removable can be removed to exercise the limb, thus they prevent muscle wasting and stiffness.

4. **Immobilization of soft tissue injuries and dislocations** Splints or casts made of plaster of Paris can be used in the immobilization of soft tissue injuries and joint dislocations to allow for soft tissue healing and minimizing the movement and pain in the initial period.

5. **Fabrication of prostheses** A positive cast of the limb has to be made for fabrication of approximate sized prostheses. This consists of use of plaster of Paris to make a mold of the limb. Into this the desired material is poured to create the negative cast. This procedure is time consuming and needs considerable expertise.

6. **Postoperative immobilization**

Methods of Plaster application

Three techniques of plaster application have been described :

1. *Skin-tight cast* was advocated by Bohler where the plaster is directly applied to the skin without use of any padding

2. *Bologna cast* was advocated by Sir John Charnley. Unlike Bohler's method, generous amounts of cotton padding are applied to the limb and compressed by the plaster bandage with "appropriate amount of tension". The application of plaster bandages with tension is demanding and thus followed the "contemporary" method of plaster application often referred to as "the third way".

3. *Third way* In this method the plaster is applied without tension over a single layer of cotton wadding which is applied over a stockinette.

Several precautions have to be taken while applying a plaster of paris cast. It must be emphasized that faulty plaster application may result in disastrous consequences.

• Plaster should be applied over a layer of cotton wool. Well-padded casts are less prone to cause circulatory impairment.

• The plaster should be applied in a single direction preferably distal to proximal. The encircling turns of plaster bandages must not be pulled tightly and should be applied so that the subsequent turn overlaps the preceding turn by one-half. The plaster should not be encircled more than once at a given time at the same place except near the plaster ends and near joints to enable uniform application. Care should be taken to avoid ridges and irregularities to minimise the chances of a plaster sore. Appropriate bridges should be used near joints to prevent vascular compromise.

Note The rolled plaster bandages should be thoroughly immersed in water until air bubbles stop rising. At this point the bandage is held with one end in each hand and gently squeezed. The first 2 to 3 inches of the bandages should be unwrapped before wetting to avoid struggle to look for the end of bandage after wetting.

Ideally 8-inch bandages are used for the thigh, 6-

inch bandage for the leg and 4-inch bandage is for the forearm and hand.

One must remember that

A good looking plaster may not always be well applied.

A bad looking plaster "can never be well applied".

- Acute injuries are best managed by plaster slabs. The use of plaster casts should generally be avoided in the acute setting. A complete cast should never be used in the presence of swelling or circulatory impairment.

- The patient should be advised to keep the limb elevated for 24-48 hours after plaster application. A careful vigil is maintained for the development of any swelling, increased pain, loss of pulse, cyanosis, numbness or anesthesia. These clinical features suggest circulatory compromise and should be carefully explained to the patient. In the presence of any such features the plaster is immediately slit open or bivalved and all the cotton removed till the skin. If the patient is sent home after plaster application all precautions should be explained and the patient is advised to report immediately to the hospital in the presence of any of the above features.

Persistent pain should never be ignored. It always suggests some problem and one must not hesitate to slit or bivalve the plaster.

- Presence of burning, itching or pain in a localized area associated with discharge and/or foul smell under the plaster should raise the suspicion of a plaster sore.

  In these cases a window is made to inspect the underlying skin.

Thickness of the casts The POP cast could be about ¼ inch thick. Upper extremity casts require less plaster as compared to the lower extremity casts.

Funtional cast bracing was devised by Sarmiento. Functional cast bracing consists of the use of cast braces to immobilize the fracture, at the same time allowing movement of the nearby joint. This method accepts some amount of mal-reduction of the fracture site. It consists of

- Use of a tightly fitting cast to immobilize the fracture.

- Early encouragement of movement and function of the extremity.

The advantages of this method are that muscles acting in a closed compartment generate hydraulic pressure which is predominantly directed inwards towards the fracture site, thus immobilizing the fracture. Some movement is allowed at the fracture site which promotes osteogenesis. Movement of the limb leads to improved vascularity. Muscle wasting and joint stiffness is prevented.

The classic example for functional cast bracing is the patellar tendon bearing cast of Sarmiento, which is very useful in the treatment of the fractures of the tibia.

Although cast-bracing has a useful place in the conservative management of fractures, some caution has to be used while using this method in acute setting. It is best used in conjunction with the other methods of treatment. A functional cast is best applied once the fracture is sticky (3–6 weeks). This would prevent displacement of the fracture.

Complications of Plaster Casts

Improper application of plaster casts can lead to several complications.

These include:

1. **Plaster sore** Pressure sores may develop from localized increase in pressure. The causes include too tight cast, formation of ridges or irregularities on the under surface of the cast, wedging of a wet plaster, inadequate padding of bony prominences, broken plaster, and foreign bodies introduced by the patient between the plaster and the limb.

2. **Skin blisters** Plaster blisters usually occur within 24 hours of injury and signify increased severity of trauma. They are caused by the post traumatic edema of the cuticle. The exudate is usually hemorrhagic. The plaster blister when present should be punctured and painted with antiseptic/antibiotic preparation.

3. **Purulent dermatitis** results from application of skin tight cast usually in atopic individuals, or in those who have developed a plaster sore, the secretions from which lead to allergic skin reaction. Extensive windowing or even removal of cast may be required for the care of the skin.

4. **Reactionary edema** is usually seen in the initial 48 hours following plaster application and it is best prevented by advising limb elevation and active movements of the digits.

5. **Nerve palsy** can occur due to pressure rise that is caused by swelling of the limb following plaster application.

   The common peroneal nerve is particularly vulnerable to pressure (near neck of fibula) by an improperly padded above knee cast. It is imperative that the motor and sensory functions in the distal part of the extremity are assessed from time to time.

6. **Circulatory embarrassment** Both arterial and venous occlusion may occur due to increasing swelling, especially with vascular injury or a tightly applied cast. This is especially true of supracondylar fractures of humerus in children, which are widely displaced (with/without vascular injury). The resultant ischemia may lead to gangrene of part or whole of the distal extremity. Vascular status should be evaluated from time to time. Presence of diminished capillary return, absence of pulse, cold limb, edema and paralysis of muscles all indicate vascular compromise and should be attended to promptly. "At the first sign of circulatory compromise the plaster and every layer of cotton beneath it, must be cut till the skin is exposed widely in the gap".

7. Loss of fracture reduction may occur. Charnley has classified fractures into 3 types based on their stability with plaster management. Type 1 fractures are transverse and inherently stable with closed management in plaster. Type 2 fractures are potentially stable against shortening (oblique fractures with <45° angulation to the long axis of bone). Type 3 fractures have no stability against shortening (>45° oblique, spiral and comminuted fractures). Type 2 and 3 fractures are prone to displacement and loss of reduction may occur following treatment with plaster immobilization alone.

8. Muscle wasting, weakness and stiffness of joints may occur following prolonged immobilization. This along with disuse osteoporosis and swelling in the distal extremity is referred to as "*Fracture disease*"

9. Miscellaneous complications resulting from prolonged plaster immobilization include, disuse osteoporosis, hypostatic pneumonia (more so in the elderly), renal calculus formation, deep vein thrombosis etc.

   Patients treated in spinal jackets may develop pernicious vomiting caused by obstruction of the third part of duodenum due to constriction of the superior mesenteric vessel the so-called *Cast Syndrome*. Cast syndrome can occur acutely or in a sub acute form called Wilkie's syndrome. The other causes of cast syndrome include hip spica application, spinal instrumentation, correction of spinal deformity, burns, visceroptosis etc. Treatment is conservative with elimination of oral intake, decompression of upper G.I. tract by Ryle's tube aspiration and monitoring of serum electrolyte levels. Severe cases not responding to treatment warrant removal of plaster cast or even the spinal (internal) fixation. Laparotomy to divide ligament of tietz or to perform gastro jejunostomy may be required in extreme cases.

Removal of plaster can be accomplished either by plaster cutting shear or an electric saw. Plaster removal should be done with care to avoid damage to the underlying skin. The use of elastic supportive bandage like elastocrepe is recommended following removal of the plaster in order to prevent the development of persistent and recurrent edema.

Fiber Glass Casts have been introduced and are especially useful for immobilizing soft tissue injuries. These casts are made up of a variety of materials like cotton, rayon or fiberglass impregnated with poly urethane-prepolymers. The prepolymer is methylene biphenyl disocyanate (MDI). These casts have very short setting time (2–4 hours as compared to 24–48 hours for plaster of Paris cast), are stronger, very light and cosmetically more acceptable. They are also more radiolucent than POP casts. The method of application differs from that of conventional casts. The plaster is not generally immersed in water, handling is slightly more difficult than the plaster of paris. Generous "tucks" cannot be made, stockinette should always be used and gloves should be used for the application of these casts.

Splints and Traction

Splints and traction are the alternative methods to plaster for the conservative management of fractures. The use of splints for the immobilization of fractures dates back to ancient times.

Traction is another important treatment modality in orthopedic practice.

The main *indications* for use of traction are:

1. *To achieve reduction* of fractures and dislocations eg. Fracture/dislocations of cervical spine, dislocation of hip etc.

2. *To maintain fracture reduction* Some fractures are so unstable that maintenance of reduction in a plaster cast may not be possible. Sometimes the use of plaster of Paris may not be feasible eg. in cases of fractures with burns, compound fractures, fractures with severe soft tissue injury and/or swelling. In these cases traction is necessary to maintain fracture reduction.

3. *Prevention and correction of deformities* Traction is useful in the prevention and correction of joint deformities e.g. correction of flexion contracture of hip and knee, treatment of scoliosis etc.

   Agnes-Hunt Traction is a unique method for correction of flexion deformity of hip.

4. *To keep inflammed joint surfaces apart* as in the treatment of septic arthritis/tuberculosis of hip and knee, in order to relieve "night cries" and prevent development of deformity and/or pathologic dislocation.

5. *Relief of pain* In chronic conditions like cervical/lumbar spondylosis, prolapsed lumbar/ cervical intervertebral disc pain relief and immobilization can be achieved by the use of intermittent traction.

Methods of Traction

Traction and Counter Traction

For any traction to be maximally effective there should be a force directed in the opposite direction which is known as counter traction. Counter traction can be from a fixed point on the patient's body (fixed traction) or can be provided by the body weight (by modifying the position of patient's bed), acting in the opposite direction (sliding traction).

Fixed Traction is most commonly employed with the help of a Thomas splint eg. Fixed traction on a Thomas splint for the treatment of a fracture of shaft of the femur. In this the resistance of ring of the Thomas splint against the pelvis prevents the splint from moving down, while adhesive tapes are used to pull the limb downwards.

The drawback of fixed traction is that it cannot be used to achieve fracture reduction. It can only be used for maintenance of reduction and, for splinting the limb during transfer of the patient from one place to another.

Sliding or Balanced Traction In this method the traction is provided by a weight hung over a pulley at the end of the extremity, which pulls on the limb by means of an adhesive traction or steinmann pin. The counter traction is provided by the body weight sliding away from the splint. This method can be used to achieve as well as to maintain reduction of fracture eg. in the treatment of fracture of femur the traction can be applied with a Thomas splint and counter traction by the body weight (by elevating the foot end of the bed).

Methods of application of Continuous Traction

Continuous traction may be required for the treatment of unstable fractures, fractures, which are subjected to large muscular forces e.g. fractures of the femur. This can be applied by two ways. Traction can be applied to the skin directly or directly to bone by means of pins passed into it. Traction methods have their share of complications especially those related to prolonged immobilization like muscle wasting, joint stiffness, hypostatic pneumonia, DVT, thromboembolism etc.

Skin Traction is applied by using adhesive strapping or foam rubber strips to the limb held in place by circular turns of crepe bandage. Skin traction is applied through a weight attached to a cord passing through the distal end of the strapping. The maximum weight that can be used with skin traction is 6.7 kg. Greater weights lead to skin problems like skin necrosis or skin sloughing. Skin traction is less effective than skeletal traction in achieving traction on bone. The force is dissipated in distraction of skin and soft tissues. Hence, it is not a very good method to maintain fracture reduction. The role of skin traction in adults is more to relieve pain and muscle spasm (e.g. fractures of neck of femur) and post operative traction (following hemi / total replacement arthroplasty of hip). It can be used to maintain reduction of pediatric fractures. In fact it is easy to use and simple and is the standard method of traction in children.

Precautions should be taken to pad the bony prominences like the fibular neck and to avoid excessive pressure while applying traction.

The disadvantages with use of skin traction are:

1. It cannot be used for prolonged periods, in the presence of injured skin, or in patients with allergic skin lesions.

2. Some patients may be allergic to the adhesive agent.

3. Excessive amount of weights cannot be used. (> 6.7 kg)

4. Risk of skin necrosis and sloughing is present.

5. The traction may become loose and needs repeated readjustments.

6. Improperly applied skin traction may lead to nerve palsies e.g. common peroneal nerve palsy.

Skeletal Traction is useful in achieving and maintaining fracture reduction. It is superior to skin traction and is the most commonly employed traction method in adults. Continuous skeletal traction may be indicated, where it is necessary to maintain a sustained pull to neutralize strong muscle forces and maintain normal length of the bone. This is especially true in cases of conservatively treated fractures of femur. Skeletal traction is usually applied by using either a Steinmann pin or Denham's pin. Steinmann pin is usually smooth, while a Denham pin has threads in its central portion providing better purchase on the bone. Denham pin is commonly employed in elderly osteoporotic patients in whom skeletal traction is needed. K-wires (usually pretensioned using K-wire tensioner) are used in children to apply skeletal traction. Pretensioning greatly increases the stiffness of the K-wire and prevents pin loosening.

The Method of Pin Insertion During application of skeletal pin aseptic precautions should be taken. The pin is applied usually under local anesthesia. In children care should be taken not to damage the growth plate. Damage to neurovascular structures can be avoided by careful selection of entry site and proper pin application. Some of the commonly employed sites for skeletal traction are:

1. *Upper tibial* The pin should be passed from lateral to medial to avoid the lateral popliteal nerve.

2. *Supra malleolar* (*lower tibial*) The pin is passed from medial to lateral carefully avoiding injury to the great saphenous vein.

3. *Calcaneal pin* is passed from the medial to lateral side-avoiding injury to the posterior tibial neurovascular bundle.

4. *Supra condylar* or lower femoral traction is employed rarely for the treatment of fracture shaft femur. It is more commonly employed intraoperatively to give traction during interlocking nailing of the femur. The pin is passed from the medial to the lateral side.

Some Common Lower Limb Tractions

1. *Perkin's Traction* In this type of traction either skeletal or skin traction is applied. The limb usually rests on a pillow and is not supported by any splint.

2. *Hamilton Russell Traction* is used for fracture neck of femur or fracture shaft femur. This is essentially a skin traction without use of any splint to support the limb. After below knee skin traction is applied, a sling is placed under the knee, which keeps the hip and knees slightly flexed. A cord attached to the sling passes through pulleys at the end of the bed through which weight is suspended. The foot end is elevated, and the body weight provides counter traction. A single weight serves the double purpose of supporting the limb and exerting continuous traction.

3. *Gallows or Bryant's traction* is used in the treatment of femoral fractures in children under 2 years of age. In this method both the lower limbs are suspended by means of above knee skin traction. The cords are tightened so that the buttocks are just lifted off the cot. The counter traction is provided by the weight of the child.

The knees should be slightly flexed by means of

back splints to minimize risk of vascular insult.

The reason for use of this method are:

(a) In children till 2 years the flexors, abductors and external rotators are stronger than their antagonists as a result of which the proximal fragment is flexed, abducted and externally rotated. This method aligns the distal fragment to the proximal fragment.

(b) Children tolerate this method quite well.

In children above 2 years use of this method is fraught with the risk of vascular compromise and hence, should be avoided.

4. *Ninety-Ninety Traction* This method can be used in the treatment of femoral fractures with extensive soft tissue injuries and/or burns and in some subtrochanteric fractures of femur. It is also used for the correction of severe flexion deformities of the knee (to prevent posterior subluxation of tibia during correction).

In this method, the hip and knee are kept in 90 degrees of flexion.

One steinmann is passed either through the distal femur or proximal tibia while the other pin is passed through the calcaneum or lower tibia. Through the first pin the thigh is suspended overhead by appropriate pulley arrangement, while traction to the leg is applied through the second pin.

5. *Agnes Hunt traction* is a special method devised for the correction of flexion deformity of hip. The unaffected limb is placed in a single hip spica with the hip and knee flexed to 90°. The affected limb is placed in a Thomas splint and traction is applied to the limb. The splint is gradually lowered thus correcting the flexion deformity of hip.

Methods of Skull Traction

1. *Crutch field, Blackburn or Garden-Wells tongs* can be used to apply skull traction in the treatment of unstable cervical spine injuries. Counter traction is provided by the body weight by elevation of the head end of the bed. The head is shaved and drill holes are made in case of crutch field tongs with a special drill bit, which has a stop preventing penetration of more than 4mm. Garden Wells tongs can be directly screwed on without pre-drilling.

2. *Halo traction* (Fig. 31.1) can be halo-pelvic or halo-femoral. This modified method of skull traction is most commonly employed for the treatment of scoliosis deformity of spine. It is also useful in patients with fracture of atlas, axis (C_1/C_2) and in post surgical patients of atlanto-occipital fusions. Halo consists of a metal ring which is fixed to the skull by means of four pins pasing through the outer table of skull. The anterior pins are placed in frontal bone superior and lateral to the supra orbital ridge so that ring margin lies about 0.5 cm above the lateral margin of the eyebrows. Posterior pins are placed posterior and superior to the external ear so that the margin of ring lies above the ear. Diagonally opposite pins are tightened simultaneously to ensure that the ring is centered. After care of halo traction is very important. Complication of the halo traction include cranial nerve palsies (especially VI cranial nerve) and degeneration of cervical vertebral joints. The daily monitoring of cranial nerve function and rest of neuro muscular system is important. Periodic x-rays of cervical spine (lateral views) should be taken. Overdistraction is suggested by prominence of the sternomastoids, excessive distraction of the

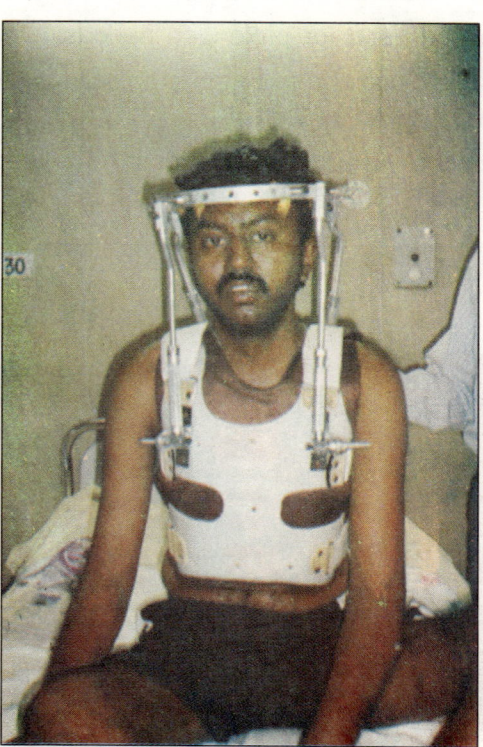

Fig. 31.1. Halo traction

cervical vertebrae and/or paralysis of the lateral gaze (lateral rectus palsy due to VI nerve dysfunction).

Pelvic rings are applied by passing threaded pins into the ilium on either side. A distractor with four rigid upright bars (with threaded portion) is used to connect the two portions. Distraction is done gradually to achieve correction of deformity. As an alternative to pelvic ring a plaster cast may be applied. In case of halo femoral traction, the femoral traction is by means of (two) supracondylar pins.

Precautions during Skeletal Traction

The patient should be monitored daily to look for development of sores, direction of traction, position of fracture fragments, and development of any neurovascular deficit. Traction should be adjusted so that the patient is comfortable. Isometric muscle excercises should be commenced as soon as possible to avoid muscle wasting.

Advantages of skeletal traction

- Large amounts of weight can be used (1/10 of body weight)
- The limb can be observed daily, and dressing can be done .
- Can be used for prolonged periods.
- Use of special attachments allows for mobilization of adjacent joints.
- It can be used in the presence of injured skin.

Disadvantages of Skeletal Traction

- Pin loosening, infection of the pin tract, rarely causing osteomyelitis.
- Damage of neurovascular structures, and/or growth plate can occur if the pin is passed without proper care.
- Should be used with caution in osteoporotic bone.
- Complications of prolonged immobilization like pressure sore, hypostatic pneumonia, DVT and thrombo embolism may result and should be carefully looked for.

Splints are devices used to support the limb while traction is applied. The two most commonly used splints are the Thomas splint and Bohler Braun splints.

1. **Thomas splint** (Fig. 31.2) It was devised by Hugh Owen Thomas. It is the most common splint used for lower limb fractures. It consists of a padded metal ring connected to two iron bars at either end of the ring. The outer bar is longer than the inner bar and makes an angle of 120° with the ring. Distally the two iron bars are connected by means of "W" shaped iron bar. There is a flare outward about 2" on the outer bar which allows for the greater trochanter. The splint is available in different sizes and length. It is important to use an appropriately sized splint for each case.

   A Pearson knee flexion attachment (also made

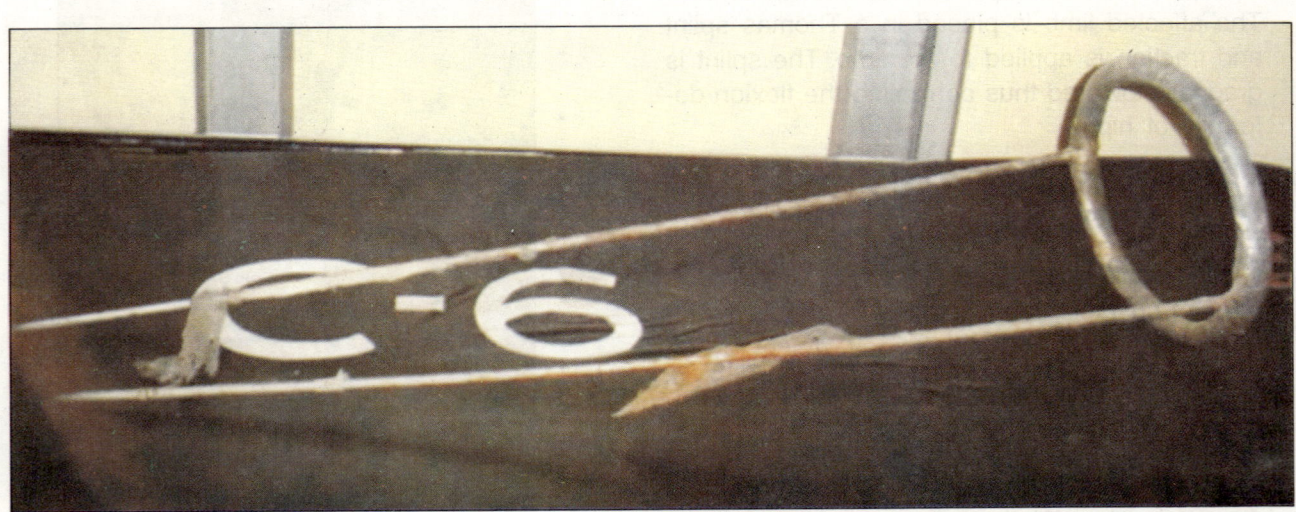

Fig. 31.2. Thomas splint

of 2 iron bars connected distally) can be attached to the Thomas splint to allow for knee flexion.

2. **Bohler-Braun splint** (Fig. 31.3) is used in the treatment of supracondylar fractures of the femur, injuries of knee, leg and foot. It is not commonly used as it is bulky and it is difficult to apply counter traction.

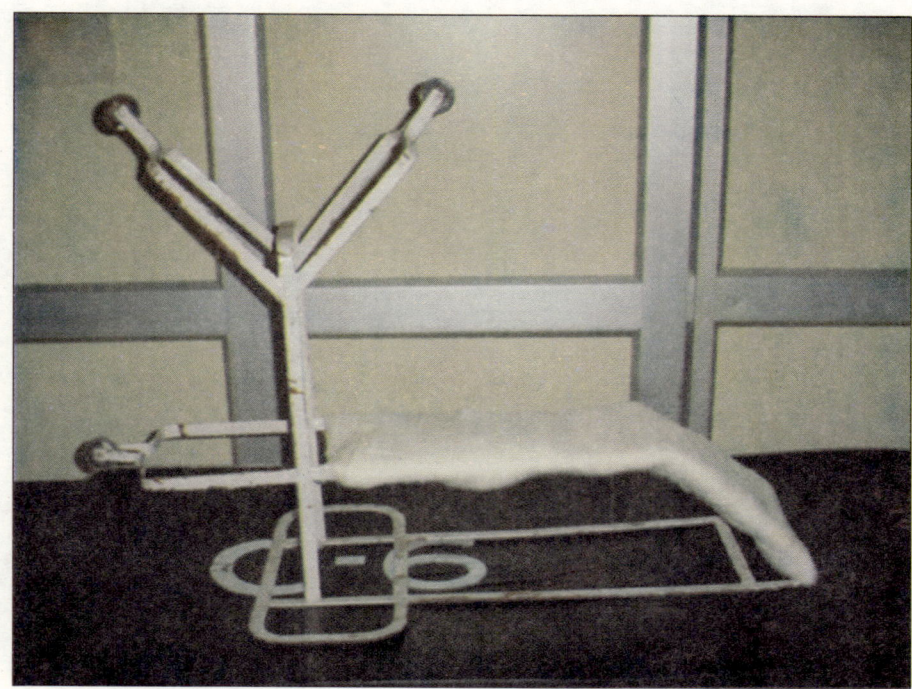

Fig. 31.3. Bohler-Braun splint

Index